Textbook of
Blood Banking
and Transfusion
Medicine

Textbook of
Blood Banking
and Transfusion
Medicine

Second Edition

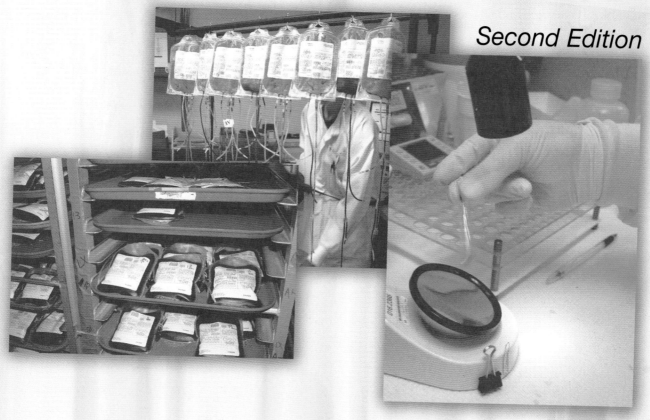

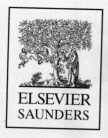

ELSEVIER
SAUNDERS

Sally V. Rudmann,
PhD, MT(ASCP)SBB, CLS

Professor and Director
Medical Technology Division
The Ohio State University
Columbus, Ohio

ELSEVIER
SAUNDERS

The Curtis Center
170 South Independence Mall West, 300E
Philadelphia, Pennsylvania 19106-3399

TEXTBOOK OF BLOOD BANKING AND TRANSFUSION MEDICINE
SECOND EDITION
Copyright © 2005, 1995 by Elsevier

0-7216-0384-X

NOTICE

Blood banking is an ever-changing field. Standard safety precautions must be followed, but as new research and clinical experience broaden our knowledge, changes in treatment and drug therapy may become necessary or appropriate. Readers are advised to check the most current product information provided by the manufacturer of each drug to be administered to verify the recommended dose, the method and duration of administration, and contraindications. It is the responsibility of the treating physician, relying on experience and knowledge of the patient, to determine dosages and the best treatment for each individual patient. Neither the Publisher nor the editor assume any liability for any injury and/or damage to persons or property arising from this publication.

Previous edition copyrighted 1995

International Standard Book Number 0-7216-0384-X

Publishing Director: Andrew Allen
Managing Editor: Mindy Hutchinson
Developmental Editor: Ellen Wurm
Publishing Services Manager: Jeffrey Patterson
Senior Project Manager: Mary Stueck
Senior Designer: Teresa McBryan

Printed in United States of America

Last digit is the print number: 9 8 7 6 5 4 3 2 1

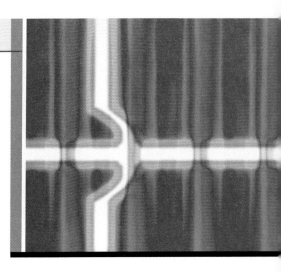

I would like to dedicate this book to my students, past, present, and future.

It is from their struggles to learn, their comments and inquiries, their successes, and their failures that I have derived many, if not all, of the ideas for the content, the format, and the presentation of this book.

They have been and continue to be my inspiration.

Contributors

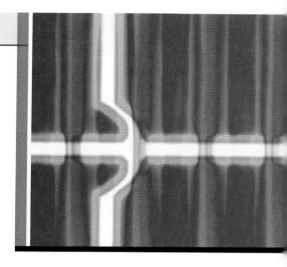

Linda Aldridge, MT(ASCP)SBB
Blood Bank Manager
City of Hope National Medical Center
Duarte, California
Compatibility Testing

Dorothy A. Bergeron, MS, CLS(NCA)
Associate Professor and Program Director
Department of Medical Laboratory Science
University of Massachusetts Dartmouth
North Dartmouth, Massachusetts
Component Preparation

Kerry Burright-Hittner, BS, MT(ASCP)SBB
Reference/QC Supervisor
American Red Cross, Midwestern Region
Omaha, Nebraska
Resolving ABO Typing Discrepancies and Other Typing Problems

Suzanne H. Butch, MA, CLDir
Chief Technologist
Blood Bank and Transfusion Service
University of Michigan Hospitals and Health Centers
Ann Arbor, Michigan
*Safety; Quality Control, Quality Assurance, Quality
Improvement, and Peer Review; Record Keeping and Computers*

Susan M. Cotter, DVM
Diplomate American College of Veterinary Internal
    Medicine (Oncology and Internal Medicine)
Distinguished Professor
Department of Clinical Sciences
Tufts University, School of Veterinary Medicine
North Grafton, Massachusetts
Expert Opinion: Veterinary Transfusion Medicine

C. Guillermo Couto, DVM, dip. ACVIM (Oncology
    and Internal Medicine)
Professor
Chief of the Clinical Oncology Hematology and
    Transfusion Medicine Services
Veterinary Teaching Hospital and Department of Veterinary
    Clinical Sciences
College of Veterinary Medicine
Member of the OSU Comprehensive Cancer Center
The Ohio State University
Columbus, Ohio
Expert Opinion: Veterinary Transfusion Medicine

Kay Doyle, PhD, MT(ASCP)
Professor and Program Director
Clinical Laboratory Science/Medical Technology Program
Department of Health and Clinical Sciences
University of Massachusetts Lowell
Lowell, Massachusetts
Blood Component Preservation and Storage

Deborah T. Firestone, MA, MT(ASCP)SBB
Clinical Assistant Professor
Department of Clinical Laboratory Sciences
School of Health Technology and Management
State University of New York at Stony Brook
Stony Brook, New York
Component Therapy; Adverse Effects of Blood Transfusion

Joy L. Fridey, MD, MBA
Director of Transfusion Medicine
City of Hope National Medical Center
Duarte, California
Donor Screening and Blood Collection

George Garratty, MD, FRCPath.
Scientific Director
American Red Cross Blood Services, Southern California
Los Angeles, California
*Expert Opinion: Do We Have to Worry About Not Detecting
Antibodies to Low-Incidence Antigens*

Lawrence T. Goodnough, MD
Professor of Pathology and Medicine
Stanford University
Stanford, California
Expert Opinion: Recombinant Erythropoietin in Surgery

Gerald A. Hoeltge, MD
Head, Section of Transfusion Medicine
The Cleveland Clinic Foundation
Cleveland, Ohio
Expert Opinion: The Technology of Patient Identification

Robert L. Jones, MD, MBA
President, New York Blood Center
New York, New York
Expert Opinion: Lessons for Disaster Preparedness after September 11

Candace E. Kay, MS, MT(ASCP), SI, BB
Coordinator, Program Development Training
Donor Aphersis Center
Department of Transfusion Medicine
City of Hope National Medical Center
Duarte, California
Donor Screening and Blood Collection

Larry C. Lasky, MD
Associate Professor of Pathology and Internal Medicine
The Ohio State University
Columbus, Ohio
Expert Opinion: Collection and Expansion of Blood-Forming (Hematopoietic) Stem Cells from Cord Blood

Elizabeth Kenimer Leibach, EdD, MS, CLS, MT(ASCP)SBB
Chair and Associate Professor
Department of Biomedical and Radiological Technologies
Medical College of Georgia
Augusta, Georgia
Fundamentals of Genetics: Blood Bank Applications; Immunology: Review and Applications

Mary A. Lieb, MT(ASCP)SBB
Consultant
Quality Source by Blood Systems
Scottsdale, Arizona
Compatibility Testing

Maria Lukas, BS, ASCP(BB)
Quality Improvement Consultant
Cincinnati Children's Hospital and Medical Center
Cincinnati, Ohio
Hematopoietic Stem Cells and Cellular Therapy

Kathleen K. Nicol, MD
Clinical Assistant Professor
Director of Transfusion Services
The Ohio Statue University
Columbus, Ohio
Children's Hospital
Columbus, Ohio
Transfusion Issues in Selected Patient Populations

Christine Pitocco, MS, MT(ASCP)BB
Clinical Assistant Professor
Stony Brook University
Stony Brook, New York
Component Therapy; Adverse Effects of Blood Transfusion

Karen Rodberg, MBA, MT(ASCP)SBB
Director, Immunohematology Reference Laboratory
American Red Cross, Southern California Region
Los Angeles, California
Antibody Identification

Patricia L. Strohm, BS, MT(ASCP)SBB
Blood Bank Manager
Forum Health
Northside Medical Center
Youngstown, Ohio
Hemolytic Disease of the Fetus and Newborn

Brian Susskind, PhD, dABHI
Director, Transplantation Immunology Division
Hoxworth Blood Center
Associate Professor of Surgery
University of Cincinnati Medical College
Cincinnati, Ohio
The HLA System

Susan L. Wilkinson, EdD, MT(ASCP)SBB
Associate Director and Associate Professor
Hoxworth Blood Center
University of Cincinnati Medical Center
Cincinnati, Ohio
The ABO and H Blood Group Systems; Secretor and Soluble ABH Antigens, and The Lewis, I, P, and Globoside Blood Group Systems; The Rh Blood Group System; Other Blood Groups; Autoimmune and Drug-Induced Immune Hemolytic Anemias

Robert M. Winslow, MD
Adjunct Professor
University of California, San Diego
San Diego, California
Expert Opinion: Blood Substitutes 2004

Reviewers

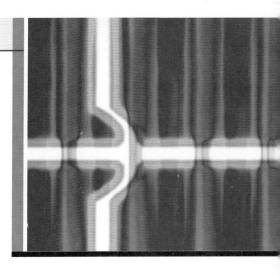

Virginia Hughes, MS, MT(ASCP)
Assistant Lecturer
Department of Medical Technology
College of Health Sciences
University of Wyoming
Laramie, Wyoming

Shirley J. Noble, MS, MT(ASCP)
Instructor
Medical Laboratory Technician Program
Southeast Community College
Lincoln, Nebraska

Anne T. Rodgers, PhD, MT(ASCP)
Associate Professor
Medical Laboratory Technology Program
Dalton State College
Dalton, Georgia

Acknowledgments

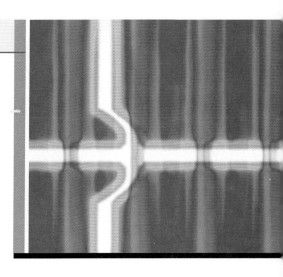

I would like to thank those individuals whose behind-the-scenes contributions made this book possible. A special thanks to the American Red Cross, Blood Services, The Ohio State University Hospital Transfusion Service, and Childrens' Hospital in Columbus, Ohio for their patience and willingness to help me gather photographic materials for the book. A special thanks goes to my colleagues Janelle Chiasera and Michele Suhie who provided assistance and support throughout the process and who picked up the pieces for me when I was preoccupied with writing. I would also like to thank my editor, Ellen Wurm, for her persistence, her encouragement, and her support.

I would also like to thank those who through their support, their love, and their patience helped make this book possible—my husband Jim Barlow, my son Daniel, my grandchildren Keegan, Connor, and Anna, and my canine companion for 16 years, Terra (now deceased). A special thank you to my son Stephen, who provided countless hours of editorial assistance, offering the dual perspectives of a recent student and a blood banker.

I will always remember with gratitude my own teachers who stimulated my desire to learn and encouraged me with the example of their own scholarship and who instilled in me a love of blood banking and of teaching. A particular thank you to Delores M. Mallory, Dr. Nancy Bigley and Dr. Charles R. McFarland for helping me to learn and to love learning.

Sally V. Rudmann, PhD, MT(ASCP)SBB, CLS

Preface

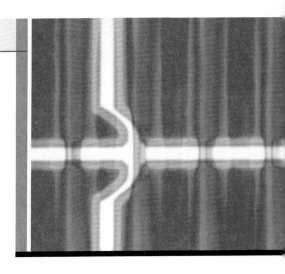

AUDIENCE

This book was designed to be used as a textbook rather than solely as a scientific or technical reference. Every attempt was made to sequence material in such a way as to organize learning and provide a logical hierarchical approach to content. The book was created with the student and the instructor in mind, and in this way the editor and the contributors believe that it is unique. The intent was to provide basic blood banking theory, technical practice considerations, regulatory guidelines, related transfusion medicine, and advanced concepts sequenced in such a way as to facilitate learning and retention. The major audience for this text is students in medical technology (clinical laboratory science) education programs. The incorporation of both advanced and basic concepts make this text useful for a diverse audience, including those in medical laboratory technician programs as well as SBB and resident education. Because of its pragmatic practice orientation, the book also is useful as a reference and review resource for the blood bank professional.

The book is divided into content-related sections, some of which are written by a single author to provide consistency and continuity. This approach minimizes the fluctuations in style and content that are characteristic of most multiple-contributor publications. *Textbook of Blood Banking and Transfusion Medicine* contains a number of special pedagogical features designed to enhance the teaching/learning process. It was the intent of the contributors to provide a text that would be practical, organized, interesting, and fun to use.

FEATURES

The book contains a number of unique features that address the needs of students and instructors.

- **Margin Definitions:** Important terms are defined in the margins next to where they appear. Such definitions provide an easily accessed resource for the student and yet do not interfere with the flow of the narrative. Their prominence in the margins provides a helpful study guide for students.
- **Margin Notes:** These messages are located in the margins throughout the text and provide the student with reinforcement for important concepts, a reminder of some previously discussed topic, an alternate view of the principle, and/or a cross reference to another source of related information within the text.
- **Expert Opinions:** Within sections of the book, experts in the field of immunohematology have contributed essays on areas of research interest or of new and advancing technologies in the field. These are included to provide current information and to stimulate interest.
- **Objectives:** Each chapter is preceded by a list of behavioral objectives. These provide the expected learning outcomes and are useful for students as well as instructors.

- **Multiple-Choice Study Questions:** At the end of the book is a set of registry-like multiple-choice questions that are tied to the behavioral objectives at the beginning of the chapter. Students can use these questions as self-assessment tools to measure learning outcomes.
- **Chapter Outlines/Summaries:** Each chapter is preceded by an outline of the content to be addressed. So, too, each chapter contains a brief summary of the important points contained within. Both of these features are useful for instructors and students because they provide a rapid overview of the chapter content.
- **Glossary of Terms:** An alphabetical list of all terms defined in the text are given in one convenient location. Over 300 terms are included.
- **Suggested Readings:** Resources for further study that would be useful to both students and instructors are provided at the end of the chapter.
- **Up-to-date References:** Each chapter contains recent articles published in the field as well as older articles of historical/developmental interest and importance.

Contents

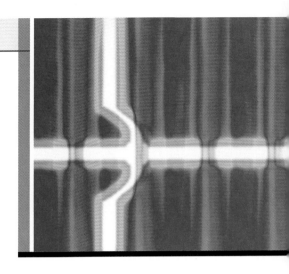

SECTION FIVE
Transfusion Therapy

SECTION SIX
Clinical Considerations

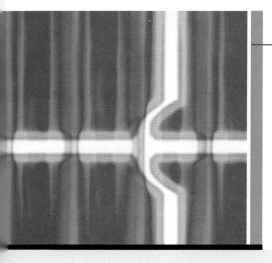

Basic Science Review

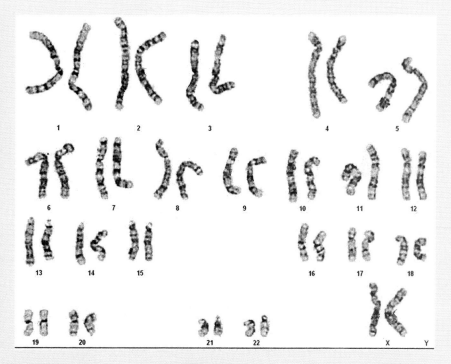

Blood banking and transfusion medicine are applied sciences and rely on a number of basic sciences for their theoretical framework. Students of blood banking need to be grounded in the basic natural and physical sciences and in immunology and genetics to achieve a broad understanding of immunohematology content.

Genetics, the study of inheritance, provides the necessary background for understanding the principles of blood group inheritance, patterns of inheritance, and population genetics. Blood bank applications of this science include the determination of genotype and phenotype frequencies in the population, calculations of the number of units that must be screened to find compatible blood, and the interpretation of parentage testing results. Molecular genetics has further expanded our ability to explain, at the molecular level, those phenomena that we have historically described serologically.

Immunology is the very basis of blood banking, since the science of immunohematology is concerned primarily with blood group alloantigens and their respective antibodies. Knowledge of the nature of the immune response is central to the development and selection of appropriate serological techniques for pretransfusion problem solving, the selection of appropriate components for transfusion, and the interpretation of adverse immunologic responses to transfusion.

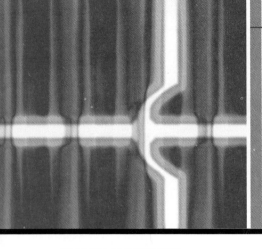

CHAPTER ONE

Fundamentals of Genetics: Blood Bank Applications

Elizabeth Kenimer Leibach[*]

[*]*The author would like to recognize the contributions of Stephanie Summers to this chapter in the previous edition.*

LEARNING OBJECTIVES

After reading and studying this chapter, the student should be able to:

1. Define the following genetics terms:
   pedigree chart
   incomplete dominance
   gene
   homozygous
   genotype
   dominance
   codominance
   diploid
   mitosis
   pedigree chart
   autosomal
   linkage
   polymorphic
   allele
   heterozygous
   phenotype
   recessiveness
   incomplete dominance
   haploid
   meiosis
   proband/propositus
   X-linked
   blood group antigens
   intron
   exon
   genomics
   proteomics
   single nucleotide polymorphism (SNP)
   polymerase chain reaction (PCR)
   knockout gene
   Southern blotting
   Northern blotting

2. Correctly use the terms in Objective 1 in written and oral discussions of inheritance in general and specific applications to blood group inheritance.

3. Describe the major concepts of mendelian genetics, including the following:
   Law of Independent Segregation
   Law of Independent Assortment

4. Briefly describe mitosis and meiosis.

5. Construct and interpret a pedigree chart using the symbols described in this chapter.

6. Describe four patterns of inheritance. For each pattern, draw an example of a pedigree of that type of inheritance.

7. Briefly describe linkage and give examples from blood group genetics.

8. Briefly describe what is meant by the term position effects and give one example from blood group genetics that illustrates this phenomenon.

9. Given the necessary data, calculate gene, genotype, and phenotype frequencies in the population. Given the frequency of blood group antigens in the population, calculate the number of units of blood that must be screened for a given transfusion.

10. Briefly define the term polymorphic and describe the impact of blood group polymorphisms on human blood group systems.

11. Discuss applications of molecular techniques in recombinant antibody production, nucleic acid analysis in the blood supply, and molecular antigen typing.

12. Briefly describe PCR, DNA sequencing, and microarray hybridization analysis, DNA-based methods holding promise for widespread applications in clinical blood banking.

13. Discuss the usefulness of molecular techniques in expanding knowledge related to structure, genetics, and function of blood group–associated antigens.

The primary objective of this chapter is to introduce clinical laboratory science students to the principles, language, and methods of human genetics and to indicate some of its actual and potential applications in blood banking. The chapter has three sections: mendelian genetics, population genetics, and molecular genetics. Because each section is deserving of an entire book, the information provided here is intended only to lay a foundation of knowledge upon which detailed and specialized information can be built. It is hoped that this chapter and its bibliography will make the literature of genetics accessible to readers requiring further information.

MENDELIAN GENETICS: TENETS OF HEREDITY

The basic techniques of genetic analysis were established well over 100 years ago by the Augustinian monk Gregor Mendel. By crossing strains of peas differing in a single phenotypic trait, Mendel deduced that the traits resulted from single genetic factors. (These factors are the **genes**, although Mendel never used that

Gene: Composed of deoxyribonucleic acid (DNA); the basic unit of inheritance.

term.) Mendel's experiments prepared the way for modern genetic research. The results of his experiments and the theory he formulated to explain them were published in 1865. For 35 years these results were overlooked, and his theory was unappreciated and poorly disseminated among scientists. The turn of the twentieth century marked an important date for the science of heredity and genetics, for it was in 1900 that Mendel's work was rediscovered.

Three investigators—Correns, von Tschermak, and deVries—working independently, made some remarkable discoveries about the nature of inheritance. In each case, their work substantiated the work done by Mendel 35 years earlier. The rediscovery and confirmation of Mendel's research, in the more receptive climate of the twentieth century, altered the course of research and prepared the way for tremendous advances in our knowledge of heredity and genetics.

Law of Independent Segregation

Mendel made a series of crosses between pairs of strains of true-breeding peas that differed by only a single inherited characteristic or trait, such as tall versus short plants or round versus wrinkled seeds. The first series of progeny, called the first filial generation (F_1), resembled only one of the two parental strains. For example, in the cross of tall with short plants, all of the progeny were tall (Fig. 1-1). The trait that is expressed in the F_1 (tall) is called the *dominant trait*, and the one that is not expressed (short) is the *recessive trait*. Mendel then crossed the F_1 plants with themselves. He recovered the next generation, the second filial or F_2 generation, and recorded the **phenotype** of each plant. He found many plants with the dominant trait and others with the recessive trait. Moreover, he recognized that the number of progeny closely approximated 75% dominant and 25% recessive, a 3:1 ratio of dominant to recessive plants.

Phenotype: The inherited traits that are expressed in an individual.

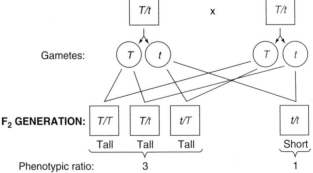

Fig. 1-1 Diagrammatic illustration of Mendel's Law of Independent Segregation. The inheritance of a single characteristic—plant height—is shown. The dominant gene is represented by *T* (tall) and its recessive allele by *t* (short). *(From Crispens CG: Essentials of Medical Genetics. Philadelphia, JB Lippincott, 1971, p 3.)*

Mendel concluded that hereditary factors exist that cause each of the two phenotypic traits. A factor for each parental trait had to be present in the F₁ plants, even though these plants resembled only one parent, because the F₁ plants subsequently produced both types of plants. Furthermore, the factors must be discrete entities whose inherent characteristics are preserved in the F₁ plants even in the presence of an alternative factor. This is the Law of Independent Segregation (see Fig. 1-1).

In essence, Mendel's first law states that the hereditary characteristics are determined by particulate units or factors. These factors occur in pairs in an individual, creating a **diploid genotype,** but in the formation of germ cells (gametes) these entities are segregated so that only one member of the pair is transmitted through any one gamete (**haploid** genotype). When male and female gametes unite, the double number of factors is restored in the offspring. Substituting the word *gene* in place of *factor,* the statements read almost as if Mendel had known of the existence of chromosomes and the physical basis of heredity at the time he performed the experiments.

Diploid: The condition of having two sets of chromosomes (maternal and paternal). The somatic cells of higher organisms are diploid.

Genotype: The genetic makeup of an individual.

Haploid: The condition of having one set of chromosomes (maternal or paternal). The sex cells (gametes) of higher organisms are haploid.

Law of Independent Assortment

Mendel's work with monohybrids established that a 3:1 ratio is to be expected from a cross of two monohybrids. A question that occurred to Mendel was how two or more pairs of factors might behave in relationship to one another when followed at the same time in a cross. His further studies followed the behavior of two pairs of alleles and led to the formation of Mendel's second law.

From his monohybrid crosses, Mendel knew that the color of the pea seeds can be either yellow or green and that the factor for yellow *(Y)* is dominant to green *(y).* When plants homozygous for yellow seeds are crossed with those having green seeds, the F₂ generation contains the yellow and green phenotypes in a ratio of 3:1.

Mendel designed an experiment that crossed a pure-breeding tall plant with yellow seeds *(TTYY)* and a pure-breeding short plant with green seeds *(ttyy).* From Mendel's first law, we expect two factors for each characteristic to be present in each parent. The F₁ dihybrid receives one factor for each character from each one of the parents and has a genotype *TtYy.* The F₁s are all found to be tall plants with yellow seeds. The question that now arises is, "What will happen when the F₁ dihybrids are followed further?" Will the factors for yellow and tall stay together through later generations because they were together in one of the original parents? The same question arises for green and short.

Mendel examined these questions by performing a dihybrid test cross. The F₂ offspring resulting from this test cross are of four types. These results indicate that the dihybrid forms four different types of gametes. This in turn means that the factors for seed color and plant height behave independently. This is the Law of Independent Assortment. Fig. 1-2 is a diagram of this concept.

Knowing that any dihybrid individual forms four different kinds of gametes in equal proportions, we can depict diagrammatically what to expect in a dihybrid cross. The Punnett square method is used to bring together the gametes from both parents in all possible combinations (Fig. 1-3). When all possible combinations are counted and categorized, we obtain four different phenotypic types in a ratio of 9:3:3:1. This classic dihybrid ratio is so fundamental to genetic studies and so frequently encountered that we must be able both to recognize it and to predict the phenotypes to be expected from a cross of any two dihybrids.

Incomplete Dominance and Codominance

Although Mendel noted **dominance** and **recessiveness** among the pairs of alleles he studied, he did not say that dominance must always apply. *Dominant* and *recessive* are often used as terms of convenience, but, strictly speaking, they are not very precise. Sometimes the heterozygous phenotype is intermediate between the two

Dominance: Expression of inherited trait when the allele is present in either the homozygous or heterozygous form.

Recessiveness: Expression of inherited trait only when the allele is present in the homozygous form.

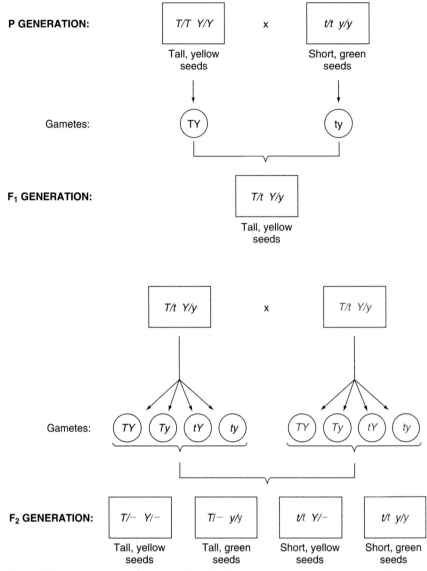

P GENERATION: T/T Y/Y x t/t y/y

Tall, yellow seeds   Short, green seeds

Gametes: TY   ty

F₁ GENERATION: T/t Y/y

Tall, yellow seeds

T/t Y/y x T/t Y/y

Gametes: TY Ty tY ty   TY Ty tY ty

F₂ GENERATION: T/– Y/–   T/– y/y   t/t Y/–   t/t y/y

Tall, yellow seeds   Tall, green seeds   Short, yellow seeds   Short, green seeds

Fig. 1-2 Diagrammatic illustration of Mendel's Law of Independent Assortment. The inheritance of two characteristics—plant height and seed color—is followed through the F₂ generation. Tall *(T)* is dominant over short *(t)*; yellow seed color *(Y)* is dominant over green seed color *(y)*. *(From Crispens CG: Essentials of Medical Genetics. Philadelphia, JB Lippincott, 1971, p 5.)*

Homozygous: Pertaining to the condition that exists when the two alleles for a given trait are the same.

Heterozygous: Pertaining to the condition that exists when two alleles for a given trait are different.

Incomplete dominance: The condition in which the products (traits) of both alleles are expressed but the effect of one allele is stronger than that of the other.

Allele: Any alternate form of a gene that can occupy a given chromosomal location (locus). Each individual inherits one allele from the mother and one from the father, making up a homologous pair for each trait.

homozygous phenotypes. For example, the cross between a pure-breeding red snapdragon and a pure-breeding white variety produces F₁ progeny of the intermediate pink color. If these F₁ progeny are crossed among themselves, the resulting F₂ progeny contain red, pink, and white flowers. In this case it is possible to distinguish **heterozygotes** from **homozygotes** by their phenotype. When dealing with humans, the term **incomplete dominance** is used to refer to situations in which both alleles are expressed but the effect of one **allele** appears greater than that of the other. The blood disorder known as sickle cell anemia, a condition in which an abnormal hemoglobin is present, illustrates this point very well.

For the sake of convenience, let us represent the alleles responsible for the normal and the sickle cell hemoglobin as "*A*" and "*a*," respectively. Superficially *AA* and *Aa* individuals appear the same (disease free), in contrast to the homozygotes, *aa*, who present an abnormal phenotypic picture (sickle cell disease). We might

		MALE			
Gametes		(TY)	(Ty)	(tY)	(ty)
FEMALE	(TY)	T/T Y/Y Tall, yellow seeds	T/T Y/y Tall, yellow seeds	T/t Y/Y Tall, yellow seeds	T/t Y/y Tall, yellow seeds
	(Ty)	T/T y/Y Tall, yellow seeds	T/T y/y Tall, green seeds	T/t y/Y Tall, yellow seeds	T/t y/y Tall, green seeds
	(tY)	t/T Y/Y Tall, yellow seeds	t/T Y/y Tall, yellow seeds	t/t Y/Y Short, yellow seeds	t/t Y/y Short, yellow seeds
	(ty)	t/T y/Y Tall, yellow seeds	t/T y/y Tall, green seeds	t/t y/Y Short, yellow seeds	t/t y/y Short, green seeds

9	:	**3**	:	**3**	:	**1**
Tall, yellow seeds		Tall, green seeds		Short, yellow seeds		Short, green seeds

Fig. 1-3 The use of a Punnett square for determination of genotypes and phenotypes expected among the progeny obtained from crosses that involve more than one pair of genes. *(From Crispens CG: Essentials of Medical Genetics. Philadelphia, JB Lippincott, 1971, p 7.)*

conclude that absolute dominance pertains. However, the heterozygotes, *Aa,* are actually somewhat different from *AA* homozygotes. They may be identified when their blood is examined microscopically, because a certain percentage of their red blood cells can be made to sickle by a test that subjects the cells to certain agents capable of reducing the oxygen tension in the immediate environment. Although this effect in the body of a heterozygote would be very unusual, the allele for sickle cell hemoglobin is not completely recessive.

A frequently encountered term more directly applicable to blood banking is **codominance.** Codominance implies that a definite product or substance controlled by each allele can be identified. The genetic factors that govern human blood types are, as a rule, codominant alleles. Each controls the formation of a different red blood cell protein or antigen. For example, in the Kidd blood group system, the red cells of a Jk^aJk^b individual have Jk^a and Jk^b antigens, customarily designated as Jk(a+b+). The Jk^a allele produces the Jk^a antigen; the Jk^b allele produces the Jk^b antigen. Neither allele is dominant to the other. The individual with a red cell phenotype of Jk(a+b+) is a heterozygote and has the alleles for both the Jk^a and Jk^b antigens. Both of the proteins produced by these alleles, Jk^a and Jk^b, are easily detected. This is a clear-cut case of codominance between a pair of alleles.

The distinction between incomplete dominance and codominance depends on our ability to detect in the heterozygote distinct substances controlled by each member of the allelic pair. Is the allele for normal hemoglobin incompletely dominant to the sickle hemoglobin allele, or are they codominant? In the sense that the normal allele results in a heterozygote who has normal red blood cells except for those that sickle under test conditions, the allele appears to be an incomplete dominant. However, refined techniques demonstrate that two different proteins, normal hemoglobin controlled by the gene, *A,* and sickle cell hemoglobin controlled by

Codominance: Inherited traits that are expressed whether the allele is present in the homozygous or heterozygous form.

its allele, are present in the blood. Based on this criterion, the alleles are codominant. The choice of words depends on the level at which we describe the phenotype of the heterozygote; it also depends on the techniques available to us to detect chemical differences. The normal and the sickle cell allelic pair may be described as incomplete dominant at one level of reference (small percentage of sickling) or as codominant at another (presence of two specific protein products).[1,2]

Human Chromosomes

A principal reason for the original failure to appreciate Mendel's discovery was the absence of firm facts about the behavior of chromosomes during **meiosis** and **mitosis.** This knowledge was available, however, when Mendel's laws were rediscovered and it was seized on in 1903 by the American, Sutton. In his classic paper, *The Chromosomes in Heredity,* he emphasized the importance of the fact that the diploid chromosome group consists of two morphologically similar sets and that, during meiosis, every gamete receives only one chromosome of each homologous pair. He then used this fact to explain Mendel's results by the assumption that genes are parts of the chromosome. He postulated that the yellow and green seed genes are carried on a certain pair of chromosomes and that the tall and short genes are carried on a different pair. This hypothesis immediately explains the experimentally observed 9:3:3:1 segregation ratio. Although Sutton's paper did not prove the chromosomal theory of heredity, it was immensely important because it brought together for the first time the independent disciplines of genetics (the study of breeding experiments) and cytology (the study of cell structure).

Somatic Cell Division: Mitosis

The basic, self-sustaining unit of any living organism is the cell. Complex organisms are made up of very large numbers of cells. In the case of humans, the number is estimated to be on the order of 100,000 billion.[3] All of these cells are derived from just one original cell, the fertilized egg. Of course, many different types of cells are present in a human. The presence of different cell types means that when they divide they must have the ability to reproduce their own special characteristics. This ability to reproduce, like from like, is the essence of living matter.

Mitosis is the name given to the period in a normal cell's lifetime when it divides and ensures that the two newly formed cells contain genetic information identical to that in the parent cell. During most of a cell's life, its chromosomes exist in a highly extended linear form. The duplication of chromosomes occurs chiefly when they are in this extended state.

During mitosis, the chromosomes, having already duplicated, condense into compact bodies and become clearly visible. Mitosis is conventionally divided into four major stages: prophase, metaphase, anaphase, and telophase. The four stages of mitosis are defined by the state of the chromosomes. During the remainder of a cell's life cycle, it is said to be in interphase. The behavior of a typical chromosome during these stages is illustrated schematically in Fig. 1-4.

Gametes and Meiosis

The mixing of hereditary endowments is accomplished by the fusion of germ cells, or gametes (for example, egg and sperm), and their entire sets of chromosomes. Two haploid cells (gametes), one from each parent, fuse to form a diploid cell, the zygote. During the process of gametogenesis, meiosis occurs. The main function of meiosis is to reduce the diploid chromosome complement to a haploid complement. Meiosis occurs in two divisions: The first results in the pairing of duplicated homologous chromosomes, and the second separates replicated chromatids. Four haploid cells result.

Meiosis must satisfy one further important requirement: The chromosome complements of parent and offspring must be equivalent. This means that the

---

Meiosis: Cell division and replication that result in the formation of haploid gametes (eggs and sperm), which carry either the maternal or paternal genetic information.

Mitosis: Cell division and replication that result in the formation of two diploid daughter cells with exactly the same genetic information as the parent cell.

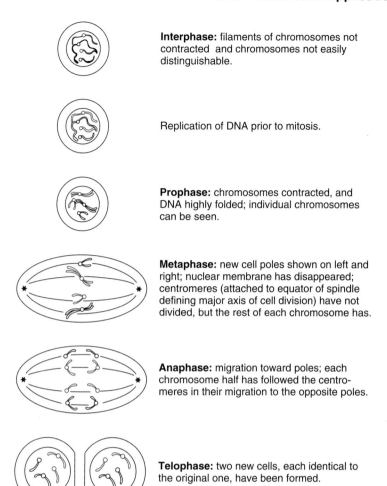

Interphase: filaments of chromosomes not contracted and chromosomes not easily distinguishable.

Replication of DNA prior to mitosis.

Prophase: chromosomes contracted, and DNA highly folded; individual chromosomes can be seen.

Metaphase: new cell poles shown on left and right; nuclear membrane has disappeared; centromeres (attached to equator of spindle defining major axis of cell division) have not divided, but the rest of each chromosome has.

Anaphase: migration toward poles; each chromosome half has followed the centromeres in their migration to the opposite poles.

Telophase: two new cells, each identical to the original one, have been formed.

Fig. 1-4 Mitosis. Diagrammatic representation of mitosis in a hypothetical organism that has one pair of short chromosomes and one pair of long chromosomes.

reduction in chromosome number cannot be arbitrary. Meiosis must ensure that the gametes receive one member of each pair of homologous chromosomes. In this way, fertilization restores the normal diploid chromosome complement.

Two major features of meiosis distinguish it from mitosis:

1. Halving of the number of chromosomes. Meiosis involves two cell divisions with only a single chromosome duplication. This leads to a reduction by one half of the number of chromosomes in the gamete.
2. Pairing. Duplicated homologous chromosomes, behaving as a unit, pair with each other during the first division of meiosis and then separate to opposite poles.

This behavior of homologous pairs of chromosomes ensures that each gamete contains just one member of each homologous pair.

As is true for mitosis, each meiotic division has four periods: prophase, metaphase, anaphase, and telophase. The process of meiosis is illustrated diagrammatically in Fig. 1-5. As in mitosis, the chromosomes are already duplicated by the time they become visible at the start of the first meiotic division. The metaphase of the first meiotic division is also preceded by pairing of the duplicated homologues. The immediate products of the first meiotic division are two cells, each containing a diploid chromosome set. However, each homologous pair of chromosomes in one of these cells is a pair of either maternally or paternally originated chromosomes.

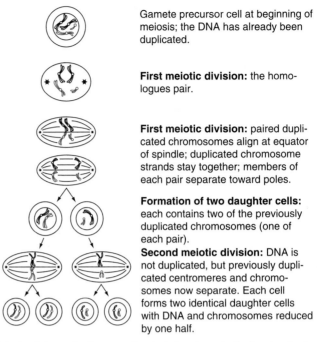

Gamete precursor cell at beginning of meiosis; the DNA has already been duplicated.

First meiotic division: the homologues pair.

First meiotic division: paired duplicated chromosomes align at equator of spindle; duplicated chromosome strands stay together; members of each pair separate toward poles.

Formation of two daughter cells: each contains two of the previously duplicated chromosomes (one of each pair).

Second meiotic division: DNA is not duplicated, but previously duplicated centromeres and chromosomes now separate. Each cell forms two identical daughter cells with DNA and chromosomes reduced by one half.

Fig. 1-5 Meiosis. Schematic diagram of meiosis in a hypothetical male who has one pair of identical autosomes and one dissimilar XY pair.

The second meiotic division is similar to ordinary mitosis except that it is not preceded by chromosome duplication. Thus this second division halves the number of chromosomes. In this division each of the two products of the first division produces identical daughter cells with half the usual number of chromosomes.

Each of the four products of a single meiosis in the male usually becomes a sperm. Each female meiosis, however, produces only one ovum or egg, which develops at random from one of the four meiotic products. The other three products remain in the periphery of the cell and form polar bodies.

Patterns of Inheritance

Inheritance patterns of genetic traits that are of primary interest to blood bankers are the same as those for other human genetic traits. The pedigree patterns described in the following section show that inheritance of traits depends on two factors: (1) whether the gene responsible is on an autosome or on the X chromosome and (2) whether the trait is dominant—that is, expressed even when the gene is present on only one chromosome of a pair—or recessive—expressed only when the gene is present on both chromosomes. Thus four basic transmission patterns are possible in humans: autosomal recessive, autosomal dominant, X-linked recessive, and X-linked dominant. All antigenic markers routinely evaluated in the blood bank are inherited by one of these mechanisms.

Pedigree Charts

Mechanisms of gene transmission are essentially the same in humans as in other animals. However, for obvious reasons, controlled studies of selected matings cannot be performed in humans. Therefore, the analysis of inheritance requires very different approaches when humans are studied. One fact in our favor is the enormous size of the human population. This fact makes it likely that the cross has occurred and that the results are available for study. Because variant traits are often deleterious and come to the attention of health care professionals, it is possible to document specific information with the affected individuals and their immediate families. Examination of family histories is an important approach in the study of human patterns of inheritance. The analysis of these family histories, or pedigrees, is used to determine the pattern of gene transmission.

Constructing a Pedigree Chart

Geneticists working on the inheritance of blood-related antigens have borrowed liberally from classic genetics. Standardized rules, symbols, and notations for constructing and interpreting **pedigree charts** have been adapted to blood banking genetics.

In the analysis of human gene transmission, the starting point is often the identification of an affected individual, called the **propositus** or **proband,** followed by the construction of a genetic history, or pedigree, of the individual's family. The pedigree chart has a specific form to facilitate the identification of and relationship between each individual in the study. By convention, each generation is displayed on a different level, and standard symbols are used to denote sex, zygosity, and other pertinent information about each family member. Symbols used in constructing a pedigree chart are shown in Fig. 1-6.

Once the molecular basis of an inherited disorder is understood, it is possible, using chemical procedures, to detect persons who are carriers of the defective gene. A complete and accurate analysis of any lineage depends on a thorough understanding of elementary genetic principles and the laws of mathematical probability. In addition to these basic concepts, little more than common sense is needed to avoid certain common pitfalls often overlooked in hasty interpretations.

Examining a Pedigree

Before examining any pedigree, it is essential to realize that some histories do not provide enough information to permit definitive statements to be made. It is just as important to know that an interpretation is impossible in one case as it is to know that a precise answer can be given in another. These points are illustrated in the following discussion.

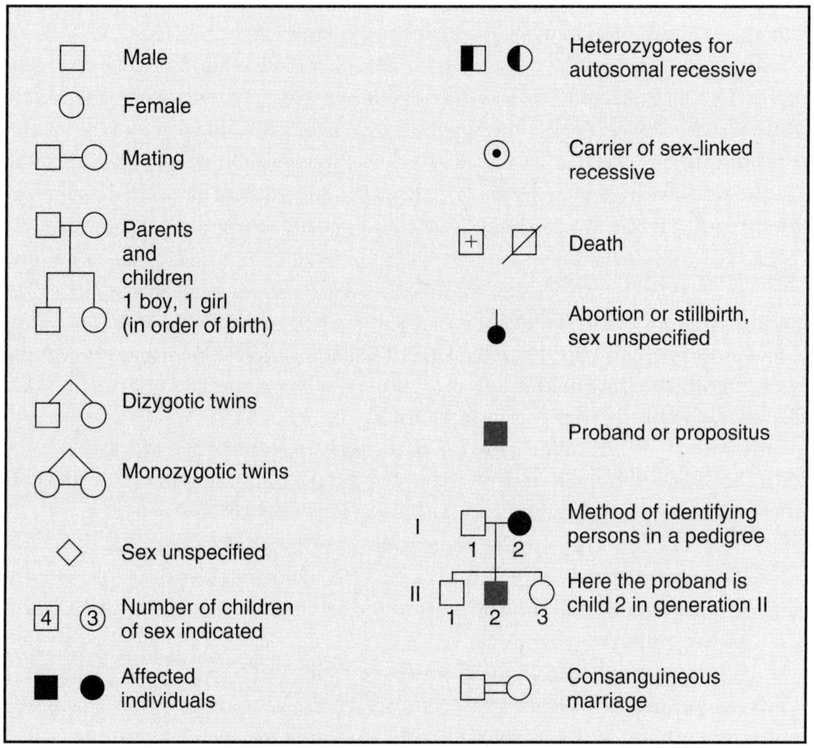

> **Pedigree chart:** A diagrammatic method of illustrating the inheritance of genes within a given family.
>
> **Proband/propositus:** The individual being studied in a pedigree, such as the individual with a certain disease or other inherited trait of interest.

Fig. 1-6 Symbols commonly used in pedigree charts.

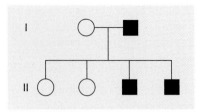

Fig. 1-7 Small family pedigree.

When presented with a pedigree, one should attempt to determine whether the trait follows a dominant or recessive pattern of inheritance. At the same time, we should ask if the expression of the trait seems to be influenced by the sex of an individual. Suppose we are given the pedigree in Fig. 1-7 with no additional information and are requested to comment on it.

We note that the male parent expresses a particular trait and that one half of the offspring, both sons, also show it. Can we say with any degree of certainty how the condition is inherited? The answer is emphatically "No!" The reason becomes obvious if we allow *"A"* to represent any dominant and *"a"* its recessive allele. Assuming that the trait results from a homozygous recessive condition, the genotype of the male parent must be *"aa"* and that of the female parent *"Aa."* An interpretation is possible on this basis. But another conclusion is equally feasible, if we assume that the trait is due to a dominant allele and that the male parent is the heterozygote, *"Aa";* the female parent would then be homozygous recessive, *"aa,"* for the normal condition.

All three males and none of the females in the pedigree express the trait; therefore, the responsible gene might be sex-influenced, sex-limited, or sex-linked to the X or Y chromosome. Because an argument can be made for each one of these possibilities, nothing about the inheritance of the trait can be stated definitely from this pedigree standing by itself. Those who argue that the sex of the individual is influencing the expression of the trait should realize that too few people are represented in the pedigree to draw that conclusion. Elementary probability tells us that theoretical ratios can become distorted by chance factors when we work with small samples. The fact that only males in this pedigree show the trait may reflect nothing more than chance. Not enough people are involved to indicate anything about the relationship of the trait to the sex of the individual. Therefore a valid response to a question about this pedigree is that more information is needed before any definitive statement regarding inheritance and gene transmission can be made.

Autosomal Inheritance

Recall that genes at the same locus on a pair of homologous chromosomes are alleles. An individual who inherits identical alleles at that locus on both chromosomes is homozygous. In the heterozygous condition, the alleles present at that locus on each chromosome are nonidentical.

Autosomal inheritance shows a characteristic pattern that is easy to recognize in both the dominant and recessive condition. The following are criteria for autosomal dominant inheritance:

1. The trait appears in every generation.
2. The trait occurs with equal frequency in males and females.
3. On the average, the trait is transmitted by an affected person to half of his or her children.
4. Unaffected family members do not transmit the trait to their children.

Most blood group antigens fit into this category. When two alleles are present, both traits are expressed and are said to be codominant. Fig. 1-8 presents a pedigree showing a typical pattern of autosomal dominant inheritance.

Autosomal inheritance: Alleles that are carried on any autosome (except the X or Y sex chromosome).

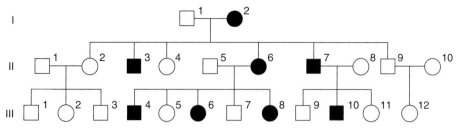

Fig. 1-8 Family pedigree showing typical autosomal dominant inheritance.

An autosomal recessive trait is expressed only in homozygotes who have received the recessive gene from both parents. The following are the criteria for autosomal recessive inheritance:

1. The trait characteristically appears only in siblings, not in the parents or other relatives.
2. On the average, one fourth of the siblings are affected.
3. The parents of the affected child may be consanguineous.
4. Males and females are equally likely to be affected.

Parents of affected children who lack the trait must necessarily be carriers, that is, heterozygous for the gene whose presence is not phenotypically apparent. When a recessive gene is rare, related persons are more likely to carry the same rare gene than are unrelated persons. Fig. 1-9 presents a pedigree showing a typical pattern of autosomal recessive inheritance.

X-Linked Inheritance

Dominant and recessive traits may be determined by genes on the X chromosomes. When the gene products of sex-linked (X-linked) genes are studied in females, the phenotype or expression of dominant and recessive traits is the same as that for autosomal genes because females have two X chromosomes. In contrast, males have one X chromosome and one Y chromosome, and most of the genetic material on the X chromosome in males does not have an analogous region on the Y chromosome. Males are said to be **hemizygous** for the X chromosome. As a result, the expression of X-linked genes that specify a dominant trait is effectively the same in males and females but is quite different for recessive traits. An X-linked recessive trait is expressed by all males who carry the gene but by females only if they are homozygous. Consequently, X-linked recessive diseases such as hemophilia are almost entirely restricted to males.

The following are the criteria for **X-linked** dominant **inheritance:**

1. Affected males transmit the trait to all their daughters and none of their sons.
2. Affected heterozygous females transmit the trait to half their children of either sex.

Hemizygous: Used to describe the genetic material on the X chromosome of the male for which there is not equivalent material on the Y chromosome.

Sex-linked (X-linked) inheritance: An allele that is carried on the X chromosome.

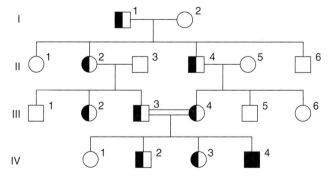

Fig. 1-9 Family pedigree showing autosomal recessive inheritance.

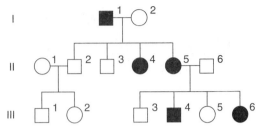

Fig. 1-10 Family pedigree showing typical X-linked dominant inheritance.

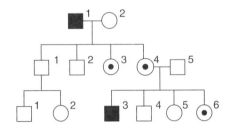

Fig. 1-11 Family pedigree showing typical X-linked recessive inheritance.

3.   Affected homozygous females transmit the trait to all their children.
4.   In rare X-linked dominant disorders, females are more often affected but are usually heterozygous and have a variable, less severe expression.

An example of an X-linked dominant trait in blood group genetics is the Xg^a blood group.

The following are the criteria for X-linked recessive inheritance:

1.   The incidence of the trait is much higher in males than in females.
2.   The trait is transmitted from an affected male through all his daughters to, on the average, half of each of their sons.
3.   The trait is never transmitted directly from father to son.
4.   The trait is transmitted from a carrier female to one half of her daughters (carriers) and one half of her sons (affected).

Hemophilia A is the classic example of an X-linked recessive disease. Figs. 1-10 and 1-11 present pedigrees showing typical patterns of X-linked dominant and recessive inheritance.

Linkage and Position Effects
Linkage

Linkage: The tendency of genes that are located in close proximity on a chromosome to be associated in inheritance.

Genes close together on the same chromosome tend to be inherited together; they are said to be linked or in **linkage.** According to Mendel's Law of Independent Assortment, genes that are not allelic assort independently of one another. Linkage is a major exception to this law; if two loci are linked—that is, if they are on the same chromosome and not too far apart—alleles at those loci do not assort independently but are transmitted together to the same gamete. Many blood group genes, such as *M, N, S, s* and *K, k, Kp^a, Kp^b, Js^a, Js^b*, appear to be linked. The classic way to detect linkage is by observing the simultaneous transmission of nonallelic genes through successive generations of families. Examination of such pedigree charts is a major tool in gene mapping, which is the assignment of genes to specific chromosomal locations. Since 1968 the rate of progress in gene mapping has been transformed by means of new technologies: chromosome banding, somatic cell hybridization, recombinant DNA technology, gene sequencing, PCR, and the development of computer programs to cope with the mass of information accumulated.[4]

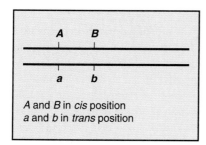

Fig. 1-12 Gene position on a chromosome pair.

Close analysis of family studies usually demonstrates linkage or independent assortment. However, the situation becomes more difficult if crossover occurs during meiosis, resulting in recombinants. Recombination is the formation of new combinations of linked genes by the exchange of genetic information between paired chromosomes. These recombinant events occur randomly along the length of the chromosome. The closer two loci reside along the chromosome, the less likely it is that a crossover will occur between them. Additional information on recombinants and gene mapping may be found in most standard genetics textbooks.

Position Effects

Two arrangements of pairs of linked genes are possible, as shown in Fig. 1-12. The genes on the same chromosome are said to be in coupling or cis position, whereas those on the opposite chromosome of a pair are in repulsion or trans position. This terminology is particularly useful in the Rh blood group system; for example, the E antigen produced by the *DcE (R^2)* gene *(D in cis position to E)* is quantitatively weaker than E antigen produced by the *dcE (r")* gene.

POPULATION GENETICS: GENE POOL DISTRIBUTIONS

During World War I, Hirszfeld and Hirszfeld discovered that different groups of people had different ABO group distribution. This discovery was the beginning of population genetics—the study of the distribution of genes in populations and how the frequency of genes and genotypes is maintained or changed. A basic understanding of population genetics, probability, and simple algebra is important in blood banking. These concepts are used in parentage testing and clinical situations such as predicting the likelihood of finding blood compatible with a serum that contains multiple antibodies directed toward red blood cell antigens.

Equilibrium Frequency of Genes in Populations

For any gene locus, in a population with random mating, the genotype frequencies are determined by the relative frequencies of the alleles at that locus. Every population is characterized by a set of gene frequencies for each blood group system. In the short term, over a period of a few generations, these frequencies change very little. Four main causes exist for gene frequency change: mutation, natural selection, genetic drift, and linkage equilibrium.

Mutation

Mutation is constantly taking place in genetic systems. It is, however, a rare event, with any one gene being affected in only about one in a million reproductive cells. Mutation is a change in the hereditary material of an organism. This change may involve the chromosome (chromosomal mutation) and include alterations such as deletions and inversions. Mutations also affect individual genes (point mutations). They involve a change, by the substitution or alteration of single nucleotide pairs, in the base sequence of a DNA molecule.

Natural Selection

A changed gene appears in substantial numbers of members of a population only if the substitution gives its carrier some advantage over those with the unchanged gene. One example of natural selection is the gene for hemoglobin A and its partial replacement in many African populations by an allelic gene, hemoglobin S. Homozygotes for the S gene have the disease sickle cell anemia, but the gene, despite this apparent selection against it, persists at a high level. The explanation for this phenomenon is now known to be that heterozygotes for hemoglobins A and S are much more resistant to malaria than are persons with only hemoglobin A. The result is a balance between selection by malaria and selection by sickle cell anemia, so that the population settles down to a hemoglobin S frequency related to the local incidence of malaria.

Genetic Drift

In small isolated populations the frequency of many of the blood group genes differs widely from those found in the larger population from which they descended. In any population, individual families may show chance variations in the frequency of offspring of different blood groups. For instance, a pair of AO and OO parents should have equal number of AO and OO children, but they may, by chance, have other proportions. In a large population family variations balance each other, but in small populations random events substantially affect overall ratios. The long-term effect, as long as the population remains small, is a gradual erratic drift of gene frequency.

Linkage Equilibrium

In blood group systems, such as Rh, MNSs, Kell, and human leukocyte antigen (HLA), which have three or more closely linked loci, changes occur in the frequencies of haplotypes. Normally, linked loci should be in equilibrium; that is, the relative proportions of the possible combinations should be determined only by the population frequencies of the alleles of the loci. Linkage equilibrium is maintained over time because crossover distributes the alleles at one locus so that ratios between the frequencies of combinations of the genes at a second closely linked locus are the same as the ratios between the total frequencies for these genes in the population.

Two causes are possible for a lack of linkage equilibrium (linkage disequilibrium). Either selection is favoring those haplotypes found in excess of equilibrium levels, or the population is the result of recent mixing of two or more separate populations. Linkage disequilibrium is particularly obvious for alleles at some of the HLA loci, and this phenomenon is thought to underlie the association of HLA and disease, creating a selection in favor of certain HLA haplotypes. Additionally, linkage disequilibrium in the HLA system is important in parentage studies, because haplotype frequencies in the relevant population make transmission of certain gene combinations more likely than others.

Phenotype Frequencies

Blood typing procedures performed in laboratories establish phenotypes. Phenotype frequencies are determined by testing red blood cells from a large random sample of individuals of the same race. The percentage of positive or negative reactions is calculated. For a given blood group system, all the possible phenotype frequencies should equal 100%. For example, if the red blood cells from 10,000 Caucasian blood donors are tested for the K antigen with anti-K, 900 blood samples produce positive reactions. The remaining 9100 blood samples produce negative reactions. Thus, the frequency for the K-positive phenotype is 9%. Conversely, the frequency for the K-negative phenotype is 91%. If blood is needed for a patient with anti-K, 91%, or approximately 9 in 10, of ABO-compatible units of blood should be compatible.

Gene Frequencies

In 1908, a British mathematician, G. H. Hardy, and a German physician, W. Weinberg, proposed independently a theory of gene distribution in a population. This theory, known as the Hardy-Weinberg law, states in algebraic form that the relative proportion of genotypes with respect to a given locus remains constant (or in equilibrium) in a population as long as mating is random. The Hardy-Weinberg law is one of the most useful tools in the study of population genetics because of its application in problem solving. It permits estimation of gene frequencies from phenotype frequencies observed in a sample, and reciprocally the determination of genotype and phenotype frequencies of a population from the gene frequency.

The Hardy-Weinberg equilibrium is expressed in algebraic terms as the expansion of the binomial equation: $p^2 + 2\,pq + q^2 = 1$. Thus, if two alleles, *A* and *B*, have gene frequencies of p and q, the homozygotes and heterozygotes are present in the population in the following proportions:

$$AA = p^2 \quad AB = 2\,pq \quad BB = q^2$$

It is worth noting that for two alleles, only one gene frequency is needed, for example p, because q can be calculated using the binomial equation $p + q = 1$.

Example 1

Problem: Determine the gene frequencies of alleles *K* and *k* from the observation that 9% of blood samples are K+.

Given: In the Hardy-Weinberg equation, $p^2 + 2\,pq + q^2 = 1$,

$$p = \text{frequency of } K \text{ gene}$$
$$q = \text{frequency of } k \text{ gene}$$
$$p^2 = \text{frequency of } KK$$
$$2\,pq = \text{frequency of } Kk$$
$$q^2 = \text{frequency of } kk$$

Therefore:

$p^2 + 2\,pq$ = frequency of the K antigen (K+), which was given above (9% or 0.09)

Solve for q:

$$p^2 + 2\,pq + q^2 = 1$$
$$q^2 = 1 - (p^2 + 2\,pq)$$
$$q^2 = 1 - 0.09$$
$$q^2 = 0.91$$
$$q = 0.95$$

Because the frequencies of allelic genes must equal 1.00,

$$p + q = 1$$
$$p = 1 - q$$
$$p = 1 - 0.95$$
$$p = 0.05$$

Therefore:

The gene frequency of *K* gene (p) is 0.05 and the gene frequency of *k* gene (q) is 0.95.

Example 2

Assuming that there are three possible genotypes, *KK, Kk,* and *kk,* determine the genotype frequencies from the gene frequencies, *K* = 0.05; *k* = 0.95.

Given: Using the Hardy-Weinberg equation, $p^2 + 2\,pq + q^2 = 1$,

$$p = \text{frequency of } K = 0.05$$
$$q = \text{frequency of } k = 0.95$$

Therefore:

$$p^2 = (0.05)^2 = 0.0025 = \text{frequency of } KK$$
$$2\,pq = 2(0.95)^2 = 0.095 = \text{frequency of } Kk$$
$$q^2 = (0.95)^2 = 0.90 = \text{frequency of } kk$$

Probability

Genetic transmission from parent to child is much like tossing coins. In both, two results are possible: The coin turns up heads or tails; the parent transmits one or the other of each pair of alleles. In either case, the outcome is determined by chance.

Statisticians define probability, the mathematical expression of chance, as the ratio of the number of occurrences of a specified event to the total number of all possible events. The probability that a child whose father is of blood group AB will receive the A allele rather than the B allele is as follows:

Possibility of A

Total number of possibilities = one in two (1/2) or 50% (0.5)

Therefore:

The chance that a child whose parents are both of blood group AB will receive the A allele from each parent is the product of the two probabilities as follows:

$$(0.5)(0.5) = 0.25 \text{ (one in four or 25\%)}$$

The probabilities of receiving the A allele from each parent are independent events; the occurrence of one event has no influence on the occurrence or nonoccurrence of the other event. As illustrated, the chance of these events occurring together is the product of the chances of each one occurring by itself.

The blood bank applications of this simple but important principle are numerous. Perhaps one of the most useful is the case of a patient who has multiple blood group antibodies and it is necessary to estimate the number of units of blood that will have to be screened with that patient's serum to find units of blood negative for the appropriate antigens.

For example, if a patient has anti-c and anti-K, how many ABO-compatible units of blood must be tested to find two units of the appropriate phenotype?

Given:

Antigen frequencies: c negative = 20% (0.20)
K negative = 91% (0.91)

Therefore:

To calculate the frequency of the combined phenotype of these independent events, multiply the individual frequencies.

$$0.20 \times 0.91 = 0.18 \text{ (18\%)}$$

It follows then that in 100 units of blood, approximately 18 are negative for both antigens. If only five ABO-compatible units are available, it is unlikely that two units of blood will be found that are negative for both antigens without the assistance of the local blood supplier.

When two events are mutually exclusive—that is, the occurrence of one event prevents the occurrence of the other—the probability of either event occurring is obtained by adding the probabilities of each event.

Example: Consider this simplified paternity case.

Alleged Father	Mother	Child	Possible Type of Biologic Father
A	O	A	A or AB

The frequencies of phenotypes for A and AB are 0.44 and 0.04, respectively. To calculate the frequency of either of these mutually exclusive events occurring, add the individual frequencies.

$$0.44 + 0.04 = 0.48 \ (48\%)$$

The alleged father (group A) cannot be excluded. However, 48 out of every 100 men could equally be the biologic father. Obviously, additional testing is needed before an interpretation can be made regarding this hypothetical case.

MOLECULAR GENETICS: MOLECULAR BASIS OF HEREDITY

A gene may be defined as a unit of heredity. In the last few years, remarkable progress has been made in our knowledge of the structure and function of genes at the molecular level. The major properties of genetic molecules are replication, a requirement for passing hereditary information from generation to generation; mutation, a requirement for the genetic variability necessary for evolution; and functional complexity, a requirement for the production of the enormous range of inherited physical characteristics or phenotypes found in humans.

The state of knowledge of protein and nucleic acid chemistry in the 1930s greatly influenced early beliefs about the chemical nature of the genetic material. In brief, proteins were known to be highly complex polymeric molecules, whereas nucleic acids were thought to be comparatively simple. Therefore, many geneticists favored proteins as the major component in genetic material. In the early 1950s, working with bacteria, Hershey and Chase confirmed the role of DNA as the carrier of hereditary information.[5] In 1953, Watson and Crick put forth their hypothesis of the chemical structure of the gene.[6] Their hypothesis illustrated the chemical complexity necessary for genetic material and provided a mechanism for self-duplication and mutation.

The Nucleic Acids

The nucleic acids, deoxyribonucleic acid (DNA) and ribonucleic acid (RNA), are macromolecules composed of three types of units: a five-carbon sugar (deoxyribose in DNA, ribose in RNA), a nitrogen-containing base, and a phosphate. The bases are of two types, purines and pyrimidines. DNA contains two purine bases, adenine (A) and guanine (G), and two pyrimidines, thymine (T) and cytosine (C). In RNA, uracil (U) replaces thymine. A schematic diagram of DNA is shown in Fig. 1-13.

DNA and the Genetic Code

Genetic information is stored in DNA by means of a code in which three adjacent bases (a triplet) constitute a codon, the coding for a specific amino acid. For a three-base code, 64 combinations are possible. These 64 codons define the genetic code. As might be expected, the sequence of codons in the coding sequences of the DNA molecule represents successive amino acids of a corresponding polypeptide. A gene, as the basic unit of inheritance, is the sequence of DNA codons required for production of this functional polypeptide.

RNA—Transcription and Translation

Genetic information is stored in DNA in the chromosomes within the cell nucleus. The transfer of this information is accomplished through a group of intermediary macromolecules composed of RNA. The link between DNA and protein synthesis is RNA. The relationship of DNA to RNA to polypeptide is referred to as the central dogma of molecular genetics.

As already noted, the primary structure of RNA is similar to that of DNA, except that RNA contains a different sugar, ribose, and the base uracil in place of

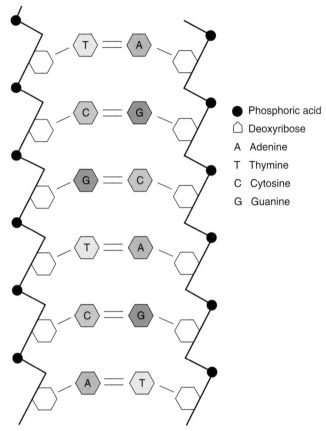

Fig. 1-13 Schematic diagram of DNA.

● Phosphoric acid
⌂ Deoxyribose
A Adenine
T Thymine
C Cytosine
G Guanine

thymine. Three specialized forms of RNA each serve specific functions: messenger RNA (mRNA), ribosomal RNA (rRNA), and transfer RNA (tRNA). Messenger RNA is the material from which proteins are made, ribosomal RNA is the structure on which proteins are made, and transfer RNA is the molecule that places the amino acids in proper sequence.

The process by which the genetic information of DNA is transferred to RNA has been termed transcription, is mediated by an RNA polymerase, and occurs in the cell nucleus. It involves the synthesis, according to the base-pairing rules, of a complementary single strand of mRNA on one of the two strands of a DNA molecule. At it simplest, genes are transcribed into mRNA, which will code for specific polypeptides. However, the vast majority of genes are interrupted by one or more noncoding regions called **introns.** These intervening sequences are initially transcribed into mRNA but are later excised from the mature mRNA message. Introns alternate with coding sequences, or **exons,** that ultimately encode the sequence of the polypeptide chain.

Once formed, mRNA moves from the cell nucleus to the cytoplasm, where it becomes associated with cytoplasmic organelles known as ribosomes. The process of translation of protein synthesis takes place in the cytoplasm and is the process by which genetic information transcribed in mRNA directs the sequence of amino acids during polypeptide chain synthesis.

Ribosomes, which are complex structures made up of proteins and rRNA, are easily dissociated into two subunits. The lighter of these has an attachment site for mRNA, whereas the heavier has two attachment sites for tRNA. The ribosome brings together the mRNA and tRNA and functions as the site of protein synthesis. Ribosomal RNA attaches to the mRNA and moves along it one triplet at

Intron: Gene segment that is initially transcribed but is then removed from within the primary RNA transcript by splicing together the sequences (exons) on either side of it.

Exon: Transcribed region of a gene that is present in mature messenger RNA.

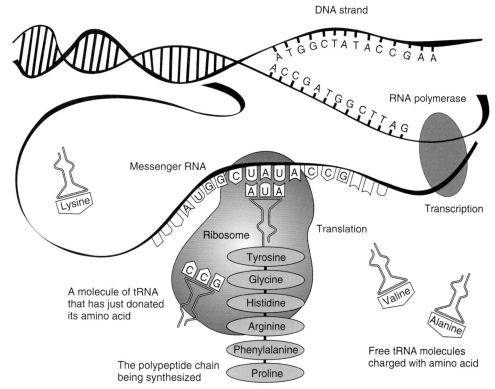

Fig. 1-14 Schematic of protein synthesis. Strands of messenger RNA (mRNA) are formed on a DNA template in the nucleus. The mRNA travels to the cytoplasm, where it attaches to a ribosome. A tRNA–amino acid complex, whose anticodon triplet matches the codon triplet being "read" (translated) on the mRNA, fits into place against the mRNA. As the mRNA strand is translated, the tRNA molecules are cleaved from the attached amino acids. The amino acids are joined together by peptide bonds to form the protein molecule encoded in the original DNA strand.

a time. At each triplet position (codon), the corresponding tRNA, already charged with an amino acid, enters the ribosome and aligns its complementary sequence (anticodon) with the current triplet being read on the messenger. The amino acid on the end of the tRNA is then transferred to the growing polypeptide. Thereafter, amino acids are added, one at a time, by the same process until the polypeptide chain is completed (Fig. 1-14).

Biosynthesis of Blood Group Antigens

Blood group antigens are chemical structures embedded in or protruding from the red blood cell membrane. Additionally, structures similar to red blood cell antigens are found in body fluids. Antigens found in this form are referred to as soluble blood group substances. Both forms of blood group antigens are under genetic control. The proteins produced by genes combine with other polypeptides, lipids, or oligosaccharides to form complex antigenic molecules. Alternatively, the protein coded for by the genes may be an enzyme called a transferase. The three most common forms of blood group antigens are glycoproteins, glycolipids, and proteins.

Glycoproteins are polypeptide chains with oligosaccharides (sugars) attached. The ABH and Lewis antigens of the saliva (soluble blood group substances) are glycoproteins. In these systems, the function of blood group genes is to synthesize transferases that construct the oligosaccharide portion of the antigen. The antigens of the MN blood group system (see Chapter 6) also are glycoproteins, but these

Blood group antigens: Membrane chemical structures capable of inducing the production of antibody in foreign hosts. Red cell antigens differ among members of the species (alloantigens); therefore individuals can produce antibodies directed against antigens on transfused red cells. This is the basis for much of the science of immunohematology.

Refer to Chapters 3 through 6 for an indepth discussion of the blood group antigen systems.

antigens are part of the red blood cell membrane. The specificity of the M and N antigen is related to the amino acid sequence of the protein portion (glycophorin A) of the molecule. In other words, the *M* and *N* genes control the terminal amino acid sequence of glycophorin A rather than the sugars that are attached.

From a structural point of view, the best-characterized glycolipids with blood group reactivity belong to the ABO, Hh, Ii, and P systems (see Chapters 3 and 4). Glycolipids are composed of oligosaccharides and lipids. The genetic control of glycolipids rests in the production of transferases, adding specific sugars to the lipid portion of the molecule. Moreover, for a given ABH specificity, the terminal sugars carrying blood group activity are identical to those described previously for secreted glycoproteins (soluble blood group substances).

Those antigens that are almost entirely protein are embedded in the red blood cell membrane. The most studied of these structures are the molecules that carry the Rh antigens (see Chapter 5). The protein nature of the Rh antigens indicates that they are probably the direct product of their corresponding genes.

Polymorphisms in Blood

The ABO blood group system, discovered by Karl Landsteiner in 1900, was the first genetic polymorphism defined in humans. Since that time blood groups have played a prominent role in the study of human polymorphisms. More than one third of the human genetic loci that have been studied have been found to be **polymorphic.**[7] Examples include the major blood group systems, a variety of red cell enzymes and serum proteins, and the cellular antigens encoded by the major histocompatibility locus. *Polymorphism* is defined as the occurrence of two or more alleles for a given locus in a population, where at least two alleles appear with frequencies of more than 1%. Because of their ready classification into different phenotypes, relatively simple mode of inheritance, and different frequencies in different populations, blood groups are useful genetic markers in family and population studies and in linkage analysis.

A significant proportion of the population is heterozygous, and, considering the amount of genetic polymorphism, the opportunity for new combinations of alleles is staggering. For example, using an estimate of 6.7% for the average heterozygosity in humans, the calculated number of possible combinations of alleles is so large that any two persons (except monozygotic twins) are highly unlikely to have exactly the same set. Assuming that there are 100,000 loci in the human, the 6.7% figure indicates that a person would be heterozygous at approximately 6700 loci and could potentially produce 26,700 types of gametes. As the number of polymorphic systems used increases (red blood cell antigens, platelet antigens, HLA antigens), the number of individuals who appear to be identical becomes smaller and the idea of genetic solitude becomes more understandable: Each individual is unique.

Molecular DNA-based techniques in common use today allow for the demonstration of these polymorphisms at the single base pair level. Detection of these **single nucleotide polymorphisms (SNPs)** and determination of their significance is the basis of molecular antigen typing in blood banking.

MOLECULAR APPLICATIONS IN BLOOD BANKING

The ability to discriminate between different forms of a gene is key in all human genetics research. Genetic markers are of enormous practical use in mapping genes to particular chromosome regions; prenatal diagnosis of genetic disease; evaluation of risk for adult-onset diseases such as coronary artery disease, cancer, and diabetes; parentage testing; tissue typing for organ and tissue transplant; and forensic applications establishing the identity of perpetrators in criminal investigations.

Polymorphic: Describes a population that contains two or more phenotypes.

Single nucleotide polymorphism (SNP): A polymorphism in DNA sequence consisting of variation in a single base.

surfaces again as an ideal model not only because of all the available comparative serology and genetics related to blood group systems but because RBCs provide natural "knockouts" (null states) for the study of function.[17,18]

Historically, blood group antigens were described and identified when alloantibodies in the sera of immunized individuals were detected by agglutination. Through the years, this detailed codification of reaction characteristics and significance was taught as the body of knowledge related to transfusion serology. The development of PCR has made it possible to use DNA-based methods to assay blood group alleles directly. Current research focuses on assessment of the significance of blood group alleles in blood banking by comparing information from molecular genetics studies to observed serologic reactions and transfusion outcomes.

Molecular Genetics Methods

Molecular techniques for antigen typing holding promise for future widespread clinical applications are PCR in combination with restriction fragment length polymorphism analysis (PCR-RFLP), sequence-specific PCR (SS-PCR), real-time PCR, DNA sequencing, and DNA microarray analysis.[19]

PCR-RFLP restriction enzyme digestion is commonly used for genomic DNA fingerprinting and for applications in antigen typing. Large probes (sequence-specific oligonucleotides) are used to select and amplify large portions of the genome. Amplified sequences are digested with restriction enzymes and the products are analyzed by Southern blot. This technique is time-consuming, requires post-PCR analysis, and can be problematic because large portions of the genome are amplified and contaminating DNA will be amplified as well.

SS-PCR will partly overcome issues of contamination because a gene-specific sequence or even an allele-specific sequence is used as primer. Only DNA complementary to that sequence will be targeted and amplified. In addition, this technique does not require the use of Southern blotting. Amplified sequences are separated by gel electrophoresis.

In real-time PCR, a fluorescein-based PCR is performed in a device that detects the amplified products at each round of amplification. This method is relatively rapid and requires no post-PCR analysis. However, at the present time, the equipment is expensive and technically complex to operate.

DNA sequencing methods utilize specific tags attached to primers that can then be analyzed in instruments such as a mass spectrometer or pyrosequencer. The actual DNA sequence is reported and unexpected sequences are readily identified. Even though the technology is potentially semiautomated, it is too expensive, time-consuming, and technically complex to have clinical applicability currently.

Microarray (DNA chip) hybridization analysis could be used to potentially allow for the screening of all blood group–associated polymorphisms in a single reaction. In this method, microdots (microarrays) of immobilized DNA representing blood group–associated SNPs are fabricated by high-speed robotics onto glass or nylon substrates. Sample DNA, produced by PCR using fluorescein-labeled probes, is added and hybridized to the microarray. After hybridization, the alleles present are detected by fluorometry. This technique has great potential for high throughput in an automated platform and thus great applicability in massive donor red cell antigen screening.

Clinical Applications of Molecular Techniques

Theoretically, once a gene is shown to encode a protein that carries a blood group antigen, molecular genotyping and subsequent matching of recipient and donor for clinically significant polymorphisms could virtually eliminate the risk

Knockout gene: Gene that has been disrupted usually by recombinant DNA technology; used as a model for investigation of the function and interactions of the normal counterparts of the disrupted gene.

Summary 1-1

Applications of Molecular Antigen Typing in Blood Banking

Typing patients who have been recently transfused, who are at risk for hemolytic disease of the newborn,[a] or who have a positive direct antiglobulin test[b]

Typing patients with weak antigen expression

Typing donors for antibody identification panels[c]

Screening for antigen-negative donors

Resolving ABO and Rh typing discrepancies[d]

Tissue typing

Parentage testing

Forensic testing

Determining the origin of lymphocytes in stem cell transplant and graft-versus-host disease

[a]Refer to Chapter 16 for a discussion of hemolytic disease of the newborn (HDN)
[b]Refer to Chapter 2 for a discussion of the direct antiglobulin test (DAT)
[c]Refer to Chapter 12 for a discussion of antibody identification
[d]Refer to Chapter 13 for information regarding the resolution of serologic problems

Refer to Chapter 16 for a discussion of hemolytic disease of the newborn and Chapter 2 for a discussion of the direct antiglobulin test (DAT). A positive DAT is a serologic finding in most cases of autoimmune hemolytic anemia. Refer to Chapter 17 for a discussion of autoimmune hemolytic anemia.

of transfusion alloimmunization. In addition, molecular genotyping can be accurately applied in the massively or chronically transfused individual, in the presence of a positive direct antiglobulin test (e.g., **autoimmune hemolytic anemia, hemolytic disease of the newborn**), and to resolve ABO and Rh typing discrepancies. DNA-based techniques for molecular genotyping can also be used to antigen-type reagent cells for antibody identification panels. These techniques are particularly useful in situations where antibody availability is rare or performance weak. Applications of DNA-based techniques are given in Summary 1-1.

Future Directions in Molecular Techniques

Currently, molecular techniques are not in common use in blood banks because of several problematic technical areas. First, quality of DNA may be compromised in clinical samples. For instance, automated analysis of specimens results in carryover contamination among sequential samples in some systems (e.g., automated blood typing, automated crossmatching). Also, different DNA collection sites may yield different results. For instance, buccal samples may differ from peripheral white blood cells because of stem cell transplant, or even pregnancy. DNA analysis from urine may differ from buccal samples because of kidney transplant and the presence of sequestered donor cells. Many of the techniques under evaluation require specialized instrumentation, and the associated costs for reagents, training, and regulation restrict their use. The most critical need to be addressed in implementation of molecular techniques is the lack of information linking SNP to clinical significance. Identification of modifying and regulator polymorphisms, as well as all SNP of significance in blood group systems, is not complete. Therefore interpretation of molecular genotyping can be inaccurate in some ethnic groups. For instance, in the great majority of $Rh_0(D)(-)$ black individuals, the genome would carry a grossly intact *RHD* gene (*RHDψ*), but the gene *RHDψ* is not expressed. If genotyping interpretation is based on the presence of the gene only, this analysis would yield a false positive.[20]

Information obtained from molecular techniques compared with hemagglutination studies will continue to increase knowledge related to structure, genetics, and function of blood group–associated antigens. Genes encoding significant blood group antigens could be expressed by transfection in heterologous systems, such as mammalian cell lines. Then, in theory, panels of cells expressing these individual antigens could be prepared for development of automated, objective antibody detection and identification methods, such as enzyme-linked immunosorbent assay (ELISA) or solid phase red cell adherence. Soluble forms of cloned antigens could be prepared, or genes could be engineered to produce soluble antigens, for use in antibody inhibition/identification studies. Among the most promising routes of research is the elucidation of the biologic functions of blood group antigens. These analyses compare gene products of normal red cells with those of null states such as Rh null. Characterization of the functions of antigens could provide opportunity for new drug development, therapeutic modalities, or even surrogate compatibility testing. Molecular methods also hold promise for direct allelic analysis of platelet-specific antigens and are particularly useful in thrombocytopenic states when platelets sufficient for serologic assay are difficult to obtain.[19]

CHAPTER SUMMARY

1. Mendel's laws, which form the cornerstone of the science of genetics, were derived from his experiments with peas, in which he crossed pure lines differing in one or more clear-cut characteristics and followed the progeny of the crosses for at least two generations. The laws he derived from the results of his experiments may be stated as follows:
   a. Law of Independent Segregation. Members of a single pair of genes are not found in the same gamete but instead segregate and pass to different gametes.
   b. Law of Independent Assortment. Members of different gene pairs assort to the gametes independently of one another.
2. Two kinds of cell division occur—mitosis and meiosis. Mitosis is the period of a cell's lifetime when it divides and ensures that two newly formed cells are precisely identical to the parent cell. Meiosis occurs only once in a life cycle and results in the production of gametes.
3. Four basic patterns of inheritance are seen in humans: autosomal recessive, autosomal dominant, X-linked recessive, and X-linked dominant. All antigenic markers routinely evaluated in the blood bank are inherited by one of these mechanisms.
4. The Hardy-Weinberg law states in algebraic form that the relative proportion of genotypes remains constant (or in equilibrium) in a population as long as mating is random. It permits determination of genotype and phenotype frequencies of a population from the gene frequency.
5. Genetic information is stored in DNA by means of a code in which three adjacent bases constitute a codon. The sequence of codons in the DNA molecule represents successive amino acids,

which are polymerized into long polynucleotide chains.
6. Blood group antigens are inherited characteristics. The three most common forms of blood group antigens are glycoproteins, glycolipids, and proteins. Because products of gene action are proteins, genetically determined carbohydrate antigens have an intermediate step. This intermediate step usually requires an enzyme to add the carbohydrate to the protein or lipid portion of the molecule.
7. Numerous polymorphisms are known in the components of human blood, especially in the antigens of red cells. Red cell antigens are useful genetic markers in family and population studies and in linkage analysis. The detection and characterization of SNP is the basis of molecular DNA–based techniques.
8. Current molecular genetics research efforts cluster around the production of recombinant DNA diagnostic and therapeutic agents, detection of nucleic acid evidence of infection in the blood supply, and molecular techniques for antigen detection.
9. Various types of PCR, including PCR-RFLP, SS-PCR, real-time PCR, DNA sequencing methods, and microarray DNA hybridization analysis, are the molecular methods holding the most promise for widespread clinical applications in blood banking.
10. Applications of molecular techniques are the focus of intense research in clinical blood banking. Information obtained from the comparison of molecular techniques to hemagglutination studies will continue to increase knowledge related to structure, genetics, and function of blood group–associated antigens.

REFERENCES

1. Klug WJ, Cummings MR: Concepts of Genetics. Columbus, OH, Charles E. Merrill, 1983.
2. Thompson JS, Thompson MW: Genetics in Medicine, 4th ed. Philadelphia, WB Saunders, 1986.
3. Bodmer WF, Cavalli-Sforza LL: Genetics, Evolution, and Man. San Francisco, WH Freeman, 1976.
4. Fristrom JW, Clegg MT: Principles of Genetics, 2nd ed. New York, WH Freeman, 1988.
5. Hershey AD, Chase M: Independent functions of viral protein and nucleic acid in growth of bacteriophage. J Gen Physiol 36:39-56, 1952.
6. Watson D, Crick FHC: Molecular structure of nucleic acids: A structure for deoxyribose nucleic acid. Nature 171(4356): 737-738, 1953.
7. Gelehrter TD, Collins FS: Principles of Medical Genetics. Baltimore, Williams & Wilkins, 1990.
8. Siegel DL: Diagnostic and therapeutic applications of phage display technology. In Stowel C, Dzik W (eds): Emerging Technologies in Transfusion Medicine. Bethesda, MD, American Association of Blood Banks, 2003.
9. Emery AE: An Introduction to Recombinant DNA. New York, John Wiley & Sons, 1984.
10. Weinberg RA: The molecules of life. In Piel J (ed): The Molecules of Life. New York, WH Freeman, 1985.
11. Watson JD, Tooze J, Kurtz DT: Recombinant DNA: A Short Course. New York, WH Freeman, 1983.
12. Pogo AO, Miller KS, Chaudhuri A, et al: The cloning of blood group genes. In Edwards-Moulds J, Tregellas WM (eds): Introductory Molecular Genetics. Washington, DC, American Association of Blood Banks, 1986.
13. Brecher ME (ed): AABB Technical Manual, 14th ed. Bethesda, MD, American Association of Blood Banks, 2002.
14. Saito Y: Bacteria detection techniques. In Stowell C, Dzik W (eds): Emerging Technologies in Transfusion Medicine. Bethesda, MD, American Association of Blood Banks, 2003.
15. Reid ME, Lomas-Francis C: Molecular approaches to blood group identification. Curr Opin Hematol 9:152-159, 2002.
16. Reid ME: Applications of molecular biology techniques to transfusion medicine. Semin Hematol 37(2):166-176, 2000.
17. Avent ND: Molecular biology of the Rh blood group system. J Pediatr Hematol 23(6):394-402, 2001.
18. Lee S, Russo DCW, Reiner AP, et al: Molecular defects underlying the Kell null phenotype. J Biol Chem 276(29):27281-27289, 2001.
19. Demomme G, Lomas-Francis C, Storry JR, et al: Approaches to blood group molecular genotyping and its applications. In Stowell C, Dzik W (eds): Emerging Technologies in Transfusion Medicine. Bethesda, MD, American Association of Blood Banks, 2003.
20. Avent ND, Reid ME: The Rh blood group system: A review. Blood 95(2):375-387, 2000.

FURTHER READINGS

Birge EA: Bacterial and Bacteriophage Genetics. New York, Springer-Verlag, 2004.

Brecher ME (ed): American Association of Blood Banks (AABB) Technical Manual, 14th ed. Bethesda, MD, American Association of Blood Banks, 2002.

Biological Sciences Curriculum Study (BSCS) Staff: Basic Genetics, 4th ed. Dubuque, IA, Kendall Hunt, 2000.

Connor JM Ferguson-Smith MA: Essential Medical Genetics, 5th ed. Oxford, Blackwell Science, 1997.

Dzik W, Stowell C: Emerging Technologies in Transfusion Medicine. American Association of Blood Banks, 2003.

Ellard S, Turnpenny P: Emery's Elements of Medical Genetics, 12th ed. New York, Churchill Livingstone, 2005.

Harwell L: Genetics: From Genes to Genomes, 2nd ed. Boston, McGraw-Hill Higher Education, 2004.

Horwitz M: Basic Concepts in Genetics: A Student's Survival Guide. New York, McGraw-Hill Health Profession Division, 2000.

Jaiwl PK, Singh RP (eds): Applied Genetics of Leguminosae Biotechnology (Focus on Biotechnology). Norwell, MA, Kluwer Academic, 2004.

Klug WS: Concepts of Genetics, 7th ed. Upper Saddle River, NJ, Prentice Hall, 2003.

Nussbaum RL, McInnes RR, Willard HF: Thompson and Thompson's Genetics in Medicine, 6th ed. Philadelphia, WB Saunders, 2001.

Omoto CK: Genes and DNA: A Beginner's Guide to Genetics and Its Applications. New York, Columbia University Press, 2004.

Pasternack JJ: An Introduction to Human Molecular Genetics: Mechanisms of Inherited Diseases. New York, Wiley-Liss, 1999.

Pogo AO, Chaudhuri A: The Duffy Protein: A Malarial and Chemokine Receptor. Semin Hematol 37(2):122-129, 2000.

Race RR, Sanger R: Blood Groups in Man, 6th ed. London, Blackwell Science, 1975.

Snustad DP, Simmons MJ: Principles of Genetics. 3rd ed. New York, Wiley, 2003.

Strachan T: Human Molecular Genetics. New York, Wiley-Liss, Oxford, BIOS Scientific Publishers, 1996.

Telen MJ: Red Blood Cell Surface Adhesion Molecules: Their Possible Roles in Normal Human Physiology and Disease. Semin Hematol 37(2):130–142, 2000.

Watson JD: Molecular Biology of the Gene. 5th ed. San Francisco, Pearson/Benjamin Cummings, Cold Spring Harbor Laboratory Press, 2004.

Watson JD: A Passion for DNA: Genes, Genomes, and Society. Cold Spring Harbor, NY, Cold Spring Harbor Laboratory Press, 2000.

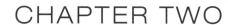

CHAPTER TWO

Immunology: Review and Applications

*Elizabeth Kenimer Leibach**

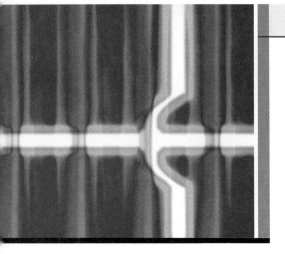

LEARNING OBJECTIVES

After reading and studying this chapter, the student should be able to:

1. List and define the three overall functions of the immune system.
2. Briefly describe the components of the immune system, including a discussion of the origin and function of the monocyte-macrophage cells, B cells, T cells, and natural killer (NK) cells.
3. Define the following terms and use them correctly in written and oral discussion of the immune system as it relates to immunohematology:
defense
surveillance
reticuloendothelial system
T lymphocytes
T-cell receptors
MHC molecules (HLA antigens)
MHC restriction
lymphokines
primary response
affinity
specificity
constant region
hypervariable region
prozone
postzone
hemolysis
direct antiglobulin test
antigen
antigenic determinants
cross-reaction
autologous
humoral immunity
homeostasis
pluripotential cell
macrophage clearance
B lymphocyte
isotype switching
clonal selection
anamnestic response
avidity
immunoglobulin
variable region
elution
equivalence

The author would like to recognize the contributions of Stephanie Summers to this chapter in the previous edition.

agglutination
sensitization
indirect antiglobulin test
immunogenicity
immunodominant
allogeneic
cell-mediated immunity
apoptosis
antigen-presenting cell
antibody repertoire

4. Compare and contrast innate immunity and adaptive immunity.

5. Define the term antigen and describe the common characteristics of antigen molecules that contribute to immunogenicity.

6. Discuss the role of the cellular immune response in delayed hypersensitivity and cell-mediated cytotoxicity (viral resistance and allograft rejection).

7. Discuss the mechanism of the humoral immune response.

8. Compare and contrast the characteristics of the primary antibody response with the secondary (anamnestic) response, including time from antigen challenge to antibody production, antibody titer, antibody class, and antibody affinity and avidity.

9. Describe the basic immunoglobulin structure.

10. Describe the structural and functional characteristics of the five immunoglobulin classes and any implications these may have in immunohematology.

11. Discuss the clinical significance of blood group antibodies.

12. Discuss the importance of the complement system to blood banking.

13. Briefly describe the structure of the red cell membrane, including implications for blood banking.

14. Discuss the following methods used in the detection of antigen-antibody reactions: agglutination, hemolysis, gel column technology, and solid-phase adherence.

15. Discuss in detail the two stages of the agglutination reaction and factors that can affect each phase.

16. Given a tube with red cell agglutination, grade the agglutination using the scheme provided in the chapter.

17. Compare the direct and indirect antiglobulin tests.

Defense: Immunologically mediated resistance to infection.

Homeostasis: That function of the immune system which removes effete or damaged self-components, such as aged red cells.

Surveillance: That function of the immune system which detects and destroys mutant cells, thus providing protection from malignancy.

Antigen: A substance capable of eliciting an immune response and reacting specifically with the product of that response.

Antibody: An immunoglobulin molecule produced in response to stimulation by a specific antigen and capable of responding to the antigen that elicited its production.

Pluripotential cell: A bone marrow cell capable of differentiation into many different cell types.

Reticuloendothelial system (RES)/Mononuclear phagocytic system (MPS): A group of cells having in common the ability to sequester substances such as inert particles and vital dyes. Included in this system are the fibroblasts of the bone marrow; macrophages; endothelial linings of the liver, spleen, and bone marrow; and reticular cells of the lymphatic system.

Antigen-presenting cells (APCs): Cells that process antigen into peptides and display complexes of MHC molecules and peptides on their surfaces.

Monocyte-macrophage: Monocytes are phagocytic leukocytes produced in the bone marrow. Monocytes are transported to the tissues, such as lung, liver, and spleen, where they develop into macrophages.

The concepts of immunology are derived primarily from the study of resistance to infection. Contributions to immunology come from both the basic sciences (biochemistry, developmental biology, genetics, pharmacology, and pathology) and the study of clinical entities (allergy, infectious diseases, organ transplantation, rheumatology, immune deficiency diseases, and oncology).

In the modern view, immunologic responses serve three functions—**defense, homeostasis,** and **surveillance.** At its most basic level, the discipline known as *immunology* involves identification and definition of **antigens** by means of their specific **antibodies.** It is the basic discipline on which the applied science of blood banking is based. This chapter explores the components of the immune system and the immunologic responses appropriate to immunohematology. A bibliography is included for study in greater detail.

THE IMMUNE SYSTEM

The immune system is one of the human body's most fascinating groups of organs, tissues, and cells. It reacts to a great variety of stimuli—from bee stings to heart transplants. It protects the body by responding to a nearly constant invasion of microbes and viruses, which, if left unchecked, would produce disease. The cells of the immune system are also responsible for a broad range of inflammatory responses, which are recognized as signs or symptoms of disease. The control of immunity and inflammation is one of the great challenges for future medical research.

Components of the Immune System
Cells and Tissues of the Immune System

The immune system of humans consists of a number of organs and several different cell types that have evolved to recognize non-self antigens accurately and specifically. **Pluripotential cells,** whose descendants, the lymphopoietic stem cell and hematopoietic stem cell, are located within the bone marrow, fetal liver, and yolk sac of the fetus, give rise to both inflammatory and immune cell lines. Progeny of these stem cells differentiate into red blood cells, white blood cells, megakaryocytes, and phagocytic cells (Fig. 2-1). This collection of cellular elements is distributed strategically throughout the tissues and lines the lymphatic and vascular channels as well. Immune system cells are housed within the blood, body tissues, thymus, spleen, liver, lymph nodes, and those body tracts exposed to the external environment—respiratory, gastrointestinal, and genitourinary (Fig. 2-2). This ubiquitous immunologic cell, tissue, and organ system is called the **reticuloendothelial system (RES).** Other terms such as **mononuclear phagocytic system (MPS)** provide equivalent terminology to describe the cells, tissues, and organs of the immune system. Both terms are now widely used.[1] Cells of the RES travel continuously through the fluids, tissues, and solid organs of the system. This movement facilitates direct contact between antigen and immune cell—a basic requirement for the immune response.

Monocyte-Macrophage Cell System and Other Antigen-Presenting Cells

Appreciation for the diversity of cells in the monocyte-macrophage system is increasing. **Monocyte-macrophage cells** (Box 2-1) derive from the hematopoietic stem cell in the bone marrow. Bone marrow stem cells produce blood monocytes, which circulate to sites of inflammation or migrate to various tissues. Monocytes that leave the bloodstream for the tissues further differentiate into tissue macrophages. Tissue macrophages are found throughout the body but are especially prominent in the liver and spleen; in peritoneal, pleural, and synovial fluids; and in lymph nodes, tonsils, and gut-associated lymphoid tissues.

A large variety of antigens and receptors have been identified on the surface of macrophages. These may be grouped as cell receptors and cell recognition mole-

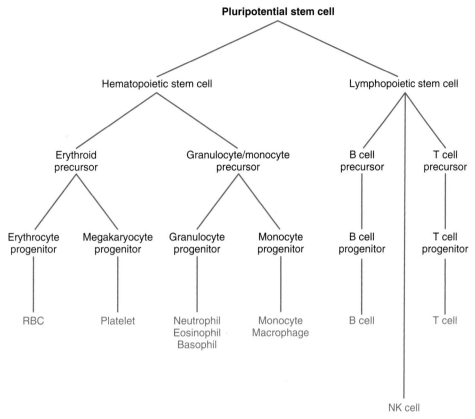

Fig. 2-1 Cells of the immune system.

cules, which have been characterized immunologically and also structurally by monoclonal antibodies. Both cell receptors and recognition molecules are significant in blood banking.

An important cell surface receptor of macrophages is the receptor for the Fc portion of the immunoglobulin molecule. Cells coated with immunoglobulin can attach to macrophages when the Fc portion of the immunoglobulin comes in contact with the Fc receptor on the surface of the macrophage. In this way many kinds of cells—autologous, microbial, transplanted, or transfused—may be removed from the circulation by macrophages. Variation in the intensity of **macrophage clearance** may be important in the variation in severity of certain autoimmune diseases or the variation in destruction of allogeneic transfused cells.

Macrophage clearance: The ability of macrophages to remove antibody-coated cells via the Fc receptor.

Tissue macrophages also possess a receptor for one of the portions of the third component of complement, C3b. Cells or microorganisms to which complement has become attached can be removed from the circulation by phagocytic macrophages in a manner analogous to the result of immunoglobulin interaction with the Fc receptor. Some blood group antibodies are capable of complement activation, resulting in complement-coated cells. These cells are susceptible to C3b receptor–mediated destruction by macrophages.

A second major group of cell surface recognition molecules found on macrophages are those of the **major histocompatibility complex (MHC),** which function in antigen recognition. Macrophages express both class I (HLA-A, HLA-B, HLA-C) and class II (HLA-DP, HLA-DQ, HLA-DR) antigens. MHC class I molecules are important in the presentation of processed antigen derived from intracellular sources such as replicating viruses or antigenic transformation resulting from cancer. Class II molecules are important in the presentation of processed antigen taken up from the extracellular environment, for example,

MHC molecules: Major histocompatibility complex molecules, either class I or class II. Also called *histocompatibility locus antigens* (HLAs).

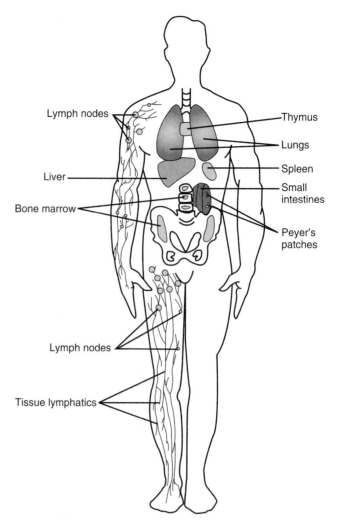

Fig. 2-2 Major organs and tissues of the reticuloendothelial system.

T lymphocytes (T cells): Thymus-dependent lymphocytes that originate from lymphoid stem cells, differentiate under the influence of thymus hormones, are characterized by cell-surface antigens, and are primarily responsible for cell-mediated immunity.

B lymphocytes (B cells): Bursa-dependent lymphocytes that are the precursors of antibody-producing plasma cells and are primarily involved in humoral immunity. B-cell maturation takes place predominantly in the bone marrow, and the cells are characterized by the presence of surface immunoglobulin.

bacteria. In addition, class II MHC antigen expression on macrophages plays an important role in transplantation immunity, in presentation of antigen to helper **T lymphocytes,** and in the development of hypersensitivity.[2] Macrophages, along with dendritic cells and **B cells,** function as "professional" antigen-presenting cells (APCs) with the purpose of triggering naïve T-cell activation. These three APCs express MHC class II molecules and characteristically present antigens of extracel-

Box 2-1	Functions of Monocyte-Macrophage Cells

Phagocytosis
  Microbes
  Aged erythrocytes
  Antibody/complement–coated cells
  Tumor cells
Inflammation
  Secretion of chemicals of inflammation
Immunity
  Antigen presentation to T cells
  Release of chemical substances (interleukin-1, interferon)
  Stimulation of transplantation responses

lular origin to helper (CD4) T cells. Extracellular antigens are taken up and processed by the APC, and then antigen-derived peptides are presented in complex with MHC class II molecules on the surface of the APC. A helper CD4 T cell will recognize its specific peptide:MHC class II complex on the APC, bind, and undergo stimulation of its effector functions. The APC types differ in their means of antigen uptake, their MHC class II expression, the types of antigens they present, and their location within the body. Macrophages specialize in presenting bacterial antigens, and dendritic cells present viral antigens. B cells present soluble antigens such as bacterial toxins. In the case of macrophages, stimulation of helper CD4 T cells results in effector functions, including interleukin production, that increase macrophage phagocytic capacity. Stimulation of CD4 T cells by B cells results in CD4 T-cell effector functions that regulate proliferation and antibody production in that specific B-cell clone.

On the other hand, MHC class I molecules are expressed by most cell types because all human cells are subject to infection by intercellular pathogens. This class of recognition molecule is involved in stimulating cytotoxic T-cell effector functions leading to **apoptosis** of cells infected with intracellular pathogens such as viruses and perhaps intracellular allergens internalized by endocytosis. Internalized antigen is processed by the infected cell and antigen-derived peptides presented in complex with MHC class I molecules on the cell surface. A cytotoxic CD8 T cell will recognize its specific peptide:MHC class I complex on the cell surface, bind, and undergo production of its effector functions leading to apoptosis (programmed cell death) of the infected cell.[3]

Apoptosis: A mechanism of controlled cell death in which cells are induced to degrade themselves from within.

T Lymphocytes (T Cells)

T lymphocytes derive from lymphopoietic stem cells in the bone marrow. Precursor cells leave the marrow and travel to the thymus gland (hence the term T cell), an organ located in the chest beneath the breastbone. The cells develop further in the thymus and are released into the circulation as mature T cells. Approximately 75% to 80% of lymphocytes in the blood are T cells. The different kinds of T cells are named according to their respective functions: natural killer (NK) cells (involved in innate immunity and discussed later), helper T cells (divided into two subgroups), and cytotoxic T cells.

A great deal has been learned about surface proteins on T cells. A listing of the better-known cluster determinants (CDs) or antigens recognized by monoclonal antibodies is given in Table 2-1. Of these antigens, the CD4 and CD8 antigens deserve special attention because their detection and quantitation are widely used in clinical medicine.

In broad functional terms, CD4-positive cells enhance and promote the action of other immune cells and are called helper CD4 T cells; CD8-positive cells have

TABLE 2-1 Selected Examples of T-Cell Antigens (Cluster Determinants)	
Antigen	Association
CD1	T cells; thymic antigen
CD2	T cells; recognizes LFA-3 adhesion molecules of APCs and binds to sheep RBCs
CD3	T cells; signaling complex associated with T-cell receptors
CD4	Helper T cell; recognizes MHC class II molecules of APC
CD8	Cytotoxic T cell; recognizes MHC class I molecules of APC
CD28	T cells; interacts with B7 costimulatory molecules to promote T-cell activation

APC, Antigen-presenting cell; CD, cluster determinant; LFA, lymphocyte function-associated antigen; MHC, major histocompatibility complex; RBC, red blood cell.

generally suppressive or cytotoxic effects and are called cytotoxic CD8 T cells. Based on these broad functions, T cells were recognized to participate in the regulation of cellular immune response, as well as humoral (antibody) immune response. As further research continued, the concept of a normal balance between CD4 T cells and CD8 T cells emerged. With the ability to rapidly quantitate the relative proportions of regulatory T-cell subsets using monoclonal antibodies and flow cytometry, abnormalities of this balance could be determined in a large number of diseases by measuring the ratio of CD4 to CD8 T cells and comparing this ratio to that in normals.[4,5] Analysis of blood T-cell subsets has shown that approximately 65% of T cells have the helper CD4 phenotype, and approximately 35% of T cells have the cytotoxic CD8 phenotype. Therefore, the CD4:CD8 ratio in the healthy, immunocompetent individual is about 2:1.

As indicated, T cells participate in an array of immune functions. These effector functions can be divided into two major categories, regulatory and cytotoxic, and, defined as such, are mediated by cytokines and cytotoxins, respectively. Regulatory activity by T cells is of two varieties: up-regulation (activation, or amplification) and down-regulation (inhibition). Both kinds of regulation, effected by cytokines secreted by stimulated T cells, can act locally on another type of cell (i.e., B cells, macrophages) or other T cells (paracrine action), or on the cell that made them (autocrine action). The cytoplasmic tails of most cytokine receptors are associated with protein kinases, which are activated on cytokine binding. Through a short signaling pathway, genes are activated in the target cell, which ultimately results in the target immune cell response.

The second functional category of T-cell activity is the exclusive domain of the cytotoxic CD8 T cell. Since intracellular pathogens (or antigens) are inaccessible to antibodies and other immune system proteins, the function of CD8 T cell–secreted cytotoxins is to kill cells terminally overwhelmed with infection. Cells targeted by cytotoxins die through apoptosis, which not only prevents pathogen replication but also pathogen spread to neighboring, vulnerable cells.

CD4 T cells can be further subdivided into T_H1 cells and T_H2 cells (where "H" is helper). T_H1 cells secrete cytokines that mainly activate macrophages; T_H2 cells primarily assist B cells in antibody production. Both types of CD4 T cells direct actions that help eliminate extracellular pathogens by either up-regulating B cell production of antibody that can fix complement or opsonize pathogens (or both) or activating macrophages to effectively facilitate pathogen elimination.[3]

B Lymphocytes (B Cells)

B lymphocytes derive from lymphopoietic stem cells and develop through a number of stages (see Fig. 2-1). B lymphocytes are so named because they were originally discovered in experiments on chickens, which showed that the cells developed from stem cells in an organ called the bursa of Fabricius. In humans, B-cell (bursa-cell) development occurs in the bone marrow.

B cells are the most important cells of the humoral immune response. B cells and the plasma cells that develop from them make immunoglobulin (antibody), the soluble, variable antigen-specific protein secreted in response to infection. B cells circulate in the blood, where approximately 15% of lymphocytes are B cells. Like T cells, B cells circulate from the blood to lymphatic organs and return to the bloodstream via lymphatic ducts. B cells, like other immune cells, exist in a resting form and an activated form. Activated B cells have been triggered to begin antibody production and undergo a process called clonal expansion (Fig. 2-3). Clonal expansion, in this application, involves the commitment of a B cell to the production of one kind of antibody (e.g., production of immunoglobulin G [IgG] with specificity for the Fy^a red blood cell antigen) and the proliferation of that particular cell line.[6] This process generates many B cells that are committed to production of the same antibody. Regulation of the process of clonal expansion

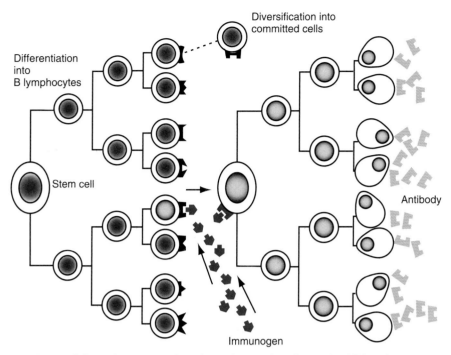

Differentiation into B lymphocytes

Diversification into committed cells

Stem cell

Antibody

Immunogen

Fig. 2-3 Schematic representation of clonal expansion of committed B lymphocytes.

and antibody production is of vital importance to the proper functioning of the immune system. Collectively, an individual's ability to make a vast array of antibody specificities is known as the **antibody repertoire** and is thought to be as high as 10^{16}.[3]

Many surface proteins have been recognized on B cells and can be grouped, like macrophages and T cells, into cell recognition molecules and cell receptors. However, the unique expression of surface immunoglobulin characterizes B-cell receptors; each B cell expresses only one type of surface immunoglobulin. When triggered to produce antibody, the specificity of the surface immunoglobulin determines the specificity of the antibody produced. Therefore, the surface immunoglobulin on the B cell serves as the receptor for the particular antigen to which that B cell reacts.

As stated, the primary function of B cells is to make antibody. For certain antigens, binding to the B-cell surface immunoglobulin is sufficient to induce clonal expansion and antibody production. However, in most cases, the trigger for B-cell antibody production also requires the presence of helper T cells. These helper T cells secrete cytokines that bind to specific B-cell receptors and induce clonal expansion and antibody production.

The majority of B cells express surface μ-chain immunoglobulins (see immunoglobulin later in this chapter). Once activated, these cells differentiate into IgM-secreting plasma cells. On continued antigen selection and subsequent direction by T_H2 cytokines, the B cell frequently changes immunoglobulin (Ig) class of its heavy chain. This process is known as **isotype switching** and can result in the production of IgG, IgA, or IgE heavy chains. In blood banking, production of clinically significant antibodies usually involves an IgM-to-IgG switch. During isotype switching, B cells with highest antigen affinity are selected for differentiation and antibody production in a process known as affinity maturation. Taken together, isotype switching and affinity maturation result not only in the generation of memory B cells with IgG surface immunoglobulin but account for the fact that a secondary or anamnestic antibody response usually results in the production of high-affinity IgG antibody.

Antibody repertoire: The total variety of antibodies made by an individual.

Isotype switching: A change in isotype expression by B cells from IgM to IgG secretion with continuous antigen stimulation.

Natural killer (NK) cells: The population of lymphocytes that carry neither T nor B cell markers.

Azurophilic: The ability to stain with blue aniline dyes.

Innate immunity: The nonspecific ability of the host to respond to injury or potential infection.

Adaptive immunity: The ability of the immune system to specifically respond to antigenic challenge; that is, the ability to discriminate between self and non-self. Adaptive immunity can be divided into cellular and humoral immunity.

Natural Killer Cells (NK Cells)

A relatively small proportion of lymphocytes that do not consistently carry markers of either T or B cells have been identified in the blood. Collectively these represent a third population of lymphocyte called **natural killer (NK) cells.** The structure of these cells is typical of a large granular lymphocyte that has abundant cytoplasm and easily recognizable **azurophilic** granules. The greatest interest in NK cells focuses on their function. Without apparent antigenic stimulation, these cells have the capacity to lyse and destroy a wide variety of cells unwanted by the host. NK cells therefore represent an early defense against cells that become infected with virus or undergo malignant transformation.[7] Their function, with some important distinctions, is similar in many ways to that of cytotoxic T cells. However, NK cells do not rearrange their receptor or effector function genes for increased specificity in response to antigenic stimulation. Another important distinction is that the NK cell cytotoxic actions are general responses to inflammation and infection and are not guided by immunologic memory. Given these characteristics, NK cells are considered part of **innate immunity,** rather than **adaptive immunity.**

Individuals who lack NK cells suffer from persistent viral infections even though they have normal adaptive immune responses. Because NK cells represent the first line of defense in the immune system, research has focused on mechanisms that control and maintain adequate NK cell activity.[6] NK cells are up-regulated by selected interferons (α and β), interleukins (IL-12), and tumor necrosis factor (TNF-α). NK cells also express cell surface receptors for MHC class I molecules, present on healthy cells. Binding of MHC class I by NK cells inhibits effector actions of NK cells and is thought to be the mechanism by which NK cells are prevented from attacking healthy cells carrying self MHC class I markers. Viral-infected cells often lose MHC class I expression as a result of evolved viral mechanisms and therefore become susceptible to NK cell attack. The actions of the cytokines named previously, as well as NK cell sensitivity to MHC class I status, activate NK cells to either overcome infection or contain it until CD8 cytotoxic T cells can be developed.[3]

The Immune Response

An immune response consists of two parts: the innate immune response (nonspecific) and the adaptive immune response (cognate and specific). Phagocytosis, cytotoxic mechanisms, and inflammation are the processes of the innate immune response. Discrimination and memory are the hallmarks of adaptive immunity.

Innate Immunity

The exterior of the human body is an effective barrier to most infectious agents. However, if an organism penetrates an epithelial surface, it encounters phagocytic cells of the RES. Their function is to nondiscriminantly engulf particles, internalize them, and destroy them. Further, NK cells participate in cytotoxic activities independent of antigen recognition and stimulation. These separate noncognate components of innate immunity act together to arrest or contain an immune challenge until the adaptive immune response develops.

Inflammation is the body's reaction to injury or infection. During the initial response, elements of the immune system are directed to the injured or infected site. Three things occur during this response:

1. Increased blood supply to the area
2. Increased capillary permeability
3. Migration of leukocytes into the surrounding tissue

These three events manifest themselves in the symptoms we recognize as inflammation: pain, heat, redness, and swelling.

Adaptive Immunity

Adaptive immunity, a capacity present only in vertebrates, has the unique characteristics of specificity, recognition, memory, and specific reactivity. The ability to recognize and discriminate between "self" and "non-self" is established early in embryogenesis. Encounter with non-self or foreign material initiates adaptive changes that result in either the production of antibodies, called the humoral response, or a cell-mediated response, which reflects actions of a T-cell subset.

The separation of adaptive immunity into cellular and humoral arms is artificial (albeit useful for teaching purposes). A great deal of interaction exists between these two systems. Although immunohematology is concerned primarily with the causes and effects of humoral immunity, the production of antibodies is closely intertwined with cellular components of immunity. Many cell populations act to enhance, suppress, and modulate the processes we recognize as the immune response. Therefore, it is necessary for the blood bank technologist to have an understanding of both humoral and cellular immunity.

Diversity and Specificity of the Adaptive Immune Response

The diversity of the response of B and T cells to immune challenge is the result of a genetic mechanism unique to the immunoglobulin and T-cell receptor genes, respectively. In the genome of lymphocytes, both the antigen-binding (variable) regions and the constant regions of the immunoglobulin (Ig) and T-cell receptor (TCR) chains are encoded in a series of separate gene segments. To produce functional cell surface markers (that is, Ig in B cells and TCR in T cells), gene rearrangement of this germ-line configuration must occur that places variable-region genes in close proximity to constant-region genes for transcription as a unit. This process of gene rearrangement in lymphocytes is known as somatic recombination and results in the production of many alternative forms of cell surface receptors. As a population, then, human immune system lymphocytes make millions of different immunoglobulins and **T-cell receptors** expressing unique, idiotypic specificities with affinity for a multitude of different pathogens or antigens, in general.

T-cell receptors: Highly variable antigen receptor of T cells usually made up of α and β subunits.

On immune challenge, only a very small portion of lymphocytes will have receptors that recognize the antigen and bind it strongly enough to be activated to divide and differentiate into effector cells. This recognition and binding of antigen gives rise to **clonal selection** and clonal expansion in which a family of lymphocytes all expressing the same immunoglobulin or T-cell receptor is created. The use of a small fraction of the total lymphocyte repertoire in this fashion ensures both the economy and specificity of the adaptive immune response. Clonal selection and expansion in a B-cell population are illustrated in Fig. 2-3.

Clonal selection: Adaptive immune responses derive from a single antigen-specific lymphocyte that proliferates in response to antigen.

Early in fetal development during maturation in the bone marrow (for B cells) and thymus (for T cells), lymphocytes, randomly generated by somatic recombination, expressing receptors for autologous ("self") fetal structures are destroyed. This negative selection of potentially self-reactive lymphocytes ensures that the remaining pool of circulating lymphocytes is self-tolerant, or nonresponsive to normal components of the body.[3]

Antigens

An antigen is a substance capable of eliciting an immune response when introduced into an immunocompetent individual or host to whom it is foreign. This immune response consists of the production of antibody, the development of cell-mediated immunity, or both. Whereas antibodies, products of the humoral immune response, can bind directly to native, extracellular antigens, T cells, involved in the cell-mediated immune response, can bind only antigens processed into small peptide subunits by antigen-presenting cells (APCs). Antigens must be processed and then assembled into complexes with MHC molecules on the APC surface before presentation to T cells. Normally, antigens must be foreign to the host and have molecular weights greater than 10,000. Smaller molecular structures, known as haptens, can elicit an immune response when they are coupled with a larger carrier protein. Antigens capable of eliciting an immune response without prior coupling with a carrier molecule are called immunogens. Several factors other than the intrinsic properties of the antigen contribute to the **immunogenicity** of a molecule (Box 2-2).

Portions of the three-dimensional structure of every immunogen (antigen) contain surface groupings known as **antigenic determinants,** or **epitopes.** Epitopes are multivalent and consist of up to seven sugars or amino acids, which may be linear or brought into apposition by the tertiary (conformational) structure of the molecule. The sugar or amino acid in the epitope that binds most strongly to antibody is called the **immunodominant** group.

Multivalent antigens may elicit antibodies of different specificities, each directed to a different epitope. Because a given antigen generally bears several different antigenic determinants or epitopes, it is possible for otherwise unrelated antigens to possess a common epitope. Some antibody molecules produced in response to one antigen may therefore react with other antigens having the common determinant (termed **cross-reactivity**).

Considerable structural diversity exists among antigens. Blood group antigens are chemical structures embedded in or protruding from red cells, white cells, and platelets. The three most common forms of blood group antigens are glycoproteins (HLA system), glycolipids (ABH, Lewis, Ii, and P blood group systems), and proteins (Rh, MNSs blood group systems). Broadly speaking, antigens may be classified into two major types: **exogenous** and **endogenous** (Table 2-2). As blood

Immunogenicity: The degree to which an antigen is capable of eliciting an immune response; also called *antigenicity*.

Antigenic determinant/epitope: That portion of the antigen molecule with which antibody can combine.

Immunodominant group: The portion of the epitope or antigenic determinant that binds most strongly with the antibody. The immunodominant group gives the antigen its specificity.

Cross-reactivity: The quality of broad specificity and the ability to react with more than one antigenic determinant or epitope.

Exogenous/endogenous: Exogenous means "outside" and endogenous means "within." An endogenous disease, for example, arises from circumstances within the organism.

Box 2-2	Factors Influencing the Immune Response to an Antigen (Immunogenicity)

1. Nature of immunogen molecule
   Protein content
   Size and shape
   Solubility
   Molecular complexity
   Foreignness
2. Dose
   Low—moderate—high
3. Route of entry
   IM, SC → lymph nodes
   IV → spleen
   Oral → Peyers patches
   Inhalation → bronchial lymphatic tissue
4. Addition of substances with synergistic effects
   Adjuvants
   Other antigens
5. Genetic factors
   Individual differences
6. Other factors
   Age
   Environment
   Nutrition
   Individual health status

IM, Intramuscular; IV, intravenous; SC, subcutaneous.
Adapted from Chapel H, Haeney M: Essentials of Clinical Immunology, 2nd ed. Boston, Blackwell Scientific, 1988, p 7.

TABLE 2-2 Classification of Antigens

Exogenous	Microbes, pollen, drugs
Endogenous	
Xenogenic (heterologous)	Forssman antigen
Autologous	Damaged or mutant cells
Allogeneic	Blood group antigens
	Leukocyte antigens
	Platelet antigens
	Immunoglobulin antigens

bankers, we are concerned primarily with antigens defined as **allogeneic** or **homologous** (from another human) and autologous (self). These antigens are important in pregnancy, transfusion, and transplantation.

Cellular Immunity

The term **cell-mediated immunity (CMI),** or **cellular immunity,** was originally coined to describe localized reactions to organisms, usually intracellular pathogens, mediated by lymphocytes and phagocytes rather than by antibody production (humoral immunity). However, it is now often used in a more general sense for any response in which antibody plays a subordinate role. The series of reactions involved in this type of immunity seems to be characteristically associated with effector–target cell interactions involved in (1) delayed hypersensitivity; (2) transplantation immunity; and (3) tumor rejection. In each of these situations, antigen is either intracellular or architecturally inaccessible, making the antigen-antibody reaction, characteristic of the humoral response, relatively inefficient. In contrast, cellular reactions appear to be effective in the elimination of such sterically inaccessible antigens. CMI does not occur as the result of a single action but is an event orchestrated by macrophages and other APCs, several subsets of T cells, and the cytokines produced by these cells. T cells and macrophages play major roles in CMI. The effector T cells involved include cytotoxic CD8 T cells and subsets of helper CD4 cells, T_H1 and T_H2.

CMI was first described through the delayed-type hypersensitivity reaction. In delayed-type hypersensitivity (DTH or type IV), the CD4 T_H1 cell responsible for the DTH response is activated, followed by a delay of many hours, allowing for the synthesis of **lymphokines** (cytokines produced by lymphocytes) and the effects of these lymphokines to occur. Table 2-3 lists the major T-cell lymphokines.

Allogeneic/homologous: Referring to antigens that are from the same species but are antigenically distinct. Blood group antibodies can be formed when an individual receives red cells from another individual that carry allogeneic antigens. Antibodies made to these alloantigens are known as alloantibodies.

Cell-mediated immunity (CMI)/cellular immunity: Immune responses mediated by T lymphocytes either as a result of direct cytotoxicity or through the liberation of lymphokines.

Lymphokines: A general term for those soluble mediators of the immune response, other than complement and antibody, that are secreted by sensitized lymphocytes on contact with antibody.

TABLE 2-3 T-Cell Lymphokines

Lymphokine	Activity
Interleukin-2 (IL-2)	Stimulates T-cell proliferation
Type-1 interferons (INF-α, INF-β)	Block spread of viruses to uninfected cells
Interferon γ (INF-γ)	Activates macrophages
Chemotactic factor (CF)	Attracts macrophage to area
Migration inhibition factor (MIF)	Localizes macrophage
B-cell growth factor (IL-9)	Stimulates B-cell division
Interleukin-3 (IL-3)	Stimulates T-cell division
Skin release factor (SRF)	Promotes inflammation
Interleukin-4 (IL-4)	Promotes B-cell growth and differentiation
Colony stimulating factors (CSFs)	Stimulate growth of specific cell lines

Delayed-type hypersensitivity is manifested by an inflammatory reaction at the site of antigen accumulation and reaches its peak in 24 to 48 hours. Memory T cells are generated after exposure to the foreign antigen. The tuberculin skin test and the allergic response to poison ivy are familiar examples of delayed-type hypersensitivity. (See more type IV hypersensitivity discussion to follow.)

Cell-mediated cytotoxicity is important in lysis of virus-infected cells and rejection of allograft and tumor cells. Antigen is presented to the cytotoxic CD8 T cell by an APC. The CD8 T cell recognizes antigen by means of class I MHC antigens (HLA-A, HLA-B, and HLA-C).[8] Helper CD4 T cells amplify the reaction. Helper T cells are activated by interleukin-1 (IL-1) produced by APCs (macrophages), and they in turn secrete IL-2, which, among other activities, enhances proliferation of CD8 T cells. After this, cytotoxic T cells bind to target cells and cause lysis. These cells are the effectors of allograft rejection and graft-versus-host disease. Memory CD8 T cells are generated, with an anamnestic response occurring on rechallenge.

Other cytotoxic cells involved in the cell-mediated immune response are the NK cells, part of the innate immune response. These cells, discussed earlier in this chapter, are able to attach to target cells and cause cell death. The cytotoxic activity of these cells, though, does not depend on antigenic specificity, MHC expression, or previous exposure. Less mature cells such as fetal cells are more susceptible to this type of cell-mediated cytolysis, as are abnormal cell populations such as tumor cells and virus-infected cells.

Humoral Immunity

Humoral immunity is mediated by a group of lymphocytes that differentiate in bone marrow and are referred to as B lymphocytes or B cells. Antibody is a product of B-cell elements and is either cell bound or secreted. Antibody has the capability of reacting with the specific immunogen or antigen responsible for its production. In humans, antibody is associated with five major classes of proteins, the immunoglobulins, that can be differentiated from one another on the basis of size, biologic function, biochemical properties, and serologic activity. These five classes of immunoglobulins are discussed in detail later in this chapter.

The immunologic reaction may involve other humoral factors that can augment or amplify the response. One example is the complement system, in which a variety of factors (proteins), both cell bound and soluble, come into play and set the stage for protective and, in some cases, detrimental events. The complement system is described later in this chapter.

In discussing potential mechanisms of antibody formation, two points should be addressed: antigen recognition and activation of B cells to produce antibody. Antigens enter the human body in a variety of ways, including eating, breathing, injection, and injury. The potential antigen becomes immunogenic only after processing or presentation. Interaction between antigen and receptor cell is a complex process. Most antigens undergo some degree of chemical or physical modification for optimal exposure of specific epitopes. Cells that process antigen are called antigen-presenting cells (APCs) and are frequently macrophages, although other cells (monocytes, histocytes, dendritic cells, Langerhans cells) may function as APCs (Fig. 2-4). APCs are found in highest concentration in the lymph nodes and spleen but are present in all tissue. The continuous circulation of lymphocytes through the RES brings idiotypically specific cells into contact with APCs, where they may recognize the processed antigen.

Antibody production involves at least three types of cells: macrophages (acting as APCs), B cells, and T cells. Antigens that stimulate this type of response are referred to as T-dependent antigens. Some antigens, particularly polysaccharides, are capable of activating B cells to produce antibody independent of T-cell help and are referred to as T-independent antigens. In general, antibody produced to T-independent antigens is IgM, which correlates with the fact that antibody to polysac-

Humoral immunity: Immunity mediated by antibodies.

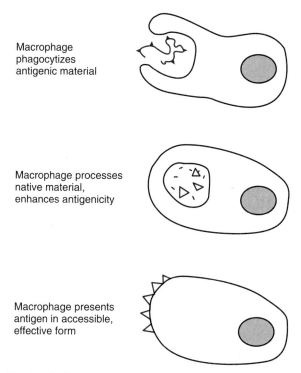

Macrophage
phagocytizes
antigenic material

Macrophage processes
native material,
enhances antigenicity

Macrophage presents
antigen in accessible,
effective form

Fig. 2-4 Antigen processing by antigen-presenting cell (APC).

charide blood group antigens is predominantly IgM. For purposes of this discussion, the T-dependent response serves as the model.

Most antigens are ingested by an APC, processed, and presented on the outer surface of that cell, where they may be recognized by appropriate T cells or B cells.[2] The helper CD4 T_H2 cell has on its surface complexes of receptors for foreign antigen and class II (DR) MHC antigens. MHC antigens are also located on the surface of the APC. The helper T cell recognizes foreign antigen when T-cell class II MHC antigens match the class II MHC antigens present on the APC. The requirement for histocompatibility between the APC and the helper T cell is referred to as **MHC restriction.**

When the T_H2 cell reacts with the presented foreign antigen along with the MHC antigen, a series of changes occurs. The APCs secrete cytokines such as IL-1, which up-regulates CD4 T cells and activates vascular epithelium to increase access of effector cells. The activated helper T cells in turn begin to secrete lymphokines. These changes allow the helper T cell to proliferate. At this point B cells are activated by the helper T cells.

The activation of B cells has two phases: proliferation and differentiation. The role of proliferation is to expand the number of cells capable of reacting with antigenic substances that have been introduced into the individual. Proliferation has two consequences: (1) increase in the number of cells that may differentiate into antibody-secreting cells and (2) production of cells with immunologic memory. The proliferative phase of B-cell response is driven, at least in part, by a T_H2 lymphokine designated B-cell growth factor (IL-9). During this process, B cells appear to require direct interaction with a T_H2 cell. T-cell help is antigen specific; that is, only helper T_H2 cells that have responded to antigen presented by macrophages can subsequently help B cells already committed to that antigen. Direct cooperation between B cells and T cells is also restricted by class II MHC antigens. This requisite B cell–T cell interaction does not occur if the lymphocytes are incompatible at the DR region.[9] B cells are further stimulated by another T_H2 lymphokine, B-cell differentiating factor (IL-6), and undergo clonal expansion to produce

MHC restriction: T-cell receptors recognize antigen only when bound to a particular form of MHC molecule.

genetically identical daughter cells. Some of the B cells differentiate into antibody-secreting cells, the plasma cells; others become memory B cells and enter the circulation.[10]

Primary and Secondary Immune Responses and the Generation of Antibody Diversity

The immune events, humoral and cellular, that occur when an immunocompetent host encounters an antigen for the first time are the **primary immune response.** In addition to measurable immune products, the primary immune response generates memory cells. These memory cells contribute to the immune events, either humoral or cellular, that occur on second or subsequent exposure to an antigen—the **anamnestic (secondary) immune response.**

Antibody production occurs in four phases following antigen challenge: (1) a lag phase when no antibody is detectable; (2) a log phase in which the antibody titer rises logarithmically; (3) a plateau phase during which the antibody titer remains steady; and (4) a decline phase during which antibody levels gradually decline as a result of catabolism and decreased production (Fig. 2-5). Examination of the responses following primary and secondary antigenic challenge shows that the responses differ in several major respects:

1. Time. When the host first encounters a particular antigen, days, weeks, or even months may elapse before the appearance of detectable antibody or cell-mediated activity; this is called the lag phase. The anamnestic response becomes apparent more rapidly, with increased antibody levels detectable in a matter of hours. The result is a shorter time period or lag phase between antigen exposure and detectable antibody during the secondary immune response.

2. Antibody titer. The plateau levels of antibody are much greater in the secondary immune response. During cell proliferation in the primary response, memory cells are generated, resulting in a greater pool of potential antibody-forming cells. Thus reintroduction of the same antigen stimulates a relatively large population of cells to differentiate and produce antibody at a

Primary immune response: The characteristics of the immune response to the first or primary antigen presentation.

Anamnestic (secondary) immune response: The characteristics of the immune response to a second or subsequent exposure to a specific antigen. This response differs in a number of ways from the typical first (primary) response.

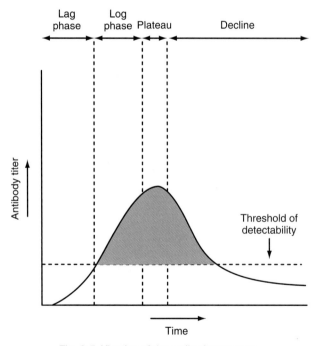

Fig. 2-5 Kinetics of the antibody response.

more rapid rate of synthesis, at a higher peak titer, and with a longer period of persistence.

3. Antibody class. Two classes of antibody are made in the primary immune responses. The earliest and predominant antibody is the IgM class. Within 2 to 3 weeks, IgM antibody levels decline and IgG antibodies are found in the circulation. In the secondary immune response, the memory B cell responds to antigenic stimulation, resulting in a predominantly IgG class of antibody. This isotype switching from IgM to IgG antibody production is mediated by T_H2 lymphokines that induce isotype switching by stimulating transcription from switch regions located at the beginning of heavy chain, constant-region genes in dividing B cells.[3] In most T-dependent immune reactions, lymphokines induce daughter cells to switch to IgG production, and some of these become memory cells. Not all antigen binding results in this IgM-to-IgG switch, however. Memory cells do not develop from B cell clones that direct IgM production.[10]

4. Antibody **affinity** and **avidity**. Antibodies formed early in the primary immune response usually have low affinity for their respective antigens. The affinity of antibody for antigen is greatly increased in the secondary immune response. In addition to increases in affinity, an increase also occurs in avidity, or the strength of the antibody-antigen bond. As a consequence of these changes, the cross-reactivity of a given antibody also increases, probably owing to the fact that high-affinity antibodies can react with closely related antigenic determinants more readily than with their low-affinity counterparts. Antibody affinity and avidity should not be confused with antibody **specificity.** Specificity is the unique, reproducible configuration that restricts antibody interaction to an antigen of complementary configuration. Because antibody production is the response to a specific antigenic determinant, both primary and secondary immune responses demonstrate specificity.

The characteristics of primary and secondary antibody responses are schematically represented in Fig. 2-6.

IMMUNOGLOBULINS

Immunoglobulins are a structurally similar group of glycoproteins synthesized by plasma cells with the help of T cells and secreted into the plasma. On exposure to appropriate antigens, plasma cells proliferate and synthesize immunoglobulins capable of specifically combining with the original antigen—a functional characteristic referred to as antibody activity. The immunoglobulin molecule has two functionally distinct parts: One part determines antigen-binding specificity (antigen-binding site), and the other part links antigen to the effector functions that eventually cause the bound antigen to be eradicated. Although immunoglobulins are not capable of direct destruction of antigenic substances, the final in vivo consequence of this antigen-antibody interaction is, with notable exceptions, elimination of the antigen or antigen-coated cell from the body.

The entire process usually involves two interdependent events. First is the highly specific binding of antigen with antibody-combining sites of immunoglobulin molecules, which serves to selectively localize and limit the immunologic assault to the offending antigen. Second is conformational change of the immunoglobulin molecule, which exposes receptor sites capable of complement activation. Antibody-antigen interaction may trigger other major host defense systems, that is, mast cells and phagocytic cells, in a highly controlled and selective manner.

The degree of binding specificity manifested in antigen-antibody interactions is determined by the three-dimensional configuration (tertiary structure) of the immunoglobulin molecule. Therefore we begin with a discussion of structural characteristics of various immunoglobulin classes and relate these characteristics to their functional activities.

Affinity: The degree of fit between an antigen and an antibody.

Avidity: The strength of the bond between an antigen and its respective antibody.

Specificity: The configuration of an antibody that results in its reaction only with the unique antigenic determinant that elicited its response.

Immunoglobulins: Any of the structurally related glycoproteins that function as antibodies. Immunoglobulins are divided into five classes based on their structure and function.

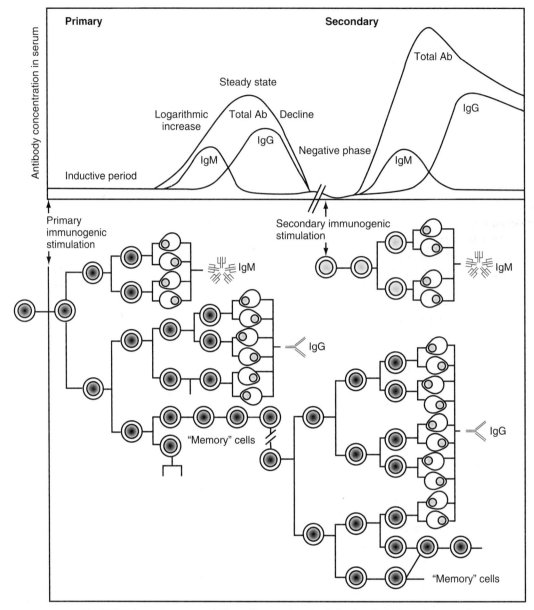

Fig. 2-6 Schematic representation of humoral and cellular events in the primary and secondary immune responses. *(Adapted from Bellanti JA: Immunology III. Philadelphia, WB Saunders, 1985, p 120.)*

Immunoglobulin Structure

All immunoglobulin molecules have a common structure consisting of four polypeptide chains, two large and two small, arranged as shown in Fig. 2-7. The large polypeptide chain, termed the heavy chain or H chain, contains approximately 440 amino acids; the smaller one is termed the light chain or L chain and has approximately 220 amino acids. The four chains are connected by disulfide bonds and held together by noncovalent hydrophobic bonds. This four-chain unit is called the Ig monomer. Immunoglobulin molecules consisting of 2, 3, or 5 monomers are described as dimers, trimers, or pentamers, respectively. Human immunoglobulins have been assigned to five classes based on primary structure of their respective heavy chains; these are IgG, IgA, IgM, IgD, and IgE; the respective heavy chains are gamma (γ), alpha (α), mu (μ), delta (δ), and epsilon (ε). There are two types of light chains, kappa (κ) and lambda (λ). Each type of light chain occurs

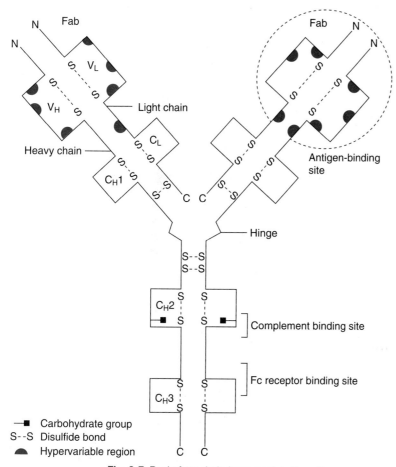

Fig. 2-7 Basic four-chain immunoglobulin unit.

in association with each kind of heavy chain. Any immunoglobulin may therefore be designated by its heavy chain and light chain composition. For example, an IgG molecule has the formula $\gamma_2\kappa_2$ or $\gamma_2\lambda_2$. Differences within the H chain type allow subdivision of Ig classes into subclasses. IgG has four subclasses, designated IgG1, IgG2, IgG3, and IgG4; IgA and IgM each have two subclasses; IgD and IgE appear to be uniform within their class.

Immunoglobulin monomers have only H and L chains, but an additional component called the joining, or "J," chain is found in polymeric immunoglobulins such as IgM and IgA. This is a short polypeptide chain of approximately 120 amino acids and seven to eight carbohydrate residues for a molecular weight of about 15,000. The J chain is synthesized by plasma cells engaged in the production of IgM and IgA immunoglobulins and initiates polymerization by binding basic Ig units through a disulfide bridge. The J chain is added to the polymerized immunoglobulin before leaving the plasma cell.

Disulfide bonds join light chains to heavy chains and link the two H chains at approximately their midpoints. The area surrounding the disulfide bonds that links the two H chains has considerable flexibility and is called the hinge region. Flexibility in this region allows the molecule to change shape while interacting with antigen epitopes located at irregular intervals.

Proteolytic cleavage of the basic structural unit has delineated important functional regions. Papain digestion breaks the Ig monomer at a point just above the hinge region, resulting in three fragments (Fig. 2-8). Two fragments (Fab) are identical, each containing a light chain and a portion of the heavy chain. Each Fab fragment contains one antibody-combining site. The third fragment (Fc), which contains the remaining heavy chain, is the region that determines functional properties not directly related to antigen binding, such as complement activation and placental transport. Pepsin cleavage, which breaks the H chain below the hinge region, results in one large fragment that includes both antigen-binding sites (see Fig. 2-8). This large fragment, F(ab)2, is capable of binding with two epitopes simultaneously. The remainder of the H chain is degraded into small fragments with no immunologic activity.

Heavy and light chains have regions called domains. Serologic and biologic actions of antibodies result from the amino acid sequence within these domains. From the carboxyl terminus (COOH) of the heavy chain to midway through the Fab fragment and homologous light chain region, the amino acid sequence is remarkably constant in all Ig classes. These domains constitute the constant region. In the remaining heavy and light chain domains the amino acid sequence is highly variable. These domains constitute the variable region of the Ig molecule. Variable domains of H and L chains are denoted V_H and V_L, respectively. Some areas of the **variable domain** show great variability in amino acid sequence composition (hypervariable regions) and provide the framework for antigen recognition. The same nomenclature is used for **constant domains,** C_H and C_L. Light chains have only one constant domain; α, δ, and γ H chains have three constant domains (C_H1, C_H2, C_H3); ε and μ chains have an additional domain, C_H4.[6] Table 2-4 summarizes the different functions ascribed to the domains of IgG. The biologic and functional differences among antibody classes reflect properties of the constant domains.[11]

In spite of basic similarities, immunoglobulins as a group are remarkably heterogeneous, owing to differences in amino acid sequence, number of structural units, and total carbohydrate content. Such variations account for differences in molecular size, charge, and antigenic determinants, all of which serve as the basis for classifying immunoglobulins.

Immunoglobulin Superfamily

Immunoglobulin domains were first described in antibodies. However, very similar structures, known generally as immunoglobulin-like domains, have now been found in other cell-surface proteins, for example, the T-cell receptors, TCRα and TCRβ, and intracellular adhesion molecules (ICAMs) pivotal to T-cell migration through epithelium. These structures collectively, together with immunoglobulins, are known as the immunoglobulin superfamily.[3]

Constant and variable domains or regions: Portions of the immunoglobulin and T-cell receptor molecules that have constant amino acid sequences are known as *constant regions,* and those with variable amino acid sequences are known as *variable regions.* Portions of the variable regions have extreme variability. These hypervariable regions give the antibody molecule its specificity for a particular antigen.

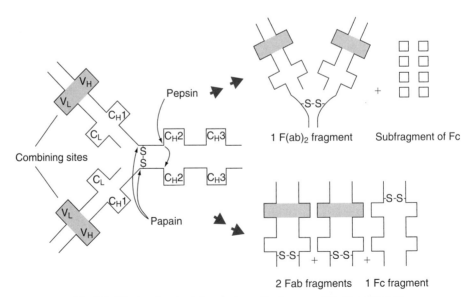

Fig. 2-8 Effects of proteolytic agents on the immunoglobulin monomer.

TABLE 2-4 Functions of the Domains of the IgG Molecule

Domain	Function
$V_H + V_L$	Antigen recognition
$C_H1 + C_L$	Binds C4b fragment
	"Spacers" between Ag binding and effector functions
C_H2	Complement fixation (Clq)
	Catabolism control
C_H3	Interaction between Fc-receptor on macrophages and monocytes
$C_H2 + C_H3$	Binds to *Staphylococcus aureus* protein A, Fc receptor on placental syncytiotrophoblast, neutrophils, and K cells

Specific Immunoglobulins

Five distinct classes of immunoglobulin molecule are recognized in humans and constitute approximately 20% of plasma proteins. These differ from each other in size, charge, amino acid composition, and carbohydrate content. Table 2-5 lists some of the properties of each class of immunoglobulin.

IgG Class

IgG is the most abundant immunoglobulin class in human serum, contributing 70% to 80% of circulating immunoglobulin. IgG exists only as a monomer (two γ heavy chains and two light chains, either κ or λ), with a molecular weight of approximately 150,000. Serum levels vary from 700 to 1500 mg/dL in normal individuals, but IgG is also distributed throughout the extravascular fluid compartment. Antibodies of this class are produced in response to a wide variety of antigens, including bacteria, viruses, and red and white blood cell alloantigens, and they are the major antibody of the secondary immune response. These immunoglobulins provide an essential defense system directed toward the elimination of soluble and particulate antigens that have gained access to the internal environment. They are necessary for efficient phagocytosis of particulate antigens by means of Fc receptors on macrophages and other cells. Toxin antigens, such as diphtheria toxin, are neutralized when combined with specific IgG antibodies. IgG is the only immunoglobulin class to cross the placenta from mother to fetus, providing immune protection to the neonate. In rare cases, transmission of maternal IgG antibody has harmful effects. The most conspicuous example is the condition called

TABLE 2-5 Physical and Biologic Properties of Human Immunoglobulin Classes

	IgG	IgA	IgM	IgD	IgE
H chain class	γ	α	μ	δ	ε
H chain subclasses	4	2	2	None	None
Constant domains	3	3	4	3	4
Exist as polymer	No	Yes	Yes	No	No
Molecular weight	150,000	160,000	900,000	180,000	190,000
Serum concentration (mg/dl)	1500	350	200	3	0.05
Carbohydrate (%)	3	8	12	13	12
Serum half-life (days)	23	6	5	2–8	1–5
Present in secretions	No	Yes	No	No	No
Antibody activity	Yes	Yes	Yes	No	Yes
Complement fixation	Yes	No	Yes	No	No
Cross placenta	Yes	No	No	No	No
Usual serologic characteristics	Nonagglutinating	Nonagglutinating	Agglutinating	?	?

Refer to Chapter 16 for an in-depth discussion of hemolytic disease of the newborn.

Complement: A system of at least 25 functionally related serum proteins that cause immune cytolysis and other biologic activities.

hemolytic disease of the newborn, which affects fetal red blood cells. The serologic behavior and characteristics of IgG antibodies make them one of the most clinically significant in blood banking.

Most blood group antigens capable of eliciting an immune response result in the production of IgG antibodies. These antibodies are detected by serologic test procedures based on their reaction characteristics, such as reactivity at 37° C, **complement** activation, indirect agglutination, and hemolysis. Much of routine blood banking involves serologic test procedures designed to detect and identify IgG antibodies. IgG can be further subdivided into four subclasses: IgG1, IgG2, IgG3, and IgG4. Each subclass has distinctive functional characteristics. Some of the major characteristics of IgG subclasses are summarized in Table 2-6.

IgA Class

IgA is the dominant immunoglobulin of external secretions—tears, saliva, colostrum, and gastrointestinal, bronchial, and nasal mucosal secretions. Serum IgA circulates as a monomer (two α heavy chains and two light chains, either κ or λ), but the secreted forms are largely dimers. IgA has two subclasses—IgA1 and IgA2—which may occur in both serum and secretory IgA.

Secreted IgA has, in addition to the J chain present in polymerized immunoglobulin, a glycoprotein called the secretory piece, and the total secretory IgA has a molecular weight of approximately 390,000. The secretory piece is formed in epithelial cells and is required for active transport of IgA across mucosal membranes. The presence of the secretory piece appears to protect the immunoglobulin from digestion by enzymes. Although IgA does not bind complement and has no bactericidal effect, it is thought to play an important role in the localization of certain infectious agents.

From a blood banking perspective, some antibodies to IgA can cause severe, life-threatening anaphylactic transfusion reactions. These reactions occur in individuals who are IgA deficient and make antibody to IgA. These antibodies then react with all immunoglobulins of the IgA class present in blood products transfused. Once identified, these individuals must be transfused with blood products that lack IgA.

IgM Class

IgM characteristically exists as a pentamer of five basic immunoglobulin units, each of which has two μ heavy chains and two light chains, either κ or λ, as well as a short additional polypeptide chain, the J chain. IgM has two subclasses—IgM1 and IgM2.

The disulfide bonds of the J chain are easily cleaved by reduction with 2-mercaptoethanol or dithiothreitol, separating the five subunits. This treatment destroys both hemolyzing and direct agglutinating activity of IgM antibodies and is a useful blood bank technique.

TABLE 2-6 Characteristics of IgG Subclasses				
	IgG1	IgG2	IgG3	IgG4
Percent of total IgG	60–70	15–25	4–8	2–5
Serum half-life (days)	23	23	8	23
Complement fixation	Yes	Yes*	Yes	No
Cross placenta	Yes	Yes	Yes	Yes
Fc receptor on				
Macrophages	Yes	No	Yes	No
Neutrophils	Yes	Yes	Yes	?
Gm groups present	Yes	Yes	Yes	No

*Less efficient than IgG1 and IgG3.

IgM constitutes approximately 10% of total serum immunoglobulin and is the first class of immunoglobulin produced as the fetal immune system matures. Additionally, it is the predominant class of antibody in the early stages of a primary immune response. Many, but not all, blood group antibodies that are capable of agglutinating antigen-positive red blood cells suspended in saline, in tests performed at 22° C, are IgM. IgM (and IgD) are the major immunoglobulins expressed on the surface of B cells. Owing to its size (molecular weight of 900,000), most IgM (1) is confined to the bloodstream with very little in the tissues; (2) does not cross the placenta; and (3) readily combines with antigen on dispersed particles, causing visible agglutination. The typical pentameric IgM molecule has 10 antigen-binding sites; however, owing to steric restriction, only five are functional at any given time. In spite of this apparent limitation, IgM antibodies are potent agglutinators that activate complement very efficiently.

IgD Class

IgD molecules consist of two δ heavy chains and two κ or two λ chains linked by disulfide bonds. It is a minor component of serum immunoglobulins, found only in trace amounts in the serum. It exists as a monomer slightly larger than IgG.

Little is known about the biologic function of serum IgD. Most IgD is present as membrane immunoglobulin on B cells and may serve as a receptor for antigen. No blood group antibodies have been reported to belong to this class.

IgE Class

IgE exists as a monomer (two ε heavy chains and two light chains, either κ or λ) at very low concentrations in serum. It has the shortest half-life, highest fractional catabolic rate, and lowest synthetic rate of all the immunoglobulin classes. Virtually all of the body's IgE molecules are bound to specialized tissue granulocytes called mast cells or their circulating equivalent, basophils. Basophils and mast cells have membrane receptor sites for the Fc (C_H4) of IgE. Combination of the IgE molecule with its specific antigen triggers the basophil or mast cell to release histamine and other vasoactive substances from its granules. The clinical effects of IgE-mediated reactions include increased vascular permeability, skin rashes, respiratory tract constriction (wheezing), and increased secretions from epithelium (tears and runny nose). These effects are consistent with allergic-type reactions (type I hypersensitivity, discussed in the following section).

Clinical Significance of Immune System Reactions

Immune system reactions, primarily protective in nature, can produce deleterious effects in some individuals predisposed through repeated antigen exposure, immunologic memory, and genetic makeup to react to molecules generally considered innocuous. These types of immune reactions, which include transfusion incompatibilities, can be categorized into four groups of hypersensitivity reactions (types I through IV).[3]

Type I hypersensitivity reactions result from the binding of antigen to antigen-specific IgE on the surface of mast cells (primarily) and basophils. Antigen-IgE binding causes degranulation and release of mediators such as histamine and other inflammatory peptides. This category encompasses the continuum of reactions from simple allergies to life-threatening anaphylactic shock and is represented by such well-known maladies as pollen, drug, food, and venom allergies. Important in transfusion medicine is the rare but clinically serious IgA–anti-IgA anaphylactic reaction, described previously, that can occur in IgA-deficient individuals with IgA antibodies who are transfused with blood products containing IgA.

Type II hypersensitivity reactions result from the binding of antibody to antigens, either integral or adsorbed to the membrane, found on cell surfaces. Hemolytic disease of the newborn, autoimmune disorders involving red cells, drug-related hemolytic anemia, and transfusion reactions caused by blood group antibodies, described previously, are examples of this type of hypersensitivity.

Type III hypersensitivity reactions result from the physiologic reactions to immune complexes formed by soluble antigens and the antibodies bound to them. These complexes activate complement and polymorphonuclear cells and thus produce local inflammatory responses at the sites of complex formation. Serum sickness, caused by serum protein–antibody complexes, is an example of this type of immune reaction. When nonhuman animal proteins, such as horse antitoxins, are given therapeutically, serum sickness is a potential risk. Hyperacute solid organ rejection is also an example of type III hypersensitivity.

Type IV hypersensitivity reactions differ from types I through III in that the effector molecules are products of T cells versus antibodies produced by B cells. As previously discussed, the mechanism for type IV hypersensitivity involves the development of T_H1 cell-mediated inflammation at the site of antigen accumulation. Acute rejections of solid organ transplants, as well as graft-versus-host reactions, are examples of this type of hypersensitivity.[3]

Refer to Chapter 15 for a more complete discussion of adverse reactions to transfusion.

The clinical significance of blood group antibodies is evaluated by their ability to produce a transfusion reaction or hemolytic disease of the newborn. The term **transfusion reaction** is used to describe any unfavorable response by a recipient to the infusion of blood or blood products. Such reactions include hemolysis, decreased cell survival, anaphylaxis, urticaria, graft-versus-host disease, posttransfusion purpura, alloimmunization, bacterial contamination, and disease transmission. Some adverse effects can be prevented; others cannot. Not all transfusion reactions are associated with red cell destruction following in vivo formation of antigen-antibody complexes; however, those that have such association are among the more serious.

Refer to Chapters 3 through 6 for a more complete discussion of blood group systems.

At least 26 different **blood group systems** have been recognized in humans, each system consisting of a gene locus specifying antigens appearing on the red cell surface.[12] An individual with a particular blood group can recognize cells carrying different blood group antigens and produce antibodies to them. Transfusion of blood products into a recipient who has antibodies to those antigens may produce a transfusion reaction. The severity of the reaction depends on a number of factors, including the characteristics of the immunoglobulin involved. For example, antibodies to the ABO system antigens are usually of the IgM class; they cause complement activation and intravascular hemolysis. Other red cell antigens induce IgG antibodies, which may activate type II hypersensitivity mechanisms and cause accelerated red cell destruction. Symptoms of red cell destruction may include fever, low back pain, nausea and vomiting, circulatory shock, anemia, jaundice, and acute tubular necrosis of the kidneys. Transfusion reactions to incompatible blood products may develop immediately in previously sensitized individuals or over days or weeks in unsensitized individuals (note that some individuals may never mobilize an immune response to transfused blood products).

Antigen-antibody–mediated transfusion reactions to other components of blood, including leukocytes and platelets, may also occur, although their consequences are not usually as severe as reactions to red blood cells. As mentioned earlier, transfusions have additional adverse effects such as disease transmission. The topics of transfusion reactions and the adverse effects of transfusion are broad and complex.

THE COMPLEMENT SYSTEM

The complement system is an integral part of the body's immune system. It is composed of more than 25 glycoproteins with varying electrophoretic mobilities that circulate in plasma in an inactive form. The complement system plays a role in both innate and adaptive immunity. In the innate response, the complement system can be activated by acute-phase recognition molecules such as mannose-binding protein, which results in complement binding to bacterial cell surfaces. Complement receptors on the surface of macrophages then bind to the complement-coated organisms and phagocytosis is triggered. In the adaptive immune response, complement proteins can be activated by two independent pathways, termed the classic pathway and the alternative pathway. The biologic consequences are similar for both pathways.

Complement was first described as a factor present in the plasma, necessary for the lysis of antibody-coated cells, such as bacteria and red blood cells. This remains the best-known function of the system. A second function is to mediate opsonization, a process in which foreign cells are prepared for phagocytosis. A third function of the complement proteins is the generation of peptide fragments that regulate features of the inflammatory and immune responses.[13] Activation of the complement system results in a cascade of interaction of the complement proteins, leading to the generation of products that have important biologic activities. The major biologic consequences of these activities are opsonization, immune adherence, and chemotactic and anaphylatoxic activity. To the blood bank technologist, complement is important in two major areas: (1) Some antigen-antibody complexes cause sufficient quantities of complement to be bound to red blood cells to complete the activation cycle, causing hemolysis; and (2) antigen-antibody complexes initiate complement binding in a way that allows for demonstration of the existence of such complexes by the use of serologic techniques and antiglobulin serum. Because many of the proteins of complement are unstable and heat labile, in blood bank testing it is necessary to use fresh serum to ensure adequate quantities of viable complement.

The Classic Pathway
Proteins of the Classic Pathway

Eleven components summarized in Table 2-7 participate in complement activation by the classic pathway. They are all glycoproteins and constitute 5% of total serum protein. They are numbered C1 to C9; unfortunately, the components do not react in orderly numerical sequence. Most components are globulins with molecular weights of 100,000 to 200,000 and consist of one or two polypeptide chains joined by disulfide bonds. The major exceptions are C4 with three peptide chains and C1 with its unique structure of three subcomponents.

TABLE 2-7 Components in the Classic Pathway of Complement Activation

Complement Component	Cleavage Fragment	Function
C1		
C1q		Complexes with antibody Fc region
C1r		Complexes with C1q and activates C4 and C2
C1s	C1s	
C2	C2a, C2b	C2b complexes with C4b to form C3 convertase
C3	C3a, C3b C3c, C3d	C3b binds to membrane
C4	C4a, C4b C4c, C4d	See C2 above
C5	C5a, C5b	C5b binds to membrane
C6		
C7		Attack sequence
C8		
C9		

The complement cascade, like the coagulation cascade, requires the presence of cations, both calcium and magnesium. Activation of the classic pathway is almost always initiated by immunoglobulin. One molecule of IgM bound to the membrane is necessary to activate the complement system, but two IgG molecules in close proximity are needed. The process involves protein-to-protein interactions, usually proteolytic cleavage, such that removal of part of the complement molecule leaves the residual portion enzymatically or biologically active. Cleavage of most components generates a small fragment, which enters the surrounding plasma, and a larger fragment, which attaches to the cell surface and continues the reaction sequence. The major controls on the system are inhibitory proteins (C1 and C3 inhibitors), spontaneous decay of enzymatically active proteins, and rapid clearance of active fragments. Activation is divided into three phases: recognition phase, activation phase, and attack phase.

Recognition Phase

The C1 complement protein complex is a unique feature of the classic complement cascade that leads to C3 conversion. C1 is, in fact, a complex of three subcomponents named C1q, C1r, and C1s. Receptors on the CH2 domain (Fc region) of immunoglobulin G molecules bind to heads of the C1q hexamer structure (Fig. 2-9). C1q is the only complement protein that reacts directly with the immunoglobulin molecule. C1r and C1s complex with C1q to form a trimolecular complex of C1q, C1r, and C1s that requires calcium for its integrity. At this point, C1r and C1s develop enzymatic activity. The function of C1r is to cleave C1s. C1s cleaves the next two components in the sequence, C4 and C2, to initiate the activation phase.

Activation Phase

Activated C1s cleaves C4 and C2, beginning the activation phase (see Fig. 2-9). C4 is divided first, resulting in two fragments, C4a and C4b. C4a is a small, free-floating fragment with modest anaphylatoxic effect. C4b, a large fragment, binds to the target cell surface. C4b decays rapidly, and those molecules that do not collide with cell membrane in time become inactive and no longer can participate in the complement activation sequence.

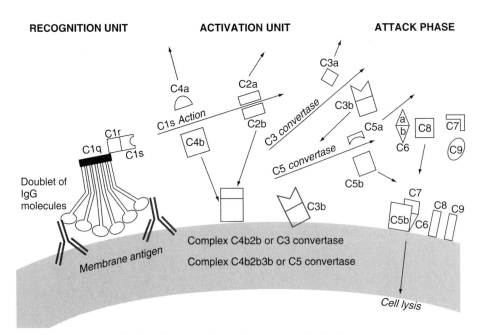

Fig. 2-9 Classic pathway of complement activation.

Activated C1s also cleaves C2 into two fragments, C2a and C2b, when C2 is in complex with C4b. C2a is released into the surrounding fluid, and C2b remains bound to C4b. Both calcium and magnesium ions are required for the complement sequence to reach the C4b,2b point. The bimolecular complex C4b,2b is a protease that cleaves C3 and therefore is called C3 convertase. A single C4b,2b complex has the ability to activate large numbers of C3 molecules, but only about 10% become bound to the target cell. Cleavage of C3 by C3 convertase generates two important peptides, C3a, a powerful anaphylatoxin, and C3b, which attaches to the target cell surface near the C4b,2b complex. C3b is actually a complex of C3c and C3d. On some occasions C3b binds to target membrane, whereas on others only C3d reaches the cell surface.

The component or components of C3 that reach or remain on the cell surface are important to the immunohematologist. First, depending on which component is present, the complement-coated cells may be prematurely removed from circulation in vivo. C3b protein on cellular surfaces mediates phagocytosis by appropriately primed cells, such as macrophages, that possess C3b receptors. Second, in vitro detection of bound C3 in laboratory testing is affected and depends on the C3 component on the cell surface.

Continuing the classic sequence, the C4b,2b,3b complex (also called C5 convertase) splits the C5 peptide into C5a and C5b and is the last enzymatic step in the classic pathway of complement activation. C5a is another anaphylatoxin released into the surrounding fluid. C5b attaches to the cell membrane and is the nucleus for the formation of the membrane attack complex.

Attack Phase

Once membrane bound, C5b binds C6 and C7 by adsorption. This trimolecular complex attaches to the cell membrane and binds C8 and a variable number of C9 molecules (see Fig. 2-9). The components C5b, C6, C7, C8, and C9 make up the terminal membrane attack unit. This multimolecular unit becomes embedded in the cell membrane and forms a central pore or hole, which results in a change in membrane permeability. Thus the membrane loses its ability to retain cellular contents and prevent entrance of extracellular material such as water. This loss of cellular integrity results in rapid cell death and lysis, probably owing to changes in osmotic pressure within the cell.[14]

The Alternative Pathway

The four normal serum proteins that participate in the alternative pathway of complement activation are summarized in Table 2-8. Two additional proteins, factor H and factor I, participate as regulators. The factors participating in the activation process are globulins of high molecular weight, which form an alternative reaction pathway for the conversion of C3 to C3b. Proteins of the alternative pathway perform activities roughly analogous to those in the classic pathway but are usually non-antibody triggered. In this pathway any one of a wide variety of substances can initiate complement activation. The list of triggers for the alternative pathway includes, but is not limited to, bacterial polysaccharides and lipopolysaccharides, endotoxins, cobra venom, trypsin-like enzymes, and aggregates of IgA and IgG4 that do not activate C1. Classic pathway components C1, C4, and C2 do not participate in the alternative pathway of complement activation. Like the classic pathway, the alternative pathway generates a fluid-phase C3a and a surface-bound C3b and eventuates in C5 convertase, but the initiating events are very different. The alternative pathway is rarely initiated by blood group antibody and therefore is of minimal significance in blood banking.

Regulation of the Complement Cascade

Activation of the complement cascade results in a complex series of molecular events with potent biologic consequences. Accordingly, modulating mechanisms

TABLE 2-8 Factors of the Alternative Pathway of Complement Activation

Factor	Function
Factor B	C3 proactivator
Factor D	Proactivator convertase
Properdin (factor P)	Stabilizes molecular complex
C3	Substrate for C3 convertase

are necessary to regulate complement activation and to control the production of biologically active split products.

The first mechanism by which the activity of many activated complement components is modulated is spontaneous decay. An example of this mechanism is the short half-life of the enzymatically active complexes C4b,2b. Additionally, active fragments are rapidly cleared from the body.

A second type of regulator mechanism involves specific control proteins that modulate the activity of certain complement components at critical activation steps. The first of these, C1 inhibitor, blocks the activities of C1r and C1s. Factor H functions to down-regulate C3 cleavage by accelerating the dissociation of factor B from C3b in the alternative pathway, thereby destroying the activity of the alternative pathway C3 convertase. Factor I (C3b/C4b inactivator) in the presence of certain cofactors can inactivate C3b and C4b. Because it modifies the reactive portions of both C3b and C4b, it affects both the classic and alternative pathways. Factor I cleaves the large C4b and C3b proteins into a small, biologically inert free fragment designated "c" and a residual large fragment called "d" that remains bound to the membrane but is unable to activate other complement proteins. Finally, a number of proteins act to control the membrane attack sequence. The most abundant are the S proteins, which are thought to be structurally similar to the membrane attack unit and act by competing for the binding of C5b67 complexes.[13]

THE RED BLOOD CELL MEMBRANE

The red blood cell membrane forms a boundary between the interior of the cell, containing its highly concentrated solution of hemoglobin, and the plasma. In addition to serving as a barrier, the membrane contains pumps and channels for the movement of sodium, potassium, calcium, and oxidized glutathione, and it facilitates the transport of glucose and other small molecules. It is responsible for the biconcave shape and structural integrity of the erythrocyte.

Of importance to the immunohematologist, the antigenic determinants of most blood group antigens are on the red blood cell membrane. Their accessibility to antibody for cross-linking to produce in vitro agglutination indicates that they are surface-oriented antigen components. The following is a brief summary of red blood cell membrane structure as it relates to serologically detectable blood group antigens.

The most generally accepted structural model was described in 1972 by Singer and Nicolson.[15] According to this model, the red blood cell membrane is a fluid mosaic consisting of a lipid framework arranged in a double layer in which globular proteins float and move (Fig. 2-10). The lipid structure possesses both hydrophobic and hydrophilic groups. These molecules form a duplex structure, with the hydrophobic lipid groups on the inner surface facing each other and the hydrophilic polar-head groups in direct contact with the outer aqueous medium (plasma). The lipids of the cell membrane play an important role in its organization and its exchange with plasma. Glycosphingolipids are essential to immunohematology because they bear all the currently known lipid red blood cell group antigens: A, B, H, I, i, P, Pk, and P1. Others, such as Lewis

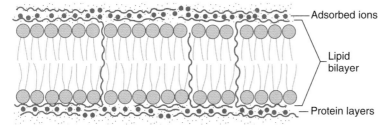

Fig. 2-10 Schematic representation of the fluid mosaic model. The polar head groups of the phospholipids face the cytoplasmic and plasma environments, whereas their acyl tails are enmeshed to form the lipophilic membrane core.

glycosphingolipids, originate from the plasma and are adsorbed by the red blood cell membrane.[16]

In addition to the lipid portion, the membrane has a relatively large number of protein components. The majority are inserted deeply into the bilipid layer and protrude into the surrounding plasma, whereas others lie on the interior surface of the lipid layer. Within the red blood cell cytoplasm are a number of proteins that complex with each other to form the cytoskeleton. These peripheral proteins include polypeptide 1 and 2 (spectrin), 4, 5 (actin), and 6 (glucose 3-phosphate dehydrogenase). Spectrin and associated polypeptides make up the major portion of the skeleton and are responsible for red blood cell shape, deformability, and possibly the stabilization of the lipid bilayer.[17]

Integral proteins are firmly anchored in the lipid bilayer. They include polypeptides 3 and 7 and glycophorins. Band 3 crosses the lipid bilayer several times and is the major membrane-penetrating protein attaching to proteins of the red cell cytoskeleton. Other integral proteins of special significance to immunohematology are glycophorin A (GPA), also known as the MN sialoglycoprotein (MN-SGP), and glycophorin B (GPB), also known as the Ss sialoglycoprotein (Ss-SGP). MN-SGP provides an additional point of attachment of the spectrin complex to a transmembrane protein. This protein accounts for most of the negative electrical charge of red blood cells and carries MN antigens as well as several lectin receptors. Ss-SGP is a transmembrane protein that is not anchored in the spectrin complex. Some researchers believe that although it is embedded in the membrane bilayer, it may not actually span the membrane. Ss-SGP carries the antigens 'N,' S, s, and U[16] (Fig. 2-11). The net effect of this highly orchestrated series of protein interactions and specific membrane bilayer binding is to produce a strong, flexible skeletal network capable of supporting and providing remarkable physical integrity.

ANTIGEN-ANTIBODY REACTIONS

The union of antibody with its specific antigen depends on the structure and charge of the molecule. The common example of complementary fit is the analogy to a lock and key, in that the antigen fits into the antibody like a key fits into a lock. Of equal importance is the electrical charge of the molecules: Opposite charges on antigen and antibody create attraction forces. Binding of antibody by its specific antigen follows the law of mass action, which exhibits two fundamental characteristics—specificity and reversibility. Reversibility permits dissociation of immune complexes; with the result that antibody may be separated from its antigen at the red blood cell surface. Such a dissociation is called **elution.** Once blood group antigen and antibody have made contact, they are held together by physical forces. These forces are weak intermolecular, noncovalent interactions: electrostatic forces, hydrogen bonds, hydrophobic effects, and van der Waals forces. These attractive forces vary in strength with changes in pH, ionic strength, temperature, and nature of the solvent.

Elution: The process by which bound antibody is removed from red cells.

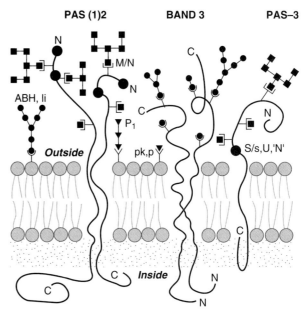

Fig. 2-11 Diagrammatic illustration of membrane bilayer and supporting skeleton showing some blood group antigens associated with membrane components.

The interaction of antigen with antibody is a reversible bimolecular reaction that follows the law of mass action according to the following equation:

$$[Ag] + [Ab] \underset{k_2}{\overset{k_1}{\rightarrow}} [AgAb]$$

Simply stated, the law of mass action means that blood group antibodies and their antigens bind to each other until a dynamic equilibrium is reached in which as many bonds are formed as are disrupted. Under optimal conditions, the expression of these interactions is usually represented as a standard bell-shaped curve. This concept is graphically illustrated in Fig. 2-12, in which antigen in increasing concentration is added to aliquots of antibody at a constant concentration.

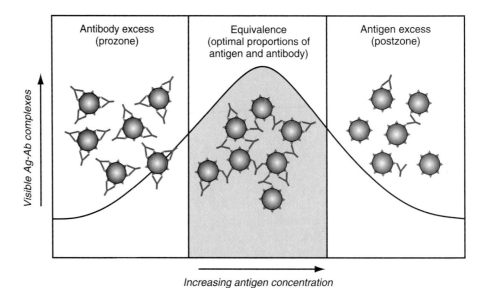

Fig. 2-12 Antigen-antibody binding as a function of the concentration of reactants.

When antibody excess (termed **prozone**) is present, visible aggregates are minimal because individual antibodies compete for the few antigen epitopes available. When antigen sites and antibody molecules are approximately equal, the formation of antigen-antibody complexes is optimal and visible aggregates are seen (zone of **equivalence**). As antigen concentration increases, a state of antigen excess (termed **postzone**) is reached, the formation of antigen-antibody complexes is again minimal, and visible aggregates are not seen because free antigen sites bind with an individual antibody molecule rather than simultaneously engaging several different antibody molecules.

Detection of Antigen-Antibody Reactions

The union of antigen and antibody gives rise to a series of reactions, which is the domain of serology. The type of reaction observed depends on the physical state of the antigen (soluble or particulate) and the physical conditions of the test environment. Once antibody has been formed, it can be serologically detected in a number of ways. Some of the common methods include **agglutination,** precipitation, **hemolysis,** immunofluorescence, radioimmunoassay (RIA), enzyme-linked immunosorbent assay (ELISA), acrylamide gel column technology, and solid phase adherence. Several of these methods are compared in Table 2-9 and are briefly described in the following sections.

Agglutination

Agglutination is the formation of aggregates of particles, such as red blood cells, that bear antigenic determinants on their surface that combine with antibodies present in the test serum. The mechanism of agglutination is the formation of antibody bridges that connect the antigenic determinants of adjacent cells. Agglutination can be observed through both direct techniques (ABO grouping) and indirect techniques (antiglobulin procedures). The method can be performed in standard serologic (10 × 75 mm or 12 × 75 mm) tubes, in

Prozone: The condition of antibody excess in which few agglutinates form.

Equivalence: Optimal antigen-antibody concentrations that facilitate the development of visible agglutinates.

Postzone: The condition of antigen excess in which few agglutinates form.

Agglutination: The clumping together of antigen-bearing cells (such as red blood cells) in the presence of specific antibody.

Hemolysis: The disruption of the red cell membrane with the subsequent loss of cellular contents. Immune hemolysis is the result of the binding of complement on the cell membrane in conjunction with the binding of antibody to a red cell antigen.

TABLE 2-9 Antihuman Globulin Definitions

Reagent	Definition*
Polyspecific (rabbit polyclonal)	Contains anti-IgG and anti-C3d; may contain other anticomplement and other anti-immunoglobulin antibodies
Polyspecific (rabbit/murine monoclonal blend)	Contains rabbit antihuman IgG and murine monoclonal anti-C3b and C3d
Anti-IgG	Contains anti-IgG with no anticomplement activity (not necessarily gamma chain specific)
Anti-IgG (heavy chain)	Contains only antibodies reactive against human gamma chains
Anti-C3d and anti-C3b (rabbit polyclonal)	Contain only antibodies reactive against the designated complement component(s), with no anti-immunoglobulin activity
Anti C3d (murine monoclonal)	Contains only antibodies reactive against the designated complement component, with no anti-immunoglobulin activity
Anti-C3b, C3d (monoclonal)	Contain only antibodies reactive against the designated complement component, with no anti-immunoglobulin activity

*As defined by the Food and Drug Administration: Code of Federal Regulations 21 CFR 660.

microwell plates, in gel columns, and on glass tiles (ABO forward grouping only).

An antibody is said to be agglutinating when it is capable of producing red cell agglutination in saline. Conversely, an antibody is said to be nonagglutinating when its binding to the red cell is not sufficient to agglutinate red cells in saline suspension. Agglutination is one of the most common procedures used in immunohematology; it is discussed in more detail later in this chapter.

Hemolysis

Hemolysis represents destruction of the red blood cell membrane through the action of complement proteins that are activated by the reaction of specific antibody to a surface antigen. Hemolysis is a positive result in tests for red cell antibody, indicating the presence of a complement-activating antibody. Antibody-mediated hemolysis does not occur in the absence of complement or in plasma when a calcium-chelating agent (such as EDTA) is present.

Acrylamide Gel Column Technology

Acrylamide gel column technology is based on the agglutination reaction. In this technology, agglutination reactions take place within microtubes and are interpreted relative to size of the agglutinates and the degree of migration through the column after a standard time of centrifugation. Cells and serum (if needed) are added to the top of the column and allowed to react to form agglutinates. On centrifugation, agglutinates migrate through the gel relative to size. Larger agglutinates (stronger reactions) remain at the upper part of the column whereas smaller agglutinates (weaker reactions) migrate farther through the column. Unsensitized red cells spin through the column into a button on the bottom of the microtube to form a negative reaction. Gel columns with embedded antisera (e.g., anti-A, anti-IgG) are available, as well as columns without antiserum. Gel technology methods for red cell antigen typing, antibody detection and identification, and crossmatching are available in semiautomated or automated configurations.[18]

Solid Phase Adherence

Solid phase adherence methods are used to detect and identify antigen or antibody.[19] These methods consist of chemically modified microplates that are coated with antibody or monolayers of cellular material (red blood cells). When antibody is applied to the sides of the microplate well, cells are added, and if the appropriate antigen is present on the cells, they adhere to the sides of the well. If no antigen-antibody reaction occurs, the cells settle to the bottom of the well. This method permits the detection or typing of cells for specific antigen.

When reagent cells are applied to pretreated microplate wells, serum is added, incubated, and washed free. Indicator cells (IgG-coated cells) are added. Again, an antigen-antibody reaction (positive reaction) is indicated if the coated cells adhere to the side of the well. If the coated cells settle to the bottom of the well, no antigen-antibody reaction has occurred (negative reaction). The system is designed to detect and identify predominantly IgG antibodies to antigens carried on reagent red blood cells but can be applied to detection of antibodies to platelets. Solid-phase red cell adherence methods have been automated to form the basis of a random-access, "walk-away" analyzer available for antigen typing, antibody detection and identification, and crossmatching.

Methods Based on Agglutination

Although much of the following discussion applies to all antigen-antibody reactions, the focus is predominantly on agglutination, the end point for most test methods involving red cells and blood group antibodies. Numerous variables influence these reactions. Understanding these variables, their effect on antigen-antibody reactions, and how they can be manipulated to obtain the optimal test conditions is essential.

Stages of Reaction

Agglutination occurs in two distinct stages, and different variables influence each stage. In the first stage, referred to as **sensitization,** the antibody attaches to the corresponding antigen site on the red blood cell membrane. The second stage, referred to as agglutination, is the formation of bridges between the sensitized red cells to form a lattice structure and create visible clumps of red cells. Although the distinction of a two-stage process is useful for didactic purposes, the two steps actually proceed simultaneously, and agglutination begins before the first step reaches completion.

Sensitization: The binding of antibody or complement components to a red cell antigen, the first phase of the agglutination reaction.

First Stage

Sensitization is a dynamic reaction in which antibody associates with and dissociates from its specific antigen. Sensitization occurs only when specific antigen and antibody are present simultaneously. Even when the necessary elements are present, characteristics of the antibody and the reaction conditions influence the rate and magnitude of sensitization. The bonds holding the antigen-antibody complex in apposition dissociate and reassociate at different but progressively decreasing rates until equilibrium is reached; that is, the rate of association (k_1) equals the rate of dissociation (k_2). The reaction is thus in a state of relatively stable but dynamic equilibrium. As mentioned earlier, the equilibrium constant is affected by numerous variables. This first stage of agglutination can be manipulated by concentration of antigen, concentration of antibody, and conditions of the test environment such as pH, ionic strength, temperature, and time. Altering the physical conditions of agglutination tests can influence the rate of sensitization.

Antigen-Antibody Ratio

The sensitivity of blood grouping tests depends on the number of antibody molecules bound per red cell. If the quantity of antibody present in the test is increased, the amount of antigen-antibody complex formed also increases. For routine blood grouping tests, increasing the serum-to-cell ratio results in a larger number of antibodies bound per cell, more antigen-antibody complexes, and a stronger observed reaction.

pH

The reactivity of the majority of blood group antibodies is optimal at a pH of 6.5 to 7.5. For routine blood bank procedures, a pH of 7.0 should be used.

Ionic Strength

The Na^+ and Cl^- ions in normal saline cluster around and partially neutralize the charges on antigen and antibody molecules. This ionic cloud or cluster hinders the association of antibody with antigen. By decreasing the ionic strength in the reaction mixture, this shielding effect is reduced. Additionally, by lowering the salt concentration of the reaction mixture, the rate at which antigen-antibody complexes are formed is increased. Low ionic strength solutions (LISS) are frequently used in blood banking procedures as an enhancement agent to reduce the ionic strength of the mixture and increase the rate of antigen-antibody association.

Temperature

Blood group antibodies differ with respect to their optimal thermal activity and show reactivity over a restricted temperature range. Cold antibodies, generally IgM, show optimal reactivity at lower temperatures (4° to 27° C); on the other hand, warm antibodies, generally IgG, react best at 37° C.[20,21] Antibodies that react in vitro only at temperatures below 37° C usually are considered to have no clinical significance and rarely cause red cell destruction.

Time

Antigen-antibody reactions have an optimal time of incubation that favors maximal binding of antibody to antigen. Short incubation periods may not allow for significant amounts of antibody to be bound; prolonged incubation may result in dissociation of antibody from antigen. Enhancing agents such as LISS increase the amount of antibody uptake and therefore decrease the incubation time needed to reach equilibrium.

Second Stage

The second stage of agglutination is the formation of bridges between the sensitized red blood cells to form the latticework that results in visible aggregates or "clumps" of red blood cells. However, once red blood cells are sensitized, agglutination is not guaranteed. Agglutination is influenced by the characteristics of the antibody molecule, number and location of antigen sites, and electrostatic repulsion forces.

Immunoglobulin Class

As discussed earlier, considerable differences exist in the physical characteristics of IgG and IgM molecules. The IgG monomer, which is 250 Ångström units long, often fails to agglutinate red blood cells after sensitizing surfaces that express the appropriate antigen. The IgM pentamer, with a diameter of about 1000 Ångström units, is far more effective in inducing agglutination. This difference in size and number of antigen-binding sites offers a reasonable explanation for the observed reaction patterns of IgG and IgM antibodies.

Antigen Sites

Other variables to consider are the number and location of antigen sites on the red blood cell membrane. If antigen sites are sparsely distributed on red blood cell surfaces or if they are present in relatively low numbers, antibody molecules attached to one site may fail to encounter epitopes on another cell. The result is a lack of lattice formation and therefore no visible agglutination. Additionally, antigen mobility and membrane flexibility may play a role in the agglutination stage of the antigen-antibody reaction.

Electrostatic Repulsion Forces

In addition to antibody characteristics and antigen site location and number, the second stage or lattice formation depends on overcoming the electrostatic repulsion forces of red blood cells.[22] The distance between two red blood cells in saline suspension does not depend solely on their net surface charge. Ions in solution orient themselves around the red blood cell so as to form a diffuse double layer or cloud. The difference in charge density between the inside and the outside of the ionic cloud creates an electrostatic potential known as the *zeta potential*. The zeta potential is the major determining factor of the repulsion effects of two adjacent red blood cells. By reducing the zeta potential, red blood cells come closer together and may permit agglutination. The zeta potential may be reduced by (1) treatment of red blood cells with proteolytic enzymes, for example, papain and ficin, and (2) use of various colloidal diluents, for example, albumin, polyethylene glycol (PEG), polybrene, and polyvinylpyrrolidone (PVP), that change the dielectric constant of the aqueous electrolyte solution. The net result is that electrostatic repulsion forces are overcome and the cells can approach each other, permitting the coupling of antigen with antibody. Centrifugation is a physical process used to increase proximity of antibody and antigen-bearing cells, thereby facilitating antigen-antibody binding.

Reading and Interpreting Agglutination Reactions

Most routine procedures performed in the blood bank depend on agglutination or hemolysis (or both) as the end point. In serologic testing, the hemolysis or agglutination that constitutes the visible end point must be described accurately and consistently. Immediately after centrifugation, the supernatant is observed for hemolysis and the red cell button is gently dispersed to observe for agglutination. The manner in which red cells are dislodged from the bottom of the test tube affects detection of agglutination. The test tube should be held at an angle so that the fluid sweeps across the cell button as the tube is gently tilted. Gentle tilting should be continued until there is an even suspension of red cells or agglutinates. In positive reactions, the agglutinates break away from the cell button, whereas in negative reactions the free red cells trail or "smoke" away from the cell button.

The strength of agglutination observed with each red cell sample must be recorded as the test is read. All technologists in a laboratory should use the same interpretation scheme and notation. The following system is widely used:

4+	One solid aggregate
3+	Several large agglutinates
2+	Medium-sized agglutinates, clear background
1+	Small agglutinates, turbid background
w+	Tiny agglutinates, turbid background
0	No agglutination or hemolysis
PH	Partial hemolysis
H	Complete hemolysis, no red cells remaining
mf	Mixed field, some agglutinated red cells and some free red cells

For maximum reproducibility, a light source and an optical aid should be used. Microscopic readings are not routinely used in blood banking but may be helpful in distinguishing rouleaux from agglutination. Rouleaux formation is pseudoagglutination in which red cells adhere to each other on their flat surfaces, giving a "stack of coins" appearance. This nonimmunologic adherence of red cells to one another is frequently due to high concentrations of globulin in the serum. Patients with multiple myeloma, as well as those who have received dextran as a plasma expander, frequently demonstrate rouleaux formation in blood grouping tests. Rouleaux are dispersed by adding saline to the reaction. This procedure is known as the saline replacement technique. True red cell agglutination is not dispersed by this technique.

Antiglobulin Procedures

In some cases, a short antibody molecule such as IgG can sensitize red blood cells but cannot produce agglutination, even when the various manipulations described previously are employed. The small size of the antibody molecules makes them unable to overcome the forces that cause red blood cells to repel one another and form cross-linked bridges that connect cells. In 1945, Coombs and colleagues[23] described a test for detecting these nonagglutinating, coating (sensitizing) antibodies. Later, the same test was used to demonstrate coating of red blood cells with complement components. This test is known as the *antiglobulin test*.

The antiglobulin test is performed in two ways: (1) the **direct antiglobulin test (DAT)** and (2) an **indirect antiglobulin test (IAT)**. The DAT is a diagnostic procedure used to detect antibody or complement (or both) bound to red blood cells in vivo. The IAT is used to detect in vitro reactions between antibody and red cell antigens. For example, the DAT is useful for the detection of IgG-sensitized red blood cells in an infant suspected of having hemolytic disease of the

Direct antiglobulin test (DAT): A one-step test used to identify red blood cells that have been sensitized with antibody or complement in vivo.

Indirect antiglobulin test (IAT): A two-step test used to determine if antibody reacts with antigen on red blood cells in vitro.

newborn; the IAT is useful for the detection of unexpected blood group antibodies in the serum of a potential transfusion recipient.

The principle of the test is straightforward. Human serum contains immunoglobulins and complement proteins. When human serum or purified protein components are injected into a suitable laboratory animal, usually a rabbit or goat, they act as immunogens to the animal, invoking an immune response that results in the production of antibodies directed against the human globulin—thus the term *antihuman globulin* (AHG). The animals are bled, and unwanted antibodies such as antispecies, anti-A, anti-B, and anti-H are removed by adsorption. The serum is then diluted to the point that the AHG reacts optimally with the corresponding protein. AHG reacts with human globulin molecules either bound to red cells or free in the test serum. To avoid neutralization by free globulin molecules, red cells are washed to remove unbound globulin before testing with AHG. Washed red cells coated with human globulin are agglutinated by AHG. The strength of the reaction is roughly proportional to the amount of globulin coating the red cells.

AHG reagent is available from several commercial suppliers. The Food and Drug Administration (FDA) Center for Biologics Evaluation and Research has established definitions for a variety of AHG reagents.[24] As shown in Table 2-10, two types of AHG reagent are available, polyspecific and monospecific. Polyspecific AHG reagent contains both anti-IgG and anti-C3d. A monospecific AHG reagent is specific either for complement components C3b and C3d or for IgG. In reagents with specificity for IgG proteins, the antibody is directed against antigenic sites on the heavy chain of the immunoglobulin.

Recently a new approach to the production of AHG reagents and other blood banking antisera has become commercially feasible. Monoclonal antibodies, produced from a clone of a single cell and specific for a single antigen, can be produced in large quantity using hybridoma technology. Briefly, this process involves the fusion of a normal mouse spleen cell that produces the antibody desired with an abnormal cell from a mouse that has myeloma. In culture, these hybrid cells produce clones that grow rapidly and produce large quantities of the desired antibody. Hybridoma cells may be injected intraperitoneally into mice, where they induce the effusion of large quantities of antibody-rich fluid into the peritoneal cavity. After a suitable time the mouse ascitic fluid is harvested for manufacture into blood bank reagent. The technique is schematically shown in Fig. 2-13. Advantages of monoclonal reagents are consistency from lot to lot and, theoretically, greater specificity. This last point, however, can also be argued to be a disadvantage of monoclonal reagents, because they are sometimes so narrow in their specificity that reaction strength suffers or many varieties of monoclonal antibodies are needed to detect all the variations seen in human immune responses.

TABLE 2-10 Comparison of Blood Bank Methods			
Feature	Tube	Gel	Solid Phase
End point	Agglutination	Agglutination	Immune adherence
Indicator	DA/AHG*	AHG†	AHG-RBC‡
Wash step	Yes	No	Yes
Stability	30 minutes	2–3 days	2 days
Process steps	11-14	4	5-8
Special equipment required	No	Yes	Yes
Automation available	No	Yes	Yes

*Direct agglutination and antiglobulin reaction.
†Antiglobulin reaction.
‡AHG-sensitized indicator cells.
AHG, Antihuman globulin; DA, direct agglutination; RBC, red blood cell.

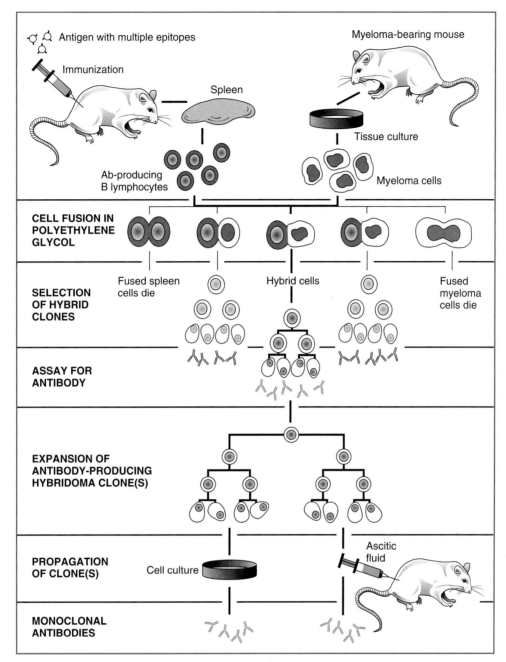

Fig. 2-13 Schematic representation of the hybridoma technique for the production of monoclonal antibody.

CHAPTER SUMMARY

1. The immune system of humans consists of pluripotential cells whose descendants include both inflammatory and immune cell lines. Progeny of these stem cells differentiate into red cells, white cells, megakaryocytes, and phagocytic cells.

2. An antigen is a substance capable of provoking an immune response when introduced into an immunocompetent host to whom it is foreign. Encounters with foreign material initiate adaptive

changes that result in either production of antibodies (humoral response) or a cell-mediated response.

3. The immune events that occur when an immunocompetent individual encounters a foreign antigen for the first time constitute the primary immune response. The immune events that occur on second or subsequent exposure constitute the secondary or anamnestic immune response. Primary and secondary immune responses differ with respect

to response time, antibody titer, class, affinity, and avidity.

4. All immunoglobulin molecules have a common structure consisting of four polypeptide chains (two H chains and two L chains) connected by disulfide bonds and held together by noncovalent hydrophobic bonds. Human immunoglobulins are categorized into classes according to the H chain expressed. The immunoglobulin classes are IgA, IgG, IgM, IgD, and IgE.

5. Blood group antibodies considered to be clinically significant are usually IgG or IgM class immunoglobulins.

6. Activation of the complement system is important in blood banking in two major ways: (1) increased red cell destruction by phagocytosis or hemolysis and (2) detection of antigen-antibody reactions through red cell–bound complement components.

7. Hemagglutination is the most common method used in blood banking for the detection and identification of blood group antigens and antibodies.

Hemagglutination occurs in two stages: (1) sensitization and (2) formation of a lattice structure resulting in visible clumps of red cells.

8. A number of variables affect each stage of hemagglutination:

Stage One	Stage Two
Temperature	Electrostatic repulsion
pH	Ig class
Incubation time	Antigen sites
Ionic strength	
Ag-Ab ratio	

9. Antiglobulin test procedures, both direct and indirect techniques, have wide application in the blood bank. The direct antiglobulin test is a diagnostic procedure used to demonstrate in vivo coating of red cells with antibody or complement. The indirect antiglobulin test is used to demonstrate in vitro reactions between red cell antigens and coating antibodies.

REFERENCES

1. Holborow EJ, Reeves WG (eds): Immunology in Medicine, 2nd ed. New York, Grune & Stratton, 1983.
2. Unanue ER: Antigen-presenting function of the macrophage. Annu Rev Immunol 2:395-428, 1984.
3. Parham P: The Immune System. London, Current Trends, 2000.
4. Geha RS, Rosen FS: Immunoregulation of T-cell defects. Immunol Today 4:233-236, 1983.
5. Fauci AS, Macher AM, Longo DL, et al: Acquired immunodeficiency syndrome: Epidemiologic, clinical, immunologic and therapeutic considerations. Ann Intern Med 100:92-106, 1984.
6. Bellanti JA: Immunology: Basic Processes, 2nd ed. Philadelphia, WB Saunders, 1985.
7. Ferrarini M, Grossi CE: Definition of the cell types within the "null lymphocyte" population of human peripheral blood. Semin Hematol 21:270-286, 1984.
8. Goldfarb RH: Cell-mediated cytotoxic reaction. Hum Pathol 17:138-145, 1986.
9. Tada T: Help, suppression, and specific factors. In Paul WE (ed): Fundamental Immunology. New York, Raven Press, 1984.
10. Smith KA: Lymphokine regulation of T cell and B cell function. In Paul WE (ed): Fundamental Immunology. New York, Raven Press, 1984.
11. Henry JB (ed): Clinical Diagnosis and Management by Laboratory Methods, 18th ed. Philadelphia, WB Saunders, 1991.
12. Reid ME, Rios M, Yazdanbakhsh K: Applications of molecular biology techniques to transfusion medicine. Semin Hematol 37(2):166-176, 2000.
13. Frank MM: Complement and kinin. In Stites DP, Terr AI: Basic and Clinical Immunology. Norwalk, CT, Appleton & Lange, 1991.
14. Chapel H, Haeney M: Essentials of Clinical Immunology, 2nd ed. London, Blackwell Scientific, 1988.
15. Singer SJ, Nicolson GL: The fluid mosaic model of the structure of cell membranes. Science 175:720-731, 1972.
16. Salmon C, Cartron JP, Rouger P: The Human Blood Groups. Chicago, Year Book, 1984.
17. Shohet SB, Beutler E: The red cell membrane. In Williams WJ, Beutler E, Erslev AJ, Lichtman MA: Hematology, 4th ed. New York, McGraw-Hill, 1990.
18. Brecher ME (ed): AABB Technical Manual, 14th ed. Bethesda, MD, American Association of Blood Banks, 2002.
19. Plapp FV, Rachel JM, Beck ML, et al: Blood antigens and antibodies: Solid phase adherence assays. Lab Management 22:39-46, 1984.
20. Issitt PD: Antibodies reactive at 30° centigrade, room temperature and below. In Butch SH, Beck M (eds): Clinically Significant and Insignificant Antibodies. Arlington, VA, American Association of Blood Banks, 1979.
21. Garratty G: Clinical significance of antibody reactive optimally at 37° C. In Butch SH, Beck M (eds): Clinically Significant and Insignificant Antibodies. Arlington, VA, American Association of Blood Banks, 1979.
22. Pollack W, Hager HJ, Reckel R, et al: A study of the forces involved in the second stage of hemagglutination. Transfusion 5:158-183, 1965.
23. Coombs RRA, Mourant AE, Race RR: A new test for the detection of weak and "incomplete" Rh agglutinins. Br J Exp Pathol 26:255-266, 1945.
24. The Code of Federal Regulations. Title 21 CFR 660.55. Washington, DC, US Government Printing Office, 2004.

FURTHER READINGS

Abbas AK: Cellular and Molecular Immunology. Philadelphia, WB Saunders, 1997.

Abbas AK: Basic Immunology: Functions and Disorders of the Immune System. Philadelphia, WB Saunders, 2001.

Florido M, Goncalves AS, Gomes MS, Appelberg R: CD40 is required for the optimul induction of protective immunity to *Mycobacterium avium*. Immunology 111(3):323-327, 2004.

Hall SS: A Commotion in the Blood: Life, Death, and the Immune System. New York, Henry Holt, 1998.

Hayday AC, Pennington DJ, Giuggio VM: Genomics and immunology. Semin Immunol 15(4):201-208, 2003.

Heyman B: The immune complex: Possible ways of regulating the antibody response. Immunol Today 11:310-313, 1990.

Leffell MS, Donnenberg AD, Rose NR (eds): Handbook of Human Immunology. Boca Raton, FL, CRC Press, 1997.

Moynihan J, Kruszewska B, Madden K, Callahan T: Sympathetic nervous system regulation of immunity. J Neuroimmunol 147(1-2):87-90, 2004.

Notarangelo LD, Giliani S, Mazzolari E, Gulino AV: Primary immune deficiencies unravel the molecular basis of immune response. Rev Clin Exp Hematol 7(1):84-111, 2003.

Parr MD, Messino MJ, McIntyre W: Allogeneic bone marrow transplantation: Procedures and complications. Am J Hosp Pharm 48:127-137, 1991.

Paul WE (ed): Immunology: Recognition and Response. New York, WH Freeman, 1990.

Remick DG, Friedland JS (eds): Cytokines in Health and Disease. New York, Dekker, 1997.

Rich RR (ed): Clinical Immunology: Principles and Practice. London, New York, Mosby, 2001.

Roitt IM: Roitt's Essential Immunology, 9th ed. Oxford, Malden, MA, Blackwell Science, 1997.

Rosen FS: Case Studies in Immunology: A Clinical Comparison. New York, Garland, 2001.

Rydberg L, Breimer ME, Brynger H, Samuelsson BE: ABO incompatible kidney transplantation: Qualitative and semiquantitative studies of the humoral immune response against different blood group A antigens. Transplantation 49:954-960, 1990.

Sheehan C: Clinical Immunology: Principles and Laboratory Diagnosis. Philadelphia, Lippincott, 1997.

Stites DP, Terr AI: Basic and Clinical Immunology, 7th ed. Norwalk, CT, Appleton and Lange, 1991.

Trowsdale J, Parham P: Mini-review: defense strategies and immunity-related genes. Eur J Immunol 34(1):7-17, 2004.

van Boven M, Weissing FJ: The evolutionary economics of immunity. Am Nat 163(2):277-294, 2004.

Virella G (ed): Medical Immunology, 5th ed. New York, Dekker, 2001.

von Rood JJ, Claas HJ: The influence of allogeneic cells on the human T and B cell repertoire. Science 243:1388-1393, 1990.

Walker RH (ed): Technical Manual, 11th ed. Bethesda, MD, American Association of Blood Banks, 1993.

Williams WJ, Beutler E, Erslev AJ, Lichtman MA: Hematology, 4th ed. New York, McGraw-Hill, 1990.

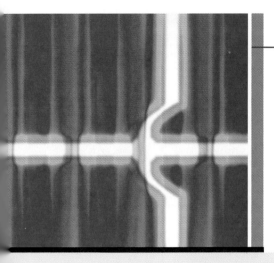

Blood Group Serology

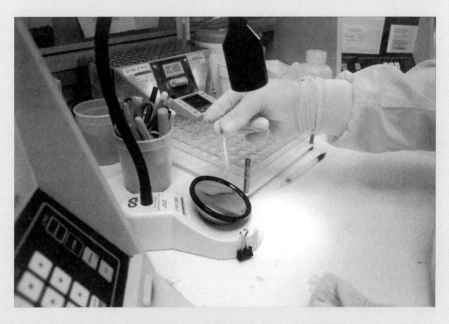

At the beginning of the twentieth century Karl Landsteiner made the observation that the blood of his colleagues, when mixed together, resulted in visible agglutination and hemolysis. As a result of these early experiments, Landsteiner identified three of the four phenotypes of the ABO blood group system. This system remains the most important in transfusion medicine. Since this early discovery, the science of red blood cell immunology has continued to expand. Currently researchers have identified approximately 300 antigen substances on the surface of the red cell, and the list continues to grow. As we expand our knowledge we continue to refine theories of blood group inheritance and biochemistry. The theoretic base continues to grow and to change with new discoveries and advancing technology. Molecular techniques have provided us with an important tool elucidating our understanding of the blood groups, their relationships, and their inheritance.

Understanding of the blood groups, their inheritance, and their biochemistry is fundamental to the practice of transfusion medicine and to the technology of blood group serology. Expanded knowledge enables the practitioner and the research scientist to develop more sensitive methods of antibody detection and identification and also facilitates the selection of appropriate components for transfusion.

Applications of this knowledge include antibody identification and prediction of clinical significance; identification of the causative agents of hemolytic disease of the newborn, autoimmune hemolytic anemia, drug-induced hemolysis, and other hemolytic events; elucidation of the structure of the red cell membrane; identification of disease association; prediction of the probable success of organ transplantation; investigation of adverse reactions to transfusion; submission of evidence in forensic medicine; and determination of the relative probability in cases of disputed paternity.

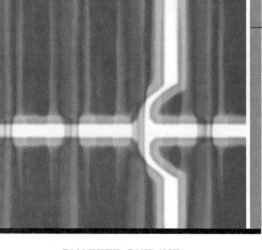

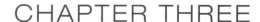

CHAPTER THREE

The ABO and H Blood Group Systems

Susan L. Wilkinson

LEARNING OBJECTIVES

After reading and studying this chapter, the student should be able to:

1. Briefly describe the events leading to the discovery of the ABO blood groups.
2. Discuss the inheritance and biochemistry of the ABH antigens.
3. Differentiate type 1 and type 2 precursor chains.
4. Given an ABO phenotype, determine possible ABO genotype(s).
5. Given information regarding the ABO genotype of parents, determine the possible ABO genotypes of offspring and the probability of each.
6. Describe why ABH antigen expression is diminished in newborns.
7. Describe the biochemical and serologic characteristics of the ABO antibodies.
8. Explain why the ABO blood group is the most significant of all blood group systems.
9. Describe the range of possible reactions that would be expected if an A_2 person's blood was tested with anti-A, anti-B, anti-A,B, anti-A_1 lectin, A_1, B, and A_2 cells.
10. List ABO blood groups in order from most to least with respect to the amount of H antigen present on the red cells.
11. Define the term subgroup and give three examples of ABO subgroups.
12. Identify the two phenotypes that result from hybrid transferases.
13. Describe the inheritance and serologic findings associated with the classic Bombay phenotype.
14. Briefly describe the para-Bombay phenotypes.
15. List six red cell–associated causes of ABO typing discrepancies.
16. List six serum-associated causes of ABO typing discrepancies.
17. Given a set of serologic reactions in which the ABO forward and reverse reactions do not match, give a possible explanation for these results.

Karl Landsteiner first described the ABO blood group system in 1900.[1] Even though the significance of the discovery was not fully appreciated at the time, it served as the beginning of blood banking and transfusion medicine. As we now know, the single most important test performed is the determination of the ABO group of both donors and recipients. Failure to determine an accurate ABO typing result has been responsible for both morbidity and mortality in the blood recipient population.

Landsteiner's early studies involved testing the red cells and sera from himself and six associates and noting the presence or absence of agglutination. In this initial investigation, three ABO groups were observed. These included A, B, and O. Group A red cells possessed an A antigen and demonstrated anti-B in the serum that agglutinated group B red cells. The serum from individuals with group B red cells (and therefore the B antigen) contained anti-A and caused agglutination of the group A red cells. The third ABO group, group O, appeared to have no antigens on the red cell, yet had serum that contained antibodies to both the A and B antigens. The last ABO group, group AB, in which red cells possess both the A and B antigens and lack all ABO antibodies in the serum, was discovered by two of Landsteiner's associates, von Descatello and Sturli, in 1902.[2] A summary of expected ABO typing results is presented in Table 3-1.

Even before the discovery of the **Bombay phenotype,** some serologic evidence suggested that group O red cells expressed an antigen that was more weakly expressed on A, B, or AB red cells. Following the discovery of the Bombay phenotype and the initial biochemical configuration for soluble ABO, H, and Lewis antigens, it became clear that another locus termed *H* and the final product of the genes at that locus, H antigen, were necessary for the expression of normal ABO antigens. The amount of H antigen varies, depending on the ABO group inherited. These variations are summarized in Fig. 3-1.

The ABH and related antigens are ubiquitous in humans, and recent biochemical studies have proposed the term histo-antigens for these carbohydrate structures.[3] It is emphasized in this chapter and the next that a discussion on ABO includes not only the *ABO* and *H* loci but other loci that include *SE, LE, P,* and *I.* The products of the genes at all of these loci are various **transferase** enzymes. These enzymes "transfer" specific carbohydrates to preformed structures to confer antigen specificity.

The ABH antigens of the red cell membrane are found partly as glycolipids but primarily as glycoproteins. In addition to being present on the red cell membrane, these antigens may also occur in the secretions as glycoproteins. The presence of ABH antigens in the secretions depends on the inheritance of at least one *Se* gene at the *secretor (SE or FUT2) locus.*

Bombay phenotype: The rare inheritance of two *h* genes at the *Hh* locus and the subsequent lack of the H antigen. Such individuals are unable to express other ABO antigens. True Bombay individuals also have mutant alleles at the *Se* locus.

Transferase: An enzyme that transfers chemical groups from one compound to another. *A* and *B* gene products are glycosyltransferases, meaning that they transfer sugars. These sugars are responsible for ABO blood group specificity.

Secretor: An individual who secretes ABH antigen substances into body fluids such as saliva and plasma. Secretor status is inherited.

TABLE 3-1 Expected Reactions for ABO Groups

RED CELLS			SERUM			INTERPRETATION
Anti-A	Anti-B	Anti-A,B	A₁ Cells	A₂ Cells	B Cells	ABO Group
0	0	0	4+	4+	4+	O
4+	0	4+	0	0	4+	A
0	4+	4+	4+	4+	0	B
4+	4+	4+	0	0	0	AB

Greatest $\longrightarrow$ Least

O, A$_2$, A$_2$B, B, A$_1$, A$_1$B

Amount of H antigen

Fig. 3-1 Variation in H antigen.

GENETICS AND BIOCHEMISTRY

Type 1 and Type 2 Structures

Throughout this chapter and the next, antigens and preantigen structures are described as either type 1 or type 2 structures. These designations refer to the linkages found between the terminal sugars galactose and *N*-acetylglucosamine. In type 1 structures, the linkage is described as beta (β)1-3. In type 2, the linkage is β1-4. The number 1 carbon of d-galactose is linked to the number 3 carbon of *N*-acetylglucosamine in type 1 structures and to the number 4 carbon of *N*-acetylglucosamine in type 2 structures. Type 2 structures are characteristically associated with integral red cell membrane antigens as glycolipids. **Type 1 and type 2 structures** are found as glycoproteins in body fluids and on cell surfaces. These structures are characterized in Fig. 3-2.

H Locus

The *H* locus has been assigned to chromosome 19 (19q13.3) and is linked to the *SE (secretor)* and *LU (Lutheran)* loci.[4] The two major alleles at the *H* locus are designated *H* and *h*. *H* (also described as the *FUT1* gene) produces the transferase enzyme **2-alpha(α)-fucosyltransferase,** which transfers fucose to type 2 paragloboside (or lacto-*N*-neotetraosylceramide), binding to galactose through an alpha (α)1-2 linkage on the red cell membrane to produce H antigen (Table 3-2). As described later in this chapter, the H antigen acts as an acceptor of the transferase enzymes produced by *A* and *B* genes. The *h* gene is described as an amorph and was thought to produce no detectable product.

Studies have shown that the *h* gene represents a number of different and unique mutations of the *H(FUT1)* gene.[5-7] These mutations may be the result of nucleotide substitutions (missense and nonsense mutations) that lead to unusual amino acid sequences that result in events such as stop codons or frameshifts. For example, a change from guanine to cytosine at nucleotide 1047 in the *H* gene results in the production of the amino acid cysteine instead of tryptophan at position 349 of the H transferase enzyme.[5] Such genetic events lead to the production of a gene product without fucosyltransferase functionality or, occasionally, weak fucosyltransferase activity.

The inheritance of two *h* genes, or two mutated *H(FUT1)* genes, at this locus results in the Bombay phenotype or the para-Bombay phenotype, which are described in more detail later in this chapter. People of the Bombay phenotype are unable to produce H antigen and therefore, even in the presence of normally inherited *A* or *B* genes, are unable to produce A or B antigen. Para-Bombay individuals may lack ABO antigens on their red cells or may express them very weakly on their red cells. With the advent of molecular methods to evaluate these

---

Type 1 and type 2 structures: Precursor substances and antigens in the ABO system differentiated by the type of linkage between terminal carbohydrates (see Fig. 3-2).

2-α-fucosyltransferase: The product of the *H* gene that transfers fucose to type 2 chains on the red cells to produce H antigen.

Type 1

β1-3 β1-3

Gal —— GlcNAc —— Gal — R

Type 2

β1-4 β1-3

Gal —— GlcNAc —— Gal — R

Fig. 3-2 Type 1 and type 2 oligosaccharide structures. Gal, galactose; GlcNAc, *N*-acetylglucosamine.

TABLE 3-2 Products of *H, A,* and *B* Genes

Gene	Gene Product	Sugar Transferred by Enzyme	Terminal Oligosaccharide Antigen Structure
H	2-α-fucosyltransferase	Fucose	Gal$\frac{\beta1\text{-}3 \text{ or } \beta1\text{-}4}{}$GlcNAc——Gal—R, α1-2 Fuc
A	3-α-*N*-acetylgalactosaminyl-transferase	*N*-acetylglactosamine	GalNAc$\frac{\alpha1\text{-}3}{}Gal\frac{\beta1\text{-}3 \text{ or } \beta1\text{-}4}{}$GlcNAc—Gal—R, α1-2 Fuc
B	3-α-galactosyltransferase	Galactose	Gal$\frac{\alpha1\text{-}3}{}Gal\frac{\beta1\text{-}3 \text{ or } \beta1\text{-}4}{}$GalNAc—Gal—R, α1-2 Fuc
O	None	None	

Fuc, Fucose; Gal, galactose; GalNAc, *N*-acetylgalactosamine; GlcNAc, *N*-acetylglucosamine.

unusual phenotypes, it has become clear that these classifications represent many variations and both Bombay and para-Bombay individuals represent very heterogeneous groups at the molecular level. The reader is encouraged to consult several references that go into much more detail about these complex findings.[5-9]

ABO Locus

The *ABO* locus is found on the long arm of chromosome 9 (9q34.1-q34.2) and is linked to the *AK1* (adenylate kinase) locus and the *NP* (nail-patella syndrome) locus.[10] The *ABO* gene consists of seven exons, and exons 6 and 7 are responsible for encoding the ABO glycosyltransferases.[11] The three major alleles at this locus are described as *A, B,* and *O.* The *A* and *B* genes are responsible for the production of **3-α-*N*-acetylgalactosaminyltransferase** and **3-α-galactosyltransferase,** respectively. The transferase enzyme produced by the *A* gene transfers *N*-acetylgalactosamine and the enzyme produced by the *B* gene transfers galactose to preformed carbohydrate structures. Once transferred, these structures confer A or B antigen specificity (see Table 3-2). This preformed structure, as stated earlier, is the H antigen, and the inheritance of at least one *H* gene is necessary for normal ABO group expression. The *O* gene is believed to be an amorph, producing no detectable product. Therefore individuals who inherit two *O* genes express only H antigen on their red cells. This explains why group O red cells demonstrate more H antigen than the red cells of other ABO groups.

Molecular assays have shown that genetic variability exists as to how the group O phenotype arises. A common allele for group O individuals, termed *O¹*, contains a nucleotide deletion that results in a product that lacks enzymatic activity.[10] Another allele, identified as *O²*, also produces a product without enzymatic activity.[12]

Following the cloning of the ABO genes,[10] it was shown that the A and B transferase proteins differ only by four amino acids at positions 176, 235, 266, and 268 in a total of 354 amino acids. These amino acid substitutions are shown in Table 3-3. Group O cDNA is identical to group A cDNA except for a single base nucleotide deletion that results in a frame shift and an enzymatically inactive protein, producing no transferase. This is the common *O¹* allele. This finding supports the concept that the *A* gene is the ancestral gene for *O.* The *O* gene does produce a protein, but that protein is enzymatically nonfunctional.

Fucose, *N*-acetylgalactosamine, and galactose are also referred to as the **immunodominant sugars** for the H, A, and B antigens, respectively. These terminal sugars confer H, A, and B antigen specificity. The products of the *ABO* genes are expressed in an **autosomal codominant** fashion. For example, an individual who inherits both an *A* and a *B* gene expresses both gene products and is group

3-α-*N*-acetylgalactosaminyltransferase: Transfers the sugar *N*-acetylgalactosamine (GalNAc) to the H antigen, conferring group A specificity.

3-α-galactosyltransferase: Transfers the sugar galactose to the H antigen, conferring B blood group specificity.

Immunodominant sugar: The terminal sugar that confers ABO antigen specificity.

Autosomal codominant: A pattern of inheritance in which alleles are located on autosomes and are expressed whenever present. Since *A* and *B* are autosomal codominant, if both are inherited both A and B antigens will be expressed (group AB). Refer to Chapter 1 for a discussion of inheritance patterns.

TABLE 3-3 Amino Acid Substitutions in A and B Transferases

Phenotype	AMINO ACID NUMBER			
	176	235	266	268
A	Arg	Gly	Leu	Gly
B	Gly	Ser	Met	Ala

Ala, Alanine; Arg, arginine; Gly, glycine; Leu, leucine; Met, methionine; Ser, serine.

AB. An individual who is group B could have inherited two *B* genes or a *B* and an *O* gene. Family studies would therefore be needed to determine the actual genotype. Genotypes and resulting possible phenotypes are noted in Table 3-4. Phenotype frequencies vary across various racial groups. For example, the B phenotype is more common in blacks than in whites.[13]

Although the three major alleles at the *ABO* locus have been the focus of discussion to this point, many more alleles at this locus have been described and have been classified as subgroups of both A and B, often presenting in the laboratory as aberrant ABO typings. Exons 6 and 7 of the *ABO* gene are responsible for encoding the ABO glycosyltransferases.[11,14-17] It is within these two exons that nucleotide substitutions or deletions have been detected, resulting in the various ABO aberrations or polymorphisms that are described at the serologic level. These polymorphisms produce aberrant transferases that result in unique and diminished levels of A and B antigens on the red cell. The most common subgroup is that associated with an *A* gene. It is well established that both A_1 and A_2 subgroups give rise to group A individuals without aberrant typings. Subgroups for both groups A and B are discussed, as are the differences between the A_1 and A_2 phenotypes. The more

TABLE 3-4 ABO Groups of the Offspring of Different ABO Matings

Mating Phenotypes	Mating Genotypes	Offspring Possible Phenotypes (and Genotypes)
A × A	AA × AA	A (AA)
	AA × AO	A (AA or AO)
	AO × AO	A (AA or AO) or O (OO)
B × B	BB × BB	B (BB)
	BB × BO	B (BB or BO)
	BO × BO	B (BB or BO) or O (OO)
AB × AB	AB × AB	AB (AB) or A (AA) or B (BB)
O × O	OO × OO	O (OO)
A × B	AA × BB	AB (AB)
	AO × BB	AB (AB) or B (BO)
	AA × BO	AB (AB) or A (AO)
	AO × BO	AB (AB) or A (AO) or B (BO) or O (OO)
A × O	AA × OO	A (AO)
	AO × OO	A (AO) or O (OO)
A × AB	AA × AB	AB (AB) or A (AA)
	AO × AB	AB (AB) or A (AA or AO) or B (BO)
B × O	BB × OO	B (BO)
	BO × OO	B (BO) or O (OO)
B × AB	BB × AB	AB (AB) or B (BB)
	BO × AB	AB (AB) or B (BB or BO) or A (AO)
AB × O	AB × OO	A (AO) or B (BO)

rare subgroups of both A and B that are discussed demonstrate diminished levels of antigen on the red cells.

ABH ANTIGENS

Although ABH antigens have been detectable as early as 5 to 6 weeks' gestation, weaker expression of ABH antigens is expected when evaluating the erythrocytes of newborns. Indeed, adult levels of ABH antigen expression are not observed until approximately 2 to 4 years of age. The apparent reason for this diminished expression of ABH antigens on newborn red cells is the lack of complexity of the antigenic structures themselves.[18] This is described as the transformation from linear carbohydrate structures (less complex) to more branched (complex) carbohydrate structures as the individual grows older. Several different structures have been described for the A, B, and H antigens. These include the less complex or more linear structures designated A^a, B_I, and H_1; the more complex structures A^b, B_{II}, and H_2; and the most branched or most complex structures A^c, A^d, B_{III}, H_3, and H_4.[19,20] A characterization of linear and branched H antigen is shown in Fig. 3-3. As can be seen, the branched structure has multiple antigenic epitopes, compared with a single epitope on the more linear structure. Studies have demonstrated that A^a, A^b, H_1, and H_2 antigens, or those that are more linear, have equivalent levels in adult and newborn erythrocytes. Conversely, A^c, A^d, H_3, and H_4, the more branched structures, are low or absent from red cells of the newborn.[18] It is proposed that the branched and more complex ABO structures extend from the surface of the erythrocyte membrane to a greater extent than do those antigenic structures that are more linear.

ABO ANTIBODIES
Origin and Development of ABO Antibodies

In adults, anti-A or anti-B (or both) is present in the serum when the corresponding ABO antigen is genetically absent from the red cells. At birth, ABO antibodies are generally absent, although there has been documentation of ABO antibody synthesis in utero. Between 3 and 6 months of age, ABO antibody pro-

Refer to Chapter 13 for a discussion of the investigation of ABO typing discrepancies and other serologic problems.

Historically blood group antigens and their respective antibodies have been described serologically. The development of molecular techniques has elucidated the reason for many of these serologic patterns.

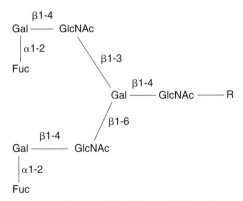

Fig. 3-3 Linear versus branched H antigen. Fuc, Fucose; Gal, galactose; GalNAc, *N*-acetylgalactosamine; GlcNAc, *N*-acetylglucosamine.

duction begins, and this production peaks at approximately 5 to 10 years of age. In adults, advancing age may be associated with diminished antibody levels. ABO antibody production appears to be influenced by both environmental and genetic factors. Evidence for an environmental influence was established during experiments with chickens, which produce an antibody similar to anti-B.[21] Chickens that were raised in a sterile environment failed to produce anti-B. However, chickens that were fed a diet rich in a particular strain of *Escherichia coli,* known to have galactose residues on its surface, produced high-titered anti-B. Chickens fed their normal diet in their normal environment produced expected levels of anti-B. Although similar experiments have not been done in humans, it is postulated that bacterial organisms in the external environment and the internal environment (digestive tract) provide an opportunity for exposure to numerous carbohydrate structures that are present on the surfaces of these organisms. Following exposure to these carbohydrate antigens, and based on the person's genetically determined ABO group, ABO antibody production then occurs. Although ABO antibodies are thought of as naturally occurring, some exposure to antigen must take place for antibody production to occur. The presence of these carbohydrate antigens in the environment most likely serves as the immunizing event.[22]

Immunoglobulin Class

Anti-A and anti-B in group B and group A individuals, respectively, tend to have a greater IgM component. However, IgG and IgA are also well represented. Anti-A,B in group O individuals, however, tends to be predominantly IgG, although IgM and IgA components are also present.[13,23] Whether the ABO antibodies are IgG or IgM, they are very efficient at activating complement.[24] As discussed earlier, the branching structures of these antigens, facilitating accessibility for antibody, probably play a role in complement activation. Their ability to activate complement makes the ABO antibodies clinically important. If major ABO-incompatible blood is transfused, the ability of the recipient's ABO antibodies to activate complement causes intravascular lysis of red cells that may precipitate such consequences as **disseminated intravascular coagulation** and acute renal failure in the recipient. Initial signs of an acute hemolytic transfusion reaction may include fever, chills, chest pain, hemoglobinuria, flushing, hypotension, back pain, and pain at the infusion site. Generalized bleeding at the surgical site may be the first indication of an acute reaction in anesthetized recipients. Whenever an acute hemolytic reaction is suspected, the transfusion must be stopped immediately and a thorough transfusion reaction investigation begun. These potential consequences make ABO typing the most important test performed in the blood bank.

Anti-A,B in Group O

The ABO antibodies found in the serum of group O individuals are not simply a mixture of anti-A plus anti-B. An antibody, designated anti-A,B, is also present and behaves quite differently. For example, if anti-A,B is **adsorbed** onto and **eluted** from group A red cells, the resulting eluate reacts not only with A cells but also with B cells, although usually not as strongly. In contrast, the same studies repeated using a mixture of anti-A plus anti-B yield an eluate that reacts only with A cells.[25] Anti-A,B appears to contain additional antibodies directed to shared determinants on the A and B antigens.

ABO Antibodies in Transfusion Therapy

In most transfusions, blood components that are ABO identical to the recipient are issued. However, in certain circumstances, ABO-compatible but not identical components may be issued. For red cell transfusions, group O red cells, which lack the A and B antigens, may be transfused to all other ABO groups. Although this

Disseminated intravascular coagulation (DIC): A condition associated with the activation of the coagulation cascade within the vasculature. DIC causes fibrin deposition in the microcirculation and consumption of platelets and fibrinogen. The major complication of DIC is clinical bleeding.

Refer to Chapter 15 for a discussion of the serology and management of hemolytic transfusion reactions.

Adsorption: The attachment of specific antibody to the red cell surface via the binding with specific antigen; for example, A cells adsorb anti-A from solution. Adsorption is a blood bank technique in which cells and plasma are mixed and antibody is adsorbed onto the red cell surface.

Elution: The process by which adsorbed antibody (on the red cell surface) is removed and returned to solution. Elutions can be performed by a number of physical and chemical procedures.

is not a common practice, it is the reason group O donors are referred to as *universal donors*. Group O recipients can receive only group O red cells. Conversely, a group AB recipient can receive all other ABO group red cell components because anti-A and anti-B are absent. This is why group AB recipients are sometimes referred to as *universal recipients*. Group AB red cell components are infused only into group AB recipients. Group A and group B red cells are usually transfused only into ABO-identical recipients. However, both can be transfused to an AB recipient. For the transfusion of plasma components, AB plasma may be infused into any recipient. Conversely, group O plasma is usually infused only into group O recipients. Group A and group B plasma are usually infused into ABO-identical recipients.

ABO SUBGROUPS
Subgroups of A
A_1 and A_2

As stated earlier in this chapter, at least two genes at the ABO locus appear to result in a normal, nondiscrepant group A phenotype. These have been identified as the A_1 and A_2 genes, but it is known that at least four different polymorphisms at the genetic level give rise to what is considered the A_2 phenotype.[17,26] Although all genes produce *N*-acetylgalactosaminyltransferase, quantitative and qualitative differences are observed with these genes.[23,27,28] These two phenotypes are best differentiated using the anti-A_1 **lectin** extracted from the seeds of *Dolichos biflorus*. This reagent is further discussed in the section on ABO reagents, and its reactivity with A_1 and A_2 red cells is summarized in Table 3-5. A_2 and A_2B individuals can produce anti-A_1. Approximately 4% of all A_2 individuals have naturally occurring anti-A_1 in their serum. In A_2B individuals, up to 25% may have anti-A_1. Although such individuals produce anti-A_1, if enough adsorptions are performed, A_2 cells can eventually adsorb anti-A_1 to completion. The amount of H antigen found on these cells is quite different. A_2 cells have increased levels of H antigen, second only to that noted on group O red cells. A_1 red cells have substantially less H antigen. This finding suggests a more efficient conversion of H antigen to A antigen by the product of the A_1 gene.[27] Consistent with this finding, many more copies of the A antigen occur on A_1 cells than on A_2 cells. Approximately 1 million copies have been reported on cells that express the product of an A_1 gene and only about 250,000 copies on those cells that express the product of an A_2 gene.[28] The transferase enzymes produced by these genes also seem to differ. The A_1 gene transferase reacts optimally at a pH of 5.6, requires Mn^{2+} and Mg^{2+} ions, and demonstrates a high Michaelis constant (Km) value for its affinity to H antigen. The A_2 transferase reacts optimally at a pH of 7.5, requires only Mg^{2+} ions, and demonstrates a low Km value for its affinity to H antigen.[27]

Other Subgroups of A

A number of other subgroups of A have been described. These appear to result from the inheritance of rare alleles at the ABO locus and include A_{int}, A_3, A_x, A_m, A_{end}, A_{el}, A_{bantu}, and A_{finn}. The serologic characteristics of these phenotypes are shown in Table 3-5. Except for A_{int} and A_3, many A subgroup red cells are weakly reactive or nonreactive when tested with human anti-A. The amount of H antigen expressed is usually equivalent to that seen with group O red cells. In some subgroups, the presence of A antigen is demonstrable only if adsorption and elution studies are performed. In these studies, commercial anti-A is adsorbed onto the red cells believed to be a subgroup of A. Following sufficient washing of the red cells with saline, an eluate is prepared, using an elution method that optimizes the recovery of ABO antibodies. The eluate is then tested for anti-A. If anti-A is recovered, the presence of A antigen on the red cells is confirmed. If monoclonal anti-A is being used, weak reactions may not always

Lectin: Any of a group of plant substances capable of binding specifically with antigen substances (sugars) on the surface of red blood cells, resulting in agglutination. *Dolichos bifloris,* for example, is a lectin with anti-A_1 specificity.

TABLE 3-5 Serologic Characteristics of Different Subgroups of A

| | REACTIONS WITH | | | | | | |
Subgroup	Human Anti-A	Anti-A,B	Anti-A₁*	Anti-H	Monoclonal Anti-A	Substance(s) In Saliva if Secretor	Anti-A₁ In Serum
A₁	++++	++++	++++	+ʷ	++++	A and H	No
A₂	++++	++++	0	+++	++++	A and H	4%
A_int	++++	++++	++	+++	++++	A and H	No
A₃	++ mf	++ mf	0	++++	++++	A and H	Few
Aₓ	0/+ʷ	+/++	0	++++	+++	H	Usually
A_m	+ʷ	+ʷ	0	++++	NT	A and H	No
A_end	+ʷ	+ʷ	0	++++	NT	H	No
A_el	0	0	0	++++	0	H	Few
A_bantu	+ʷ	+ʷ	0	++++	++	H	Usually
A_finn	+ʷ	+ʷ	0	++++	NT	H	All

Dolichos biflorus.
mf, Mixed field; NT, not tested.

be noted when evaluating A subgroup red cells, including the Aₓ phenotype. Many monoclonal reagents have been blended to ensure that some A subgroup red cells are readily detected. Although monoclonal reagents detect some subgroups, other subgroups continue to be weakly reactive or nonreactive with these monoclonal reagents (see Table 3-5). Some subgroups of A have a naturally occurring anti-A₁ in the serum, whereas others do not. This information is also summarized in Table 3-5. If the subgroup under investigation is also a secretor, soluble H antigen or both soluble H and A antigens are present in the saliva (see Table 3-5). Soluble ABH antigens are more extensively discussed in the next chapter. Although it is sometimes possible to determine an individual's precise subgroup, more often it is not an easy task. Some subgroups, such as Aₓ, can be fairly obvious if human antisera are used. To facilitate categorization, saliva studies may be useful, as may family studies.

As discussed earlier for A₁ and A₂ phenotypes, studies have shown that the subgroups are a result of genetic mutations in the exon structures (particularly exon 7) of the *ABO* genes.[17,26,29] These changes in nucleotides give rise to unique amino acid sequences in the A transferase and confer the unique serologic findings that qualify as different A subgroups. Those subgroup phenotypes that have been evaluated at the molecular level demonstrate many polymorphisms. Subgroups that appear to be identical serologically, such as the Aₓ phenotype, have been shown at the molecular level to arise because of at least six unique mutations in the *A* gene.[29] These mutated genes produce aberrant transferases, conferring unique ABO-related serologic findings.

Subgroups of B

As described for A, subgroups of B have been reported. Again, reactions of red cells with anti-B are weak and variable. Serum may contain anti-B, and saliva, if the individual is a secretor, demonstrates either soluble H antigen or soluble H and B antigens. Four categories for B subgroups are summarized in Table 3-6. As discussed for subgroups of A, adsorption and elution with anti-B may be necessary to demonstrate the presence of the B antigen.

As discussed under A subgroups, molecular analyses have occurred with B subgroups.[29] As anticipated, molecular studies have once again confirmed nucleotide changes in primarily exon 7 of the *ABO* gene, giving rise to unique B transferases.

TABLE 3-6 Subgroups of B

	Anti-A	Anti-B	Anti-A,B	Substance in Saliva
B$_3$	0	1+^{mf}	2+^{mf}	B and H
B$_m$	0	0	0/+^{w}	B and H
B$_x$	0	0/+^{w}	0/2+	H
B$_{el}$	0	0/+^{w}	0/+^{w}	H

mf, Mixed field.

Clinical Significance of ABO Subgroups

Subgroups of A and B may have clinical relevance. If a subgroup is unrecognized for what it is, the error usually results in the sample being identified as group O. In the case of a recipient, the consequences of such an error would be minimal. However, in the case of a donor, the error could have significance. If a subgroup of A, for example, were labeled group O and then transfused to a group O recipient, the anti-A,B of the recipient might cause the early destruction of the transfused red cells.

Hybrid Transferases

Several phenotypes, described as *cis*-AB and B(A), appear to arise from hybrid transferases that encode both A and B antigen specificity.[15,30,31] In the *cis*-AB phenotype, red cells have equivalent amounts of A and B antigen. In the B(A) phenotype, the red cells express more B antigen and diminished amounts of A antigen. In a similar fashion as mentioned for both A and B subgroups, changes in exon 7 of the *ABO* gene give rise to unique transferases that are capable of transferring both galactose and N-acetylgalactosamine to H antigen. The amino acid sequences for these unique transferases have revealed amino acid substitutions at positions 176, 234, 235, 266, and 286 (Table 3-7).

THE BOMBAY PHENOTYPE
Classic Bombay

As mentioned previously, this phenotype arises when two *hh* genes (or two inactive alleles of *H* or *FUT1*) are inherited at the *H* locus. Numerous genetic mutations of the *H* or *FUT1* gene have been described.[5,7,8] Because these individuals are unable to convert type 2 paragloboside to H antigen since they cannot produce the corresponding fucosyltransferase, they are unable to make A or B antigens, even though these individuals have inherited two genes at the *ABO* locus.[23,28] In addition, Bombay individuals also have mutant alleles at the *SE(FUT2)* locus and cannot produce fucosyltransferase to produce H, A, or B antigens in the secretions.[32] Because these individuals are deficient in H, A, and B antigens, they produce anti-H, anti-A, and anti-B as naturally occurring antibodies. On initial testing, Bombay red cells appear to be group O. Their red cells are nonreactive with anti-A, anti-B, and anti-A,B, whereas their serum reacts with A$_1$ and B cells. However, their serum

TABLE 3-7 Amino Acid Substitutions in Hybrid Transferases

Phenotype	AMINO ACID NUMBER				
	176	234	235	266	268
cis-AB	Arg	Pro	Gly	Leu	Ala
cis-AB	Gly	Pro	Ser	Leu	Ala
B (A)	Gly	Pro	Gly	Met	Ala
B (A)	Gly	Ala	Ser	Met	Ala

Ala, Alanine; Arg, arginine; Gly, glycine; Leu, leucine; Met, methionine; Pro, proline; Ser, serine.

also reacts with antibody-screening cells and all normal group O cells tested, because of the presence of anti-H. These antibodies preclude individuals from being transfused with other than Bombay red cells.[28] O_h is used to identify the Bombay phenotype. If it is possible to determine ABO genes that the individual inherited but is unable to express, the phenotype is written O_h^A, O_h^B, or O_h^{AB}.

Para-Bombay

Individuals who are para-Bombay (like Bombay) also have mutant alleles at the *H* or *FUT1* locus but normal genes at their *SE* or *FUT2* locus.[6,7,33] Even with an abnormal *H* gene, some para-Bombays demonstrate minute quantities of ABH antigens on their red cells, regardless of whether they possess them in their secretions. Other para-Bombays fail to demonstrate ABH antigens on their red cells. But as expected, they may or may not express ABH antigens in the secretions, based on the genes inherited at the *SE* or *FUT2* locus. Para-Bombay serum will also contain anti-H.

The para-Bombay category is a broad one, and the literature is replete with complex and conflicting descriptions for such individuals. Part of the complexity for this category arises because two loci are involved (*H* or *FUT1* and *SE* or *FUT2*) and alleles at these loci may be functional, weakly functional, or nonfunctional. The reader is encouraged to review Reid and Lomas-Francis[8] and Spitalnik and Spitalnik[9] for further detail on para-Bombay phenotypes.

ABO REAGENTS
Routine ABO Reagents

Although anti-A, anti-B, and anti-A,B from human sources are readily available, most blood group reagent manufacturers are producing monoclonal sources for these ABO typing reagents. Although not required, some facilities do use anti-A,B in routine ABO typing. Other routine ABO reagents include reagent red cells (human) that may be packaged as A_1 and B cells or as A_1, A_2, and B cells. A_2 red cells are optional for reverse ABO typing.

Use of routine ABO reagents is fairly straightforward, as is the interpretation of ABO grouping results. ABO forward groupings, or the assessment of recipient or donor red cells, seek to determine the presence or absence of A and B antigens by testing red cells with anti-A, anti-B, and anti-A,B (optional); ABO reverse groupings, or the assessment of recipient or donor serum or plasma, seek to determine the presence of ABO antibodies. Manual ABO forward and reverse groupings are usually performed using a tube method, although slide ABO groupings may also be done. The manufacturer's directions should be consulted for specific red cell and ABO antisera proportions and for appropriate spin times and speeds. Interpretations of ABO forward groupings are described in Table 3-1.

Lectins

Lectins are extracts from plants (seeds) or animals that have the ability to combine with simple sugars. Two such lectins have been useful in the blood bank relative to the ABO system.[23,28] The lectin from the seeds of *Dolichos biflorus* is used as a source of anti-A_1. This lectin binds with the simple sugar N-acetylgalactosamine. The lectin from the seeds of *Ulex europaeus* is used as a source of anti-H. This lectin binds with the simple sugar fucose.

ABO DISCREPANCIES

An ABO discrepancy implies that the forward, or red cell, ABO grouping does not agree with the reverse, or serum, ABO grouping. As stated earlier in this chapter, an accurate ABO grouping is the most important test performed in the blood bank. Mistyping either a donor or an intended recipient can lead to transfusion with ABO-incompatible blood. As stated earlier, ABO antibodies are extremely efficient at complement activation and result in in vivo hemolysis. The clinical consequences of this in vivo red cell destruction can be significant and may even result in the death of the recipient. It is important to identify an ABO discrepancy, to ascertain the cause, and then to resolve that discrepancy to facilitate transfusion therapy.

ABO discrepancies can be categorized on the basis of causes that are primarily red cell mediated and those that are primarily serum mediated. The various causes of ABO discrepancies are listed in Box 3-1 and described in the following sections.

Red Cell Mediated
Subgroups of A or B

In these discrepancies, the forward ABO grouping appears as a group O, but the reverse grouping appears as a group A or B. This type of discrepancy is best resolved by adsorbing and eluting anti-A or anti-B from the red cells in order to prove the presence of diminished antigen. Saliva studies, if the individual is a secretor, may also be useful, as may family studies.

Genetic Chimera

The term **chimera** means multiple cell populations. Genetically, this can arise because of anastomosis, or joining, of dissimilar tissues in twins during early embryonic life. Because the graft occurs early, tolerance to the graft is ensured. Dispermic chimerism can also account for a genetic chimera. Here, two sperm fertilize a single egg, giving rise to what is also called generalized tissue mosaicism. The forward ABO grouping may appear to be group O, for example, and the reverse grouping, A. If the graft were indeed group A and the host group O, this is what might be observed. Resolution for chimeras can include cell separation studies of the two cell populations. The reader is referred to Judd[34] for various separation methods.

The term cell-mediated discrepancies refers to some characteristics of the red cells (added, missing or altered) that cause aberrant typing results. Serum-mediated discrepancies, on the other hand, result from substances in the serum that similarly cause aberrant results.

Chimera: An individual who has more than one cell population from different sources. In the blood bank, chimerism may result in multiple red cell populations with differing antigens thus resulting in discrepant cell typing.

Box 3-1   ABO Grouping Discrepancies

I. Red cell mediated
1. Subgroups of A or B
2. Genetic chimera
3. Artificial chimera
    a. Blood transfusion
    b. Bone marrow and stem cell transplantation
4. Polyagglutination
    a. Tn activation
    b. Acquired B antigen
5. Substances in plasma or serum
    a. Excess blood group substance
    b. Dyes
    c. Wharton's jelly
6. Positive direct antiglobulin test
7. Reagents

II. Serum mediated
1. Subgroups of A or B
2. Alloantibodies that include anti-M, anti-Le[a], anti-P$_1$
3. Autoantibodies that include anti-I, anti-IH
4. Rouleaux
5. Transfusion of non–ABO identical plasma products
6. Age
7. Disease
8. Reagents

Artificial Chimera

Blood transfusion, bone marrow and stem cell transplantation, and fetal/maternal bleed can result in multiple cell populations that have the potential to manifest as ABO discrepancies. Patient history and perhaps cell separation studies are the best ways to address these types of discrepancies.

Polyagglutination

Two types of **polyagglutination** routinely cause a cell-mediated ABO discrepancy—Tn activation and acquired B. In Tn activation, the alkali-labile tetrasaccharides of glycophorin A and B fail to incorporate both a galactose residue and a sialic acid residue. This allows a now terminal *N*-acetylgalactosamine molecule to react with anti-A, resulting in an acquired A antigen, or Tn activation. Resolution includes the identification of Tn-activated red cells and repeat testing with enzyme-premodified cells. The acquired B phenomenon occurs only with A_1 red cells. Here, a deacetylase enzyme produced by certain microbes has the ability to remove the acetyl group from the *N*-acetylgalactosamine, resulting in galactosamine. Galactosamine has the ability to cross-react with anti-galactose (anti-B), giving the cells the appearance of a B antigen. Cells then forward type as AB and reverse type as A. Resolution involves ascertaining that cells do have the acquired B antigen. Such cells can be reacetylated with the use of acetic anhydride. Refer to Judd[34] for specific procedures.

Substances in Serum or Plasma

Some substances in plasma may inhibit the expected reaction in an ABO forward typing. This primarily includes the secretion of excess AB substances, as can occur in certain tumors. In this situation, blood typing antibody combines with soluble blood group substance, precluding it from reacting with the appropriate antigen on the red cells. This type of ABO discrepancy is not observed with washed red cells. Other substances in the plasma actually cause false-positive reactions with ABO typing reagents and red cells and include such antibodies as anti-acriflavin (dye used in some anti-B reagents). In this type of ABO discrepancy, immune complexes form and support red cell agglutination. This type of reaction is not detected when red cells are washed with normal saline. Wharton's jelly (hyaluronic acid), a contaminant of cord blood, can also cause incorrect ABO forward typing. Here, the newborn appears as an AB. However, because reverse groupings are not performed on newborns, there is no built-in quality assurance check on the ABO typing. Because of this, it is a common laboratory policy to more closely evaluate group AB cord blood typings. Wharton's jelly can usually be removed by washing the red cells in saline. However, on occasion, hyaluronidase must be added to negate the "agglutinating" effects of the jelly.[23,34]

Positive Direct Antiglobulin Test

Although rare, cells may be so heavily sensitized with antibody that red cells spontaneously agglutinate when tested with anti-A or anti-B, appearing to forward type as AB. In these circumstances, a saline control is also positive. Removal of antibody with heat, chloroquine, or ZZAP (cystein-activated papain and DTT) may be useful in resolving this type of discrepancy. The reader is referred to Judd[34] for appropriate methods.

Reagents

Rarely, the ABO reagent being used may contain an antibody defining a low-incidence antigen and the red cells being ABO tested just happen to express that low-incidence antigen. Such a sample may forward type as A and reverse group as O if the antibody defining the low-incidence antigen is in the anti-A. This type of reaction is not seen when using monoclonal ABO reagents.

Polyagglutination: A condition in which red cells are agglutinated by a large percentage of human sera regardless of blood types but not agglutinated by autologous serum. Most forms of polyagglutination are due to the exposure of some hidden receptor on the surface of the red cell.

Serum Mediated
Subgroups of A or B

Although mentioned under cell-mediated discrepancies, subgroups may also manifest primarily as a serum discrepancy because of the presence of anti-A_1 or anti-B. These usually appear to forward type as a group O but reverse group as an A or B. Again, resolution would be done primarily as discussed previously for subgroups.

Alloantibodies

IgM alloantibodies such as anti-Le^a, anti-P_1, anti-M, and anti-N may cause a serum-mediated discrepancy because the reverse ABO grouping cells, in addition to expressing their A or B antigens, also express the antigen to which a room temperature alloantibody is directed. The forward grouping might clearly be group A, but now the reverse grouping appears to be group O. Antibody identification studies are needed, followed by the selection of A or B cells that lack the other antigen. Repeat testing with these cells should resolve the discrepancy.

Autoantibodies

On occasion, potent autoantibodies such as anti-I or anti-IH may be responsible for serum-mediated discrepancies in which the forward grouping could be A and the reverse group, O. Serum containing such antibodies should be autoadsorbed to remove these antibodies and the reverse grouping repeated using autoadsorbed serum.

Rouleaux

Patients with abnormal globulins may induce rouleaux of red cells, which may appear as agglutination. The forward grouping may appear as A but the reverse as O. If unwashed red cells are tested, the forward typing may appear as AB. Saline replacement tests should resolve these discrepancies.

Transfusion of Non–ABO-Identical Plasma Products

Patients receiving platelets and fresh frozen plasma that are non–ABO identical may have such a discrepancy. For example, a group B receiving group O platelets may demonstrate both anti-A and anti-B in his or her serum. The patient's transfusion history is the best approach to dealing with this problem.

Age

As stated earlier, newborns do not express their respective ABO antibodies. If this concept is forgotten, ABO discrepancies result. Serum from aged patients may also cause a serum-mediated discrepancy because they may have a decline in their ABO antibody levels. Patient history may be helpful in both of these situations in which the reverse grouping is likely to be AB.

Disease

Hypogammaglobulinemia or agammaglobulinemia can cause serum-mediated ABO discrepancies. An AB reverse grouping is the likely outcome. Patient history is helpful in these situations.

Reagents

Deterioration of reagent red cells can occur if products are not adequately stored or used after the manufacturer's outdate.

CHAPTER SUMMARY

1. The single most important test performed on blood donors and recipients is the ABO grouping. This is because antibodies to the ABO antigens absent from the red cells are routinely present. These antibodies have the ability to hemolyze incompatible red cells.

2. Several genetic loci interact with the *ABO* locus. These include the *H, SE, LE, I,* and *P* loci. The products of genes at these loci are transferase enzymes. These enzymes transfer sugars to other oligosaccharides to confer antigen specificity.

3. H antigens serve as the precursor material for the A and B antigens. Group O individuals demonstrate only H antigen, because the *O* gene appears to be an amorph.

4. If two *h* genes are inherited, H antigen is not produced and, consequently, neither are A or B antigens. Individuals who inherit two *h* genes (and two nonfunctional *SE* genes) are referred to as the Bombay phenotype.

5. In adults, anti-A or anti-B (or both) is present in the serum when the corresponding antigen is absent from the red cells. These antibodies are generally absent at birth and are produced as a result of exposure to carbohydrate structures in the environment.

6. Normal group A individuals are either A_1 or A_2. Additional genes at the ABO locus are responsible for the rare subgroups of A and B that have been described.

7. When the red cell ABO grouping is not identical to the serum ABO group, an ABO discrepancy exists. ABO discrepancies may be red cell or serum mediated. Resolution of ABO discrepancies is critical.

REFERENCES

1. Landsteiner K: Zur Kenntnis der antifermentativen, lytischen und agglutinierenden Wirkungen des Blutserums und der Lymphe. Zbl Bakt 27:357-362, 1900.
2. von Decastello A, Sturli A: Uber die Isoagglutinine im Serum gesunder und kranker Menschen. Munchen Med Wochenschr, 1090-1095, 1902.
3. Clausen H, Hakomori S: ABH and related histo-blood group antigens; immunochemical differences in carrier isotypes and their distribution. Vox Sang 56:1-20, 1989.
4. Reguigne-Arnould I, Faure S, Chery M, et al: Physical mapping of 49 microsatellite markers on chromosome 19 and correlation with the genetic linkage map. Genomics 87:458-461, 1996.
5. Wagner FF, Flegel WA: Polymorphism of the h allele and the population frequency of sporadic nonfunctional alleles. Transfusion 37:264-290, 1997.
6. Yu LC, Yang YH, Broadberry RE, et al: Heterogeneity of the human H blood group α1-2 fucosyltransferase gene among para-Bombay individuals. Vox Sang 72:36-40, 1997.
7. Kaneko M, Nishihara S, Shinya N, et al: Wide variety of point mutations in the H gene of Bombay and para-Bombay individuals that inactivate H enzyme. Blood 90:839-849, 1997.
8. Reid ME, Lomas-Francis C: The Blood Group Antigen FactsBook, 2nd ed. London, Academic Press, Elsevier, 2004.
9. Spitalnik PF, Spitalnik SL: Human carbohydrate blood group systems. In Simon TL, Dzik WH, Snyder EL, et al (eds): Rossi's Principles of Transfusion Medicine, 3rd ed. Philadelphia, Lippincott Williams and Wilkins, 2002.
10. Yamamoto F, Clausen H, White T, et al: Molecular genetic basis of the histo-blood group ABO system. Nature 345: 229-233, 1990.
11. Seltsam A, Hallensleben M, Kollmann A, et al: Systematic analysis of the *ABO* gene diversity within exons 6 and 7 by PCR screening reveals new *ABO* alleles. Transfusion 43: 428-439, 2003.
12. Yamamoto F, McNeill PD, Yamamoto M, et al: Molecular genetic analysis of the ABO blood group system: 4. Another type of O allele. Vox Sang 64:175-178, 1993.
13. Brecher M (ed): Technical Manual, 14th ed. Bethesda, MD, American Association of Blood Banks, 2002.
14. Ogasawara K, Yabe R, Uchikara M, et al: Different alleles cause an imbalance in A_2 and A_2 B phenotypes of the ABO blood group. Vox Sang 74:242-247, 1998.
15. Yamamota F, McNeill PD, Yamamoto M, et al: Molecular genetic analysis of the ABO blood group system: 3. A_x and B(A) alleles. Vox Sang 64:171-174, 1993.
16. Yamamota FI, McNeill PD, Yamamoto M, et al: Molecular genetic analysis of the ABO blood group system: 1. Weak subgroups: A^3 and B^3 alleles. Vox Sang 64:116-119, 1993.
17. Olsson ML, Chester MA: Heterogeneity of the blood group A_x allele: Genetic recombination of common alleles can result in the A_x phenotype. Transfus Med 8:231-238, 1998.
18. Hakomori S: Blood group ABH and Ii antigens of human erythrocytes: Chemistry, polymorphisms and their developmental change. Semin Hematol 18:39-62, 1981.
19. Fukuda MN, Hakomori S: Structures of branched blood group A–active glycosphingolipids in human erythrocytes and polymorphism of A- and H-glycolipids in A_1 and A_2 subgroups. J Biol Chem 257:446-455, 1982.
20. Clausen H, Levery SB, Kannagi R, Hakomori S: Novel blood group H glycolipid antigens exclusively expressed in blood group A and AB erythrocytes (type 3 chain H). I. Isolation and chemical characterization. J Biol Chem 261:1380-1387, 1986.
21. Springer GF, Horton RE, Forbes M: Origin of anti-human blood group B agglutinins in white leghorn chicks. J Exp Med 110:221-244, 1959.
22. Nance ST: Serology of the ABH and Lewis blood group systems. In Wallace ME, Gibbs FL (eds): Blood Group Systems: ABH and Lewis. Arlington, VA, American Association of Blood Banks, 1986.
23. Mollison PL, Engelfriet CP, Contreras M: Blood Transfusion in Clinical Medicine, 10th ed. Oxford, Blackwell Scientific, 1997.
24. Rieben R, Buchs JP, Fluckiger E, Nydegger UE: Antibodies to histo-blood group substances A and B: Agglutination titers, Ig class, and IgG subclasses in healthy persons of different age categories. Transfusion 31:607-615, 1991.

25. Dodd BE, Lincoln PJ, Boorman KE: The crossreacting antibodies of group O sera: Immunological studies and a possible explanation of the observed facts. Immunology 12: 39-52, 1967.
26. Olsson ML, Chester MA: Polymorphisms at the *ABO* locus in subgroup A individuals. Transfusion 36:309-313, 1996.
27. Topping MD, Watkins WM: Isoelectric points of the human blood group A_1, A_2 and B gene–associated glycosyltransferases in ovarian cyst fluids and serum. Biochem Biophys Res Commun 64:89-96, 1975.
28. Issitt PD, Anstee DJ: Applied Blood Group Serology, 4th ed. Durham, NC, Montgomery Scientific Publications, 1998.
29. Olsson ML, Irshaid NM, Hosseini-Maaf B, et al: Genomic analysis of clinical samples with serologic ABO blood grouping discrepancies: Identification of 15 novel A and B subgroup alleles. Blood 98:1585-1593, 2001.
30. Bennett M, Levene C, Greenwell P: An Israeli family with six *cisAB* members: Serologic and enzymatic studies. Transfusion 38:441-448, 1998.
31. Roubinet F, Janvier D, Blancher A: A novel *cis AB* allele derived from a *B* allele through a single point mutation. Transfusion 42:239-246, 2002.
32. Koda Y, Soejima M, Johnson PH, et al: Missense mutation of *FUT1* and deletion of *FUT2* are responsible for Indian Bombay phenotype of ABO blood group system. Biochem Biophys Res Commun 238:21-25, 1997.
33. Wang B, Koda Y, Soejima M, et al: Two missense mutations of H type $\alpha(1,2)$ fucosyltransferase gene (*FUT1*) responsible for para-Bombay individuals. Vox Sang 72:31-35, 1997.
34. Judd WJ: Methods in Immunohematology, 2nd ed. Durham, NC, Montgomery Scientific Publications, 1994.

FURTHER READINGS

Blood Group Antigen Gene Mutation Database:www.bioc.aecom.yu.edu/bgmut/index.htm
Brecher M (ed): Technical Manual, 14th ed. Bethesda, MD, American Association of Blood Banks, 2002.
Daniels G: Human Blood Groups, 2nd ed. Oxford, Blackwell Science, 2002.
Issitt PD, Anstee DJ: Applied Blood Group Serology, 4th ed. Durham, NC, Montgomery Scientific Publications, 1998.
Mollison PL, Englefriet CP, Contreras M: Blood Transfusion in Clinical Medicine, 10th ed. Oxford, Blackwell Scientific, 1997.
Reid ME, Lomas-Francis C: The Blood Group Antigen FactsBook, 2nd ed. London, Academic Press, Elsevier, 2004.

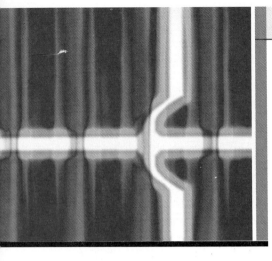

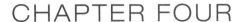

CHAPTER FOUR

Secretor and Soluble ABH Antigens

The Lewis, I, P, and Globoside Blood Group Systems

Susan L. Wilkinson

CHAPTER OUTLINE

THE *SECRETOR (SE)* LOCUS

Se and *se* Alleles
Product of the *Se(FUT2)* Gene

THE LEWIS BLOOD GROUP SYSTEM

The Lewis Antigens and the *Le(FUT3)*
and *le* Alleles
Products of the *Le(FUT3)* Gene
The Le(a–b–) Phenotype
Lewis Antibodies

INTERACTION OF *ABO, H, SE,* AND *LE*
LOCI: ANTIGENIC PRODUCTION ON THE
RED CELL AND IN THE PLASMA AND
SECRETIONS

Le, sese, H, and *ABO* Genes
Le, sese, hh, and *ABO* Genes
Le, Se, H, and *ABO* Genes
Le, Se, hh, and *ABO* Genes
lele, sese, H, and *ABO* Genes
lele, sese, hh, and *ABO* Genes
lele, Se, H, and *ABO* Genes
lele, Se, hh, and *ABO* Genes

THE I BLOOD GROUP SYSTEM

I Blood Group System Antigen and
Ii Blood Group Collection
I System Antibodies
Complex Antibodies Related to I and
Other Blood Groups

THE P AND GLOBOSIDE BLOOD GROUP
SYSTEMS AND THE GLOBOSIDE
BLOOD GROUP COLLECTION

Genetics and Biochemistry
P System Antibodies

LEARNING OBJECTIVES

After reading and studying this chapter, the student should be able to:

1. Describe the inheritance of the secretor status.
2. Given the ABO, H, and secretor genotype, determine the ABO/H antigens present on the red cells and in the secretions.
3. Briefly describe the difference between the product of the *H* gene and the product of the *Se* gene.
4. Describe the inheritance of the Lewis antigens and the products of the *Le* gene.
5. Discuss how the antigens of the Lewis blood group system differ from those of other blood groups such as ABO.
6. When provided with the ABO, H, secretor, and Lewis genotype, determine the ABO, H, and Lewis antigens present on the red blood cells and in the secretions.
7. Describe the serologic characteristics and clinical significance of anti-Le^a and anti-Le^b.
8. Differentiate between the reactivity of anti-Le^{bH} and anti-Le^{bL}.
9. Describe the serologic reactivity of anti-Le^{ab}.
10. Describe the differences between the I and i antigen structures.
11. List the serologic characteristics and clinical significance of anti-I and anti-i antibodies.
12. Briefly describe four complex antibodies that are I system related.
13. List the antigen associated with the I blood group collection.
14. List the antigens of the P and Globoside blood group systems.
15. List the antigens associated with the Globoside blood group collection.
16. Briefly describe the following phenotypes: P_1, P_2, p, P_1^k, P_2^k.
17. Describe the serologic characteristics and clinical significance of the following P system antibodies: anti-P_1, anti-P, and anti-P^k.

As stated in the previous chapter, ABH antigens are found primarily as glycoproteins and partly as glycolipids and integral to the red cell membrane. These antigens also occur as soluble glycoprotein antigens in secretions that include saliva, tears, breast milk, and seminal fluid. The presence of these soluble antigens in body secretions enabled Watkins and Morgan[1] to initially elucidate the structure of the ABH blood group antigens. The presence of ABH antigens in the secretions is controlled by the *Se(FUT2)* gene. Secreted antigens are absent when two *se* genes are inherited.

These genes, located at the *SE* locus, also interact with the *Le(FUT3)* gene at the *LE* locus. The interaction of these gene products determines the Lewis phenotypes found in the secretions and subsequently the Lewis phenotype associated with the red cell membrane. The Lewis antigens of the red cell are not an integral part of the red cell membrane but arise from Lewis glycolipids of the plasma.[2]

The I, P, and Globoside (GLOB) blood group systems are composed of antigens that are an integral part of the red cell membrane. These structures, in a similar fashion to the ABH antigens described in the previous chapter, are type 2 structures. The I antigens are both glycoprotein and glycolipid in nature, whereas the P and globoside antigens are only glycolipid.[3] The *P1* and *I* loci also interact with other loci described in this and the previous chapter. In addition, several antigens have been given blood group collection status and have been removed from blood group system status.[4] These include the P^k, LKE, and i antigens.

THE *SECRETOR (SE)* LOCUS
Se and *se* Alleles

The *SE* locus has been assigned to chromosome 19 (19q13.3) and is linked with the *H* and *LU (Lutheran)* loci.[5] The alleles at the *SE* locus include *Se(FUT2)* and *se*. *Se(FUT2)* gives rise to the autosomal dominant trait responsible for the presence of water-soluble ABH glycoproteins in secretions. Group O individuals who are **secretors** demonstrate H antigen in their secretions; A and B individuals demonstrate H and A and H and B antigens, respectively, whereas group AB individuals demonstrate H, A, and B antigens (Table 4-1). Thus, individuals with the *SeSe* or *Sese* genotype demonstrate soluble blood group substance in their secretions. These secretors are found in approximately 80% of the random population.

The *se* gene appears to produce no detectable product and is thought of as an amorph. Homozygous *se* individuals fail to secrete ABH antigens in their

Secretor: An individual who has inherited at least one *Se(FUT2)* gene, which results in the secretion of ABH antigens into body fluids. These individuals make up approximately 80% of the random population.

TABLE 4-1 ABH Antigens in Secretions

Genotype	ABH Antigens in Secretions
SeSe or Sese	Yes
sese	No

secretions. Nonsecretors, or those individuals who have inherited two *se* genes, make up approximately 20% of the random population.

It has been shown that the *se* gene can arise through a variety of genetic mutations to the *Se* gene. Some variants are caused by nonsense mutations or small deletions in the nucleotide structures of the gene that result in stop codons and truncated, nonfunctional enzymatic proteins.[6-8] Other genetic events have also led to the production of *se* genes, and the reader is encouraged to consult the excellent review by Spitalnik and Spitalnik.[9] Of interest, the entire *Se(FUT2)* gene is deleted in the classic Bombay phenotype.[10]

Product of the *Se(FUT2)* Gene

The *Se(FUT2)* gene codes for the production of an α1-2-fucosyltransferase enzyme.[11] This enzyme adds fucose in α1-2 linkage to an acceptor molecule. As stated in the previous chapter, this is the same transferase that is produced by the *H(FUT1)* gene. The *H* gene, however, preferentially adds fucose to type 2 chains, whereas the *Se* gene preferentially adds fucose to type 1 structures. Therefore, the H antigens of the red cells, which are primarily type 2 structures, arise from products produced by the *H(FUT1)* gene. The H antigens of the secretions, which are type 1 structures, arise from products produced by the *Se(FUT2)* gene. Type 2 H antigens in the secretions can also arise from the *H* gene. It is postulated that the *Se* gene is the ancestral gene of *H*.[12]

THE LEWIS BLOOD GROUP SYSTEM
The Lewis Antigens and the *Le(FUT3)* and *le* Alleles

The *LE* locus has been assigned to chromosome 19 (19p13.3).[13] The two alleles at this locus are *Le* and *le*. The *le* gene is believed to be an amorph, because it produces no detectable product. In the presence of two *le* genes, the red cell phenotype is Le(a−b−). As described for other amorphic alleles, the *le* gene arises from mutations of an *Le(FUT3)* gene where the protein material produced by the now modified gene is unable to produce functional enzyme.[14-16]

The *Le* gene behaves as an autosomal dominant characteristic. As will be discussed, the *Le(FUT3)* gene gives rise to two distinct red cell phenotypes, Le(a+b−) and Le(a−b+). The phenotype expressed depends on whether an *Se(FUT2)* gene has also been inherited.

Lewis antigen expression is minimal at birth, and most newborns type as Le(a−b−), regardless of the genes they have inherited. In whites and blacks, the Le(a+b−) phenotype occurs in approximately 22% of the random population. Approximately 72% of whites are Le(a−b+) and 6% are Le(a−b−). In blacks, the

Lewis antigens: Soluble antigens that are adsorbed onto the red cell surface and are not an integral part of the red cell membrane.

TABLE 4-2 Phenotype Frequencies for the Lewis System

Phenotype	PHENOTYPE FREQUENCY (%) White	Black
Le(a+b−)	22	23
Le(a−b+)	72	55
Le(a−b−)	6	22

Le(a−b−) phenotype is more frequent (22%) and the Le(a−b+) phenotype less frequent (55%). This is noted in Table 4-2.

Products of the *Le(FUT3)* Gene

The *Le* gene produces an α1-4-fucosyltransferase as its product. The transferase adds fucose in α1-4 linkage to an acceptor molecule on type 1 structures only. This can occur to the water-soluble glycoproteins of the secretions and the alcohol-soluble glycolipids of the plasma. Indeed, the glycolipid antigens of the plasma are responsible for the Lewis antigens that are detected on the surface of the red cell. These antigens are adsorbed onto the surface of the erythrocyte and are not an integral part of the red cell.

The products of a single *Le(FUT3)* gene can give rise to two distinct Lewis antigens if an *Se(FUT2)* gene has also been inherited. First, the *Le* gene can add fucose to **lacto-*N*-tetraose** in the secretions or to **lacto-*N*-tetraosylceramide** in the plasma to produce the Le^a antigen. The *Le* gene can also add fucose to type 1 H in the secretions and to type 1 H in the plasma, both products of the *Se* gene. This results in the Le^b antigen. These gene interactions with resulting antigens are depicted in Fig. 4-1.

Individuals who inherit an *Le(FUT3)* gene and two *se* genes have red cells of the Le(a+b−) phenotype and secrete Le^a substance in their secretions, even though they have not inherited an *Se* gene. In the presence of both *Le* and *Se* genes, Le^a and Le^b antigens are produced. However, in the plasma, less Le^a antigen is produced; there-

Lacto-*N*-tetraose: The precursor substance for the Le^a antigen in the body fluids.

Lacto-*N*-tetraosylceramide: The precursor substance for the Le^a antigen in the plasma.

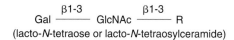

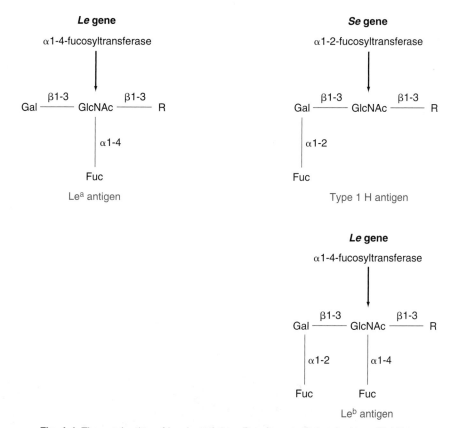

Fig. 4-1 The production of Lewis antigens. Fuc, fucose; Gal, galactose; GlcNAc, *N*-acetylglucosamine.

TABLE 4-3 Gene Interactions in the Presence of an *Le* Gene

Other Genes	Antigens in Secretions	Antigens in Plasma	Antigens on RBCs
sese, H, ABO	Le^a	Le^a	H, Le^a, A, and/or B
sese, hh, ABO	Le^a	Le^a	Le^a
Se, H, ABO	Le^a, Le^b, H, A, and/or B	↓Le^a, Le^b, H, A, and/or B	Le^b, H, A, and/or B*
Se, hh, ABO	Le^a, Le^b, H, A, and/or B	↓Le^a, Le^b, H, A, and/or B	Le^b

RBCs, Red blood cells.
*Some RBCs, particularly group O, may demonstrate some Le^a antigen.

fore, most red cells appear to lack the Le^a antigen and type as Le(a–b+). In the secretions, both Le^a and Le^b antigens are detected. This is shown in Table 4-3.

The Le(a–b–) Phenotype

As mentioned earlier, the Le(a–b–) phenotype arises from the inheritance of two *le* genes. The *le* gene is unable to produce α1-4-fucosyltransferase, and genetic studies have shown multiple mutational events to the *Le(FUT3)* gene that result in these nonfunctional alleles.[14-16] Two antibodies, anti-Le^c and anti-Le^d, have been previously described. Anti-Le^c reacted with Le(a–b–) red cells of nonsecretors (two *se* genes), and anti-Le^d reacted with Le(a–b–) red cells of secretors (at least one *Se* gene).

Anti-Le^c has been shown to be detecting lacto-*N*-tetraosylceramide, present in increased quantities on the red cells of Le(a–b–) nonsecretors, because there are neither *Se* nor *Le* genes to add fucose to this structure.[5] Anti-Le^d has been shown to be detecting type 1 H produced by the *Se* gene.[5] The lack of an *Le* gene gives rise to increased quantities of type 1 H, available to bind to the red cells of these individuals. Le^c and Le^d are not included as Lewis blood group system antigens, but are included in the Unnamed blood group collection.[17]

Lewis Antibodies
Anti-Le^a

When it was a more common practice to perform room temperature testing and samples included those of prenatal patients, anti-Le^a was a fairly common antibody. This antibody is found in the serum of Le(a–b–) secretors. Approximately 20% of Le(a–b–) secretors demonstrate this antibody.[3] The vast majority of these antibodies are IgM, but several well-documented cases of IgG anti-Le^a have also been reported. Although the majority of these antibodies are clinically insignificant, some examples of anti-Le^a, capable of activating large quantities of complement, have been considered clinically significant. In the presence of such antibodies, selection of antigen-negative units of blood is warranted. Anti-Le^a, although common in the serum of prenatal patients, is of little concern because these antibodies are IgM and newborn red cells are phenotypically Le(a–b–).

Anti-Le^b

Anti-Le^b is usually found as a less avid antibody in serum that also demonstrates anti-Le^a. Again, the antibody is seen in the serum of Le(a–b–) secretors. On occasion, anti-Le^b may be found alone. This would be expected to occur with Le(a–b–) nonsecretors and rarely with Le(a+b–) nonsecretors.[3] Most examples of anti-Le^b are IgM and poor activators of complement. Thus, for the most part, this antibody is clinically insignificant.

Two distinct forms of anti-Le^b occur. The more common form, anti-Le^{bH}, reacts preferentially with Le(b+) red cells that also demonstrate the greatest amount of H antigen. For example, anti-Le^{bH} made by a group A$_1$ individual may react strongly with group O red cells that are Le(b+) and have much H antigen, but fail to react with A$_1$Le(b+) red cells that have diminished H antigen expression.[3] The second type of anti-Le^b, called anti-Le^{bL}, reacts equally well with all Le(b+) red cells, regardless of the amount of H antigen they express.[3]

Anti-Le^{ab}

Previously called anti-Le^x, anti-Le^{ab} appears on initial testing to be anti-Le^a plus anti-Le^b, except when tested with cord red blood cells. As stated earlier, cord red cells appear to be Le(a−b−), regardless of the Lewis phenotype they will ultimately demonstrate. However, anti-Le^{ab} reacts with all cord cells that are genetically destined to be either Le(a+b−) or Le(a−b+), whereas a simple mixture of anti-Le^a plus anti-Le^b fails to react with such cord red cells. Anti-Le^{ab} appears to be directed to the disaccharide fucose in α1-4 linkage with *N*-acetylglucosamine common to both Le^a and Le^b antigenic structures (see Fig. 4-1).[17]

Other Unique Lewis Antibodies

Several unusual Lewis antibodies have been described. These are unusual because they appear to detect unique products produced when the α-fucosyltransferase of the *Le* gene uses nontraditional acceptor molecules. One such antibody has been described as anti-ALe^b or anti-A$_1$Le^b. As its name implies, this antibody reacts with A$_1$ red cells that are Le(b+). The antibody is directed to type 1 A antigen in the plasma that has also served as an acceptor molecule for fucose transferred by the *Le* gene, creating the unique structure shown in Fig. 4-2. A similar situation exists for another antibody, described as anti-BLe^b. Here again, type 1 B antigen serves as an acceptor molecule for fucose, resulting in the structure also depicted in Fig. 4-2.

INTERACTION OF *ABO, H, SE,* AND *LE* LOCI: ANTIGENIC PRODUCTION ON THE RED CELL AND IN THE PLASMA AND SECRETIONS

Based on the findings presented in this chapter and the previous chapter, the inheritance and interactions of the *ABO, H, SE,* and *LE* genetic loci can be evaluated and the expected antigens of the red cells, plasma, and secretions identified.

Le, sese, H, and *ABO* Genes

In the secretions, type 1 lacto–*N*-tetraose serves as an acceptor for the α1-4-fucose produced by the *Le* gene, producing Le^a antigen. Because no *Se* gene exists to produce type 1 H, the antigens Le^b, A, and/or B cannot be produced.

In the plasma, lacto–*N*-tetraosylceramide serves as an acceptor for the α1-4-fucose produced by the *Le* gene, producing Le^a antigen. This antigen is then adsorbed onto the red cell membrane. Le^b antigen is not produced because there is no *Se* gene and therefore no type 1 H in the plasma. The Lewis phenotype of these cells is Le(a+b−).

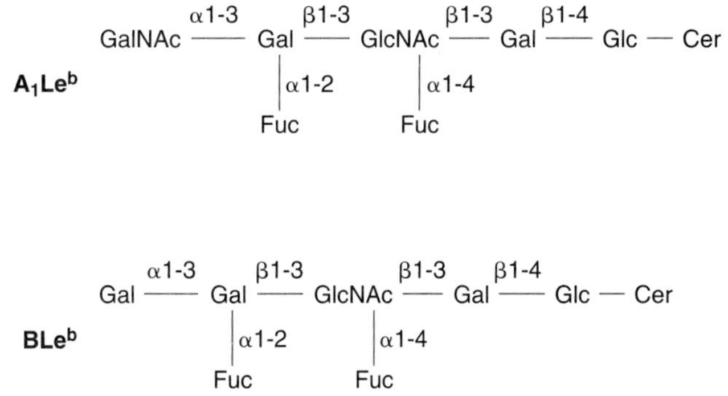

Fig. 4-2 A$_1$Le^b and BLe^b structures on the red cell. Cer, Ceramide; Gal, galactose; GalNAc, *N*-acetylgalactosamine; Glc, glucose.

As an integral part of the red cell membrane, lacto-*N*-neotetraosylceramide, or paragloboside, serves as the acceptor for the α1-2-fucose produced by the *H* gene, making H antigen. H antigen then serves as substrate for the *A* and/or *B* gene transferases to add α1-3-*N*-acetylgalactosamine and α1-3-galactose, respectively, to produce the A and/or B antigens. These genetic relationships are shown in Table 4-3.

Le, sese, hh, and *ABO* Genes

In the secretions, type 1 lacto-*N*-tetraose serves as an acceptor for α1-4-fucose produced by the *Le* gene, producing Le^a antigen. Again, because there is no *Se* gene and therefore no type 1 H antigen, the antigens Le^b, A, and/or B are absent from the secretions.

In the plasma, lacto-*N*-tetraosylceramide serves as an acceptor for α1-4-fucose from the transferase produced by the *Le* gene, producing Le^a antigen. This antigen is then adsorbed onto the red cell membrane. Le^b cannot be produced because of a lack of type 1 H. The Lewis phenotype of these cells is Le(a+b−).

In this particular genetic combination, lacto-*N*-neotetraosylceramide, or paragloboside, is produced as an integral part of the red cell membrane. However, because there is no *H* gene, H antigen is not produced. This lack of H antigen fails to provide an acceptor structure for the transferases produced by the *A* and/or *B* genes, giving rise to the Bombay phenotype in a nonsecretor. These genetic relationships are summarized in Table 4-3.

Le, Se, H, and *ABO* Genes

Because an *Se* gene is present, type 1 H is produced in the secretions, allowing the subsequent production of Le^b, A, and/or B antigens. The *H* gene also produces some type 2 H antigen in the secretions, producing additional A and/or B antigens. Le^a antigen is also produced in the secretions but is present in small quantities.

In the plasma, type 1 H is produced by the *Se* gene, allowing production of Le^b antigen. The *Le* gene is also able to produce Le^a antigen in the plasma, although not in the same quantity as Le^b. Because more Le^b is produced, this is the antigen adsorbed onto the red cell membrane in greatest quantities and is therefore the most readily detectable antigen. The Lewis phenotype of the red cells is Le(a−b+). A and/or B antigen is also produced in the plasma.

As an integral part of the red cell, H antigen is made as the *H* gene adds α1-2-fucose to lacto-*N*-neotetraosylceramide (paragloboside). This then enables the production of A and/or B antigens as described earlier. This is shown in Table 4-3.

Le, Se, hh, and *ABO* Genes

Because an *Se* gene is present, type 1 H is produced in the secretions, allowing the subsequent production of Le^b, A, and/or B-soluble antigens. Le^a antigen is also produced in the secretions.

In the plasma, type 1 H is produced because of the *Se* gene, and therefore Le^b antigen is produced. Le^a antigen is also present in the plasma, as are small quantities of A and/or B antigens. The Lewis phenotype of these red cells is Le(a−b+).

On the red cell membrane, H antigen is not produced because two *h* genes have been inherited. This also precludes the production of A and/or B antigens, giving rise to the Bombay phenotype in a secretor (Table 4-3).

lele, sese, H, and *ABO* Genes

In the secretions, only lacto-*N*-tetraose is present, as neither an *Se* nor an *Le* gene is present. In the plasma, only lacto-*N*-tetraosylceramide is present. This (also described as Le^c) is adsorbed onto the red cells, but the cells are Le(a−b−).

At the red cell membrane level, H antigen is produced. If *A* and/or *B* genes are inherited, the corresponding antigens will also be expressed. This is summarized in Table 4-4.

Iele, sese, hh, and *ABO* Genes

In this rare combination of genes, the phenotypes are as described previously, except at the red cell level, no H, A, or B antigens are produced. This is summarized in Table 4-4.

Iele, Se, H, and *ABO* Genes

In the secretions, type 1 H is produced because of the presence of an *Se* gene. Type 2 H is also produced by the *H* gene in the secretions, allowing further production of A and/or B antigens, if those genes are present.

In the plasma, the *Se* gene makes type 1 H, which is adsorbed onto cells that phenotypically are Le(a−b−) but demonstrate increased quantities of type 1 H (Le^d).

At the red cell level, H antigen is produced. If A and/or B genes are inherited, the corresponding antigens will also be expressed. This is summarized in Table 4-4.

Iele, Se, hh, and *ABO* Genes

In the event of this rare genetic combination, the secretions demonstrate type 1 H because of the *Se* gene. A and/or B (or both) type 1 antigens are also present if the genes are present.

In the plasma, type 1 H is present and adsorbed onto the surface of red cells. The red cells lack H, A, and B antigens because of the inheritance of two *h* genes. This is summarized in Table 4-4.

THE I BLOOD GROUP SYSTEM

The I blood group system was first described in 1956 by Wiener and colleagues.[18] At that time, they were testing the autoantibody from an individual with cold agglutinin syndrome with the red cells of normal blood donors. Through this testing process, 5 of 22,000 individuals were identified as being I-negative. In 1960, Marsh and Jenkins[19] described an antibody called anti-i. This antibody appeared to define what was present on the red cells of I-negative individuals, although some variation occurred in the amounts of both I and i antigens on the red cells of adults.

Another interesting finding was that cord red blood cells appeared to express more i than I antigen. However, there was a gradual change in the amounts of antigens detected over the first 18 months of life. During that time period, i antigen was gradually replaced with I antigen. At 18 months of age, infant red cells appeared to be equivalent to adult cells relative to the amounts of I and i antigens.

I Blood Group System Antigen and Ii Blood Group Collection
Genetics and Biochemistry

The I antigen was placed in a blood group system in 2002.[4] The gene responsible for the production of I resides on chromosome 6 (6p24). The product of the *I* gene is a β1-6-*N*-acetylglucosaminyltransferase. Mutations to the *I* gene have been identified and give rise to varying types of I-negative phenotypes.[20,21] The muta-

	Antigens in Secretions	Antigens in Plasma	Antigens on RBCs
TABLE 4-4 Gene Interactions in the Presence of Two *Ie* Genes			
Other Genes			
se, H, ABO	None (Le^c)	None (Le^c)	H, A, and/or B (Le^c)
sese, hh, ABO	None (Le^c)	None (Le^c)	None (Le^c)
Se, H, ABO	H, A, and/or B (Le^d)	H, A, and/or B (Le^d)	H, A, and/or B (Le^c)
Se, hh, ABO	H, A, and/or B (Le^d)	H, A, and/or B (Le^d)	None (Le^d)

tions identified result in gene products unable to produce the transferase enzyme. The I transferase adds GlcNac to i-linear structures.

In the previous chapter, linear and branched oligosaccharide structures for the H, A, and B antigens were discussed. In general, more linear structures are present on the red cells of newborns and infants, with a gradual change to branched structures that are maintained throughout adult life. As shown in Fig. 4-3, a similar situation is noted for both the i and I antigens. The i specificity is determined by a linear structure with repeating N-acetyllactosamine [Gal(β1-4)GlcNAc (β1-3)] units. The development of I depends on the addition of a branching N-acetyllactosamine unit. Consequently, it is not unexpected that newborn red cells are rich in i antigenic activity. The i antigen remain in the Ii blood group collection because its genetic basis remains undetermined. As mentioned, it resides on unbranched carbohydrate chains of repeating N-acetyllactosamine units.

I Blood Group Phenotypes

Several different phenotypes, describing the I/i antigenic composition of the red cells, have been defined and are summarized in Table 4-5.[22] The most common phenotype is I_{adult}. Rare individuals who genetically lack I are referred to as i_{adult} and typically demonstrate an apparent alloanti-I in their serum. With the advent of molecular methods to determine the basis for the genetic mutations that give rise to the I-negative phenotype, these distinctions as presented are perhaps oversimplified.[20,21] The i_{cord} phenotype is included for comparison.

I System Antibodies
Anti-I

Anti-I is a fairly common autoantibody if tests are performed at 4° C. On occasion, this IgM autoantibody may be identified if room temperature testing is performed. This antibody reacts with all (or nearly all) adult red cells but fails to react with cord red cells. Some examples of anti-I can be inhibited with saliva, human milk, or **hydatid cyst fluid.**

Although usually clinically insignificant, anti-I can be the causative autoantibody of **cold agglutinin syndrome.**[23] This may be seen in primary disease and in secondary cold agglutinin syndrome following *Mycoplasma pneumoniae* infection. For additional information on the differentiation of these autoantibodies in health and disease, see Petz and Garratty[23] and Chapter 18 of this text. As stated earlier, anti-I may also appear as an alloantibody in the serum of rare i_{adult} individuals.

Anti-i

Anti-i reacts preferentially with cord cells or i_{adult} cells. Potent examples may react to varying degrees with I_{adult} red cells. This harmless autoantibody may be found

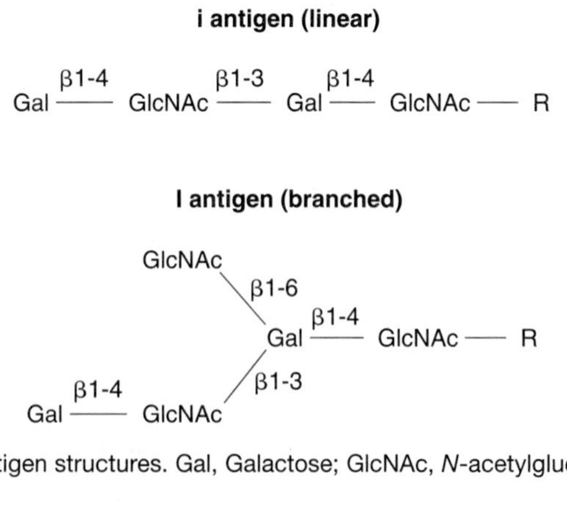

Hydatid cyst fluid: Fluid from a cyst formed from the larval form of the dog tapeworm.

Cold agglutinin syndrome: A condition resulting from the agglutination of red blood cells by a cold-reacting autoantibody. A disease associated with hemolytic anemia and/or obstruction of the microcirculation (or both).

i antigen (linear)

$$Gal \overset{\beta1\text{-}4}{\rule{1cm}{0.4pt}} GlcNAc \overset{\beta1\text{-}3}{\rule{1cm}{0.4pt}} Gal \overset{\beta1\text{-}4}{\rule{1cm}{0.4pt}} GlcNAc \rule{0.5cm}{0.4pt} R$$

I antigen (branched)

Fig. 4-3 I and i antigen structures. Gal, Galactose; GlcNAc, N-acetylglucosamine; Glc, glucose.

TABLE 4-5 Ii Phenotypes

Phenotype	I Antigen	i Antigen
I_{adult}	Strong	Weak
i_{cord}	Weak	Strong
i_{adult}	Weaker	Stronger

in the serum of individuals with **reticulosis,** myeloid leukemia, or alcoholic **cirrhosis.**[22] As with anti-I, this IgM antibody is best detected at 4° C but may be detected at room temperature.

Anti-i has been reported as the causative autoantibody of secondary cold agglutinin syndrome following infectious mononucleosis. Although not common, well-documented examples of anti-I and concomitant anti-i have been observed in patients with cold agglutinin syndrome.[23]

Anti-I^T

This IgM autoantibody reacts most strongly with cord red cells, less strongly with I_{adult} cells, and most weakly with i_{adult} red cells. IgG anti-I^T has been responsible for warm autoimmune hemolytic anemia secondary to Hodgkin's disease.[23]

Complex Antibodies Related to I and Other Blood Groups
Anti-IH

Anti-IH is found primarily as a harmless autoantibody in the serum of A_1 and B individuals but has been reported as the causative autoantibody in cold agglutinin syndrome (see Chapter 18 and reference 23). Anti-IH has been reported as the causative antibody in a hemolytic transfusion reaction.[24] Anti-IH most likely detects oligosaccharides that have acquired both the N-acetylglucosamine from the transferase product of the *I* gene and fucose from the transferase product of the *H* gene. The antibody reacts with cells that have increased quantities of both I and H. Therefore, this antibody, if made by a group A_1 individual, reacts most strongly with O and A_2 cells (strong H and I+) and least strongly with A_1 red cells (weaker H and I+). The reactions of this antibody and anti-I, anti-i, and anti-I^T are summarized in Table 4-6.

Anti-IA_1 and Anti-IB

These antibodies define additional oligosaccharides that express both the I antigen and the A or B antigen. Such antibodies fail to react with i_{adult} or cord cells that also express the A or B antigen.

Anti-IP_1

This antibody detects unique oligosaccharides that express the P_1 antigen and the I antigen. This antibody fails to react with cells that do not express both antigens.

Reticulosis: A series of disorders characterized by an increase in cells derived from the reticuloendothelial (RE) system.

Cirrhosis: Liver disease characterized by loss of normal cellular structure and fibrosis.

TABLE 4-6 Reactivity of Common I System Antibodies

Antibody Specificity	O Adult	A_2 Adult	A_1 Adult	B Adult	O Cord	O i_{adult}
Anti-I	++++	++++	++++	++++	$0/+^w$	$0/+^w$
Anti-i	$0/+^w$	$0/+^w$	$0/+^w$	$0/+^w$	++++	++++
Anti-IH	++++	+++	$0/+^w$	$0/+$	$0/+^w$	$0/+^w$
Anti-I^T	+++	+++	+++	+++	++++	+

Anti-ILe^bH

This unique antibody detects a structure that expresses the I antigen, Le^b antigen, and large quantities of H antigen.

THE P AND GLOBOSIDE BLOOD GROUP SYSTEMS AND THE GLOBOSIDE BLOOD GROUP COLLECTION

The P blood group system was discovered in 1927 when Landsteiner and Levine deliberately immunized rabbits with human red blood cells.[25] Following these immunizations, an antibody was described and named anti-P and the antigen defined by this antibody, P. In 1951, the null phenotype of the P system, or the p phenotype, was described.[26] In association with this phenotype, anti-P was described. This resulted in Landsteiner and Levine's rabbit antibody being renamed anti-P$_1$ and the antigen it defined, P$_1$. The P$_1$ antigen is the only antigen belonging to the P blood group system. An additional phenotype, P^k, was later described. The P antigen was removed from the GLOB collection in 2002 and moved to its own blood group system.[4] The antigens P^k and LKE remain in the GLOB collection.

Genetics and Biochemistry

Three different genetic loci are associated with the P and Globoside blood group systems and the Globoside blood group collection. The antigens produced by these genes are glycosphingolipid structures or oligosaccharide sequences linked to sphingolipids (ceramide) on the cell membrane. These interactions are shown in Fig. 4-4.

The gene responsible for the production of the P$_1$ antigen resides on chromosome 22 (22q11.2). The precursor for the P$_1$ antigen is paragloboside (lacto-*N*-neotetraosylceramide). The *P1* gene produces an α-galactosyltransferase that adds galactose to paragloboside, producing the P$_1$ antigen.

The *GLOB* gene, responsible for the production of P antigen, resides on chromosome 3 (3q25). The enzyme produced by the *GLOB* gene is 3-β-*N*-acetyl-galactosaminyltransferase. In fact, this transferase converts P^k antigen to the P antigen. The P^k phenotype arises because of mutations in the *GLOB* gene where changes in exons result in stop codons or frameshifts, failure to produce the transferase enzyme, and, subsequently, failure to produce the P antigen.[27]

The gene responsible for the production of the P^k antigen is found on chromosome 22 (22q13.2). This gene produces a 4-α-galactosyltransferase and converts lactosylceramide to the P^k antigen. Mutations in this *P^k* gene result in a nonfunctional galactosyltransferase and red cells with the p or null phenotype.[28] The LKE antigen appears to be dependent on the expression of terminal *N*-neuraminic acid

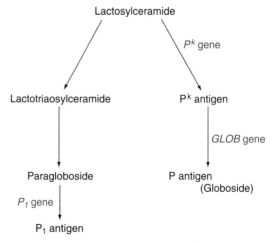

Fig. 4-4 Points of interaction for the three genetic loci of the P and Globoside blood group systems and Globoside blood group collection.

CHAPTER FOUR **Secretor and Soluble ABH Antigens**

and the expression of LKE and P^k are inversely related.[29] The P^k and LKE antigens continue to be part of the Globoside blood group collection.

P and GLOB System/Collection Phenotypes

The P blood group system and the Globoside blood group system/collection consist of three antigens that give rise to five phenotypes. The three antigens are P_1, P, and P^k. The five phenotypes are P_1, P_2, p, P_1^k, and P_2^k. These phenotypes, their relative frequencies, and the antigens associated with each phenotype are summarized in Table 4-7. The antibody or antibodies associated with each phenotype are also summarized in Table 4-7.

The P_1 Phenotype

Most individuals are of the P_1 phenotype. Red cells possess the P_1 and P antigens. P and Globoside system antibodies are not expected in the serum of P_1 individuals.

The P_2 Phenotype

Individuals who lack the P_1 antigen but express the P antigen on their red blood cells are of the P_2 phenotype. If antibody detection studies are performed at room temperature or lower, anti-P_1 is usually detectable in the serum as a naturally occurring antibody.

The p Phenotype

This phenotype represents the null phenotype of the P and GLOB blood group systems. These cells lack the P_1, P, and P^k antigens. p individuals have anti-P, anti-P_1, and anti-P^k in their serum as naturally occurring antibodies. The p phenotype is rare. Initially, the p phenotype was described as Tj(a−).[26]

The P_1^k Phenotype

The red cells of these individuals express the P_1 and P^k antigens. The high-incidence antigen, P, is missing and anti-P is present in the serum. The P_1^k phenotype is rare.

The P_2^k Phenotype

The red cells of these individuals express only the P^k antigen. The P_1 and P antigens are missing and anti-P and anti-P_1 are present in the serum. This phenotype is also rare.

P System Antibodies
Anti-P_1

Anti-P_1 is frequently found in the serum of P_2 individuals. For the most part, this antibody is clinically insignificant, although it has been reported to cause in vivo red cell destruction. This antibody may react to varying degrees with P_1 red cells, as the amount of P_1 antigen on the red cell is known to vary from person to person. This variable amount of antigen may make antibody identification a challenge if the anti-P_1 is not particularly potent. Testing at lower temperatures may aid in

TABLE 4-7 P and Globoside Blood Group Systems and Globoside Blood Group Collection

Phenotype	Frequency	Antigen(s)	Antibody
P_1	75%	P_1, P	None
P_2	25%	P	Anti-P_1
p	<1%	None	Anti-P + P_1 + P^k
P_1^k	<1%	P_1, P^k	Anti-P
P_2^k	<1%	P^k	Anti-P, anti-P_1

identification of such examples of anti-P_1. Hydatid cyst fluid and turtledove egg ovomucoid can inhibit anti-P_1.[3,22]

Anti-P

Anti-P is found in the serum of P^k individuals and as one of the antibodies produced by p individuals. Anti-P is clinically significant, and individuals with this antibody must be transfused with red cells lacking the P antigen. The presence of anti-P has been associated with spontaneous abortions in both p and P^k females.[3,22,30] This antibody is not inhibited with hydatid cyst fluid or turtledove egg ovomucoid. Autoanti-P (Donath-Landsteiner antibody) has been responsible for paroxysmal cold hemoglobinuria.[23]

Anti-P^k

Anti-P^k is one of the antibodies produced by p individuals and is considered clinically significant. Anti-P^k is inhibited by both hydatid cyst fluid and turtledove egg ovomucoid.[22]

Anti-P + P₁ + P^k

Anti-P + P_1 + P^k is the complex immune response in p individuals. These antibodies were originally thought to represent a single specificity that was described as anti-Tj^a. This antibody, albeit rare, is a potent hemolytic IgM antibody capable of causing hemolytic transfusion reactions and has been occasionally associated with hemolytic disease of the newborn. It has also been associated with early spontaneous abortions in p-negative women.[31]

CHAPTER SUMMARY

1. The alleles at the *SE* locus include a dominant allele, *Se(FUT2),* and a recessive allele, *se*. The presence of at least one *Se(FUT2)* gene permits the expression of soluble ABH antigens in the secretions. The inheritance of two *se* genes negates the presence of soluble ABH antigens in the secretions. The *Se(FUT2)* gene produces an α1-2-fucosyltransferase enzyme and type I H antigen in the secretions.

2. The alleles at the *LE* locus include a dominant allele, *Le(FUT3),* and a recessive allele, *le*. The transferase produced by the *Le(FUT3)* gene is an α1-4-fucosyltransferase.

3. Inheritance of at least one *Le(FUT3)* gene produces the Le(a+b–) or Le(a–b+) red cell phenotype. In nonsecretors (two *se* genes), only Le^a antigen is produced; consequently, red cells are Le(a+b–). In the presence of an *Se(FUT2)* and an *Le(FUT3)* gene, Le^b antigen is primarily produced and the red cell phenotype is Le(a–b+). The inheritance of two *le* genes results in the Le(a–b–) phenotype.

4. Anti-Le^a and anti-Le^b are generally considered clinically insignificant with the exception of those examples of anti-Le^a that bind complement.

5. The i antigen is enhanced on cord red blood cells and in rare individuals categorized as i_{adult}. Most individuals demonstrate normal quantities of I antigen after approximately 18 months of age.

6. Anti-I, anti-IH, and anti-i typically manifest as harmless autoantibodies. However, each specificity has been associated with cold agglutinin syndrome. Anti-I^T has been associated with warm autoimmune hemolytic anemia.

7. The P and Globoside blood group systems consist of three antigens: P_1, P, and P^k. These three antigens and their respective antibodies define five phenotypes: P_1, P_2, p, P_1^k, and P_2^k.

8. Anti-P_1 is found in the serum of many P_2 individuals and is considered clinically insignificant. p individuals produce anti-P + P_1 + P^k and this antibody is considered clinically significant. Likewise, anti-P, produced by P_1^k or P_2^k individuals, is considered clinically significant.

REFERENCES

1. Watkins WM, Morgan WTJ: Possible genetical pathway for the biosynthesis of blood group mucopolysaccharides. Vox Sang 4:97-119, 1959.
2. Sneath JS, Sneath PHA: Transformation of the Lewis groups of human red cells. Nature 176:172, 1955.
3. Mollison PL, Engelfriet CP, Contreras M: Blood Transfusion in Clinical Medicine, 10th ed. Oxford, Blackwell Scientific, 1997.
4. Daniels GL, Cartron JP, Fletcher A, et al: International Society of Blood Transfusion Committee on terminology for red cell surface antigens: Vancouver Report. Vox Sang 84:244-247, 2003.

5. Oriol R: Genetic control of the fucosylation of ABH precursor chains. Evidence for new epistatic interactions in different cells and tissues. J Immunogenet 17:235-245, 1990.

6. Yu LC, Broadberry RE, Yang YH et al: Heterogeneity of the human secretor (1,2) fucosyltransferase gene among Lewis (a+b+) non-secretors. Biochem Biophys Res Commun 222:390-394, 1996.

7. Liu Y, Koda Y, Soejima M, et al: Extensive polymorphism of the *FUT2* gene in an African (Xhosa) population of South Africa. Hum Genet 103:204-210, 1998.

8. Koda Y, Soejima M, Liu Y et al: Molecular basis for secretor type (1,2)-fucosyltransferase gene deficiency in a Japanese population: A fusion gene generated by unequal crossover responsible for the enzyme deficiency. Am J Hum Genet 59:343-350, 1996.

9. Spitalnik PF, Spitalnik SL: Human carbohydrate blood group systems. In Simon TL, Dzik WH, Snyder EL, et al (eds): Rossi's Principles of Transfusion Medicine, 3rd ed. Philadelphia, Lippincott Williams and Wilkins, 2002.

10. Koda Y, Soejima M, Johnson PH, et al: Missense mutation of *FUT1* and deletion of *FUT2* are responsible for Indian Bombay phenotype of ABO blood group system. Biochem Biophys Res Commun 238:21-25, 1997.

11. Kelly RJ, Rouquier S, Giorgi D et al: Sequence and expression of a candidate for the human secretor blood group (1,2)fucosyltransferase gene *(FUT2)*. J Biol Chem 270:4640-4649, 1995.

12. Oriol R, Danilovs J, Hawkins BR: A new genetic model proposing that the *Se* gene is a structural gene closely linked to the *H* gene. Am J Hum Genet 33:421-431, 1981.

13. Reguigne-Arnould I, Faure S, Chery M, et al: Physical mapping of 49 microsatellite markers on chromosome 19 and correlation with the genetic linkage map. Genomics 32:458-461, 1996.

14. Mollicone R, Reguigne I, Kelly RJ, et al: Molecular basis for Lewis (1,3/1,4)-fucosyltransferase gene deficiency *(FUT3)* found in Lewis-negative Indonesian pedigrees. J Biol Chem 269:20987-20994, 1994.

15. Koda Y, Kimura H, Mekada E: Analysis of Lewis fucosyltransferase genes from the human gastric mucosa of Lewis-positive and -negative individuals. Blood 82:2915-2919, 1993.

16. Elmgren A, Mollicone R, Costache M, et al: Significance of individual point mutations, T202C and C314T, in human *Lewis(FUT3)* gene for expression of Lewis antigens by the human 1,3/1,4-fucosyltransferase, FUC-TIII. J Biol Chem 269:21994-21998, 1997.

17. Reid ME, Lomas-Francis C: The Blood Group Antigen FactsBook, 2nd ed. London, Academic Press, Elsevier, 2004.

18. Wiener AS, Unger LJ, Cohen L, Feldman J: Type-specific cold autoantibodies as a cause of acquired hemolytic anemia and hemolytic transfusion reactions: Biologic test with bovine red cells. Ann Intern Med 44:221-240, 1956.

19. Marsh WL, Jenkins WJ: Anti-i: A new cold antibody. Nature 188:753, 1960.

20. Yu LC, Twu YC, Chou ML, et al: The molecular genetics of the human *I* locus and molecular background explain the partical association of the adult i phenotype with congenital cataracts. Blood 101:2081-2088, 2003.

21. Inaba N, Hiruma T, Togayachi A et al: A novel I-branching β-1,6-*N*-acetylglucosaminyltransferase involved in human blood group I antigen expression. Blood 101:2870-2876, 2003.

22. Issitt PD, Anstee DJ: Applied Blood Group Serology, 4th ed. Durham, NC, Montgomery Scientific Publications, 1998.

23. Petz LD, Garratty G: Immune Hemolytic Anemias, 2nd ed. New York, Churchill-Livingstone, Elsevier, 2004.

24. Campbell SA, Shirey RS, King KE, Ness PM: An acute hemolytic transfusion reaction due to anti-IH in a patient with sickle cell disease. Transfusion 40:828-831, 2000.

25. Landsteiner K, Levine P: Further observations on individual differences of human blood. Proc Soc Exp Biol Med 24:941-942, 1927.

26. Levine P, Bobbitt OB, Waller RK, Kuhmichel A: Isoimmunization by a new blood factor in tumor cells. Proc Soc Exp Biol 77:403-405, 1951.

27. Hellberg A, Steffensen R, Yahalom V, et al: Additional molecular bases of the clinically important p blood group phenotype. Tranfusion 43:899-907, 2003.

28. Koda Y, Soejima M, Sato H, et al: Three-base deletion and one-base insertion of the (1,4)galactosyltransferase gene responsible for the p phenotype. Transfusion 42:48-51, 2002.

29. Kooling LL, Kelly K: Inverse expression of P^k and Luke blood group antigens on human RBCs. Transfusion 41:898-907, 2001.

30. Yoshida H, Ito K, Kusakari T, et al: Removal of maternal antibodies from a woman with repeated fetal loss due to P blood group incompatibility. Transfusion 34:702-705, 1994.

31. Brecher M (ed): AABB Technical Manual, 14th ed. Bethesda, MD, American Association of Blood Banks, 2002.

FURTHER READINGS

Blood Group Antigen Gene Mutation Database: www.bioc.aecom.yu.edu/bgmut/index.htm

Daniels G: Human Blood Groups, 2nd ed. Oxford, Blackwell Science, 2002.

Issitt PD, Anstee DJ: Applied Blood Group Serology, 4th ed. Durham, NC, Montgomery Scientific Publications, 1998.

Mollison PL, Engelfriet CP, Contreras M: Blood Transfusion in Clinical Medicine, 10th ed. Oxford, Blackwell Scientific Publications, 1997.

Reid ME, Lomas-Francis C: The Blood Group Antigen FactsBook, 2nd ed. London, Academic Press, Elsevier, 2004.

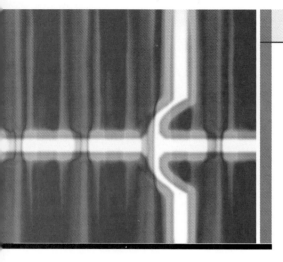

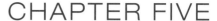

CHAPTER FIVE

The Rh Blood Group System

LW Blood Group System

Susan L. Wilkinson

LEARNING OBJECTIVES

After reading and studying this chapter, the student should be able to:

1. Describe the discovery of the antibody now known as anti-D.
2. List the five major antigens of the Rh system.
3. Indicate two reasons why the Rh system is second only to the ABO system relative to its clinical significance.
4. Compare and contrast the three systems of Rh nomenclature: Fisher-Race, Wiener, and Rosenfield.
5. Use Wiener and Fisher-Race terminology to describe Rh phenotypes.
6. Briefly describe the Rh genes, *RHD* and *RHCE,* and the inheritance of Rh antigens.
7. Briefly describe the role of *RHAG*.
8. Given the serologic results of Rh antigen typing (phenotyping), determine the possible Rh genotypes.
9. Describe the biochemical characteristics of the Rh proteins.
10. Discuss the chemical and serologic characteristics of the Rh antibodies.
11. Select appropriate blood for transfusion to patients with Rh system antibodies.
12. Briefly describe the concepts of weak D and partial D and the reasons they are different.
13. Given the anti-D testing results (including weak D on D-negative blood) from donor blood, determine whether the unit should be labeled D-positive or D-negative.
14. Compare high-protein and low-protein Rh antisera.
15. Discuss five circumstances that could result in false-positive Rh typing results.
16. Discuss four circumstances that could result in false-negative Rh typing results.
17. Define the term compound antigen and list four such antigens in the Rh system.
18. Define the term low-incidence antigen and list five such antigens in the Rh system.
19. Define the term high-incidence antigen and list three such antigens in the Rh system.
20. Define the term deletion phenotype and list four deletion phenotypes in the Rh system.

21. Describe the two genetic circumstances that give rise to the Rh$_{null}$ phenotype.
22. Describe the clinical significance of the Rh$_{null}$ phenotype.
23. Discuss the inheritance of the LW antigens, including the phenotypic association between Rh and LW antigen expression.

The Rh blood group system is one of the most complex genetic **polymorphisms** in humans. The serologic complexities and phenotypic oddities associated with this system have led to three Rh terminologies, varied theories on the genetics of this blood group system, recent data on the biochemistry of the Rh proteins, and now a full understanding of the genes responsible for those proteins. In spite of these complexities, the Rh system is applied daily in the blood center or transfusion service as both donors and recipients are tested for the presence or absence of the Rh antigen D and categorized as either D-positive (approximately 85%) or D-negative (approximately 15%).

Polymorphism: The quality of having many different forms or states. In the science of genetics, this refers to many different phenotypes.

DISCOVERY OF Rh

In 1939, Levine and Stetson[1] postulated that the cause of a case of hemolytic disease of the newborn (HDN) was maternal antibody entering the fetal circulation, leading to fetal red blood cell destruction. The causative antibody in this case of hemolytic disease was not named. In 1941, Levine and co-workers[2] published more complete data on HDN. These authors reported that the antibody responsible for this disease had the same specificity as the anti-Rh that Landsteiner and Wiener[3] produced in rabbits or guinea pigs immunized with Rhesus monkey red cells, later shown to be anti-LW. Wiener and Peters[4] also identified anti-Rh in the serum of certain individuals shown to have transfusion reactions following the administration of ABO-identical blood. Although they identified it as anti-Rh in these earliest publications, these authors were indeed describing anti-D.

In addition to the D antigen, four other antigens were soon recognized and include C, E, c, and e. These five antigens, and the antibodies that define them, account for the majority of laboratory and clinical challenges associated with the Rh blood group system.

CLINICAL SIGNIFICANCE OF Rh

Relative to transfusion therapy and blood bank practice, the Rh system becomes the most important blood group after ABO. This importance is based on the immunogenicity of the D antigen, that is, the ability of the D antigen to stimulate the production of anti-D in D-negative individuals. Production of anti-D becomes important to future transfusion therapy and, in the case of women, consequences of hemolytic disease of the newborn.

Exposure of D-negative individuals to D-positive red cells by transfusion or pregnancy is very likely to evoke an immune response. Transfusion with approximately 250 mL of D-positive red cells elicits the production of anti-D in approximately 80% of random D-negative recipients.[5] Significantly smaller amounts of red cells (approximately 1 mL) are also likely to stimulate anti-D production in 50% of D-negative recipients. In emergency situations when D-negative blood components are unavailable, recipients may be evaluated before receiving D-positive blood. Careful consideration must be given to the patient's age, gender, expected length of transfusion therapy, history of alloimmunization, and potential utilization of Rh immune globulin (RhIG) to prevent alloimmunization, before D-positive red cell–containing products are administered. Before the advent of RhIG to prevent alloimmunization to the D antigen following pregnancy, fetal D-positive cells entering D-negative maternal circulation accounted for an overall alloimmunization rate of 21%.[5]

GENETICS AND BIOCHEMISTRY OF Rh
Genetics

The *RH* locus has been assigned to chromosome 1(1p34.3-p36.13).[6] The *RH* locus is linked to the *SC (Scianna)* blood group locus. Although also located on chromosome 1, the *FY (Duffy)* locus is syntenic to *RH*. There are two adjacent genes at the *RH* locus that are responsible for Rh protein, *RHD* and *RHCE*. D-positive individuals inherit both *RHD* and *RHCE* genes, whereas D-negative persons inherit only a single *RHCE* gene from each parent. The use of *RHCE* is used in a general sense throughout this chapter to signify the Rh gene that fails to produce the antigen D. Four common genes produce the various combinations of C, E, c, and e: *RHCE, RHCe, RHcE,* and *RHce*. In addition to the Rh genes, another gene, referred to as *RHAG* (Rh-associated glycoprotein), located on chromosome 6 (6p11-p21.1), interacts with Rh protein at the red cell membrane level.[7]

The Rh genes behave as autosomal codominant alleles. Before elucidating the structure for these genes, several theories of inheritance were proposed. Perhaps more important, some of these theories contained their own Rh terminology and much of this is still used today. These previous genetic theories and terminologies will be briefly reviewed.

Fisher-Race Theory of Inheritance and Terminology

By 1943, the British workers had four antisera that appeared to detect different antigens in the Rh system.[8] Sir Ronald Fisher noted that the reactions of two of the sera were **antithetical** and proposed that the antigens recognized by these two antibodies, and therefore genes, were allelic. He named these C and c. The remaining two sera were not detecting antigens controlled by allelic genes. Fisher named those genes D and E and postulated that they had allelic forms, d and e.

Fisher and Race[9] proposed that the production of these Rh antigens was controlled by three sets of alleles whose loci were so closely linked that crossing over between them rarely occurred. These three loci were described as *D* and *d, C* and *c,* and *E* and *e*. Although we now know d does not exist, it is sometimes used in Fisher-Race terminology to denote the absence of D. Table 5-1 depicts the Fisher-Race genes and antigens as originally postulated.

Wiener Theory of Inheritance and Terminology

Alexander Wiener and his colleagues[10,11] postulated that a single gene at the *RH* locus was responsible for the production of Rh antigens. Wiener's two original genes were designated *Rh* and *rh* to describe those genes that produced $Rh_o(D)$ and those that failed to produce $Rh_o(D)$, respectively. With the discovery of additional Rh antibodies, the gene designations were modified to include additional antigen production. With time, the "h" was deleted (Table 5-2).

Antithetical genes: Genes that can reside at the same genetic locus.

TABLE 5-1 Fisher-Race Genes and Antigens

Antibodies	GENES AND ANTIGENS							
	CDe	cDE	cde	cDe	cdE	Cde	CDE	CdE
Anti-C	+	−	−	−	−	+	+	+
Anti-D	+	+	−	+	−	−	+	−
Anti-E	−	+	−	−	+	−	+	+
Anti-c	−	+	+	+	+	−	−	−
Anti-e	+	−	+	+	−	+	−	−

TABLE 5-2 Weiner's Designation for the Eight Common Rh Gene Complexes

Gene	Agglutinogen	Blood Factors
r	rh	hr′, hr″
r'	rh′	rh′, hr″
r''	rh″	rh″, hr′
r^y	rh^y	rh′, rh″
R^0	Rh$_0$	Rh$_0$, hr′, hr″
R^1	Rh$_1$	Rh$_0$, rh′, hr″
R^2	Rh$_2$	Rh$_0$, rh″, hr′
R^z	Rh$_z$	Rh$_0$, rh′, rh″

Wiener's single-gene theory further stated that the Rh gene resulted in the production of a specified agglutinogen and each agglutinogen was composed of a number of blood factors or antigens. Wiener's concept for the eight common Rh genes and their products is shown in Table 5-2.

Although neither Fisher-Race nor Wiener was correct regarding the genetics of Rh, most workers in the field continue to use a combination of their terminologies when communicating about Rh antigens, antibodies, phenotypes, and most probable genotypes. Many favor the Fisher-Race terminology over the Rh-Hr terminology of Wiener when describing Rh antigens and antibodies, such as D and C or anti-D and anti-C. However, it is convenient to describe a red cell phenotype and most probable genotype as R_1R_1 and R^1R^1 instead of D+,C+,E−,c−,e+ or DCe/DCe. The actual Rh genes for this most probable genotype would be RHDRHCe/RHDRHCe.

Rosenfield Terminology

As the complexities of the Rh system continued to increase, it became apparent that a terminology devoid of genetic implications was needed. In 1962, Rosenfield and colleagues[12] proposed a numerical terminology, which can be used to describe antigens and antibodies (Rh1 and anti-Rh1) and Rh genes. The genotype rr or cde/cde can be written as the phenotype Rh:−1,−2,−3,4,5 or as the genotype $Rh^{-1,-2,-3,4,5}$.

This terminology can be used to assign new antigens to the Rh system without any genetic implications. A summary of the 48 Rh antigens is presented in Table 5-3. It should be noted that Rh13, Rh14, Rh15, Rh16, Rh24, Rh25, and Rh38 have been removed from the Rh system.[13]

Tippett Genetic Model: The Rh Genes (*RHD* and *RHCE*) and the *RHAG* Gene

In Tippett's model,[14] two closely linked structural loci, D and $CcEe$, are proposed as the basis for Rh antigen production. Dr. Tippett worked with Dr. Race and

TABLE 5-3 Numerical and Alphabetical Designations for the Rh Blood Group System

Numerical	Alphabetical	Numerical	Alphabetical
Rh1	D	Rh29	total Rh
Rh2	C	Rh30	Go^a
Rh3	E	Rh31	hr^B
Rh4	c	Rh32	R^N
Rh5	e	Rh33	R$_o$^{Har}
Rh6	*cis* ce	Rh34	Bastiaan
Rh7	*cis* Ce	Rh35	Rh35
Rh8	C^W	Rh36	Be^a
Rh9	C^X	Rh37	Evans
Rh10	V	Rh39	C-like
Rh11	E^W	Rh40	Tar
Rh12	G	Rh41	Ce-like
Rh17	Hr$_o$	Rh42	Ce^S
Rh18	Hr	Rh43	Crawford
Rh19	hr^s	Rh44	Nou
Rh20	VS	Rh45	Riv
Rh21	C^G	Rh46	Sec
Rh22	*cis* CE	Rh47	Dav
Rh23	D^W	Rh48	JAL
Rh26	c-like	Rh54	DAK
Rh27	*cis* cE	Rh55	LOCR
Rh28	hr^H		

therefore used Fisher-Race terminology. For the eight common Rh phenotypes, two alleles are found at the first locus, *D* and *non-D*. At the second or *CcEe* locus, four alleles are needed (*ce, Ce, cE,* and *CE*). It is now known that there is only a single allele responsible for the gene producing D, and Tippett's model has been modified accordingly.

Two nearly identical genes located on chromosome 1 are responsible for the production of the Rh antigens.[15] The first gene, designated *RHD,* determines the presence of the D antigen. In D-negative individuals, this gene has been deleted. The second gene, *RHCE,* is responsible for the production of C or c and E or e. *RHCE* is used generally throughout this chapter to designate the gene responsible for the production of C or c and E or e. The alternative genes at the second locus are in fact described as *RHCE, RHCe, RHcE,* and *RHce.* Whereas D-positive individuals inherit two Rh genes from at least one parent, D-negative individuals inherit only a single Rh gene from each parent. This is shown in Table 5-4.

As stated, these genes are nearly identical.[16-19] They both produce 417 amino acids, and the D-producing polypeptide possesses 32 to 35 amino acids that are unique and responsible for the immune response and production of anti-D in D-negative individuals (Fig. 5-1). The antigens C and c differ by four amino acids at positions 16, 60, 68, and 103. Of these differences, the amino acids at position 103, which is external to the red cell membrane, appear to be the most important. For the antigen C, serine will be found, and for c, the amino acid proline is noted. The differences between E and e antigens are noted at amino acid 226. For an Rh gene producing E, the amino acid proline is present, and for e, the amino acid alanine is found (Fig. 5-2).

Each Rh gene has 10 exons. Gene conversion between *RHD* and *RHCE* is responsible for the many antigens that exist within this blood group system. These will be briefly reviewed, and the reader is encouraged to consult several excellent

TABLE 5-4 Rh Genes and Eight Common Haplotypes

First Locus	Second Locus	Haplotype	Rh Antigens
RHD	*RHCe*	R_1	D, C, e
RHD	*RHcE*	R_2	D, E, c
RHD	*RHCE*	R_z	D, E, C
RHD	*RHce*	R_0	D, c, e
—	*RHCe*	r′	C, e
—	*RHcE*	r″	c, E
—	*RHCE*	r^y	C, E
—	*RHce*	r	c, e

sources that go into much detail about the genetic basis for many of the unique antigens, phenotypes, and genotypes of this system.[20-24]

In addition to the Rh genes, the product of another gene located on chromosome 6, *RHAG* (Rh-associated glycoprotein), is necessary for Rh antigen expression because the lack thereof is responsible for one type of Rh_{null} as described later.[25] It appears that the Rh proteins produced by *RHD* and/or *RHCE* form a membrane-associated complex with the product of the *RHAG* gene. Interestingly, the *RHAG* gene has some degree of homology with *RHD* and *RHCE*. The *RHAG* gene also has 10 exons, but produces 409 amino acids.

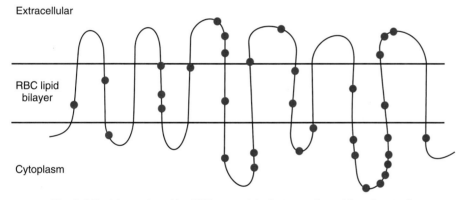

Fig. 5-1 Protein produced by *RHD* gene. ● indicates amino acids unique to D.

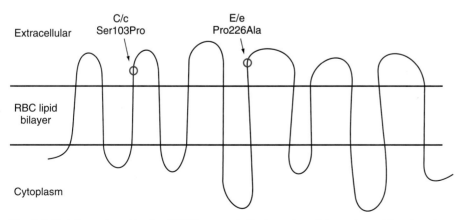

Fig. 5-2 Protein produced by the *RHCE* gene. o indicates extracellular amino acids unique to C, c, E, or e.

Glycosylated: Chemically linked with glycosyl (sugar) groups.

Biochemistry and Rh Functionality

The protein structures produced by *RHD* and *RHCE* are nonglycosylated and are linked to fatty acids (palmitate) in the lipid bilayer of the red blood cell. Each gene product spans the red cell membrane 12 times[26-28] (see Figs. 5-1 and 5-2). The protein structure produced by the *RHAG* gene is **glycosylated** and also spans the red cell membrane 12 times.[7] Based on this membrane-spanning complex formed between the products of these genes, the Rh proteins may serve a role as transporters of ammonium or other cations.[29,30]

Phenotype and Genotype

Using the five readily available Rh antisera (anti-D, anti-C, anti-c, anti-E, and anti-e), one is able to determine the Rh phenotype of the red cells being tested. Based on this phenotype and the gene frequencies for the population under study (Table 5-5), one is able to estimate the most probable Rh genotype. Family studies are the best way to establish the actual genotype, but Table 5-6 demonstrates the possible combinations for all phenotypes.

As an example, the phenotype D+,C+,E−,c−,e+ was noted following typings with Rh antisera. Based on gene frequencies, it is most likely that the genes this individual has inherited are R^1R^1 or *RHDRHCe/RHDRHCe*. However, it is possible, although less likely, that the genes inherited are R^1r' or *RHDRHCe/RHCe*. Although family studies would be necessary to determine without doubt the genes present, the most probable genotype remains R^1R^1 based on gene frequencies.

Rh ANTIBODIES

The majority of Rh antibodies are IgG and usually IgG1, IgG3, or a combination of these subclasses. However, examples of IgM Rh antibodies are documented. These IgM antibodies may be found simultaneously with IgG Rh antibodies and may reflect a rather broad immune response on the part of the antibody maker. Whereas these IgM antibodies are most often detectable in a **saline test system,** IgG Rh antibodies are most often detectable at the **antiglobulin phase** of testing. Detection of IgG Rh antibodies is often enhanced with **enzyme test methods.** It is interesting to note that although the majority of Rh antibodies are IgG1 and IgG3 (subclasses that readily activate complement), Rh antibodies rarely activate complement. Exceptional examples of Rh antibodies (anti-D and anti-C), referred to as Ripley or Ripley-like, have been described.[5,21]

The production of Rh antibodies is most often caused by transfusion or pregnancy, but well-documented cases of apparently naturally occurring Rh antibodies have also been reported. Some Rh antibodies react to a higher titer (exhibit

Saline test system: An in vitro test procedure that uses a normal (0.9% NaCl) saline medium. This system is often used to detect IgM antibodies.

Antiglobulin phase: The phase of in vitro testing that uses anti–human globulin reagent to detect in vivo or in vitro binding of IgG or complement to red cells.

Enzyme test methods: The use of proteolytic enzymes in in vitro test systems to facilitate antibody identification.

Haplotype	Rh Genes	Whites	Blacks	Native Americans	Asians
R_1	*RHD, RHCe*	0.42	0.17	0.44	0.70
r	*RHce*	0.37	0.26	0.11	0.03
R_2	*RHD, RHcE*	0.14	0.11	0.34	0.21
R_0	*RHD, RHce*	0.04	0.44	0.02	0.03
r′	*RHCe*	0.02	0.02	0.02	0.02
R″	*RHcE*	0.01	0.00	0.06	0.00
R_Z	*RHD, RHCE*	0.00	0.00	0.06	0.01
r^y	*RHCE*	0.00	0.00	0.00	0.00

TABLE 5-5 Frequencies of Common Rh Genotypes

TABLE 5-6 Rh Phenotypes and Genotypes

D	C	E	c	e	Rh Antigens	Most Likely Phenotype	Most Likely Genotype	Other Possible Phenotypes
+	+	+	+	+	C, c, D, E, e	R_1R_2	RHDRHCe/RHDRHcE	R_1r'', R_2r', R_zr, R_zR_0, R_0r^y
+	+	0	+	+	C, c, D, e	R_1r	RHDRHCe/RHce	R_1R_0, R_0r'
+	0	+	+	+	c, D, E, e	R_2r	RHDRHcE/RHce	R_2R_0, R_0r''
+	+	0	0	+	C, D, e	R_1R_1	RHDRHCe/RHDRHCe	R_1r'
+	0	+	+	0	c, D, E	R_2R_2	RHDRHcE/RHDRHcE	R_2r''
+	0	0	+	+	c, D, e	R_0r	RHDRHce/RHce	R_0R_0
0	0	0	+	+	c, e	r r	RHce/RHce	None
0	+	0	+	+	C, c, e	$r'r$	RHCe/RHce	None
0	0	+	+	+	c, E, e	$r''r$	RHcE/RHce	None
0	+	0	0	+	C, e	$r'r'$	RHCe/RHCe	None
0	0	+	+	0	c, E	$r''r''$	RHcE/RHcE	None
+	+	+	0	+	C, D, E, e	R_zR_1	RHDRHCE/RHDRHCe	R_1r^y, R_zr'
+	+	+	+	0	C, c, D, E	R_zR_2	RHDRHCE/RHDRHcE	R_2r^y, R_zr''
+	+	+	0	0	C, D, E	R_zR_z	RHDRHCE/RHDRHCE	R_zr^y
0	+	+	+	+	C, c, E, e	$r'r''$	RHCe/RHcE	$r''r$
0	+	+	0	0	C, E	r^yr^y	RHCE/RHCE	None
0	+	+	0	+	C, E, e	r^yr'	RHCE/RHCe	None
0	+	+	+	0	C, c, E	r^yr''	RHCE/RHcE	None

dosage) with red cells that carry a double dose of an Rh antigen compared with red cells that carry a single dose.

Rh antibodies are clinically significant and cause transfusion reactions and HDN. In pretransfusion testing, identification of Rh antibodies, or a previous record of Rh antibodies, necessitates transfusion with antigen-negative blood components. Although HDN due to anti-D is not frequently seen because of RhIG (see Chapter 16), examples are still encountered, as are cases of HDN due to Rh antibodies other than anti-D. Rh antibodies, because they are primarily IgG1 and IgG3, readily cross the placenta, and Rh antigens are well developed on fetal red cells.

THE D ANTIGEN, WEAK D, AND PARTIAL D

Because of its immunogenicity, the D antigen is the most clinically important antigen in the Rh blood group system. Donor and intended recipient red blood cells are routinely tested for the presence or absence of the D antigen. D-positive recipients receive D-positive blood components but may also receive D-negative blood components if inventory management necessitates such a practice. On the other hand, D-negative recipients are transfused only with D-negative blood components, except in extraordinary situations. Although D typings on the vast majority of blood samples are straightforward, some variant or weakened D typings can be encountered. These weakened typings usually manifest as D-negative on an immediate spin reading but as D-positive when an indirect antiglobulin test is completed. These variant typings are described as weak D and have previously been described as D^u. In addition, some D-positive individuals, referred to as partial D, lack part of the D antigen and can develop anti-D to those parts of the D antigen they lack. Of interest is that those missing components of the D antigen are actually "replaced" with portions of the protein produced by the *RHCE* gene.

Weak D

With the application of molecular techniques, the weak D phenotype is now more clearly understood.[31-33] This phenotype results from quantitative D epitope differences and not qualitative differences, as will be discussed for the partial D phenotypes. At least 22 different weak D phenotypes have been described, and these are designated type 1, type 2, type 3, and so forth, through type 21.[13] Type 4 is subdivided into type 4 and type 4.1. The molecular changes associated with weak D occur at the D epitopes that are found within the cytoplasm (intracellular) or those epitopes that are transmembrane, or within the lipid bilayer of the red cell (see Fig. 5-1). For example, in type 6 weak D, instead of finding the amino acid arginine at position 10, glutamine is found. Position 10 is one of the intracellular sites for a D epitope. Such a quantitative difference results in the weak D phenotype. Such quantitative differences explain why weak D individuals fail to make alloanti-D when transfused with D-positive red cells. But as donors, all apparent D-negative results at immediate spin must be tested with an indirect antiglobulin method because weak D phenotype red cells can cause the production of anti-D in transfusion recipients.[34,35]

Partial D

To explain the finding of alloanti-D in the serum of D-positive individuals, Wiener and Unger[36] proposed that the D antigen is a **mosaic,** consisting of genetically distinct pieces. Although the majority of D-positive individuals inherit *RHD* genes that produce all pieces of the D protein, some D-positive individuals inherit unique *RHD* genes that produce a D antigen that has most, but not all, epitopes or pieces of the D protein. Those D epitopes or pieces of protein that are missing are frequently replaced by corresponding portions of the *RHCE* gene, or represent unique single-point amino acid mutations.[25] It is of interest to note that these now unique amino acid sequences are responsible for the low-incidence antigens that are associated with several partial D categories.[22-25,37]

Partial D individuals are at risk, because of pregnancy or transfusion, to produce "anti-D" to the epitopes of the D antigen that they lack on their red cells. Tippett[38] described a nine-epitope model for the various partial D phenotypes, but the use of molecular analyses and monoclonal anti-D reagents has expanded this into a 30-epitope model.[39] Although beyond the scope of this textbook, the interested reader should consult several reviews for more information on this complex topic.[22-25]

Some partial D categories type as D-positive on immediate spin. However, others appear to be D-negative on immediate spin and demonstrate positive results at the antiglobulin phase of testing. Therefore, some partial D individuals appear to be of the weak D phenotype. With the increased usage of monoclonal anti-D reagents, many more partial D phenotypes are detected when tested at immediate spin. Some partial D individuals are not apparent until alloanti-D is detected in their serum. Classification requires the use of other partial D red cells, anti-D antisera produced by other partial D individuals, and highly characterized monoclonal anti-D reagents. Some partial D red cells carry unique low-incidence Rh antigens that include Goᵃ, Evans, Dᵂ, DAK, BARC, FPTT, and Rh32.

Significance of Weak D Testing

Weak D testing is required on all donor red cells that are nonreactive with anti-D in direct or immediate-spin testing.[34] Only donor red cells that are both D-negative on direct testing and demonstrate a negative test following weak D testing can be labeled D-negative. Donor red cells that test D-negative on immediate spin but positive following weak D testing must be labeled D-positive because such cells could elicit an immune response (production of anti-D) if

Mosaic: A complex antigen, such as D, that has more than a single antigenic determinant.

TABLE 5-7 Anti-D Typings and Interpretations

	IMMEDIATE SPIN		INDIRECT ANTIGLOBULIN PHASE		
	Anti-D	Rh Control*	Anti-D	Rh Control*	Interpretation
Blood donor	0	0	0	0	D-negative
	0	0	4+	0	D-positive
Blood recipient	0	0	0	0	D-negative
	0	0	4+	0	D-negative (usually)
Donor or recipient	0	0	4+	4+	Unable to interpret test

*Rh control may include anti-A or anti-B if using monoclonal (low-protein) reagents in addition to those marketed for high-protein Rh reagents. Some manufacturer's monoclonal reagents also have a unique Rh control reagent. When performing weak D testing (antiglobulin phase), a control must be included.

transfused to a D-negative recipient. The autocontrol, Rh control, or direct antiglobulin test (DAT) must also be shown to be nonreactive to validate the interpretation of the test.

The role for weak D testing in the recipient population is less clear. Many transfusing institutions have ceased to do weak D testing on recipient red cells. Rather, a negative D typing after immediate spin testing is sufficient to categorize the recipient as D-negative. But some institutions continue to do weak D testing on D-negative recipients. Although the majority of potential recipients will demonstrate a negative test following the completion of weak D testing, some individuals have a positive weak D test. However, both would generally receive D-negative blood components. Interpretations of D and weak D testing for donors and recipients are summarized in Table 5-7.

Rh REAGENTS

Although this section on Rh reagents refers primarily to anti-D typing reagents, reagent manufacturers typically also prepare Rh reagents to detect the presence or absence of the C, E, c, and e antigens. Although the use of these reagents is not routine, they may be utilized when evaluating the red cell phenotypes of both donors and patients.

Rh reagents can be thought of as those that are high-protein antisera and those that are low-protein antisera. **High-protein reagents** include "slide and rapid tube" reagents derived from human serum of immunized persons. Because of the protein added to make these antibodies react in an immediate spin test, these typings also require an Rh control test. **Low-protein reagents** include the now widely used reagents that are formulated with IgM monoclonal sources and in the case of anti-D, blended IgG monoclonal or polyclonal anti-D, or polyclonal anti-D derived from human serum, so these reagents may be used for weak D (previously described as D^u) testing. The low-protein monoclonal reagents do not require a separate Rh control test and generally rely on the ABO forward typing to control for any false-positive reactions. In the event that an individual types as group AB and D+, an Rh control is generally recommended. Based on the manufacturer's directions, this may include the use of an albumin control, or a prepackaged Rh control that contains the same chemical formulation as found in the monoclonal anti-D reagent, minus the antibody component. Each type of reagent, necessary controls, false-negative reactions, and false-positive reactions are discussed in the following sections. It must be emphasized that before using any Rh

High-protein reagents: Reagents that are enhanced by the addition of significant amounts of protein such as albumin. Such reagents are useful in the detection of IgG antibodies that may not agglutinate in saline media.

Low-protein reagents: Reagents that are not enhanced by the addition of protein. Monoclonal reagents are low-protein reagents.

reagent, the manufacturer's directions should always be consulted to determine precisely how the particular reagent should be used.

High-Protein Reagents

High-protein Rh reagents, designed for use with slide, tube, or **microplate techniques,** contain approximately 20% protein and other high molecular weight additives that enable the reagents to react rapidly at immediate spin. Because of the high protein and other additives, these reagents can cause spontaneous agglutination of certain red blood cells (particularly those with a positive direct antiglobulin test [DAT]) and give a false-positive result. Therefore, an **Rh control reagent,** consisting of everything the manufacturer has added to the Rh reagent except the Rh antibody, must be tested simultaneously before one can interpret the Rh typing result. Because additive and/or protein concentration may vary between manufacturers, the Rh control test reagent must be from the same manufacturer as the Rh antisera reagent in use. When a positive Rh test and positive Rh control test are noted, discrepancies may be resolved with the use of low-protein Rh reagents, as described in the following. Anti-C, anti-E, anti-c, and anti-e high-protein reagents are available. A negative Rh control test is also required for valid interpretation of results.

Weak D testing can be performed with high-protein anti-D using either tube or microplate methods. Again, the manufacturer's directions should be consulted for testing procedures. The Rh control test should be included and tested in a similar fashion as the weak D test, including an indirect antiglobulin phase of testing. In order to interpret the weak D test, the Rh control test must be nonreactive. In D-negative patients with a positive DAT, the weak D test cannot be determined accurately.

Low-Protein Reagents

The most recent Rh reagents to be introduced include those that are monoclonal in nature and derived from human/murine heterohybridoma sources. These monoclonal antibodies may be IgM or IgG and are suitable for slide, tube, and microplate testing. Anti-D reagents contain an IgM monoclonal antibody so that the presence or absence of the D antigen may be determined with an immediate spin test. These anti-D reagents will also include an IgG **monoclonal** or **polyclonal** component or a polyclonal anti-D derived from human serum that enables this reagent to be used for weak D testing using the indirect antiglobulin technique in tube and microplate testing. As mentioned earlier, because of the low protein content, a specific control reagent is generally not required. The manufacturer's directions may recommend the ABO forward typing as a control and, in the case of a group AB, D+ result, suggest an albumin control or manufacturer's Rh control reagent.

If using micro typing systems or gel cards to perform D testing, IgM monoclonal anti-D is contained within the gel suspension. This technology cannot be used for weak D testing. Anti-C, anti-E, anti-c, and anti-e monoclonal reagents are available. These are IgM monoclonal sources. Although many contain only a single-source clone, others may represent blends of several clones as a way to enhance reactivity.

It has been noted that some partial D red cells (particularly category VI) fail to react with the monoclonal reagents on immediate spin when other anti-D reagents (high protein) react on immediate spin. The monoclonal reagents will react with these cells in the weak D test. Such findings may cause an apparent Rh discrepancy with previous results. However, this should present no harm to an intended recipient and may actually prevent alloimmunization if the partial D individual is transfused only with D-negative red cells.

Microplate techniques: Serologic procedures that use micro well plates rather than test tubes.

Rh control reagent: The manufacturer's control that contains all of the components of the anti-D reagent except for the antibody. This reagent serves as a negative control for Rh typing.

Monoclonal/polyclonal reagents: Reagents produced in part by hybridization techniques.

Conversely, the partial D phenotype described as R_0^{Har} fails to react, or reacts only weakly, when tested with high-protein, slide, and rapid tube reagents. These partial D cells react strongly with certain IgM anti-D clones used in these low-protein reagents. Again, discrepant results may occur. In this situation, the R_0^{Har} recipient will receive D-positive red cells if transfusion therapy is needed. This may stimulate production of anti-D to the D epitopes lacking on the recipient's red cells.

False-Positive Rh Typing Results

False-positive Rh typing results can occur for several reasons, including positive DAT, rouleaux, reagent contamination, antibody to low-incidence antigen, and human error.

Positive Direct Antiglobulin Test

The most frequent cause of a false-positive Rh typing result, and probably the most frequent cause of Rh typing discrepancies in general, is spontaneous agglutination of red cells because those cells have a positive DAT. Although this is more frequently observed with high-protein reagents, some extraordinary red cells with considerable amounts of immunoglobulin on their surface may also support spontaneous agglutination in the presence of low-protein antisera. If using high-protein reagents and both the test and Rh control test are positive, retyping of the patient's red cells with low-protein reagents most often resolves any problems. On occasion, alteration of the patient's red cells with chemicals or a modified heat elution may be necessary to resolve Rh typing problems.[20]

Rouleaux

False-positive Rh typing results may also be caused by the presence of cold autoagglutinins or abnormal proteins in the patient's serum that produce **rouleaux**. The Rh control test and the Rh test are both positive. This is most likely seen with samples that are not washed in normal saline before testing. Resolution is often possible by washing the cells in saline and retesting the sample with the same Rh reagent and Rh control. Low-protein reagents may not demonstrate false-positive reactions with these types of specimens.

Rouleaux: Red cell rolls that have the appearance of a stack of coins.

Reagent Contamination

Reagent contamination may cause false-positive Rh typing results. Contamination of the dropper used in the reagent vial with other blood bank reagents may result in false-positive tests. Bacterial contamination of reagent vials may also cause false-positive test results. Development of good work habits and continued attention to detail should minimize these types of problems.

Antibody to Low-Incidence Antigen

The presence of an unidentified antibody defining a low-incidence antigen as a contaminant of a particular lot of reagent may cause a false-positive result. Here, the cells in question react with the antibody defining the low-incidence antigen. This type of reaction is unlikely to be detected unless previous results (D-negative) exist.

Human Error

Failure to follow the manufacturer's directions for appropriate use of reagents may result in a false-positive Rh type. Again, the manufacturer's directions must be followed.

Adding the wrong reagent to the test may also result in a false-positive reaction. Attention to testing procedures is of critical importance in the blood bank.

False-Negative Rh Typing Results

False-negative Rh typings can have several causes, most resulting from human error.

Human Error

A red blood cell suspension that is too heavy can result in a false-negative test result. Appropriate techniques and the manufacturer's directions should be followed when preparing cell suspensions for Rh typings.

Failure to add antisera, or the addition of the wrong antisera, can result in a false-negative reaction. Attention to testing procedures is of critical importance in the blood bank.

Failure to follow the manufacturer's directions can result in a false-negative result. Undercentrifugation or failure to incubate slide tests for the specified time can produce false-negative results.

Deterioration of the Rh reagent because of inappropriate storage can result in false-negative results. The manufacturer's directions must be followed.

Inappropriate technique may result in false-negative results. Vigorous shaking or suspending of test materials may result in false-negative findings.

OTHER Rh ANTIGENS

Compound Antigens

Compound antigens: Distinct antigens formed when two additional antigens are produced by the same gene.

Four Rh antigens, ce(f), Ce(rh$_i$), cE(Rh27), and CE(Rh22), are commonly described as **compound antigens.** This term is used to designate an antigen that arises when the two antigens are produced by the same gene. For example, the *r (RHce)* gene produces the ce(f) antigen because the gene codes for the production of both c and e antigens. Similarly, the *R$_1$ (RHDRHCe)* genotype produces the Ce(rh$_i$) antigen because the *RHCe* gene encodes for the production of both C and e. Defining the presence or absence of these compound antigens may be useful in determining the most probable genotype from a phenotype. For example, red cells that type as D+, C+, E+, c+, e+ are most likely of the R$_1$R$_2$ (CDe/cDE) and of the *RHDRHCe/RHDRHcE* genotype. However, if these cells also type as ce(f)+ and Ce(rh$_i$)−, the phenotype could be R$_Z$r (CDE/ce) or the *RHDRHCE/RHce* genotype.

Antigens of Low Incidence

Low-incidence antigens: Antigens that occur in less than 1% of the population.

Several Rh antigens of low incidence, or **low-incidence antigens,** that occur in 1% or less of the random population include C^w, C^x, Rh33, Rh32, and Go^a. The C^w and C^x antigens are antithetical to the high-incidence antigen MAR (Rh51) and are produced by *RHCe.* The molecular basis for C^w is arginine instead of glutamine at position 41. The molecular basis for C^x is threonine instead of alanine at position 36. Rh32 is a low-incidence antigen produced by the R^N gene and is antithetical to the high-incidence antigen Sec (Rh46). Rh32 is also expressed in the partial D phenotype DBT. Rh33 is produced by the partial D phenotype described as R$_0$^{Har}. Go^a is found on partial D category DIVa red cells. For more information on these antigens and other low-incidence Rh antigens, the reader is urged to consult Reid and Lomas-Francis[22] and Issitt and Anstee.[21]

Antigens of High Incidence

High-incidence antigens: Antigens that occur in greater than 99% of the population.

Rh antigens of very high incidence, or **high-incidence antigens,** have been described and include Hr, Hr$_0$, and Hr^B. These antigens are missing from Rh-deletion red cells (see the following) and some very unusual Rh phenotypes. Again, the reader is urged to consult Reid and Lomas-Francis[22] and Issitt and Anstee[21] for additional information on these and other high-incidence antigens of the Rh blood group system.

Other Antigens

Other Rh antigens include G, V, VS, hr^S, and hr^B. Rh genes that produce D or C also produce the Rh antigen G. The G antigen results when serine is found at position 103.[40] In cells that are G−, proline is found at amino acid 103. In routine antibody-identification studies, anti-G appears as anti-D + C. To determine if anti-G is present, adsorption and elution studies using r′ and R_0 cells are necessary. Rare cells that produce G but not D or C have been described. The antigens V(ce^S) and VS(e^S) are found more frequently in the black population and are associated with r, R_0, and r′^{S} haplotypes. The VS antigen arises because valine is found at amino acid 245 instead of leucine.[41] The antigens hr^S and hr^B are e-like antigens that are normally produced by all *RHCE* genes that produce e. Rare genes that produce e but not hr^S or hr^B have been described. For additional information on these and other rare Rh antigens and genes, consult Reid and Lomas-Francis[22] and Issitt and Anstee.[21]

UNUSUAL Rh GENOTYPES

D-Deletion Phenotypes

Several unusual Rh phenotypes exist which suggest that pieces of genetic material that represent the CE antigens have been deleted. These deleted phenotypes all have enhanced expression of the D antigen. Through molecular analysis, it is now known that in addition to an *RHD* gene, these individuals have inherited an *RHCE* gene that is largely replaced with material from another *RHD* gene.[23,25] These gene rearrangements represent the exact opposite of what has been described for partial D phenotypes where *RHD* is replaced with *RHCE*.

Several different types of **D-deletion** red cells have been described. These include D−− cells that fail to produce any antigens suggestive of *RHCE* and the similar D·· cells that likewise fail to produce any C/c or E/e antigens yet produce the low-incidence Rh antigen called Evans (Rh37). Several D-deletion genes produce some type of C/c antigen, and these include Dc− and DC^W−. Dc− red cells appear to be a heterogeneous group, because not all examples of this phenotype are identical. Of even greater interest is the deletion cell described as DIV(C)−. This phenotype gives rise to red cells that express not only the low-incidence antigen Go^a but also express the low-incidence antigens Rh33 and Riv(Rh45).

D-deletion phenotypes: Phenotypes that lack many Rh antigens and may result when some of the Rh genetic material is rearranged.

Rh$_{null}$ and Rh$_{mod}$ Phenotypes

The **Rh$_{null}$ phenotype** fails to demonstrate the presence of any Rh antigens and can arise through two distinct genetic events. The first type of Rh$_{null}$ occurs when the *RHAG* (Rh-associated glycoprotein) gene is absent or mutated.[25] This results in what is referred to as the more common, regulator type of Rh$_{null}$. The less frequent amorph type of Rh$_{null}$ arises from mutations to *RHCE* and deletion of *RHD*.[42] The amorph type has reduced amounts of RhAG.

In addition to the Rh$_{null}$ phenotype, a phenotype called **Rh$_{mod}$** (for modifier) has also been described. These individuals have markedly reduced amounts of Rh antigens. Genetic modifications to *RHAG* are responsible for this phenotype.

It is of interest to note that the regulator and amorph type of Rh$_{null}$ and Rh$_{mod}$ individuals experience a form of **hemolytic anemia,** suggesting that Rh antigens are necessary for normal red cell survival. This hemolytic anemia is described as Rh$_{null}$ syndrome, and **stomatocytes** are observed on peripheral blood smears from these individuals. Immunized Rh$_{null}$ individuals are at risk to produce some unusual Rh antibodies, particularly those directed to high-incidence antigens. If the immune response includes production of antibody to the Rh29 antigen (or **anti-Rh29**), transfusion therapy with other Rh$_{null}$ red cells would be required.

Rh$_{null}$ phenotype: An inherited characteristic in which none of the Rh antigens is expressed.

Rh$_{mod}$ phenotype: An inherited characteristic associated with a substantial decrease in Rh antigen expression.

Hemolytic anemia: Anemia associated with the destruction (hemolysis) of red blood cells.

Stomatocytes: Red cells with a slit-shaped rather than circular zone of central pallor.

Anti-Rh29: An antibody produced by Rh$_{null}$ patients that is frequently termed anti-"total Rh."

THE LW BLOOD GROUP SYSTEM

The LW blood group system was discovered in 1940 when Landsteiner and Wiener[3] did their classic studies immunizing rabbits and guinea pigs with Rhesus monkey red cells. The antibody produced by the rabbits or guinea pigs was called anti-Rh, although much later it became apparent that the animal anti-Rh was not identical to human anti-Rh (anti-D). Based on these findings, the animal antibody was later named anti-LW in honor of Landsteiner and Wiener.

Genetics and Phenotypic Association with Rh

The three genes assigned to the *LW* locus are *LW^a*, *LW^b*, and *LW*. The *LW^a* gene produces the LW^a antigen, an antigen of high incidence in the random population. The *LW^b* gene produces the LW^b antigen, an antigen of low incidence in the random population. The LW^a and LW^b antigens differ only by a single amino acid at position 70.[43] For LW^a, glutamine is present, and for LW^b, arginine is found. The *LW^a* and *LW^b* genes both produce the high–incidence antigen LW^ab. The *LW* gene appears to be an amorph, producing no detectable product. It has been shown that the molecular basis for the *LW* gene is caused by a deletion in exon 1 that results in a stop codon and failure to produce the LW glycoprotein.[44] The presence of two *LW* genes produces the rare LW(a–b–) phenotype. This phenotype can produce the very rare antibody, anti-LW^ab. The phenotypes associated with the possible genes at the *LW* locus are shown in Table 5-8. The *LW* locus has been assigned to chromosome 19(19p13.3).[44] The LW glycoprotein is an intercellular adhesion molecule (ICAM).[45]

Although inherited independently, a phenotypic association exists with the antigens produced by the LW genes and those antigens produced by the Rh genes. First, regardless of the LW genes an individual has inherited (*LW^a* or *LW^b*), if an individual inherits a D-producing *RHD* gene, that individual produces more LW^a and/or LW^b antigen than individuals who have inherited two non–D-producing genes (*RHCE*). Studies have shown that D-positive adults produce more LW antigen than D-negative adults.[46] Second, Rh_null red cells, whether of the amorph or regulator type, are LW(a–b–), even though it has been shown that such individuals have inherited normal LW genes. It would appear that Rh protein, and in particular that produced by the *RHD* gene, facilitates the expression of LW antigen on the red cell membrane. It is of interest to note that the LW(a–b–) phenotype has normal expression of Rh antigens.

Several other structures (see Chapter 6) on the red cell membrane that give rise to various blood group antigens also appear to interact with Rh protein. Rh_null cells (amorph or regulator) express decreased levels of glycophorin B, the structure responsible for the S, s, and U antigens. The Fy glycoprotein may also interact with Rh protein. The Fy5 antigen is absent from Rh_null cells although other Fy antigens are expressed normally.

TABLE 5-8 LW Blood Group System	
Genes	Phenotype
LW^a, *LW^a*	LW(a+b–)
LW^a, *LW^b*	LW(a+b+)
LW^b, *LW^b*	LW(a–b+)
LW, LW	LW(a–b–)

Clinical Significance of LW

LW(a−b+) or LW(a−b−) individuals are at risk to produce anti-LW^a or anti-LW^{ab}, respectively. These antibodies should be considered clinically significant. There have been reports of transient autoanti-LW^a produced by LW(a+) individuals. Some of these LW(a+) individuals have a transient loss of LW^a antigen and the autoanti-LW^a may appear to be alloantibody. Most of these antibodies have been clinically insignificant. For more detailed information on the LW blood group system, the reader is referred to Reid and Lomas-Francis.[22]

CHAPTER SUMMARY

1. Relative to transfusion therapy and blood bank practice, the Rh system is the most important blood group except for ABO. This importance is based on the immunogenicity of the D antigen and the likelihood of evoking the production of anti-D in D-negative individuals exposed to D-positive red cells.

2. The Fisher-Race, Wiener, and Rosenfield terminologies are all used to describe Rh antigens, antibodies, phenotypes, and genotypes.

3. D-positive individuals inherit two Rh genes, *RHD* and *RHCE* from at least one parent. D-negative individuals inherit only a single Rh gene, *RHCE*, from each parent.

4. The majority of Rh antibodies are IgG1 and/or IgG3 and fail to activate complement. These antibodies are clinically significant and can cause transfusion reactions and hemolytic disease of the newborn. These antibodies are most likely produced following transfusion or pregnancy.

5. In some individuals, the D antigen may demonstrate weakened expression. This weakened expression is due to either weak D or partial D. Partial D individuals are at risk to produce anti-D to the D epitopes they lack. D-negative blood donors must not demonstrate weakened expression of D.

6. Rh reagents may be classified as high-protein and low-protein reagents. High-protein reagents need an Rh control test to reliably interpret Rh typing results. The ABO forward grouping may be recommended by the manufacturer as a suitable control when using low-protein reagents.

7. Forty-eight antigens make up the Rh blood group system. Many of these antigens are of low incidence (less than 1% of the population), but many occur in more than 99% of the population.

8. Unusual phenotypes exist in the Rh blood group system and include D−− and Rh$_{null}$. D−− cells fail to express C/c or E/e antigens. Rh$_{null}$ red cells totally lack Rh antigens, and such individuals also have a compensated hemolytic anemia. Rh$_{null}$ cells are also LW(a−b−).

REFERENCES

1. Levine P, Stetson RE: An unusual case of intragroup agglutination. JAMA 113:126-127, 1939.
2. Levine P, Burnham L, Katzin EM, Vogel P: The role of isoimmunization in the pathogenesis of erythroblastosis fetalis. Am J Obstet Gynecol 42:925-937, 1941.
3. Landsteiner K, Wiener AS: Studies on an agglutinogen (Rh) in human blood reacting with anti-rhesus sera and with human isoantibodies. J Exp Med 74:309-320, 1941.
4. Wiener AS, Peters HR: Hemolytic reactions following transfusions of blood of the homologous group, with three cases in which the same agglutinogen was responsible. Ann Intern Med 13:2306-2322, 1940.
5. Mollison PL, Engelfriet CP, Contreras M: Blood Transfusion in Clinical Medicine, 10th ed. Oxford, Blackwell Scientific, 1997.
6. Cherif-Zahar B, Mattei MG, Le Van Kim C, et al: Localization of the human Rh blood group gene structure to chromosome 1p34.3-1p36.1 region by in situ hybridization. Hum Genet 86:398-400, 1991.
7. Ridgwell K, Spurr NK, Laguda B, et al: Isolation of cDNA clones for a 50Kda glycoprotein of the human erythrocyte membrane associated Rh (Rhesus) blood-group antigen expression. Biochem J 287:223-228, 1992.
8. Race RR, Sanger R: Fisher's contribution to Rh. Vox Sang 43:354-356, 1982.
9. Race RR: The Rh genotypes and Fisher's theory. Blood 3: 27-42, 1948.
10. Wiener AS, Landsteiner K: Heredity of variants of the Rh type. Proc Soc Exp Biol Med 53:167-170, 1943.

11. Wiener AS: Genetic theory of the Rh blood types. Proc Soc Exp Biol Med 54:316-319, 1943.

12. Rosenfield RE, Allen FH, Swisher SN, Kochwa S: A review of Rh serology and presentation of a new terminology. Transfusion 2:287-312, 1962.

13. Daniels, GL, Cartron JP, Fletcher A, et al: International Society of Blood Transfusion committee on terminology for red cell surface antigens: Vancouver report. Vox Sang 84:244-247, 2003.

14. Tippett P: A speculative model for the Rh blood groups. Ann Hum Genet 50:241-247, 1986.

15. Colin Y, Cherif-Zahar B, LeVan Kim C, et al: Genetic basis of the RhD-positive and RhD-negative blood group polymorphism as determined by Southern analysis. Blood 78:2747-2752, 1991.

16. Cherif-Zahar B, Bloy C, LeVan Kim C, et al: Molecular cloning and protein structure of a human blood group Rh polypeptide. Proc Natl Acad Sci 87:6243-6247, 1990.

17. Mouro I, Colin Y, Cherif-Azhar B, et al: Molecular genetic basis of the human Rhesus blood group system. Nat Genet 5:62-65, 1993.

18. Arce MA, Thompson ES, Wagner S, et al: Molecular cloning of RhD cDNA derived from a gene present in RhD-positive, but not RhD-negative individuals. Blood 82:651-655, 1993.

19. Simsek S, de Jong CAM, Cuijpers HTM, et al: Sequence analysis of cDNA derived from reticulocyte mRNAs coding for Rh polypeptides and demonstration of E/e and C/c polymorphism. Vox Sang 67:203-209, 1994.

20. Brecher M (ed): Technical Manual, 14th ed. Bethesda, MD, American Association of Blood Banks, 2002.

21. Issitt PD, Anstee DJ: Applied Blood Group Serology, 4th ed. Durham, NC, Montgomery Scientific Publications, 1998.

22. Reid ME, Lomas-Francis C: The Blood Group Antigen FactsBook, 2nd ed, London, Academic Press, Elsevier, 2004.

23. Avent ND, Reid ME: The Rh blood group system: A review. Blood 95:375-387, 2000.

24. Lomas-Francis C, Reid ME: The Rh blood group system: The first 60 years of discovery. Immunohematology 16:7-17, 2000.

25. Huang CH, Liu PZ, Chen JG: Molecular biology and genetics of the Rh blood group system. Semin Hematol 37:150-165, 2000.

26. Avent ND, Butcher SK, Liu W, et al: Localization of the C-termini of the Rh (rhesus) polypeptides to the cytoplasmic face of the human erythrocyte membrane. J Biol Chem 267:15134-15139, 1992.

27. Cherif-Zahar B, Le Van Kim C, Rouillac C, et al: Organization of the gene (RHCE) encoding the human blood group RhCcEe antigens and characterization of the promoter region. Genomics 19:68-74, 1994.

28. Agre P, Cartron JP: Molecular biology of the Rh antigens. Blood 78:551-563, 1991.

29. Marini AM, Urrestaurazu A, Beauwens R, et al: The Rh (rhesus) blood group polypeptides are related to NH_4^+ transporters. Trends Biochem Sci 22:460-461, 1997.

30. Liu Z, Peng J, Mo R, et al: Rh type B glycoprotein is a new member of the Rh superfamily and a putative ammonia transporter in mammals. J Biol Chem 276:1424-1433, 2001.

31. Wagner FF, Gassner C, Muller TH, et al: Molecular basis of weak D phenotypes. Blood 93:385-393, 1999.

32. Legler TJ, Maas JH, Blaschke V, et al: RHD genotyping in weak D phenotypes by multiple polymerase chain reactions. Transfusion 38:334-340, 1998.

33. Muller TH, Wagner FF, Trockenbacher A, et al: PCR screening for common weak D types shows different distribution in three central European populations. Transfusion 41:45-52, 2001.

34. Fridey J: Standards for Blood Banks and Transfusion Services, 22nd ed. Bethesda, MD, American Association of Blood Banks, 2003.

35. Flegel WA, Khull SR, Wagner FF: Primary anti-D immunization by weak D type 2 RBCs. Transfusion 40:428-434, 2000.

36. Wiener AS, Unger LJ: Rh factors related to the Rh0 factor as a source of clinical problems. JAMA 169:696-699, 1959.

37. Tippett P, Lomas-Francis C, Wallace M: The Rh antigen D: Partial D antigens and associated low incidence antigens. Vox Sang 70:123-131, 1996.

38. Tippett P: Rh blood group system: The D antigen and high- and low-frequency Rh antigen. In Vengeler-Tyler V, Pierce SR (eds): Blood Group Systems: Rh. Arlington, VA, American Association of Blood Banks, 1987.

39. Scott ML, Voak D, Jones JW, et al: A structural model for 30 RhD epitopes based on serological and DNA sequence data from partial D phenotypes. Trans Clin Biol 3:391-396, 1996.

40. Faas BHW, Beckers EAM, Simsek S, et al: Involvement of Ser 103 of the Rh polypeptides in G epitope formation. Transfusion 36:506-511, 1996.

41. Daniels GL, Faas BHW, Green CA, et al: The VS and V blood group polymorphisms in Africans: A serologic and molecular analysis. Transfusion 38:951-958, 1998.

42. Huang CH, Chen Y, Reid ME, Seidl C: Rh_{null} disease: The amorph type results from a novel double mutation in RHCe gene on D-negative background. Blood 92:664-671, 1998.

43. Hermand P, Gane P, Mattei MG, et al: Molecular basis and expression of the LW^a/LW^b blood group polymorphism. Blood 86:1590-1594, 1995.

44. Hermand P, Rennec PY, Rouger P, et al: Characterization of the gene encoding the human LW blood group protein in LW+ and LW− phenotypes. Blood 87:2962-2967, 1996.

45. Bailly P, Tontti E, Hermand P, et al: The red cell LW blood group protein is an intercellular adhesion molecule which binds to CD11/CD18 leukocyte integrins. Eur J Immunol 25:3316-3320, 1995.

46. Mallinson G, Martin PG, Anstee DJ, et al: Identification and partial characterization of the human erythrocyte membrane component(s) that express the antigens of the LW blood group system. Biochem J 234:649-652, 1986.

FURTHER READINGS

Cartron JP, Agre P: Rh blood group antigens: Protein and gene structure. Semin Hematol 30:193-208, 1993.

Daniels G: Human Blood Groups, 2nd ed. Oxford, Blackwell Science, 2002.

Issitt PD, Anstee DJ: Applied Blood Group Serology, 4th ed. Durham, NC, Montgomery Scientific Publications, 1998.

Mollison PL, Engelfriet CP, Contreras M: Blood Transfusion in Clinical Medicine, 10th ed. Oxford, Blackwell Scientific, 1997.

Reid ME, Lomas-Francis C: The Blood Group Antigen FactsBook, 2nd ed. London, Academic Press, Elsevier, 2004.

The Rhesus site: www.uni-ulm.de/~wflegel/RH/

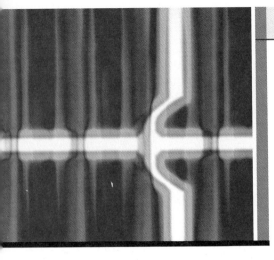

Other Blood Groups

Susan L. Wilkinson

LEARNING OBJECTIVES

After reading and studying this chapter, the student should be able to:

1. For each of the blood groups discussed in this chapter:
   Recall the major antigens in the system and write them using the appropriate nomenclature.
   Briefly discuss the inheritance of the blood group antigens.
   Identify the biochemical nature of the antigens.
   Discuss the serologic characteristics of the antibodies and their clinical significance. Briefly discuss any special testing procedures useful in the investigation of the antibodies in the systems.
2. Describe the K_0 (Kell$_{null}$) and McLeod phenotypes.
3. Briefly describe the pathology of the McLeod syndrome.
4. Briefly describe the relationship of the McLeod phenotype and chronic granulomatous disease, retinitis pigmentosa, and Duchenne muscular dystrophy.
5. Discuss the inheritance of the common antigens in the MNSs blood group system.
6. Briefly describe the relationship between the Fy antigen system and susceptibility to *Plasmodium vivax* infection.
7. Discuss the association between antibodies of the Kidd system and the incidence of delayed hemolytic transfusion reactions.
8. Discuss three genetic mechanisms leading to Lutheran null phenotypes.
9. Discuss the three types of Ge-negative red cells.
10. Describe the relationship between the Diego blood group system and the MNSs blood group system.
11. List six examples of other blood group systems.
12. Identify three high-incidence antigens that are not part of a known blood group system.
13. Identify three low-incidence antigens that are not part of a known blood group system.

THE KELL BLOOD GROUP SYSTEM
Antigens, Antibodies, and Phenotypes

The Kell blood group system was discovered in 1946 when Coombs, Mourant, and Race[1] described an antibody in the serum of Mrs. Kelleher that was responsible for hemolytic disease of the newborn (HDN). Called anti-Kell or anti-K, which is now the preferred terminology, the antigen it defined was also described as Kell or K and demonstrated a phenotype frequency of about 9% in whites. Three years later, Levine and colleagues[2] described anti-Cellano, or anti-k. This antibody detected an antigen of high frequency called k, and this appeared to be the antithetical antigen to K.

In 1957, Allen and Lewis[3] described anti-Kp^a and anti-Kp^b, antibodies that appeared to detect two antithetical antigens: Kp^a, an antigen of low frequency, and

Kp^b, an antigen of high frequency. An additional antithetical antigen to Kp^b, termed Kp^c and also of low incidence, was reported in 1979.[4] The Kell$_{null}$ or K$_0$ phenotype was described in 1957.[5] A phenotype with markedly reduced Kell antigens has also been described and is called the McLeod phenotype.[6] The Js^a antigen was described in 1958.[7] It was also noted that this antigen occurs primarily in black individuals, with a frequency of approximately 20%. The antithetical high-incidence antigen, Js^b, was described in 1963, when anti-Js^b was discovered in the serum of a black woman whose red cells were Js(a+).[8] Another pair of antibodies defining antithetical antigens in this blood group system includes K11, a high-incidence antigen, and K17, a low-incidence antigen.[9,10] The final pair of antithetical antigens is K14, an antigen of high incidence, and K24, an antigen of low incidence.[11]

An antibody defining an antigen found primarily in the Finnish population has been described. This antigen, K10 or Ul^a, occurs in about 3% of Finns. Several additional high-incidence antigens in this system have been described and include K12, K13, K18, K19, K22, TOU(K26), and RAZ(K27). Two low-incidence antigens, K23 and VLAN(K25), are also part of the Kell blood group system. Two other antigens of this system are Ku and Km, both high-incidence antigens that will be described in more detail with the K$_0$ and McLeod phenotypes. K16 is described as k-like. The 24 Kell system antigens are summarized in Table 6-1. Although the assigned system numbers go to K27, it should be noted that previously assigned K8, K9, and K15 have been removed from this blood group system.

Terminologies

As described for the Rh blood group system, the Kell system has both a numeric terminology and an alphabetic terminology. The alphabetic terminology, for the most part, is derived from letters associated with the antibody-maker's surname, or as a mechanism to denote an antithetical relationship between two antigens. Examples include K (Kelleher), k (Cellano), Js^a (Sutter), and Js^b (Matthews).

In an attempt to standardize blood group terminology, the Committee on Terminology for Red Cell Surface Antigens of the International Society of Blood Transfusion (ISBT) has proposed numeric nomenclature for all blood group systems and antigens.[12] The numeric notations for the Kell system are also summarized in Table 6-1.

Genetics and Biochemistry

The locus for the *KEL* gene has been assigned to chromosome 7(q33). The glycoprotein produced by this gene has a single pass through the red blood cell membrane. The glycoprotein is an endothelin-3–converting enzyme, capable of creating a potent vasoconstrictor.[13] K$_0$ red cells lack the glycoprotein, and McLeod red cells demonstrate diminished amounts. As will be discussed in more detail later in this chapter, there is a relationship between the Kell blood group system and the Kx blood group system. The gene responsible for Kx protein, termed *XK*, is located on the X chromosome at p21.1. In fact, the protein produced by the *XK* gene is

This chapter contains some advanced concepts that may be more appropriate for MT students. These are highlighted with a red vertical bar.

TABLE 6-1 Kell Blood Group System Antigens

Alphabetic	Numeric*	Relative Incidence	Comment
K	KEL1	Low	Antithetical to k
k	KEL2	High	Antithetical to K
Kp^a	KEL3	Low	Antithetical to Kp^b and Kp^c
Kp^b	KEL4	High	Antithetical to Kp^a and Kp^c
Ku	KEL5	High	Absent from K$_0$ cells
Js^a	KEL6	Low	Antithetical to Js^b
Js^b	KEL7	High	Antithetical to Js^a
Ul^a	KEL10	Low	
Côté	KEL11	High	Antithetical to K17
Boc	KEL12	High	
SGRO	KEL13	High	
San	KEL14	High	Antithetical to K24
k-like	KEL16	High	
Wk^a	KEL17	Low	Antithetical to K11
VM	KEL18	High	
Sub	KEL19	High	
Km	KEL20	High	Absent from K$_0$ and McLeod
Kp^c	KEL21	Low	Antithetical to Kp^a and Kp^b
NI	KEL22	High	
Centauro	KEL23	Low	
Cls	KEL24	Low	Antithetical to K14
VLAN	KEL25	Low	
TOU	KEL26	High	
RAZ	KEL27	High	

*KEL8, KEL9, and KEL15 are obsolete.

covalently linked at cysteine at position 72 to cysteine at position 347 on the glycoprotein produced by the *KEL* gene.[13]

The nucleotide changes and amino acid substitution responsible for the various Kell blood group antigens have been identified.[11] The antigens K and k differ by a single amino acid substitution that occurs at position 193. When the *KEL* gene produces the K antigen, methionine will be present and for k, threonine is detected. Amino acid changes for Kp^a, Kp^b, and Kp^c occur at position 281. When the *KEL* gene produces Kp^b, arginine is present. For Kp^a, tryptophan is produced and for Kp^c, glutamine is detected. The antigens Js^a and Js^b differ in the amino acids noted at position 597. For a *KEL* gene producing Js^a, proline is noted. For a *KEL* gene producing Js^b, the amino acid leucine is found.

Some *KEL* genes are more common in certain races than in others. The two most notable findings are the higher incidence of the gene producing the Js^a antigen in black individuals and the higher incidence of the Kp^a-producing gene in whites. If two Js^a-producing *KEL* genes are inherited, the individual lacks the high-incidence antigen Js^b and is at risk to produce anti-Js^b through pregnancy or transfusion. In a similar fashion, the person who inherits two *KEL* genes that produce Kp^a lacks the high-incidence antigen Kp^b. This information is useful when searching for units of blood that lack these high-incidence antigens or when identifying antibodies to high-incidence antigens. This is noted in Table 6-2.

The K$_0$ or Kell$_{null}$ Phenotype

The first example of this phenotype was reported by Chown and colleagues[5] when an antibody defining a previously unidentified high-incidence antigen was inves-

TABLE 6-2 Kell Blood Group System: Common Phenotypes and Frequencies

Phenotype	FREQUENCIES	
	White (%)	Black (%)
K–k+	91.0	98.0
K+k+	8.8	2.0
K+k–	0.2	Rare
Kp(a–b+)	97.7	100.0
Kp(a+b+)	2.3	Rare
Kp(a+b–)	Rare	0.0
Js(a–b+)	100.0	80.0
Js(a+b+)	Rare	19.0
Js(a+b–)	0.0	1.0

tigated. It was noted that the red cells of the antibody-maker were negative for the K, k, Kp^a, and Kp^b antigens. Interestingly, the parents of the antibody-maker were consanguineous, and one of the antibody-maker's sisters also appeared to lack all known antigens of the Kell system. Her red cells were compatible with her sister's antibody. It was postulated that these individuals had inherited two rare K_0 genes. The K_0 phenotype lacks all Kell system antigens, but red cells do express large amounts of the Kx antigen (discussed later). The **K_0 phenotype** can arise through a number of molecular events. These are summarized by Reid and Lomas-Francis.[14]

The antibody produced by K_0 individuals is called anti-Ku or anti-K5. This antibody appears to be of single specificity. Anti-K5 is considered clinically significant, and immunized K_0 individuals should be transfused with K_0 red cells.

Artificial K_0 red blood cells, useful in antibody identification studies, can be prepared by treating normal red cells with **2-aminoethylisothiouronium bromide (AET)**[15] or with **ZZAP (dithiothreitol plus cysteine–activated papain)**.[16]

The McLeod Phenotype and Kx Antigen
The McLeod Phenotype

The **McLeod phenotype** was reported by Allen and colleagues[6] in 1961. The red cells of the propositus, Hugh McLeod, showed marked depression in the expression of k, Js^b, and Kp^b. The second example of the McLeod phenotype was reported by van der Hart and colleagues.[17] In this report, the propositus also had recurrent infections, believed now to be **chronic granulomatous disease (CGD).**

CGD is a disorder of granulocyte function in which organisms are ingested but not killed. This is caused by the inability of the granulocyte to generate the superoxides that kill certain microorganisms. CGD can be caused by an X-linked mode of inheritance and an autosomal recessive mode of inheritance.[18] In the serum of the child reported by van der Hart and colleagues,[17] an unusual antibody was also noted. Termed anti-KL, the antibody actually was composed of two separable components, anti-Kx and anti-Km or anti-K20. Anti-Kx reacts most strongly with K_0 red cells, reacts more weakly with red cells of common Kell phenotype, and fails to react with McLeod red cells. Anti-Km reacts with red cells of common Kell phenotype but fails to react with K_0 or McLeod red cells.

The Genetic Locus for the McLeod Phenotype

The McLeod phenotype, described only in males, is inherited as an X-linked trait from the mother. Therefore the expression of Kx antigen is also controlled by an X-borne gene that resides at a locus now described as *XK*, located on the short arm (Xp21.1) of the X chromosome.[19] As mentioned earlier, the XK or Kx protein

K_0 (Kell_{null}) phenotype: Phenotype resulting from the inheritance of two rare *KEL* genes and associated with red cells that lack all Kell system antigens but express large amounts of Kx antigen.

2-aminoethylisothiouronium bromide (AET): A chemical that removes the activity of antigens of the Kell system (with the exception of Kx) from red cells.

ZZAP: A mixture of cystine-activated papain and dithiothreitol. Treatment of cells with ZZAP removes the activity of a number of blood group antigens. The technique is useful for the preparation of artificial K_0 cells.

McLeod phenotype: A phenotype associated with a decreased expression of Kell antigens on red cells.

Chronic granulomatous disease (CGD): An inherited disorder in which polymorphonuclear leukocytes are able to phagocytize but not kill certain microorganisms. The disease is characterized by chronic severe bacterial infections.

McLeod syndrome: The pathologic process usually associated with the McLeod phenotype, which includes hematologic, cardiac, and neurologic defects.

Acanthocytosis: An abnormal red cell morphology characterized by cytoplasmic projections resembling thorns.

Anisocytosis: An abnormal red cell morphology characterized by marked variation in red cell size.

Increased osmotic fragility: Abnormal sensitivity of red cells to lysis in various concentrations of saline.

Reticulocytosis: An abnormal increase of immature red cells (reticulocytes) in the circulation.

Haptoglobin: A mucoprotein that binds hemoglobin which has been released from lysed red cells. Haptoglobin is decreased in hemolytic disorders.

Splenomegaly: An enlarged spleen.

Creatine kinase, MM band: An isomer of creatine kinase (CK) also known as CK-3. This enzyme is present predominantly in skeletal muscle and myocardium.

Cardiomyopathy: Disease of the heart muscle.

Choreiform movements: Involuntary movement of the limbs and facial muscles.

Duchenne muscular dystrophy: A disease inherited as an X-linked trait associated with progressive degeneration of muscle fibers starting with the pelvic girdle and progressing to the shoulder girdle.

Retinitis pigmentosa: An inherited condition associated with the progressive loss of retinal response.

is covalently linked to the Kell glycoprotein.[13] The Kx protein appears to be necessary for normal expression of Kell system antigens and would explain why McLeod red cells only weakly express Kell antigens. Several genetic events give rise to the McLeod phenotype.[20] Those individuals with McLeod red cells and CGD are thought to arise because of a deletion on the X chromosome. Other McLeod phenotypes arise because of deleted nucleotides and premature stop codons, allowing for only a partial Kx protein.

McLeod Syndrome

In addition to the McLeod phenotype demonstrating unusual red cell antigens, these individuals also have a pathologic disease process called **McLeod syndrome.** The signs and symptoms of this disease include red cell morphology that demonstrates **acanthocytosis** and **anisocytosis, increased osmotic fragility, reticulocytosis,** a reduction in serum **haptoglobin** levels, and **splenomegaly.**[21,22] Individuals may also have a well-compensated hemolytic anemia. In addition, muscular anomalies with progressive deterioration may be noted, along with increased levels of **creatinine phosphokinase (isoenzyme MM). Cardiomyopathy** is also well documented, along with neurologic defects including **choreiform movements** and the absence of some tendinal reflexes.

Relationship to CGD

Some patients with X-linked CGD have red cells of the McLeod phenotype. It is believed that the genes responsible for CGD, **Duchenne muscular dystrophy (DMD),** and one form of **retinitis pigmentosa (RP)** reside on the short arm of the X chromosome at the Xp21.1 region, as does the *XK* locus.[23] Deletions at this particular area appear to be responsible for the simultaneous appearance of both CGD and the McLeod phenotype. Indeed, one unique patient with CGD, McLeod phenotype, DMD, and RP has been described.[23]

Kell System: Other Findings
Relationship with Gerbich System

Although K_0 and McLeod red cells have normal expression of Gerbich antigens, many Ge:−2,−3 red cells demonstrate weakened expression of Kell system antigens. Gerbich is genetically independent of Kell, and the Gerbich-negative phenotypes are known to arise from deletions of differing parts of the glycophorin C gene, assigned to chromosome 2 (see later in this chapter).

Cis-Modifying Genes

The presence of a *KEL* gene that produces the Kp^a antigen results in decreased expression of the k antigen. This is more marked when two Kp^a-producing *KEL* genes are present or when a Kp^a-producing gene is paired with a *KEL* gene that results in the K_0 phenotype.

K$_{mod}$ Phenotype

The K_{mod} phenotype has been used to describe phenotypes in which there is weak expression of Kell antigens but elevated expression of Kx.[24] Some of these individuals have produced an anti-K5–like antibody, and the phenotype is inherited. Several genetic events have been described that give rise to this phenotype.[14]

Kell System Antibodies
Alloantibodies and Autoantibodies

Kell system alloantibodies, particularly anti-K (anti-K1), are fairly common. This suggests that the Kell protein is fairly immunogenic. Although antibodies to k, Kp^b, and Js^b are not common because those lacking the antigen are not common, when antigen-negative individuals are challenged with antigen-positive red cells, alloantibody is often produced.

Although the majority of these antibodies are produced because of red cell transfusion or pregnancy and are IgG, naturally occurring, apparently IgM anti-K has been reported.[25] Because Kell system antibodies are primarily IgG in nature, they are considered clinically significant, and antigen-negative red cell components should be provided. One study documents the destruction of incompatible red cells transfused to a recipient with anti-Kp[b].[26] As expected, these antibodies have been reported to cause hemolytic disease of the newborn.

Kell system autoantibodies have also been reported. Specificities have included autoanti-K, autoanti-Kp[b], autoanti-K5, and autoanti-K13. Some cases have been associated with significant anemia, whereas others have failed to demonstrate increased red cell destruction. Kell system antibodies are usually detected in a 37° C/AHG or enzyme/37° C/AHG system. Examples of these antibodies remaining undetected with **low ionic strength saline (LISS)** or **LISS-polybrene** systems have been reported.[27]

THE MNSs BLOOD GROUP SYSTEM

The MN blood group system was discovered in 1927 when Landsteiner and Levine[28] deliberately immunized rabbits with human red cells. Even in 1928, Landsteiner and Levine[29] proposed that M and N were antithetical in nature and were products of alleles at a single locus. The MN blood group system was expanded in 1947 with the discovery of anti-S and anti-s in 1951.[30,31] It was also shown that the S and s antigens were antithetical and, again, the products of alleles at a single locus. It was later shown that the genetic locus where the gene responsible for the production of the S and s antigens resides is linked to the locus for the gene responsible for the M and N antigens. Both loci have been shown to be located on the long arm of chromosome 4.[32] In 1953, Wiener and colleagues[33] described an antibody, anti-U, defining a high-incidence antigen, U. One year later, Greenwalt and colleagues[34] reported that the red cells that lack the high-incidence antigen U also lack the S and s antigens, suggesting that the products of the gene responsible for the production of S and s also produce the U antigen. In 1973, it was shown that the high-incidence antigen described as En[a] is actually produced by the gene responsible for M and N antigens.[35] A number of low-incidence antigens have been assigned to this blood group system, and some are described in more detail. The blood group system also has a null phenotype, described as M[k]M[k], that produces neither MN nor Ss.[36]

Genetics and Biochemistry

The genes encoding the MNSs system antigens reside on chromosome 4 (4q28-q31). The genes at these loci are actually responsible for the production of two distinct glycophorins or sialoglycoproteins (SGPs) that are carried on the red cell membrane. These are referred to as **glycophorin A (GPA)** and **glycophorin B (GPB)**. The M and N antigens are located on GPA and the S and s antigens are located on GPB. The gene that encodes GPA is designated *GYPA* and the gene that encodes GPB, *GYPB*.[37] Of the 43 antigens assigned to the MNSs blood group system (Table 6-3), many reside on GPA or GPB and result from single nucleotide mutations, giving rise to unique amino acid sequences and low-incidence antigens.[38] Other antigens arise because of hybrid glycophorins derived from both GPA and GPB. Finally, several unusual or rare phenotypes arise because of the deletion of GPA, GPB, or both glycophorins from the red cell membrane.

GPA is a single-pass transmembrane protein consisting of 131 amino acids, and is glycosylated, or demonstrates carbohydrate-containing side-chains.[37] There are approximately 800,000 copies of GPA per red cell. GPA is divided into three segments. The outer or N-terminal end of the molecule extends into the extracellular environment of the red cell. This segment of the molecule expresses antigenic activity. Another segment extends through the lipid bilayer, and the third segment,

Low ionic strength saline (LISS): A blood banking reagent that potentiates some antigen-antibody reactions by lowering the ionic strength and thus decreasing the net charge of red cells.

LISS-polybrene: The combination of low ionic strength saline and polybrene, a polymer that brings about the agglutination of red cells.

Glycophorin A: A sialoglycoprotein produced by the *GYPA* gene.

Glycophorin B: A sialoglycoprotein produced by the *GYPB* gene.

TABLE 6-3 MNSs Blood Group System Antigens

| Alphabetic | Numeric | RELATIVE INCIDENCE | | Comment |
		White	Black	
M	MNS1	78%	74%	Antithetical to N
N	MNS2	72%	75%	Antithetical to M
S	MNS3	55%	31%	Antithetical to s
s	MNS4	89%	93%	Antithetical to S
U	MNS5	High		
He	MNS6	0%	3%	Antithetical to 'N'
Mi^a	MNS7	Low		
M^c	MNS8	Low		
Vw	MNS9	Low		Antithetical to Hut, ENEH
Mur	MNS10	Low		Higher incidence in Chinese, Taiwanese, and Thai individuals
M^g	MNS11	Low		
Vr	MNS12	Low		
M^e	MNS13			Expressed on M$^+$ and all He$^+$ RBC
Mt^a	MNS14	Low		
St^a	MNS15	Low		Higher incidence in Japanese individuals
Ri^a	MNS16	Low		
Cl^a	MNS17	Low		
Ny^a	MNS18	Low		
Hut	MNS19	Low		Antithetical to Vw, ENEH
Hil	MNS20	Low		Higher incidence in Chinese individuals
M^V	MNS21	Low		
Far	MNS22	Low		
s^D	MNS23	Low		
Mit	MNS24	Low		
Dantu	MNS25	Low		Found only in black individuals
Hop	MNS26	Low		
Nob	MNS27	Low		Antithetical to ENKT
En^a	MNS28	High		
ENKT	MNS29	High		Antithetical to Nob
'N'	MNS30	High		Antithetical to He
Or	MNS31	Low		
DANE	MNS32	Low		
TSEN	MNS33	Low		
MINY	MNS34	Low		Higher incidence in Chinese individuals
MUT	MNS35	Low		Higher incidence in Chinese individuals
SAT	MNS36	Low		
ERIK	MNS37	Low		
Os^a	MNS38	Low		
ENEP	MNS39	High		Antithetical to HAG
ENEH	MNS40	High		Antithetical to Vw and Hut
HAG	MNS41	Low		Antithetical to ENEP
ENAV	MNS42	High		Antithetical to MARS
MARS	MNS43	Low		Antithetical to ENAV

the carboxy-terminal end, extends into the cytoplasm of the red cell. The GPA that produces the M antigen (GPA^M) and the GPA that produces by the N antigen (GPA^N) differ only in the amino acids found at positions 1 and 5.[37] GPA^M demonstrates serine at the first amino acid and glycine at the fifth. GPA^N demonstrates leucine at the first amino acid and glutamic acid at the fifth. Alkali-labile oligosaccharides are found at amino acid positions 2, 3, and 4, where the amino acids serine, threonine, and threonine are found, respectively. GPAs that give rise to the M and N antigens are shown in Fig. 6-1. The deletion of exons (2-7) from the *GYPA* gene results in an absence of GPA and red cells that are termed En(a−).[37] Although these individuals produce GYB, they fail to produce the high-incidence antigens En^a and Wr^b. The En^a antigens represent segments along GPA. The Wr^b antigen is part of the Diego blood group system (see later in chapter). This antigen is not expressed because of the lack of GPA.[39] There are other En-negative cells (ENKT, ENEP, ENEH, and ENAV) that arise through different genetic mechanisms and these are described later.

GPB is also a single-pass transmembrane protein, but it consists of only 72 amino acids. This structure is also glycosylated and demonstrates approximately 200,000 copies per red blood cell. The N-terminal portion of the molecule consists of 36 amino acids, the first 26 of which are identical to the N-terminal structure of GPA^N. This finding accounts for the N-like antigen, or 'N' antigen, found on nearly all cells (see later). The carboxy-terminal end extends into the cytoplasm of the red cell. The GPB^S differs from the GPB^s in the amino acid found at position 29. The S antigen demonstrates methionine at this position, whereas the s antigens shows threonine.[40] GPB and the antigen S and s are shown in Fig. 6-1.

In a similar fashion to En^a, deletion of exons from *GYPB* results in a failure to produce GPB and a lack of the high-incidence antigen, U.[41] U− red cells lack GPB, but demonstrate normal GPA. There are some unique genes at the *GYPB* locus that give rise to red cells that express small quantities of the U antigen and are described as S−s−U+^{var}, or U variants.[42]

Four common **haplotypes** are recognized: MS, Ms, NS, and Ns. Inheritance of one haplotype is from one biologic parent, and inheritance of the additional haplotype is from the other biologic parent. Phenotypes that also include U− are shown in Table 6-4.

Haplotype: A set of alleles from a group of closely linked genes that are inherited together and are responsible for the production of a number of blood group antigens. The major antigens of the MNSs blood group system are inherited as haplotypes.

AMINO ACID POSITION	GPA^M	GPA^N	GPB^S	GPB^s
1	Ser	Leu	Leu	Leu
2	Ser ▲	Ser ▲	Ser ▲	Ser ▲
3	Thr ▲	Thr ▲	Thr ▲	Thr ▲
4	Thr ▲	Thr ▲	Thr ▲	Thr ▲
5	Gly	Glu	Glu	Glu
29	His	His	Met	Thr

▲ Alkali-labile oligosaccharide

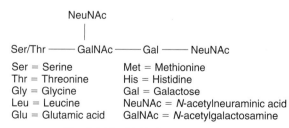

Ser = Serine
Thr = Threonine
Gly = Glycine
Leu = Leucine
Glu = Glutamic acid

Met = Methionine
His = Histidine
Gal = Galactose
NeuNAc = *N*-acetylneuraminic acid
GalNAc = *N*-acetylgalactosamine

Fig. 6-1 The M, N, S, and s antigens.

TABLE 6-4	MNSs Blood Group System: Phenotypes and Frequencies	
Phenotype	White (%)	Black (%)
M+N–S+s–	6	2.1
M+N–S+s+	14	7.0
M+N–S–s+	8	15.5
M+N–S–s–	0	0.4
M+N+S+s–	4	2.2
M+N+S+s+	24	13.0
M+N+S–s+	22	33.4
M+N+S–s–	0	0.4
M–N+S+s–	1	1.6
M–N+S+s+	6	4.5
M–N+S–s+	15	19.2
M–N+S–s–	0	0.7

Antigens and Phenotypes
Glycophorin A

M

As described in the previous section, the M antigen is expressed on GPA^M, produced by *GYPA* gene. GPA^M has serine as the first amino acid and glycine as the fifth amino acid. The amino acids at positions 2, 3, and 4, which are serine, threonine, and threonine, respectively, contain alkali-labile oligosaccharides. The M antigen is sensitive to trypsin, ficin, and papain. The antigenic structure is depicted in Fig. 6-1.

N

The N antigen is expressed on GPA^N, which is also produced by the *GYPA* gene. GPA^N has leucine at position 1 and glutamic acid at position 5. Amino acids 2, 3, and 4 are identical to those found on GPA^M. The N antigen is destroyed with trypsin, ficin, and papain. This antigenic structure is also shown in Fig. 6-1.

Low-Incidence Antigens

Several other low-incidence antigens are found on GPA and arise from single nucleotide mutations that give rise to amino acid substitutions.[38] These include Vr, Mt^a, Ri^a, Ny^a, Or, Erik, and Os^a. As an example, Vr+ red cells demonstrate tyrosine at amino acid 47 instead of the usual serine molecule that would give rise to Vr– red cells. As an additional example, Os(a+) red cells demonstrate serine at amino acid 54 instead of proline. For additional information on the molecular basis of these low-incidence antigens, consult Reid and Lomas-Francis.[14]

Glycophorin B

S

As previously described, the first five amino acids of either S- or s-derived GPB (produced by the *GYPB* gene) are identical to GPA^N. GPB^S, however, demonstrates the amino acid methionine at position 29. The S antigen is not sensitive to trypsin but is sensitive to ficin and papain. This structure is shown in Fig. 6-1.

s

The *GYPB* gene that produces GPB^s demonstrates threonine at position 29. The s antigen is insensitive to trypsin. It may or may not be sensitive to ficin and papain. The antigenic part of this structure is noted in Fig. 6-1.

Low-Incidence Antigens

Several low-incidence antigens are also present on GPB that arise through single-nucleotide mutations that result in amino acid substitutions. These include the M^V, s^D, and Mit antigens. As an example, the Mit antigen is produced when histidine is present at amino acid 35 on GPB. Mit− red cells demonstrate arginine at this amino acid.[43]

Deleted Glycophorins; Various En-negative Phenotypes
Enᵃ

As mentioned earlier, the inheritance of two *GYPA* genes that have a deletion of exons 2 through 7 results in a failure to produce GPA. These red cells lack the high-incidence antigen described as Enᵃ, but demonstrate normal GPB. Although the designation En(a−) suggests absence of a single high-incidence antigen, this is not accurate. It is now known that the term Enᵃ actually represents several amino acid segments of GPA.

ENEH, ENEP, ENAV, and ENKT

These segments or antigen sites were initially described as EnᵃTS (for trypsin sensitive), EnᵃFS (for ficin sensitive), and EnᵃFR (for ficin resistant) based on their serologic activity with anti-Enᵃ antibodies.[44] These Enᵃ antigens have now been defined based on their molecular structure and genetic evolution. Several of these phenotypes have arisen because of single nucleotide mutations and the production of low-incidence MNSs system antigens that are antithetical to the high-incidence antigen missing on GPA.[45-47] These include ENEH and its antithetical antigens Vw and Hut; ENEP and its antithetical antigen HAG; and ENAV and its antithetical antigen MARS. The final high-incidence antigen, ENKT, and its antithetical antigen Nob arise because of the insertion of five amino acids into GPA that is derived from GPB.[48]

ENEH resides on GPA that has been previously described as EnᵃTS. It is now known that when ENEH is produced, threonine is found at amino acid 28. However, when ENEH is absent, methionine (Vw) or lysine (Hut) will be found at position 28. ENEP and ENAV reside on the portion of GPA that is described as EnᵃFR. When ENEP is produced, alanine is found at amino acid 65. When absent, proline and the low-incidence antigen HAG are noted. When ENAV is produced, glutamic acid is found at amino acid 63. In its absence, lysine and the low-incidence antigen MARS is noted. ENKT resides on GPA that has been previously described as EnᵃFS. When ENKT is produced, arginine is found at amino acid 49 and threonine is found at amino acid 52. In the absence of ENKT, the low-incidence antigen Nob is produced and threonine is found at position 49 and serine at position 52.

The various En-negative individuals were evaluated initially because of unidentified antibody in their serum. It should be mentioned at this point that in addition to anti-En antibodies, these individuals also produced an antibody described as anti-Wrᵇ and, indeed, these individuals were shown to be Wr(a−b−). As is now known, the Wr antigens are part of the Diego blood group system and are inherited independently of the MNSs antigens. The very rare phenotype Wr(a+b−) has been described, and these red cells have normal GPA and are En(a+).[49] It is now known that the interaction of GPA and band 3 protein, the location for the Diego blood group system antigens, is necessary for Wr antigenic expression.[39]

U

The inheritance of two *GYPB* genes that have exons 2 through 4 deleted results in an absence of GPB and the S−s−U− phenotype. The U antigen is of high incidence and the U− phenotype is found almost exclusively in black individuals. Although the majority of S−s− individuals are truly U−, some S−s− red cells express reduced quantities of the U antigen. These are referred to as U variants or U+ᵛᵃʳ. It appears that the U+ᵛᵃʳ phenotype arises from hybrid glycophorin genes, and approximately 25% of these express the low-incidence MNSs system antigen

He.[42] There are a variety of genetic mechanisms that give rise to the He+ phenotype.[37] U− and U variant red cells express normal GPA.

Both U− and U variant red cells lack the 'N' antigen of GPB. This can present unique problems for immunized M+U− individuals, because they are at risk to produce not only anti-U but also anti-'N' and anti-N. These individuals could then be transfused only with other M+U− red cells. He+ red cells also lack the 'N' antigen and can produce anti-'N'.

As described for anti-En[a], the anti-U produced by U− and U variant individuals probably represents a heterogeneous mix of antibodies directed to different amino acid segments along GPB. In one study, anti-U antibodies were divided into those that were papain sensitive (anti-UPS) and those that were papain resistant (anti-UPR).[50] An additional study has also evaluated the antibodies made by S−s− individuals.[51] Anti-U is a clinically significant antibody.

M[k]

Neither GPA nor GPB is produced in the presence of an *M[k]* gene. It has been shown that exons 2 through 7 of the *GYPA* gene and exons 1 through 5 of the *GYPB* gene have been deleted. Individuals who inherit two such genes lack M, N, S, s, En[a], U, 'N', and Wr[b]. Therefore those individuals are at risk to produce a variety of antibodies.

Hybrid Glycophorins

Hybrid glycophorins arise during meiosis as a single, unequal crossing-over occurs between the genes that are responsible for GPA and GPB.[37] These hybrid glycophorins are unique because a portion is derived from GPA and the other portion from GPB. As would be expected, the N-terminus may be derived from GPA or from GPB. Conversely, the C-terminus may be derived from GPA or GPB. Because of the uniqueness of these structures, low-incidence antigens may be produced or red cells may lack other high-incidence antigens. When the N-terminal portion is GPA derived and the C-terminal portion GYB derived, the molecular basis is described as *GYP(A-B)*. When the N-terminal portion is GYB derived and the C-terminal portion GYA derived, the molecular basis of the gene is described as *GYP(B-A)*. Other unique hybrid glycophorins have been described that include insertion of genetic material derived from *GYPA* or *GYPB* between genetic material derived from the alternative gene. The molecular basis for these hybrid glycophorins that arise through gene conversion are described as *GYP(A-B-A)* or *GYP(B-A-B)*.[37] These hybrid glycophorins are quite complex, but several examples will be briefly described. Although now obsolete, the previously described Miltenberger subsystem and its low-incidence antigens are derived from such hybrid structures. For more information on the various hybrid glycophorins, consult Reid and Lomas-Francis.[14]

GYP(A-B) or GP(A-B)

Three glycophorins that arise through this hybrid structure will be noted here: GP.Hil (Mi.V), GP.JL (Mi.XI), and GP.TK. In the GP.Hil phenotype, two low-incidence antigens, Hil and MINY, are produced.[37] The first 58 amino acids are GPA derived, and amino acids 59-104 are GPB[s] derived. For the GP.JL phenotype, the low-incidence antigens TSEN and MINY are produced.[37] The first 58 amino acids are also GPA derived, but amino acids 59 through 102 are GPB[S] derived. Finally, GP.TK expresses the low-incidence antigen, SAT.[52] Amino acids 1 through 71 are GPA derived, and amino acids 72 through 104 are GPB derived.

GYP(B-A) or GP(B-A)

Two unique glycophorins are known to arise through this molecular basis. They are designated GP.Sch and GP.Dantu. GP.Sch produces the low-incidence antigen known as St[a] or Stones, and GP.Dantu produces the low-incidence antigen Dantu. The St[a] antigen arises when amino acid 26 from GPB joins to GPA at

Hybrid glycophorins: Abnormal glycophorins resulting from a crossover between the genes for GPA and GPB, which results in the production of a number of unique low-incidence antigens in the MNSs system.

amino acid 59.[37] For the Dantu antigen, amino acid 39 from GPB attaches to amino acid 40 or 70, derived from GPA.[37]

GYP(A-B-A) or GP(A-B-A)

The MNSs low-incidence antigens M^g (GP.M^g) and M^c arise through gene conversion and these variant glycophorins. For the M^g antigen, amino acids 1 through 4 are derived from GPA^N, amino acid 5 is derived from GPB, and the remaining amino acids through 131 are GPA derived. Asparagine is also substituted for threonine at amino acid 4, resulting in no glycosylation and altered glycosylation at amino acids 2 and 3.[53] Human and rabbit anti-M and anti-N do not detect the M^g antigen. This can have implications in paternity testing. With the M^c antigen, amino acids 1 through 4 are GPA^M derived, amino acid 5 is GPB derived, and the remaining amino acids through 131 are GPA derived.[37] Interestingly, M^c red cells react with some anti-M sera and some anti-N sera. The amino acids at positions 2, 3, and 4 are glycosylated.

GYP(B-A-B) or GP(B-A-B)

Two unique glycophorins that arise through this molecular mechanism will be described: GP.Mur (Mi.III) and GP.Bun (Mi.VI). In the GP.Mur phenotype, the first 48 amino acids are GPB derived, amino acids 49 through 57 are GPA derived, and the remaining amino acids through 103 are GPB derived. These red cells produce five low-incidence antigens: Mi^a, Mur, MUT, Hil, and MINY.[37] In the GP.Bun phenotype, the first 50 amino acids are GPB derived, amino acids 51 through 57 are GPA derived, and the remaining amino acids through 103 are GPB derived. These cells produce six low-incidence antigens: Mi^a, Mur, MUT, Hop, Hil, and MINY.[37]

MNSs Antibodies
Anti-M

Most examples of anti-M react at room temperature or lower and are considered naturally occurring antibodies. These antibodies can be both IgM and IgG and do not appear to activate complement. Many examples of anti-M exhibit dosage, or react more strongly with homozygous MM red cells than with heterozygous MN red cells. Some examples of anti-M react more strongly if tested in a medium with a pH of approximately 6.5.[54] Anti-M fails to react with ficin- or papain-premodified red cells. Some examples react with sialic acid–deficient red cells, but other examples do not.[55]

Because of these characteristics, most examples of anti-M are considered clinically insignificant. However, unusual examples of anti-M that react at 37° C and at the antiglobulin phase of testing may be clinically significant. Anti-M has rarely been responsible for hemolytic disease of the newborn.[56]

Anti-N

Virtually all examples of anti-N are IgM, naturally occurring, cold-reacting antibodies that are considered clinically insignificant. Although usually found in the sera of N– individuals, occasional examples of anti-N may be found in the sera of N+ individuals undergoing renal dialysis. The anti-N found in dialysis patients also appears to be clinically insignificant. Formation of this antibody appears to arise when patient cells are exposed to formaldehyde, causing an alteration to the normal "self" antigen, allowing the immune system to produce anti-N.[57] Anti-N fails to react with ficin- and papain-premodified red cells.

Some individuals who form anti-N are also at risk to form the clinically significant antibody anti-'N.' These individuals include those of the phenotype M+N–S–s– and the phenotypes He+M+N–S–s– or M^v+M+N–S–s–.[43,58] Although these individuals lack N, they also lack the amino-terminal end of

GPB or the 'N' antigen. Anti-'N' is IgG and reacts at 37° C and at the antiglobulin phase of testing. Anti-'N' has caused hemolytic disease of the newborn (HDN).[59]

Anti-M and anti-N Blood Typing Reagents

Although all commercial blood banking reagent companies offer anti-M and anti-N reagents, the reagent sources can be quite different. Human anti-M is available from at least one company, and another company offers only rabbit anti-M and anti-N. Monoclonal anti-M and anti-N are available, as is lectin *(Vicea graminea)* anti-N. Because of the different sources, the manufacturers' directions are quite different, and one must be aware of these differences. In addition, because of the varied sources of reagents and the segments of GPA detected, results may be different when different types of reagents are used.

Anti-S and Anti-s

The vast majority of examples of anti-S and anti-s are IgG and immune in origin. As expected, these IgG antibodies are optimally reactive at 37° C and at the antiglobulin phase of testing. Rare examples of IgM anti-S have been reported. This may be why some unique examples of anti-S react optimally at room temperature or in LISS solutions.[60] Anti-S normally does not react with enzyme-premodified S+ red cells. Anti-s may or may not react with enzyme-premodified s+ red cells. Anti-S and anti-s are considered clinically significant, and patients who demonstrate these antibodies should receive antigen-negative red cells. Examples of both anti-S and anti-s have caused HDN.

Anti-En^a

Although previously defined as several different antibodies directed to different amino acid sequences on GPA, anti-En^a antibodies tend to be IgG in nature and therefore optimally reactive at 37° C and at the antiglobulin phase of testing. These antibodies are considered clinically significant and have caused HDN. Compatible blood products for an immunized En(a−) individual require interaction with rare donor files, autologous transfusions, and/or assessment of family members for compatible products.

Anti-U

Anti-U is considered a clinically significant antibody. It is immune in origin and therefore reacts at 37° C and at the antiglobulin phase of testing. This antibody has caused HDN, and antigen-negative red cells must be used for transfusion in immunized patients. Again, rare donor registries, family members, or autologous transfusions must be considered in the presence of anti-U.

As stated earlier, some examples of anti-U are not compatible with all U− red cells. This incompatibility is due to one of two causes. First, some apparent U− cells are actually U variant cells and possess small quantities of the U antigen. Depending on the specificity of the anti-U, such cells may be incompatible. An additional concern arises in those U− individuals who are also N−. In addition to forming anti-U, they are also at risk to produce anti-N plus anti-'N.' Such immunized individuals would be compatible only with donors of other M+N−S−s− red cells.

THE DUFFY BLOOD GROUP SYSTEM

The Duffy (Fy) blood group system is composed of six antigens: Fy^a, Fy^b, Fy3, Fy4, Fy5, and Fy6. The antibody defining the Fy^a antigen was discovered in 1950 during evaluation of the serum of a hemophiliac who had received a number of blood transfusions.[61] The antithetical antigen, Fy^b, was discovered the following year during investigation of antibodies in the serum of a **multiparous** female.[62] Although

Multiparous: Having multiple pregnancies.

not a distinct antigen, a variant form of Fy^b has also been described and called Fy^x. The Fy^x antigen reacts weakly with some examples of anti-Fy^b.[63] In 1955, Sanger and colleagues[64] noted that in blacks, the Fy(a–b–) phenotype was very common and postulated that this phenotype probably represented the inheritance of two amorphic genes. It has been shown that these Fy(a–b–) cells express the Fy4 antigen. However, in rare white Fy(a–b–) individuals, the Fy4 antigen is not produced. Anti-Fy3 reacts with all cells that express the Fy^a and/or Fy^b antigens but fails to react with Fy(a–b–) red cells.[65] Anti-Fy5 is similar to anti-Fy3 but fails to react with Rh_{null} red cells that may express the Fy^a and/or Fy^b antigens. Fy6 has only been defined with monoclonal antibodies.[66]

Genetics and Biochemistry

The *FY* locus has been assigned to the long arm of chromosome 1 (1q22-q23). The *FY* gene is responsible for the production of the trans-membrane carrier molecule for Duffy glycoprotein. The Duffy glycoprotein serves as a red cell receptor for several chemokines.[67] The Fy antigens appear to play a role in susceptibility to red cell invasion by *Plasmodium vivax*.[68]

The *FY* locus is linked with the loci for antithrombin III and type 1 hereditary motor and sensory neuropathy.[69] The *FY* locus is syntenic to the *RH* locus. The difference in the Fy^a and Fy^b antigens is a result of an amino acid change at position 42 on the glycoprotein molecule. Glycine is present when Fy^a is produced, but aspartic acid is present when Fy^b is produced. Several molecular changes give rise to the aberrant Fy^b phenotype described as Fy^x.[70] Multiple molecular changes are also responsible for the Fy(a–b–) phenotype.[14] The common Fy phenotypes are summarized in Table 6-5.

Antigens and Antibodies
Fy^a and Fy^b Antigens; Anti-Fy^a and Anti-Fy^b

These Fy antigens and antibodies are frequently of concern when solving blood bank serologic problems because antibodies to these antigens are not uncommon.

The Fy^a and Fy^b antigens are destroyed by proteolytic enzymes including ficin, papain, and bromelin. These antigenic determinants are also destroyed when red cells are heated at 56° C for 10 minutes. Although antibodies to these antigens occur as sole specificities, many examples of anti-Fy^a or anti-Fy^b occur with other alloantibodies. Anti-Fy^a is seen more frequently than is anti-Fy^b. In spite of the fact that the majority of blacks lack Fy^a and Fy^b antigens, immunization to these antigens is seen less frequently than in white populations.[71] Alloimmunization to Fy^a, even in whites, is not extremely high. This is postulated to be a result of low immunogenicity for the Fy^a antigen.[58]

Detection of anti-Fy^a or anti-Fy^b usually occurs via an indirect antiglobulin technique. These IgG antibodies are also capable of activating complement. Of particular interest, weak examples of these antibodies may react only with homozygous red cells. For this reason, it is important to evaluate antibody identification studies with care, paying particular attention to the reactivity of

TABLE 6-5 Duffy Blood Group System: Phenotypes and Frequencies

| Phenotype | FREQUENCIES | |
	White (%)	Black (%)
Fy(a+b–)	18.0	0.9
Fy(a+b+)	49.0	1.3
Fy(a–b+)	34.0	22.0
Fy(a–b–)	0.01	68.0

homozygous Fy^a or Fy^b red cells compared with the nonreactivity of heterozygous red cells.

Both anti-Fy^a and anti-Fy^b are clinically significant. Patients with either of these antibodies, or those who indicate a past history of having the antibody, should be transfused with antigen-negative red cells. Both of these antibodies have been responsible for delayed transfusion reactions and HDN.

Fy3 and Anti-Fy3

Anti-Fy3 was originally described in a white Fy(a−b−) individual.[65] This immune antibody reacted with all red cells except those of the Fy(a−b−) phenotype. Anti-Fy3 has also been detected in the serum of several black Fy(a−b−) individuals and may be different from the anti-Fy3 produced by whites and that produced by a Cree Indian.[72-74] The anti-Fy3 in blacks reacted weakly, or not at all, with cord red cells that were Fy-positive, whereas the antibody produced by whites and the Cree were strongly reactive with cord red cells that were Fy-positive. The Fy3 antigen is not destroyed by treatment with proteolytic enzymes. Mild hemolytic disease of the newborn has been attributed to anti-Fy3.[65,73]

Fy4 and Anti-Fy4

When first discovered, the Fy(a−b−) phenotype in blacks was believed to represent a null phenotype. It was theorized that individuals of this phenotype had inherited two amorphic genes and produced no detectable product. This belief was modified after the discovery of anti-Fy4. Anti-Fy4 reacted with all Fy(a−b−) red cells from blacks and those Fy(a+b−) and Fy(a−b+) red cells from blacks that were heterozygous for the amorphic gene. Anti-Fy4 did not react with Fy(a−b−) red cells from whites. The Fy4 antigen is not destroyed by proteases.

Fy5 and Anti-Fy5

Anti-Fy5 is very similar to anti-Fy3. Indeed, initially it was believed to represent another example of anti-Fy3 because it failed to react with Fy(a−b−) red cells but did react with other Fy(a+) and/or Fy(b+) red cells. However, when the serum was tested with Rh$_{null}$ red cells that were Fy(a+) and/or Fy(b+), the antibody failed to react. D-deletion red cells reacted more weakly with this antibody, and the Fy(a−b−) red cells of the white woman who had made anti-Fy3 also reacted. The Fy5 antigen is not protease sensitive.

Fy6 and Anti-Fy6

Anti-Fy6 is a murine monoclonal antibody that reacts with all red cells, including Rh$_{null}$ cells, but fails to react with Fy(a−b−) red cells. The Fy6 antigen is destroyed by ficin, papain, and bromelin but is enhanced with trypsin. The Fy6 epitope is believed to play a role in the invasion of red cells by *Plasmodium vivax*.

Fy and Malaria

The relationship between the Duffy blood group system and invasion by malarial parasites was first documented by Miller and colleagues using the simian malarial parasite *P. knowlesi* that is also capable of invading human red cells.[75,76] In these studies, enzyme-treated and untreated human red cells were incubated with merozoite-infected Rhesus monkey red cells. The human cells were both Fy(a+) and/or Fy(b+) and Fy(a−b−). Invasion was high (80.3 parasitized cells per 1000) when untreated Fy(a+) and/or Fy(b+) cells were used, but invasion was quite low (2.2 cells per 1000) when Fy(a−b−) cells were evaluated. Loss of susceptibility was confirmed following enzymatic removal of the Fy antigens.

Of additional interest were several in vivo studies using *P. vivax*.[68,77,78] In the first study, five blacks and six whites who were Fy(a+) and/or Fy(b+) all contracted *P. vivax*, whereas five blacks who were Fy(a−b−) failed to develop the disease. Additional in vivo studies evaluated individuals who contracted malaria in

Vietnam. In this study, 13 of 13 blacks who had contracted the disease were also positive for either Fy^a or Fy^b or for both antigens.

> Early on, it was hypothesized that Fy^a and Fy^b were the receptors for invasion by *P. knowlesi* and *P. vivax*. However, some discrepant findings made this theory not as straightforward as it originally seemed. First, although Fy(a−b−) red cells are not invaded by *P. knowlesi*, the merozoites do attach and cause widespread deformation of the cells. This led to the proposal that although the Fy antigens are required for invasion, an additional and distinct site is required for attachment. Second, trypsin- and neuraminidase-treated Fy(a−b−) red cells could be invaded by *P. knowlesi*, and third, some New World monkeys have red cells that are susceptible to invasion by *P. knowlesi*, although they lack Fy antigens.
>
> If indeed multiple receptors for the merozoite do exist, it now seems plausible that the receptors for *P. vivax* and *P. knowlesi* are distinct.[79] The Fy3 antigen may be the receptor for invasion in nonhuman primate red cells, whereas the Fy6 receptor may be the site of invasion for *P. vivax* in human cells.[80]

THE KIDD BLOOD GROUP SYSTEM

The Kidd (Jk) blood group system was discovered by Allen and colleagues[81] in 1951 with the identification of an antibody responsible for HDN. This antibody and the antigen it defined were named Jk^a. Anti-Jk^b, the antibody defining the product of the allele of Jk^a, was discovered in 1953.[82] In 1959, the null phenotype, Jk(a−b−), and the antigen Jk3 were described. Jk3 is found on Jk(a+) and Jk(b+) red cells, but not those that are Jk(a−b−). More recently, an *In(Jk)* gene, or dominant suppressor gene, has also been described.[83,84] The Jk3 antigen is weakly expressed on these cells.

This blood group system is perhaps most noted for its association with the **delayed hemolytic transfusion reaction** (DHTR). Both anti-Jk^a and anti-Jk^b are often responsible for this consequence of transfusion therapy.

Delayed hemolytic transfusion reaction: Destruction of transfused red cells that happens days to weeks after transfusion. These reactions are difficult to identify and resolve. Anti-Jk^a is frequently associated with delayed hemolytic events. Serologic investigation of these reactions is discussed in Chapter 15.

Genetics and Biochemistry

The *JK* locus has been assigned to the long arm of chromosome 18 (18q11-q12). The product of the *JK* gene is a urea transporter molecule that spans the red cell membrane.[85] The molecular basis for Jk^a and Jk^b is differences in the amino acid found at position 280 on the urea transporter molecule. For the Jk^a antigen, aspartic acid will be present, and for Jk^b, asparagine is found. The Jk(a−b−) phenotype is rare, although it is found more frequently in Polynesian and Chinese populations, and it arises through several genetic mutations.[14] The molecular basis for the Jk3 antigen is unknown. The phenotypes and frequencies are listed in Table 6-6.

The *In(Jk)* gene, which also gives rise to an apparent Jk(a−b−) phenotype, is a dominant **suppressor gene** inherited independently of the genes at the *JK* locus.

Cells that appear to be Jk(a−b−) because of the *In(Jk)* gene actually express decreased quantities of the Jk^a and/or Jk^b antigens, as well as Jk3.

Suppressor gene: A gene that diminishes the effect of another independently inherited gene.

TABLE 6-6 Kidd Blood Group System: Phenotypes and Frequencies

	FREQUENCIES		
Phenotypes	White (%)	Black (%)	Asian (%)
Jk(a+b−)	26.3	51.1	23.22
Jk(a+b+)	50.3	40.8	49.94
Jk(a−b+)	23.4	8.1	26.84
Jk(a−b−)	<0.01	<0.01	0.9 to <0.1

> Of additional interest are the data presented by Heaton and McLoughlin[86] on the resistance to lysis that was noted with Jk(a−b−) red cells when exposed to 2M urea. This phenomenon may be the result of a defect in urea transport.[87] On a more practical note, resistance to lysis with 2M urea can be used as a screening test to identify potential Jk(a−b−) donors in those populations in which the phenotype is likely to occur. Transient Jk(a−b−) red cells have also been described.[88]

Antigens and Antibodies
Jk^a and Jk^b Antigens; Anti-Jk^a and Anti-Jk^b

One of the unique features of this blood group system is the difficulty that often surrounds the detection of Jk antibodies. Although there are adequate copies of Jk antigen per red blood cell (approximately 14,000 copies), detection of complement components activated by these IgG antibodies can be critical relative to detection. Some antibody detection systems are more sensitive in detecting anti-Jk^a and anti-Jk^b. For example, the saline/antiglobulin test is least sensitive, but techniques that include enzymes, LISS, or **polyethylene glycol (PEG)** may aid in the detection and identification of Jk antibodies.[89]

The Jk^a and Jk^b antigens, in general, are rather poor immunogens. Pure examples of anti-Jk^a are sometimes encountered, whereas pure examples of anti-Jk^b are very unusual. These antibodies are more frequently encountered in the sera of patients who have produced multiple blood group alloantibodies.[44]

Delayed Hemolytic Transfusion Reactions and Hemolytic Disease of the Newborn

Both anti-Jk^a and anti-Jk^b have been well documented as the cause of DHTR. Indeed, they are one of the most frequently encountered antibodies that cause DHTR.[44,58] Not only do these antibodies frequently cause DHTR, but they are sometimes difficult to detect. Of particular interest in evaluating these cases of DHTR is the lack of correlation between in vitro reactivity, or the strength of the antibody, and the degree of in vivo red cell destruction. On occasion, antibody removal is so rapid that posttransfusion assessment immediately following transfusion fails to detect antibody, further confounding the difficulties in identification of Kidd antibodies following DHTR. Some examples of these antibodies may react only with cells that are homozygous for the respective antigen, making identification more challenging. It may also be important to use antiglobulin reagents that contain anti-complement in addition to anti-IgG, because activated C3 may be more easily detected than IgG. IgG anti-Jk^a and anti-Jk^b are capable of causing HDN, although only mild cases of the disease have been reported.[90]

Most Kidd antibodies appear to be IgG1 and IgG3, and these antibodies are very efficient at activating complement.[44,58] Because of complement activation, removal of sensitized red cells is primarily in the liver, although occasional exceptional examples of Kidd antibodies have caused intravascular removal of antigen-positive red cells.

Jk3 and Anti-Jk3

As discussed earlier, the Jk3 antigen is produced in the presence of both the Jk^a and Jk^b antigens. It is not produced in the presence of the recessive *Jk* gene, or those mutations that result in the Jk(a−b−) phenotype. However, the *In(Jk)* dominant suppressor does appear to produce diminished quantities of Jk3.

Anti-Jk3 is the antibody produced by Jk(a−b−) individuals. Although anti-Jk^a and/or anti-Jk^b might also be produced as a part of the immune response in Jk(a−b−) individuals, anti-Jk3 behaves like inseparable anti-Jk^a plus anti-Jk^b. Anti-Jk3 has been known to cause mild HDN.[91,92]

Polyethylene glycol (PEG): A potentiating reagent used in antibody identification when weak reactions are encountered.

Autoantibodies

Autoanti-Jk^a has been documented as the causative autoantibody in both warm autoimmune hemolytic anemia and methyldopa (Aldomet)–induced hemolytic anemia.[93] Autoanti-Jk^a has also been associated with a case of chlorpropamide-induced hemolytic anemia. Autoanti-Jk3 has been described.[88] Autoanti-Jk^b in the presence of autoanti-Jk3 has also been described.

> Some of the more interesting autoantibodies associated with the Kidd system are those that appear to be LISS related because of the **parabens** added to these reagents.[94,95] Both propylparaben and methylparaben have been used as preservatives in some commercial LISS preparations. These autoantibodies were detected during routine antibody screening procedures and appeared to have no clinical significance. Judd and colleagues[94] theorized that the Jk^a antigen is altered in the presence of paraben, allowing this now-altered antigen to preferentially react with an antibody that now appears to be anti-Jk^a. The cause of the autoanti-Jk^a remains unclear. The stimulus may have been viral or bacterial in origin, because many patients had recent histories of infections. Paraben-related compounds are widely used as preservatives, so previous encounter with these substances is likely.

Parabens: Substances added to preserve reagents that may result in some discrepant serologic results.

THE LUTHERAN BLOOD GROUP SYSTEM

The Lutheran (Lu) blood group system was discovered in 1945 while evaluating the serum of a patient that contained several previously unidentified alloantibodies.[96] One new antibody was called Lutheran, the name associated with the donor whose red cells reacted with the antibody. This antibody became anti-Lu^a and the antigen it defined, Lu^a. The high-incidence antithetical antigen, Lu^b, was discovered in 1956.[97]

This system currently consists of 19 antigens with four documented pairs of antithetical antigens. These are summarized in Table 6-7. The numbers associated with this system reach 21. However, two previously associated antigens, Lu10 and Lu15, have been shown not to be part of the Lutheran system.

TABLE 6-7 Lutheran Blood Group System Antigens

Alphabetic	Numeric*	Relative Incidence	Comment
Lu^a	LU1	Low	Antithetical to Lu^b
Lu^b	LU2	High	Antithetical to Lu^a
Lu^{ab}	LU3	High	
Lu4	LU4	High	
Lu5	LU5	High	
Lu6	LU6	High	Antithetical to Lu9
Lu7	LU7	High	
Lu8	LU8	High	Antithetical to Lu14
Lu9	LU9	Low	Antithetical to Lu6
Lu11	LU11	High	
Lu12	LU12	High	
Lu13	LU13	High	
Lu14	LU14	Low	Antithetical to Lu8
Lu16	LU16	High	
Lu17	LU17	High	
Au^a	LU18	80%	Antithetical to Lu19
Au^b	LU19	50%	Antithetical to Lu18
Lu20	LU20	High	
Lu21	LU21	High	

*LU10 and LU15 are obsolete.

Additional antithetical antigens of this system include Lu6 (high incidence) and Lu9 (low incidence); Lu8 (high incidence) and Lu14 (low incidence); and Au^a and Au^b. The Au^a (Auberger) antigen has an incidence of approximately 80%, and Au^b has an incidence of 50%.

The additional antigens of the Lutheran system are all of high incidence and include Lu3, Lu4, Lu5, Lu7, Lu11, Lu12, Lu13, Lu16, Lu17, Lu20, and Lu21.[98] The Lu(a−b−) null phenotype is quite rare and can arise from three different genetic mechanisms: a recessive mode of inheritance, an independently inherited suppressor gene (*InLu*), and an X-linked genetic background.[44,58]

Genetics and Biochemistry

The *LU* locus has been assigned to the long arm of chromosome 19 (19q13.2-q13.3).[99] *LU* is linked to the *SE* locus, and this linkage group represents the first example of autosomal linkage in humans. The products of the *LU* gene are the Lutheran glycoprotein and a B-cell adhesion molecule (B-CAM). Both structures belong to the immunoglobulin superfamily.[100]

The amino acid changes responsible for the various Lu antigens have all been identified. Lu^a and Lu^b differ by amino acids found at position 77.[101] For the Lu^a antigen, histidine is present, and for Lu^b, arginine is detected. Lu8 and Lu14 differ by the amino acids detected at position 204. For Lu8, methionine is present, and for Lu14, lysine is detected. Lu6 and Lu9 differ by the amino acids found at position 275. Lu6 demonstrates serine and Lu9, phenylalanine. For the last allelic pair, Au^a and Au^b, differences are found at amino acid 539. Au^a demonstrates alanine and Au^b, threonine. For the presence or absence of the other high-incidence antigens and their amino acid changes, consult Reid and Lomas-Francis.[14]

Lutheran Null Phenotypes
InLu (Dominant Suppressor)

In 1959, the red cells of Dr. Mary Crawford, a noted immunohematologist, were shown to be Lu(a−b−).[102] As family studies were pursued, it became apparent that the genetic cause of this phenotype had to be a dominant gene at a locus other than *LU*, but able to suppress the expression of the Lutheran antigens. The Lu(a−b−) phenotype appeared in each generation, and subsequent additional families were also reported.[103,104] The dominant Lu(a−b−) red cells, however, do produce small amounts of Lutheran antigens, as shown by the ability of these red cells to adsorb and subsequently elute Lutheran antibodies. This small amount of antigen production prevents these individuals from making Lutheran alloantibodies.

Recessive

An Lu(a−b−) individual with an antibody in her serum that was compatible only with the dominant suppressor Lu(a−b−) red cells eventually was shown to be the first example of a recessive Lu(a−b−).[105] The inheritance of two null genes at the Lutheran locus *(LU)* was postulated to be responsible for this phenotype. It has been shown that a missense mutation in exon 6 of the *LU* gene results in a stop codon and failure to produce Lutheran antigens.[14] The antibody produced by recessive Lu(a−b−) individuals was described as anti-Lu3 and considered an inseparable form of anti-Lu^{a}Lu^b. The Lu3 antigen is also produced when Lu^a and/or Lu^b antigens are produced. The recessive-type Lu(a−b−) red cell neither absorbs nor elutes Lutheran antibodies.

X-Linked

The most recent type of Lu(a−b−) to be described arises as a result of inheritance of a gene on the X chromosome that inhibits the expression of the Lutheran antigens.[106] The red cells of these Lu(a−b−) individuals are similar to those of the dom-

TABLE 6-8 Lutheran Null Phenotypes

Type	Genetic Locus Involved	Comments
In(Lu) or dominant suppressor	Locus other than *LU* locus	Produce decreased quantities of Lu antigens
Recessive Lu(a–b–)	Null gene at *LU* locus	May produce anti-Lu3
X-linked Lu(a–b–)	Gene *(XS2)* on X chromosome inhibits Lu antigen expression	Produce decreased quantities of Lu antigens

inant Lu(a–b–), because small amounts of Lutheran antigen can be detected by adsorption and elution studies. However, family studies have failed to demonstrate a dominant suppressor form of inheritance and clearly demonstrate an X-borne recessive inhibitor as the cause of this unusual phenotype. The three types of Lu(a–b–) are summarized in Table 6-8.

Antigens and Antibodies

Lu^a and Lu^b are antithetical antigens. The Lu^a antigen is of lower incidence, occurring on the red cells of approximately 8% of the random population. The vast majority of red cells express the Lu^b antigen.

Anti-Lu^a is a rather uncommon antibody and may occur naturally. Anti-Lu^b, however, is usually produced following transfusion or pregnancy and is usually considered a clinically significant antibody. Mild HDN has been reported with both antibodies, because the Lutheran antigens are poorly developed on fetal cells. Mild transfusion reactions have been attributed to anti-Lu^b.

Antibodies to the remaining Lutheran antigens are rare. Those directed to the high-incidence antigens Lu3, Lu4, Lu5, Lu6, Lu7, Lu8, Lu11, Lu12, Lu13, Lu16, Lu17, Lu20, and Lu21 may be a challenge to identify. But they will all fail to react with Lu(a–b–) red cells and other red cells that lack the high-incidence antigen to which the antibody is directed. Antibodies to Au^a and Au^b are also rare. Anti-Au^a has been identified only on three instances, and each sera contained other antibodies.[107] Examples of antibodies to the remaining low-incidence antigens, Lu9 and Lu14, are also rare, but finding compatible blood in the event of transfusion is quite easy.

THE GERBICH BLOOD GROUP SYSTEM
Gerbich Antigens

The Gerbich (Ge) blood group system represents several high- and low-incidence antigens that total seven in number. However, individuals who lacked the high-incidence antigens and produced antibodies to these missing antigens were responsible for the discovery of this system in 1960.[108] The original type of anti-Ge was named for Mrs. Gerbich, one of three individuals immunized to this antigen. One year later, an additional "anti-Ge" was reported, although it became clear that this antibody-maker (Mrs. Yus) was not identical to the "Gerbich type" (Ge-type) previously described.[109] Although the serum of Mrs. Yus was compatible with the cells of Mrs. Gerbich, Mrs. Gerbich's antibody was incompatible with the Yus red cells.

In 1972, a numeric nomenclature was introduced by Booth and colleagues[87] after they identified anti-Ge1 and described the Melanesian type of Ge-negative cell. Ge1, however, has been removed from the Ge system. Ge2 was described as the antigen missing from the Yus-type Ge-negative cells, and Ge3 and Ge2 were noted

TABLE 6-9 Gerbich Phenotypes		
Historic Name	Numeric System	Frequency
Gerbich-positive	Ge:2,3,4	>99.9%
Yus-type	Ge:−2,3,4	<0.1%
Ge-type	Ge:−2,−3,4	<0.1%
Leach-type	Ge:− 2,−3,−4	Very rare

to be missing from the Ge-type Ge-negative cells. One additional phenotype has been described.[110] This phenotype, called the Leach phenotype, is also Ge:−2,−3 but is different from the Ge-type of Ge-negative red cell, because Leach phenotype cells also lack the high-incidence antigen described as Ge4. Ge4 is found on Ge-positive cells and the Ge-type and Yus-type Ge-negative cells. The four phenotypes that are now described are found in Table 6-9. As can be seen, normal Ge-positive individuals are described as Ge:2,3,4; Yus-type Ge-negative individuals are described as Ge:−2,3,4; Ge-type Ge-negative individuals are described as Ge:−2,−3,4; and Leach-type Ge-negative individuals are described as Ge:−2,−3,−4. As will be further discussed, these antigens are associated with glycophorin C (GPC) and glycophorin D (GPD).[111]

Four low-incidence antigens have been assigned to the Gerbich blood group system: Wb, Ls^a, An^a, and Dh^a.[112]

Genetics and Biochemistry

The *GE(GYPC)* gene resides on chromosome 2 (q14-q21). This gene is unique because it produces two detectable products, glycophorin C (GPC) and glycophorin D (GPD).[113,114] Gerbich antigens have been shown to reside on both GPC and GPD. Ge2 is found on GPD and Ge4 is found on GPC. Ge3 is found on both GPC and GPD.

> The Ge:−2,3,4 phenotype arises because exon 2 of the *GE* gene is deleted. The Ge:−2,−3,4 phenotype arises because exon 3 is deleted. Finally, the Ge:−2,−3,−4 phenotype arises when exons 3 and 4 are deleted. Individuals of the Leach phenotype are considered the null phenotype of the system and lack GPC and GPD.[115-118] It would appear that GPC and GPD are important in maintaining red cell shape because Leach-phenotype red cells are elliptocytic.
>
> The Wb antigen is found on GPC at amino acid 8 when serine is produced instead of the usual asparagine residue. The An^a antigen is found on GPD when serine is found at amino acid 2 instead of the usual alanine residue. Dh^a is found on GPC when the *GE* gene produces phenalanine instead of leucine at position 14. The Ls^a antigen arise because there is duplication of exon 3 of the *GE* gene.[119]

Antibodies

Gerbich alloantibodies, the majority of which are IgG, have been produced as a result of red cell exposure from transfusion and pregnancy. These antibodies have also caused mild HDN.[120] Relative to transfusion therapy, the antibodies may be clinically significant or clinically insignificant. Garratty and colleagues[121] reported one example that demonstrated increased red cell destruction in vivo, along with two examples that did not demonstrate increased red cell destruction.

Gerbich autoantibodies have also been reported as the causative agent of warm autoimmune hemolytic anemia, and specificities have included both anti-Ge2 and anti-Ge3.[93] In general, these autoantibodies failed to react with enzyme-premodified red cells. One unique autoantibody was capable of activating complement.

THE DIEGO BLOOD GROUP SYSTEM
Diego Antigens

The Diego(Di) blood group system initially included only two antigens. But new methods of system assignment have now placed a total of 21 antigens into this blood group system. There are two sets of antithetical antigens. The first includes the antithetical antigens, Di^a and Di^b. The Di^a antigen was described and named in a report of HDN.[122] The Di^a antigen is of low incidence in white and black populations but is of higher incidence in populations of Mongolian extraction. These populations include the Indians of South, Central, and North America and Japanese and Chinese populations.[44] The Di^b antigen is of high incidence. In the United States, nearly all whites and blacks are of the Di(a–b+) phenotype. The Di(a+b+) and Di(a+b–) phenotypes would be found in populations of Mongolian extraction (Table 6-10). The other pair of antithetical antigens includes Wr^a and Wr^b. Wr^a was first discovered when anti-Wr^a was responsible for HDN. Wr^a is an antigen of low incidence.[123] Wr^b is an antigen of high incidence, and only three individuals have been described who lack this antigen.[44] Most individuals are Wr(a–b+). Wr(a+b+) individuals are less common, and the Wr(a+b–) phenotype is extremely rare. The remaining antigens of the Diego blood group system are all of low incidence and include Wd^a, Rb^a, WARR, ELO, Wu, Bp^a, Mo^a, Hg^a, Vg^a, Sw^a, BOW, NFLD, Jn^a, KREP, Tr^a, Fr^a, and SW1.

Genetics and Biochemistry

The *DI* gene has been assigned to chromosome 17(q21-q22). The product of the *DI* gene is band 3 or anion exchanger 1. Band 3 is one of the major proteins of the red cell membrane and has several major functions, including maintaining structural integrity of the red blood cell, the exchange of HCO^3 and Cl anions across the red cell membrane, and stability of the lipid bilayer through interaction

TABLE 6-10 Phenotypes and Frequencies for Some Other Blood Group Systems

System	Phenotypes	Frequencies
Scianna	Sc:1,–2,3	99.7
	Sc:1,2,3	0.3
	Sc:–1,2,3	Very rare
	Sc:–1,–2,–3	Very rare
Diego	Di(a+b–)	Very rare
	Di(a+b+)	Very rare
	Di(a–b+)	100.0
Cartwright	Yt(a+b–)	91.9
	Yt(a+b+)	7.9
	Yt(a–b+)	0.2
Dombrock	Do(a+b–)	17.2
	Do(a+b+)	49.5
	Do(a–b+)	33.3
	Gy(a–)	Very rare
	Hy–	Very rare
	Jo(a–)	Very rare
Colton	Co(a+b–)	89.3
	Co(a+b+)	10.4
	Co(a–b+)	0.3
	Co(a–b–)	Very rare

with phospholipid molecules. Band 3 also interacts with glycophorin A (GPA), and this explains why cells that lack GPA (see MNSs Blood Group System) fail to express the Wr^b antigen.[39,124]

> Di^a and Di^b differ by a single amino acid at position 854 of band 3.[125] The *DI* gene that produces Di^b will express proline, whereas the gene responsible for Di^a production will demonstrate leucine. Wr^a and Wr^b also differ by a single amino acid, but at position 658.[124] The *DI* gene that produces Wr^b demonstrates glutamic acid, whereas the gene responsible for Wr^a production demonstrates lysine. The molecular basis for the remaining 17 antigens has been determined, and the reader is directed to Reid and Lomas-Francis for this information.[14]

OTHER BLOOD GROUP SYSTEMS

This section briefly reviews other blood groups that have been given system status according to the Committee on Terminology for Red Cell Surface Antigens of the International Society of Blood Transfusion.[15] The systems reviewed include Xg, Scianna (Sc), Cartwright (Yt), Dombrock (Do), Colton (Co), Cromer (Cr), and Chido/Rodgers (Ch/Rg).

Xg Blood Group System

In 1962, Mann and colleagues[126] described a red cell antigen whose presence or absence was determined by a gene on the X chromosome. This antigen was called Xg^a and the gene responsible for its production *XG*. The *XG* locus has been assigned to the long arm of the X chromosome (Xp22.3). The *XG* locus is linked to the loci for ocular albinism and retinitis pigmentosa and the gene for X-linked CGD.[23]

Because of its X-linked mode of inheritance, the frequency of the Xg^a antigen differs in females and males. For females, the frequency of the antigen is 89%. The gene behaves as an X-linked dominant trait in females, permitting individuals who are heterozygous and homozygous to express the Xg^a antigen. The frequency of the Xg^a antigen in males is only 67%. Because males inherit only one X chromosome, Xg(a+) males are considered hemizygous for the antigen. Inheritance of the *XG* gene in a male always ensures Xg(a+) daughters. The phenotypes and their frequencies are summarized in Table 6-11.

Anti-Xg^a is an uncommon antibody.[44] The antibody reacts best at the antiglobulin phase of testing and fails to react with protease-premodified red cells. The antibody does not appear to cause significant red cell destruction in vivo and has caused only serologic evidence of newborn red cell sensitization without anemia and jaundice. Autoanti-Xg^a has also been reported.[93]

> A second antigen, CD99, has been added to the Xg blood group system.[127] This antigen was first detected with a monoclonal antibody described as 12E7. The gene responsible for CD99, noted as *MIC2*, has been shown to reside on both the X (p22.2) and Y (p11.2) chromosomes.[127] On the red cells, CD99 is expressed as a qualitative polymorphism related to Xg^a. All Xg(a+) individuals have a high expression of CD99. All Xg(a−) females have a low expression of CD99, but Xg(a−) males may demonstrate either high or low expression of CD99. This variation in expression of CD99 on Xg(a−) males appears to be due to the inheritance of the gene on the Y chromosome.

TABLE 6-11 Frequencies of the Xg(a+) and Xg(a−) Phenotypes		
Phenotype	Males (%)	Females (%)
Xg(a+)	65.6	88.7
Xg(a−)	34.4	11.3

The Scianna Blood Group System

The antibody defining the high-incidence antigen in this system was described in 1962 and was initially called anti-Sm.[128] Although the antibody defining the low-incidence antigen of this system was described the following year, it was not until 1967 that the low-incidence antigen called Bu^a was shown to be antithetical to the high-incidence antigen Sm.[129] A new terminology was then devised for the system and the system renamed Scianna. The Sm antigen became Sc1 and the antibody defining the antigen, anti-Sc1. The Bu^a antigen became Sc2 and the antibody defining the antigen, anti-Sc2. On the Sc glycoprotein, it has been shown that at position 57, glycine is associated with the Sc1 phenotype and arginine is present with the Sc2 phenotype.[130] The Sc phenotypes and their frequencies appear in Table 6-10.

Nason and colleagues[131] expanded the system with their report of a unique family that was Sc:−1,−2. The propositus produced a unique antibody that was called anti-Sc3. This antibody reacted with all Sc:1,−2 and Sc:−1,2 cells and appeared to define a unique antigen, Sc3, that is produced in the presence of either an *Sc1* or *Sc2* gene. In the Sc:−1,−2,−3 phenotype, or null phenotype for the Scianna blood group system, deletions in exons 2 and 3 give rise to a truncated protein. Sc4 (Radin) was most recently added to this blood group system as a low-incidence antigen.[130] Sc:4 cells demonstrate alanine at amino acid 60 and Sc:−4 cells demonstrate proline. The *SC* locus has been assigned to the short arm of chromosome 1 (1p34) and is linked to the *RH, PGM1,* and *UMPK* loci.

Both anti-Sc1 and anti-Sc2 are rare. Although anti-Sc1 appears to be immune in origin, anti-Sc2 may, on occasion, be naturally occurring. Both antibodies are clinically significant. Anti-Sc2 has caused HDN.[132] Autoanti-Sc1 has also been described.[93] Anti-Sc3 and anti-Sc4 are also clinically significant.

The Cartwright Blood Group System

An antibody defining a previously unknown high-incidence antigen was described in 1956 by Eaton and colleagues.[133] The antibody was named anti-Yt^a (Cartwright) and the antigen it defined, Yt^a. The antibody defining the low-incidence antigen, Yt^b, was described in 1964.[134] Phenotype and antigen frequencies for this system are shown in Table 6-10. The gene, *YT,* responsible for these antigens is located on chromosome 7 (q22.1). The product of the gene is a GPI-linked glycoprotein that produces acetylcholinesterase (AchE).

Differences in the Yt^a and Yt^b antigens arise from differences in the amino acid found at position 353 on the glycoprotein structure. Histidine is found for Yt^a and asparagine for Yt^b. PNH III red cells are deficient in AchE and appear Yt(a−).[135]

Although individuals at risk to produce anti-Yt^a are uncommon, the Yt^a antigen appears to be a reasonable immunogen because anti-Yt^a is not uncommon.[44] Some examples of anti-Yt^a have been shown to be clinically significant but others have not. Anti-Yt^a and anti-Yt^b have caused subclinical HDN.

The Dombrock Blood Group System

For many years, the Dombrock system consisted of two antigens, Do^a and Do^b.[136,137] But three additional antigens, all of high incidence, have been added to the Dombrock blood group system: Hy (Holley), Gy^a (Gregory), and Jo^a.[138,139] The gene responsible for the Do glycoprotein has been assigned to chromosome 12 (p12.1-13.2). The Do protein is GPI linked and is absent from paroxysmal nocturnal hemoglobinuria (PNH) III red cells.[138,139] The Gy(a−) phenotype is the null phenotype for this blood group system and can arise by several molecular mechanisms.[140,141]

The Do[a] phenotype demonstrates aspartic acid at amino acid 265 and the Do[b] phenotype, asparagine.[142] The Hy− phenotype demonstrates valine at amino acid 108 and the Hy+ phenotype, glycine.[143] The Jo(a−) phenotype demonstrates isoleucine at amino acid 117 and the Jo(a+) phenotype, threonine.[143] The Hy− and Jo(a−) phenotypes have been found exclusively in black individuals. Hy− individuals demonstrate weakened expression of Do[b] and Gy[a]. Jo(a−) individuals demonstrate weakened expression of Do[a] and Hy. The Dombrock phenotypes and their frequencies are shown in Table 6-10.

Anti-Do[a] and anti-Do[b] are uncommon antibodies and, when encountered, are frequently present with other alloantibodies.[44] Anti-Do[a] and anti-Do[b] appear to be clinically significant.[144] Both have caused only subclinical HDN.

Anti-Hy, anti-Gy[a], and anti-Jo[a] have been responsible for shortened red cell survival following transfusion with incompatible red cells. HDN has been mild or subclinical.

The Colton Blood Group System

Studies describing an antibody, anti-Co[a], defining a high-incidence antigen called Co[a], were published in 1967.[145] The antibody defining the antithetical antigen, Co[b], was reported in 1970.[146] In 1974, Rogers and colleagues[147] described an individual whose red cells were Co(a−b−) and who produced a unique antibody, anti-Co[ab] or anti-Co3. These antisera give rise to four phenotypes: Co(a+b−), Co(a+b+), Co(a−b+), and Co(a−b−). These are shown in Table 6-10.

The gene responsible for the Co phenotypes has been assigned to chromosome 7 (p14). The trans-membrane carrier molecule produced by the *CO* gene is also known as aquaporin-1 and supports water transport. The antigens Co[a] and Co[b] arise because of amino acid changes at position 45 on the carrier molecule. Co(a+) individuals demonstrate alanine at position 45, but those that are Co(b+) demonstrate valine.[148] The Co(a−b−) phenotype arises from a variety of molecular mutations.[149,150] The location of the Co3 antigen is uncertain.

Anti-Co[a] and anti-Co[b] have caused transfusion reactions and should be considered clinically significant.[151] Anti-Co[a] and anti-Co3 have caused HDN.[152]

The Cromer Blood Group System

The Cromer blood group system is composed of eight high-incidence antigens: Cr[a], Tc[a], Dr[a], Es[a], WES[b], UMC, IFC, and GUTI, and three low-incidence antigens: Tc[b], Tc[c], and WES[a].[153,154] These antigens are located on the red cell membrane complement regulatory protein called decay-accelerating factor (DAF).[155,156] DAF is a glycoprotein that is anchored to the red cell membrane by a glycosylphosphatidyl-inositol linkage.[156]

The gene responsible for the production of DAF, named *CROM (DAF)*, is located on chromosome 1 (q32). DAF regulates the action of C3 convertase, and its absence is one of the factors associated with paroxysmal nocturnal hemoglobinuria (PNH).[157] PNH red cells either lack the Cromer-related antigens or express them only weakly.

A null phenotype for this system exists and is called the Inab phenotype or IFC−.[158] This phenotype arises through a variety of molecular mechanisms.[159] Although the red cells of this phenotype are hematologically normal, a relationship appears to exist between this phenotype and intestinal disorders, including protein-losing enteropathy.[160]

Cromer antibodies have been reported to cause transfusion reactions, but not HDN. DAF is strongly expressed on the surface of placental trophoplasts and will absorb antibodies in the Cromer system. Anti-IFC, the antibody produced by the Inab phenotype, does most certainly appear to be clinically significant.[161]

The Chido/Rodgers Blood Group System

Chido (Ch) and Rodgers (Rg) are not integral red cell membrane antigens. They represent components of the fourth complement component (C4) that are adsorbed onto the red cell from the plasma.

> The genes responsible for these complement components are located on chromosome 6 (p21.3). The *CH(C4B)* gene is responsible for C4B or Ch, whereas *RG(C4A)* is responsible for C4A or Rg. C4A and C4B are glycoproteins and are adsorbed onto the red cell membrane with C4A binding preferentially to protein and C4B to carbohydrate.[162,163]

The Ch and Rg antigens reside on the C4d structure of C4. C4-deficient individuals lack both Rg and Ch. However, Rg– individuals are not always C4A deficient and Ch– individuals are not always C4B deficient. Some individuals lacking certain Ch and Rg antigens are susceptible to a number of autoimmune disorders.[164]

> Ch has been subdivided into six high-incidence antigens: Ch1, Ch2, Ch3, Ch4, Ch5, and Ch6. Rg has been subdivided into two high-incidence antigens: Rg1 and Rg2. A ninth antigen, WH, is also part of this blood group system and is associated with the Ch:6, Rg:1,–2 phenotype. The frequency of WH is approximately 15% in the white population. The various phenotypes arise because of amino acid substitutions along the C4 structure. These are summarized in Reid and Lomas-Francis.[14]

Anti-Ch and anti-Rg have not been associated with red blood cell–related transfusion reactions, but have been associated with anaphylactic-type reactions following transfusion with plasma-containing components.[165] Anti-Ch and anti-Rg antibodies are often difficult to identify because reactions are often weak, but they can demonstrate variable reactions with different red cells. These antibodies are best identified by testing sera with C4-sensitized red cells or by inhibition with pooled sera from C4-positive individuals. Anti-Ch and anti-Rg also fail to react with enzyme-premodified red cells.[44]

Miscellaneous Blood Group Systems; Other High- and Low-Incidence Antigens and Antibodies

The JMH Blood Group System

JMH stands for John Milton Hagen, the system's first antibody producer. JMH became a blood group system after it was demonstrated that the JMH glycoprotein is identical to CDw108, and the structure was cloned.[166,167] The *JMH* locus has been assigned to chromosome 15 (q22.3-q23) and produces a single antigen. The glycoprotein bearing the JMH antigen is glycosylphosphatidylinositol (GPI) linked. Antibodies defining this high-incidence antigen are not inhibited with normal serum and fail to react with trypsin-, ficin-, or pronase-premodified red cells. The JMH antigen is absent on PNH III red cells, and anti-JMH has been shown to be clinically insignificant.

The OK Blood Group System

The OK blood group system consists of a single antigen, Okª. This high-incidence antigen is produced by a gene located on chromosome 19 (p13.3). The Ok glycoprotein is identical to the CD147 glycoprotein. The Ok(a–) phenotype arises from an amino acid change at position 92 when lysine is produced instead of glutamic acid. The few Ok(a–) individuals that have been described have been Japanese. The antibody produced by these individuals appears to be clinically significant.

The RAPH Blood Group System

The RAPH blood group system consists of a single antigen, MER2. This high-incidence antigen is produced by a gene located on chromosome 11 (p15.5). The antigen is resistant to ficin and papain treatment, but is sensitive when red cells are treated with trypsin. Anti-MER2 has not been shown to cause increased red cell destruction. Of interest, several individuals producing anti-MER2 were affected with renal disease requiring dialysis.

High-Incidence Antigens

A number of high-incidence antigens, not associated with a known blood group system or having known alleles, have been characterized. In general, these high-incidence antigens are found in more than 90% of the population. The ISBT Working Party on Terminology has categorized these as belonging to the 901 series of high-incidence antigens.[12] The reader is encouraged to consult Issitt and Anstee[44] and Reid and Lomas-Francis[14] for more information on the high-incidence antigens described here and to learn about several others not included in this review.

Vel

Anti-Vel, first described in 1952,[168] is characterized by its ability to activate complement and act as a hemolysin, even though it is primarily an IgG antibody. It has been implicated in several transfusion reactions and, for the most part, is considered clinically significant.[44]

Although the Vel antigen is of high incidence in the random population (99.9%), the expression of the antigen can be variable. Indeed, some apparent examples of Vel– red cells do adsorb and eluate anti-Vel.

Autoanti-Vel has been described in warm autoimmune hemolytic anemia.[93]

Lan (Langereis)

Anti-Lan was first described in 1961.[169] Lan+ red cells are found in more than 99.9% of the random population. Although the incidence of the Lan– phenotype is very low, the antigen is probably fairly immunogenic, because anti-Lan is not uncommon among antibodies defining high-incidence antigens.[44] Anti-Lan is IgG and considered a clinically significant antibody.

At^a (August)

Anti-At^a was first described in 1967.[170] In the random population, the incidence of At^a is greater than 99.9%. Of particular interest, the At(a–) phenotype has been demonstrated only in black individuals. The antibody is IgG and is regarded as clinically significant. Only subclinical HDN has been observed.

Jr^a (Junior)

Anti-Jr^a was first described in 1970 when a total of seven cases were reported.[44] In the random population, the incidence of the Jr^a antigen is greater than 99.9%. It is of interest to note that many of the Jr(a–) individuals who produce anti-Jr^a are Japanese.[171] Anti-Jr^a appears to be a clinically significant IgG antibody.

Sd^a (Sid)

The Sd^a antigen occurs on the red cells of approximately 96% of the random population.[172] However, the amount of antigen present on red cells can be highly variable. Some individuals express large quantities of this antigen and are considered Sd(a+++), or Cad+. Cad+ red cells are considered polyagglutinable.

Anti-Sd^a may naturally occur in the sera of individuals who are Sd(a–).[172] The immunodominant group of the Sd^a antigen is *N*-acetylgalactosamine. In urine, this structure is carried on Tamm and Horsfall glycoprotein. Thus human urine from Sd(a+) individuals can be used to inhibit anti-Sd^a.[44] Although anti-Sd^a is usually considered clinically insignificant, two cases of transfusion reactions precipitated by this antibody have been reported.[173,174]

Low-Incidence Antigens

A number of low-incidence antigens appear to have no known alleles and cannot be placed into a known blood group system. The ISBT Working Party on Terminology has placed these antigens in the 700 series of low-incidence anti-

TABLE 6-12 Low-Incidence Antigens that Remain Unassigned to Blood Group Systems or Collections

Name	Symbol
Batty	By^a
Christiansen	Chr^a
Biles	Bi
Box	Bx^a
Torkildsen	To^a
Peters	Pt^a
Reid	Re^a
Jensen	Je^a
Livesay	Li^a
Milne	
Rasmussen	RASM
Oldeide	Ol^a
	JFV
Katagiri	Kg
Jones	JONES
	HJK
	HOFM
SARA	SARAH
REIT	

gens.[12] Some of these low-incidence antigens appear in Table 6-12. The reader is urged to consult Issitt and Anstee[44] and Reid and Lomas-Francis[14] for more information on the low-incidence antigens noted in Table 6-12 and others in the 700 series. In general, these low-incidence antigens occur in less than 1% of the random population. These low-incidence antigens and the antibodies that define them are often found because they have been responsible for HDN in a specific family in which ABO HDN and HDN due to other known low-incidence antibodies could be excluded.

In addition to causing HDN, antibodies defining low-incidence antigens are sometimes found in the sera of patients with warm autoimmune hemolytic anemia, although the reason for this finding has never been understood.[93] For equally unclear reasons, some individuals produce many antibodies to low-incidence antigens. One of the better-known antisera containing antibodies defining many low-incidence antigens is Tillett, containing 13 specificities.[175]

CHAPTER SUMMARY

1. The Kell blood group system has 24 antigens. Kell system antibodies are considered clinically significant, and anti-K is frequently detected in the serum of immunized individuals.
2. The K$_0$ phenotype represents the null phenotype for the Kell system. An unusual phenotype described as McLeod weakly expresses Kell antigens.
3. The gene *(GYPA)* responsible for the MN antigens is linked to the gene *(GYPB)* responsible for the Ss antigens. The *GYPA* produces glycophorin A and *GYPB*, glycophorin B. Many of the MNSs antigens demonstrable on the red cell are the result of amino acid substitutions on glycophorin A and glycophorin B. The M, N, and S antigens are destroyed by proteases.
4. Anti-M and anti-N, for the most part, are clinically insignificant. Anti-S and anti-s are usually clinically significant.

5. Many unusual phenotypes exist in the MNS blood group system. These include individuals who lack glycophorin A (En(a–)), glycophorin B (U–), or both glycophorins (M^k). There are a number of low-incidence antigens in this blood group system.

6. Anti-Fy^a and anti-Fy^b are clinically significant alloantibodies. Anti-Fy^a is found more frequently than anti-Fy^b. The Fy(a–b–) phenotype is common in black individuals. The Fy^a and Fy^b antigens are destroyed by proteases.

7. Anti-Jk^a and anti-Jk^b are clinically significant, and either may be the causative antibody in a delayed transfusion reaction.

8. The Lutheran blood group system consists of 19 antigens.

9. The Gerbich blood group system antigens reside on glycophorin C and glycophorin D. This complex system has high- and low-incidence antigens.

10. Other blood group systems include Xg, Scianna, Diego, Cartwright, Dombrock, Colton, Chido/Rogers, and Cromer. A number of independent high- and low-incidence antigens have not been assigned system status.

REFERENCES

1. Coombs RRA, Mourant AE, Race RR: In-vivo isosensitisation of red cells in babies with hemolytic disease. Lancet 1:264-266, 1946.

2. Levine P, Backer M, Wigod M, Ponder R: A new human hereditary blood property (Cellano) present in 99.8% of all bloods. Science 109:464-466, 1949.

3. Allen FH Jr, Lewis SJ: Kp^a (Penney), a new antigen in the Kell blood group system. Vox Sang 2:81-87, 1957.

4. Yamaguchi H, Okubo Y, Seno T, et al: A "new" allele, Kp^c, at the Kell complex locus. Vox Sang 36:29-30, 1979.

5. Chown B, Lewis M, Kaita K: A "new" Kell blood-group phenotype. Nature 180:711, 1957.

6. Allen FH Jr, Krabbe SMR, Corcoran PA: A new phenotype (McLeod) in the Kell blood-group system. Vox Sang 6: 555-560, 1961.

7. Giblett ER: Js, a "new" blood group antigen found in Negroes. Nature 181:1221-1222, 1958.

8. Walker RH, Argall CI, Steane EA, et al: Anti-Js^b, the expected antithetical antibody of the Sutter blood group system. Nature 197:295-296, 1963.

9. Guevin RM, Taliano V, Waldmann O: The Cote serum (anti-K11), an antibody defining a new variant in the Kell system. Vox Sang 31(Suppl 1):96-100, 1976.

10. Strange JJ, Kenworthy RJ, Webb AJ, Giles CM: Wk^a (Weeks), a new antigen in the Kell blood group system. Vox Sang 27:81-86, 1974.

11. Lee S, Naime D, Reid M, Redman C: The *KEL24* and *KEL14* alleles of the Kell blood group system. Transfusion 37:1035-1038, 1997.

12. Daniels GL, Cartron JP, Fletcher A, et al: International Society of Blood Transfusion committee on terminology for red cell surface antigens: Vancouver report. Vox Sang 84: 244-247, 2003.

13. Lee S, Russo D, Redman CM: The Kell blood group system. Kell and XK membrane proteins. Semin Hematol 37: 113-121, 2000.

14. Reid M, Lomas-Francis C: The Blood Group Antigens FactsBook, 2nd ed. London, Academic Press, Elsevier, 2004.

15. Advani H, Zamor J, Judd WJ, et al: Inactivation of Kell blood group antigens by 2-aminoethylisothiouronium bromide. Br J Haematol 51:107-115, 1982.

16. Branch DR, Petz LD: A new reagent (ZZAP) having multiple applications in immunohematology. Am J Clin Pathol 78:161-167, 1982.

17. van der Hart M, Szaloky A, van Loghem JJ: A "new" antibody associated with the Kell blood group system. Vox Sang 15:456-458, 1968.

18. Marsh WL, Oyen R, Nichols ME, Allen FH Jr: Chronic granulomatous disease and the Kell blood groups. Br J Haematol 29:247-262, 1975.

19. Bertelson CJ, Pogo AD, Chandhuri A, et al: Localization of the McLeod locus (XK) within XP21 by deletion analysis. Am J Hum Genet 42:703-711, 1988.

20. Russo DCW, Lee S, Reid M, Redman C: Point mutations causing the McLeod phenotype. Transfusion 42:287-293, 2002.

21. Wimer BM, Marsh WL, Taswell HF, Galey WR: Hematological changes associated with the McLeod phenotype of the Kell blood group system. Br J Haematol 36:219-224, 1977.

22. Redman CM, Reid ME: The McLeod syndrome: An example of the value of integrating clinical and molecular studies. Transfusion 42:284-286, 2002.

23. Francke U, Ochs HD, de Martinville D, et al: Minor Xp21 chromosome deletion in a male associated with expression of Duchenne muscular dystrophy, chronic granulomatous disease, retinitis pigmentosa, and McLeod syndrome. Am J Hum Genet 37:250-267, 1985.

24. Marsh WL, Redman CM: Recent developments in the Kell blood group system. Transfusion Med Rev 1:4-20, 1987.

25. Morgan P, Bossom EL: "Naturally-occurring" anti-Kell (K1): Two examples. Transfusion 3:397-398, 1963.

26. Mazzara R. Lozano M, Salmeron JM, et al: Transfusion of incompatible RBCs to a patient with alloanti-Kp[b]. Transfusion 41:611-614, 2001.

27. Schultz M: Serology and clinical significance of Kell blood group system antibodies. In Laird-Fryer B, Daniels G, Levitt J (eds): Blood Group Systems: Kell. Arlington, VA, American Association of Blood Banks, 1990.

28. Landsteiner K, Levine P: A new agglutinable factor differentiating individual human bloods. Proc Soc Exp Biol 24:600, 1927.

29. Landsteiner K, Levine P: On the inheritance of agglutinogens of human blood demonstrable by immune agglutinins. J Exp Med 48:731-749, 1928.

30. Walsh RJ, Montgomery C: A new human isoagglutinin subdividing the MN blood groups. Nature 160:504, 1947.

31. Levine P, Kuhmichel AB, Wigod M, Koch E: A new blood factor, s, allelic to S. Proc Soc Exp Bio 78:218-220, 1951.

32. German J, Metaxas MN, Metaxas-Beuhler M, et al: Further evaluation of a child with the Mk phenotype and a translocation affecting the long arms of chromosomes 2 and 4. Cytogenet Cell Genet 25:160, 1979.

33. Wiener AS, Unger LJ, Gordon EB: Fatal hemolytic transfusion reaction caused by sensitization to a new blood factor U. JAMA 153:1444-1446, 1953.

34. Greenwalt TJ, Sasaki T, Sanger R, et al: An allele of the S(s) blood group genes. Proc Natl Acad Sci 40:1126, 1954.

35. Darnborough J, Dunsford I, Wallace JA: The Ena antigen and antibody. A genetic modification of human red cells affecting their blood group reactions. Vox Sang 17:241-255, 1969.

36. Metaxas MN, Metaxas-Buhler M: Mk: An apparent silent allele at the MN locus. Nature 202:1123, 1964.

37. Huang CH, Blumenfeld OO: MNSs blood group and major glycophorins: Molecular basis for allelic variation. In Cartron JP, Rouger P (eds): Molecular Basis of Major Human Blood Group Antigens. New York, Plenum Press, 1995.

38. Reid ME, Storry JR: Low-incidence MNS antigens associated with single amino acid changes and their susceptibility to enzyme treatment. Immunohematology 17:76-81, 2001.

39. Telen MJ, Chasis JA: Relationship of the human erythrocyte Wrb antigen to an interaction between glycophorin A and band 3. Blood 76:842-848, 1990.

40. Dahr W, Beyreuther K, Steinbach H, et al: Structure of the Ss blood group antigens. II. A methionine/threonine polymorphism within the N-terminal sequence of the Ss glycoprotein. Hoppe-Seylers Z Physiol Chem 361:895-906, 1980.

41. Huang CH, Johe K, Moulds JJ, et al: Delta glycophorin (glycophorin B) gene deletion in two individuals homozygous for the S−s−U− blood group phenotype. Blood 70:1830-1835, 1987.

42. Reid ME, Storry JR, Ralph H, et al: Expression and quantitative variation of the low-incidence blood group antigen He on some S−s− red cells. Transfusion 36:719-724, 1996.

43. Storry JR, Reid ME, MacLennan S, et al: The low-incidence MNS antigens M[V], s[D] and Mit arise from single amino acid substitutions on GPB. Transfusion 41:269-275, 2001.

44. Issitt PD, Anstee DJ: Applied Blood Group Serology, 4th ed. Durham, NC, Montgomery Scientific Publications, 1998.

45. Huang CH, Spruell P, Moulds JJ, Blumenfeld OO: Molecular basis for the human erythrocyte glycophorin specifying the Miltenberger class I (MiI) phenotype. Blood 80:257-263, 1992.

46. Poole J, Banks J, Bruce LJ, et al: Glycophorin A mutation Ala65→Pro gives rise to a novel pair of MNS alleles ENEP (MNS39) and HAG (MNS41) and altered Wr[b] expression: direct evidence for GPA/band 3 interaction necessary for normal Wr[b] expression. Transf Med 9:167-174, 1999.

47. Jarolim P, Moulds JM, Moulds JJ, et al: Molelular basis of the MARS and AVIS blood group antigens (abstract). Transfusion 37: S357, 1997.

48. Dahr W: Miltenberger subsystem of the MNSs blood group system. Vox Sang 62:129-135, 1992.

49. Issitt PD, Pavone GB, Wagstaff W, Goldfinger D: The phenotypes En(a−), Wr(a−b−), and En(a+), Wr(a+b−), and further studies on the Wright and En blood group systems. Transfusion 16:396-407, 1976.

50. Issitt PD, Marsh WL, Wren MR, et al: Heterogeneity of anti-U demonstrable by the use of papain-treated red cells. Transfusion 29:508-513, 1989.

51. Storry JR, Reid ME: Characterization of antibodies produced by S−s− individuals. Transfusion 36:512-516, 1996.

52. Huang CH, Reid ME, Okubo Y, et al: Glycophorin SAT of the human erythrocyte membrane is specified by a hybrid gene reciprocal to glycophorin Dantu gene. Blood 85: 2222-2227, 1995.

53. Dahr W, Beyreuther K, Gallasch E, et al: Amino acid sequence of the blood group Mg-specific major human erythrocyte membrane sialoglycoprotein. Hoppe-Seylers Z Physiol Chem 362:81-85, 1981.

54. Beattie KM, Zuelzer WW: The frequency and properties of pH-dependent anti-M. Transfusion 5:322-326, 1965.

55. Ellisor SS: Action and application of enzymes in immunohematology. In Bell CA (ed): A Seminar on Antigen-Antibody Reactions Revisited. Arlington, VA, American Association of Blood Banks, 1982.

56. Vengelen-Tyler V: The serologic investigation of hemolytic disease of the newborn caused by antibodies other than anti-D. In Garratty G (ed): Hemolytic Disease of the Newborn. Arlington, VA, American Association of Blood Banks, 1984.

57. Harrison PB, Janson K, Kronenberg H, et al: Cold agglutinin formation in patients undergoing haemodialysis. A possible relationship to dialyzer reuse. Aust N Z J Med 5:195-197, 1975.

58. Mollison PL, Englefriet CP, Contreras M: Blood Transfusion in Clinical Medicine, 10th ed. Oxford, Blackwell Scientific, 1997.

59. Telischi M, Behzad O, Issitt PD, Pavone BG: Hemolytic disease of the newborn due to anti-N.Vox Sang 31:109-116, 1976.

60. Arndt P, Garratty G: Evaluation of the optimal incubation temperature for detecting certain IgG antibodies with potential significance. Transfusion 20:210-213, 1988.

61. Cutbush M, Mollison PL, Parkin DM: A new human blood group. Nature 165:188-189, 1950.

62. Ikin EW, Mourant AE, Pettenkofer HJ, Blumenthal G: Discovery of the expected haemagglutinin, anti-Fy^b. Nature 168:1077-1078, 1951.

63. Chown B, Lewis M, Kaita H: The Duffy blood group system in Caucasians: Evidence for a new allele. Am J Hum Genet 17:384-389, 1965.

64. Sanger R, Race RR, Jack JA: The Duffy blood groups of New York Negroes. The phenotype Fy(a−b−). Br J Haematol 1:370-374, 1955.

65. Albrey JA, Vincent EER, Hutchinson J, et al: A new antibody, anti-Fy3, in the Duffy blood group system. Vox Sang 20:29-35, 1971.

66. Wasniowski K, Blanchard D, Janvier D, et al: Identification of the Fy6 epitope recognized by two monoclonal antibodies in the N-terminal extracellular portion of the Duffy antigen receptor for chemokines. Mol Immunol 33:917-923, 1996.

67. Darbonne WC, Rice GC, Mohler MA, et al: Red blood cells are a sink for interleukin 8, a leukocyte chemotaxin. J Clin Invest 88:1362-1369, 1991.

68. Miller LH, Mason SJ, Clyde DF, McGinniss MH: The resistance factor to Plasmodium vivax in blacks. The Duffy blood-group genotype, FyFy. N Engl J Med 295:302-304, 1976.

69. Guiloff RJ, Thomas PK, Contreras M, et al: Linkage of autosomal dominant type 1 hereditary motor and sensory neuropathy to the Duffy locus on chromosome 1. J Neurol Neurosurg Psychiatry 45:669-674, 1982.

70. Yazdanbakhsh K, Rios M, Storry JR, et al: Molecular mechanisms that lead to reduced expression of Duffy antigens. Transfusion 40:310-320, 2000.

71. Beattie KM: Production of anti-Fy^a in black Fy(a−b−) individuals (letter). Immunohematology 1:14, 1984.

72. Oberdorfer CE, Kahn B, Moore V, et al: A second example of anti-Fy3 in the Duffy blood group system. Transfusion 14:608-611, 1974.

73. Buchanan DI, Sinclair M, Sanger R, et al: An Alberta Cree Indian with a rare Duffy antibody, anti-Fy3. Vox Sang 30:114-121, 1976.

74. Oakes J, Taylor D, Johnson C, Marsh WL: Fy3 antigenicity of blood of newborns (letter). Transfusion 18:127, 1978.

75. Miller LH, Mason SJ, Dvorak JA, et al: Erythrocyte receptors for (Plasmodium knowlesi) malaria: Duffy blood group determinants. Science 189:561-563, 1975.

76. Miller LH, Dvorak JA, Shiroishi T, Durocher JR: Influence of erythrocyte membrane components on malaria merozoite invasion. J Exp Med 138:1597-1601, 1973.

77. Hadley TJ, Peiper SC: From malaria to chemokine receptor: The emerging physiologic role of the Duffy blood group antigen. Blood 89:3077-3091, 1997.

78. Chaudhuri A, Zbrzezna V, Johnson C, et al: Purification and characterization of an erythrocyte membrane protein complex carrying Duffy blood group antigenicity. Possible receptor for Plasmodium vivax and Plasmodium knowlesi malaria parasite. J Biol Chem 264:13770-13774, 1989.

79. Nichols ME, Rubinstein P, Barnwell J, et al: A new human Duffy blood group specificity defined by a murine monoclonal antibody. Immunogenetics and association with susceptibility to Plasmodium vivax. J Exp Med 166:776-785, 1987.

80. Horuk R, Chitnis C, Darbonne W, et al: A receptor for the malarial parasite Plasmodium vivax: The erythrocyte chemokine receptor. Science 261:1182-1184, 1993.

81. Allen FH, Diamond LK, Niedziela B: A new blood group antigen. Nature 167:482, 1951.

82. Plaut G, Ikin EW, Mourant AE, et al: A new blood group antibody, anti-Jk^b. Nature 171:431, 1953.

83. Pinkerton FJ, Mermod LE, Liles BA, et al: The phenotype Jk(a−b−) in the Kidd blood group system. Vox Sang 4:155-160, 1959.

84. Okubo Y, Yamaguchi H, Nagao N, et al: Heterogeneity of the phenotype Jk(a−b−) found in Japanese. Transfusion 26:237-239, 1986.

85. Sands JM: Molecular approaches to urea transporters. J Am Soc Nephrol 13:2795-2806, 2002.

86. Heaton DC, McLoughlin K: Jk(a−b−) red blood cells resist urea lysis. Transfusion 22:70-71, 1982.

87. Booth PB, McLoughlin K, Spark R: The Gerbich blood group system especially in Melanesians. Vox Sang 22:73-84, 1972.

88. Issitt PD, Obarski G, Hartnett PL, et al: Temporary suppression of Kidd system antigen expression accompanied by transient production of anti-Jk3. Transfusion 30:46-50, 1990.

89. Nance S, Garratty G: Polyethylene glycol: A new potentiator of red blood cell antigen-antibody reactions. Am J Clin Pathol 87:633-635, 1987.

90. Dorner I, Moore JA, Chaplin H: Combined maternal erythrocyte autosensitization and materno-fetal Jk^a incompatibility. Transfusion 14:211-219, 1974.

91. Pierce SR, Hardman JT, Steele S, Beck ML: Hemolytic disease of the newborn associated with anti-Jk3. Transfusion 20:189-191, 1980.

92. Kuczmarski CA, Bergren MO, Perkins HA: Mild hemolytic disease of the newborn due to anti-Jk3: A serological study of the family's Kidd antigens. Vox Sang 43:340-344, 1982.

93. Petz LD, Garratty G: Immune Hemolytic Anemias, 2nd ed. Philadelphia, Churchill-Livingston, 2004.

94. Judd WJ, Steiner EA, Cochran RK: Paraben-associated autoanti-Jk^a antibodies. Transfusion 22:31-35, 1982.

95. Halma D, Garratty G, Bueno R: An apparent anti-Jk^a reacting only in the presence of methyl esters of hydroxybenzoic acid. Transfusion 22:521-524, 1982.

96. Callener S, Race RR, Pagkov ZV: Hypersensitivity to transfused blood. Br Med J 2:83, 1945.

97. Cutbush M, Chanerin I: The expected blood-group antibody, anti-Lu^b. Nature 178:855-856, 1956.

98. Poole J: Review: The Lutheran blood group system 1991. Immunohematology 8:1-8, 1992.

99. Zelinski T, Coghlan G, Greenberg PH, et al: Evidence that *SE* is distal to *LU* on chromosome 19q. Transfusion 29:304-305, 1989.

100. Parsons SF, Mallinson G, Holmes CH, et al: The Lutheran blood group glycoprotein, another member of the immunoglobulin superfamily, is widely expressed in human tissues and is developmentally regulated in human liver. Proc Natl Acad Sci 92:5496-5500, 1995.

101. Parsons SF, Mallinson G, Daniels GL, et al: Use of domain-deletion mutants to locate Lutheran blood group antigens to each of the five immunoglobulin superfamily domains of the Lutheran glycoprotein: Elucidation of the molecular basis of the Lu(a)/Lu(b) and Au(a)/Au(b) polymorphisms. Blood 89:4219-4225, 1997.

102. Crawford MN, Greenwalt TJ, Sasaki T, et al: The phenotype Lu(a−b−) together with unconventional Kidd groups in one family. Transfusion 1:228-232, 1961.

103. Taliano V, Guevin RM, Tippett P: The genetics of a dominant inhibitor of the Lutheran antigens. Vox Sang 24:42-47, 1973.

104. Tippett P: A case of suppressed Lu^a and Lu^b antigens. Vox Sang 20:378-380, 1971.

105. Darnborough J, Firth R, Giles CM, et al: A "new" antibody anti-Lu^{a}Lu^b and two further examples of the gene type Lu(a−b−). Nature (Lond) 198:796, 1963.

106. Norman PC, Tippett P, Beal RW: An Lu(a−b−) phenotype caused by an X-linked recessive gene. Vox Sang 51:49-52, 1986.

107. Daniels GL, Le Pennec PY, Rouger P, et al: The red cell antigens Au^a and Au^b belong to the Lutheran system. Vox Sang 60:191-192, 1991.

108. Rosenfield RE, Haber GV, Kissmeyer-Nielson JA, et al: Ge, a very common red cell antigen. Br J Haematol 6:344-349, 1960.

109. Barnes R, Lewis TLT: A rare antibody (anti-Ge) causing haemolytic disease of the newborn. Lancet 2:1285-1286, 1961.

110. Anstee DJ, Parsons SF, Ridgwell K, et al: Two individuals with elliptocytic red cells apparently lack three minor red cell membrane sialoglycoproteins. Biochem J 218: 615-619, 1984.

111. Dahr W, Kiedrowski S, Blanchard D, et al: High frequency antigens of human erythrocyte membrane sialoglycoproteins, V. Characterization of the Gerbich blood group antigens: Ge2 and Ge3. Biol Chem Hoppe Seyler 368:1375-1383, 1987.

112. Reid ME, Spring FA: Molecular basis of glycophorin C variants and their associated blood group antigens. Transfus Med 4:139-146, 1994.

113. Colin Y, Le Van Kim C, Tsapis A, et al: Human erythrocyte glycophorin C. Gene structure and rearrangement in genetic variants. J Biol Chem 264:3773-3780, 1989.

114. High S, Tanner MJ, Macdonald EB, Anstee DJ: Rearrangement of the red-cell membrane glycophorin C (sialoglycoprotein β) gene. A further study of alterations in the glycophorin C gene. Biochem J 262:47-54, 1989.

115. Anstee DJ, Ridgwell K, Tanner MJA, et al: Individuals lacking the Gerbich blood group antigen have alterations in the human erythrocyte membrane sialoglycoproteins and

116. rearrangement in genetic variants. Biochem J 221:97-104, 1984.

116. Dahr W, Moulds J, Baumeister G, et al: Altered membrane blood group antigens. Biol Chem Hoppe Seyler 366:201-211, 1985.

117. Reid ME, Anstee DJ, Tanner MJA, et al: Structural relationships between human erythrocyte sialo-glycoprotein and abnormal sialoglycoproteins found in certain rare human erythrocyte variants lacking the Gerbich blood group antigen(s). Biochem J 244:123-128, 1987.

118. Telen MJ, Bolk TA: Human red cell antigens, IV. The abnormal sialoglycoprotein of Gerbich-negative red cells. Transfusion 27:309-341, 1987.

119. Reid ME, Mawby W, King MJ, Sistonen P: Duplication of exon 3 in the glycophorin C gene gives rise to the Ls^a blood group antigen. Transfusion 34:966-969, 1994.

120. Sacks DA, Johnson CS, Platt LD: Isoimmunization in pregnancy to Gerbich antigen. Am J Perinatol 2:208-210, 1985.

121. Garatty G, Nance S, O'Neill P: Correlation of monocyte monolayer assays and RBC survival in patients with alloantibodies of questionable clinical significance (abstract). Transfusion 25:474, 1985.

122. Levine P, Robinson EA, Layrisee M, et al: The Diego blood factor. Nature 177:40, 1956.

123. Lewis M, Kaita H, Phillipps S, McAlpine PJ: The low-incidence red cell antigen Wr^a: genetic studies. Transfusion 31:47-51, 1991.

124. Bruce LJ, Ring SM, Anstee DJ, et al: Changes in the blood group Wright antigens are associated with a mutation at amino acid 658 in human erythrocyte band 3: A site of interaction between band 3 and glycophorin A under certain conditions. Blood 85:541-547, 1995.

125. Bruce LJ, Anstee DJ, Spring FA, Tanner MJ: Band 3 Memphis variant II. Altered stilbene disulfonate binding and the Diego (Di^a) blood group antigen are associated with the human erythrocyte band 3 mutation Pro854→Leu. J Biol Chem 269:16155-16158, 1994.

126. Mann JD, Cahan A, Gelb AG, et al: A sex-linked blood group. Lancet 1:8-10, 1962.

127. Tippett P, Ellis NA: The Xg blood group system: A review. Trans Med Rev 12:233-257, 1998.

128. Schmidt RP, Griffitts JJ, Northman FF: A new antibody, anti-Sm, reacting with a high incidence antigen. Transfusion 2:338-340, 1962.

129. Lewis M, Chown B, Schmidt RP, Griffitts JJ: A possible relationship between the blood group antigens Sm and Bu^a. Am J Hum Genet 16:254, 1964.

130. Wagner FF, Poole J, Flegel WA: Scianna antigens includingRd are expressed by ERMAP. Blood 101:752-757, 2003.

131. Nason SG, Vengelen-Tyler V, Cohen N, et al: A high incidence antibody (anti-Sc3) in the serum of a Sc:−1,−2 patient. Transfusion 20:531-535, 1980.

132. DeMarco M, Uhl L, Fields L, et al: Hemolytic disease of the newborn due to the Scianna antibody, anti-Sc2. Transfusion 35:58-60, 1995.

133. Eaton BR, Morton JA, Pickles MM, White KE: A new antibody, anti-Yt^a, characterizing a blood group antigen of high incidence. Br J Haematol 2:333-341, 1956.

134. Giles CM, Metaxas MN: Identification of the predicted blood group antibody anti-Yt[b]. Nature 202:1122-1123, 1964.

135. Bartels CF, Zelinski T, Lockridge O: Mutation at codon 322 in human acetylcholinesterase (ACHE) gene accounts for YT blood group polymorphism. Am J Hum Genet 52:928-936, 1993.

136. Swanson JL, Polesky HF, Tippett P, Sanger R: A "new" blood group antigen, Do[a]. Nature 206:313, 1965.

137. Molthan L, Crawford MN, Tippett P: Enlargement of the Dombrock blood group system: The finding of anti-Do[b]. Vox Sang 24:382-384, 1973.

138. Spring FA, Reid ME: Evidence that the human blood group antigens Gy[a] and Hy are carried on a novel glycosylphatidylinositol-linked erythrocyte membrane glycoprotein. Vox Sang 60:53-59, 1991.

139. Spring FA, Reid ME, Nicholson G: Evidence for expression of the Jo[a] blood group antigen on the Gy[a]/Hy-active glycoprotein. Vox Sang 66:72-77, 1994.

140. Banks JA, Hemming N, Poole J: Evidence that the Gy[a], Hy and Jo[a] antigens belong to the Dombrock blood group system. Vox Sang 68:177-182, 1995.

141. Reid ME: The Dombrock blood group system: A review. Transfusion 43:107-114, 2003.

142. Gubin AN, Njoroge JM, Wojda U, et al: Identification of the Dombrock blood group glycoprotein as a polymorphic member of the ADP-ribosyltransferase gene family. Blood 96:2621-2627, 2000.

143. Rios M, Hue-Roye K, Oyen R, et al: Insights into the Holley-negative and Joseph-negative phenotypes. Transfusion 42:52-58, 2002.

144. Shirey RS, Boyd JS, King KE, et al: Assessment of the clinical significance of anti-Do[b]. Transfusion 38:1026-1029, 1998.

145. Heisto H, van der Hart M, Madsen G: Three examples of a red cell antibody, anti-Co[a]. Vox Sang 12:18-24, 1967.

146. Giles CM, Darnborough J, Aspinall P, Fletton MW: Identification of the first example of anti-Co[b]. Br J Haematol 19:267-269, 1970.

147. Rogers MJ, Stiles PA, Wright J: A new minus-minus phenotype: Three Co(a–b–) individuals in one family (abstract). Transfusion 14:508, 1974.

148. Smith BL, Preston GM, Spring F, et al: Human red cell aquaporin CHIP. I. Molecular characterization of ABH and Colton blood group antigens. J Clin Invest 94:1043-1049, 1994.

149. Preston GM, Smith BL, Zeidel ML, et al: Mutations in aquaporin-1 in phenotypically normal humans without functional CHIP water channels. Science 265:1585-1587, 1994.

150. Chretien S, Cartron JP, de Figueiredo M: A single mutation inside the MPA motif of aquaporin-1 found in a Colton-null phenotype. Blood 93:4021-4023, 1999.

151. Dzik WH, Blank J: Accelerated destruction of radiolabelled red cells due to anti-Colton b. Transfusion 26:246-248, 1986.

152. Joshi SR, Wagner FF, Vasantha K, et al: An *AQP1* null allele in an Indian woman with Co(a–b–) phenotype and high-titer anti-Co3 associated with mild HDN. Transfusion 41:1273-1278, 2001.

153. Lublin DM, Dompelli S, Storry JR, Reid ME: Molecular basis of Cromer blood group antigens. Transfusion 40:208-213, 2000.

154. Storry JR, Sausais L, Hue-Roye K, et al: GUTI: a new antigen in the Cromer blood group system. Transfusion 43:340-344, 2003.

155. Telen MJ, Hall SE, Green AM, et al: Identification of human erythrocyte blood group antigens on decay-accelerating factor (DAF) and an erythrocyte phenotype negative for DAF. J Exp Med 167:1993-1998, 1988.

156. Lublin DM, Atkinson JP: Decay-accelerating factor: Biochemistry, molecular biology and function. Ann Rev Immunol 7:35, 1989.

157. Medof ME, Kinoshita T, Silber R, Nussenzweig V: Amelioration of lytic abnormalities of paroxysmal nocturnal hemoglobinuria with decay-accelerating factor. Proc Natl Acad Sci 82:2980, 1985.

158. Daniels GL, Tohyama H, Uchikawa M: A possible null phenotype in the Cromer blood group complex. Transfusion 22:362-363, 1982.

159. Wang L, Uchikawa M, Tsuneyama H, et al: Molecular cloning and characterization decay-accelerating factor deficiency in Cromer blood group Inab phenotype. Blood 91:680-684, 1998.

160. Telen MJ, Green AM: The Inab phenotype: Characterization of the membrane protein and complement regulatory defect. Blood 74:437-441, 1989.

161. Smith KJ, Coonce LS, South SF, et al: Anti-Cr[a]: Family study and survival of chromium-labeled incompatible red cells in a Spanish American patient. Transfusion 23:167-169, 1983.

162. O'Neill GJ, Yang SY, Dupont B: Two HLA-linked loci controlling the fourth component of complement. Proc Natl Acad Sci 75:5165-5169, 1978.

163. Giles CM, Swanson JL: Anti-C4 in the serum of a transfused C4-deficient patient with systemic lupus erythematosus. Vox Sang 46:291-299, 1984.

164. Moulds JM: Association of blood goup antigens with immunologically important proteins. In Garratty G (ed): Immunobiology of Transfusion Medicine. New York, Deffer.

165. Westhoff CM, Sipherd BD, Wylie DE, Toalson LD: Severe anaphylactic reactions following transfusions of platelets to a patient with anti-Ch. Transfusion 32:576-579, 1992.

166. Mudad R, Rao N, Angelisova P, et al: Evidence that CDw 108 membrane protein bears the JMH blood group antigen. Transfusion 35:566-570, 1995.

167. Yamada A, Kubo K, Takeshita T, et al: Molecular cloning of a glycosylphosphatidylinsoitol-anchored molecule CDw 108. J Immunol 162:4094-4100, 1999.

168. Sussman LN, Miller EB: Un nouveau facteur sanguin "Vel." Rev Hémat 68, 1952.

169. van der Hart M, Moes M, van der Veer M, van Loghem JJ: Proceedings of the 8th Congress of the European Society of Hematology. Basel, Karger, 1961.

170. Applewhaite F, Ginsberg V, Cerena J, et al: A very frequent red cell antigen, At^a. Vox Sang 13:444-445, 1967.
171. Nakajima H, Ito K: An example of anti-Jr^a causing hemolytic disease of the newborn and frequency of Jr^a antigen in the Japanese population. Vox Sang 35:265-267, 1978.
172. Morton JA, Pickles MM, Terry AM: The Sd^a blood group antigen in tissues and body fluids. Vox Sang 19:472-482, 1970.
173. Peterman ME, Cole-Dergent J: Haemolytic transfusion reaction due to anti-Sd^a. Vox Sang 18:67-70, 1970.
174. Reznicek MJ, Cordle DG, Strauss RG: A hemolytic reaction implicating Sd^a antibody missed by immediate spin crossmatch. Vox Sang 62:173-175, 1992.
175. Contreras M, Stebbing B, Armitage SE, Lukenko A: Further data on the Pt^a antigen. Vox Sang 35:181-183, 1978.

FURTHER READINGS

Brecher ME (ed): Technical Manual, 14th ed. Bethesda, MD, American Association of Blood Banks, 2002.
Daniels G: Human Blood Groups, 2nd ed. Blackwell Science, Oxford, 2002.
Issitt PD, Anstee DJ: Applied Blood Group Serology, 4th ed. Durham, NC, Montgomery Scientific Publications, 1998.
Mollison PL, Englefriet CP, Contreras M: Blood Transfusion in Clinical Medicine, 10th ed. Oxford, Blackwell Scientific, 1997.
Reid M, Lomas-Francis C: The Blood Group Antigens FactsBook, 2nd ed. London, Academic Press, Elsevier, 2004.

VETERINARY TRANSFUSION MEDICINE

C. Guillermo Couto, DVM, dip. ACVIM, and Susan M. Cotter, DVM, dip. ACVIM

The history of veterinary transfusion medicine parallels and is intertwined with that of human medicine. As late as the end of the nineteenth century, blood was commonly transfused from one animal to another and even from animals to human patients. Although some of these transfusions appeared, at least temporarily, to be successful, Landsteiner's discovery of the human ABO blood group system opened the way for modern transfusion medicine. Over the next few years, blood group systems were identified in domestic animals. Although the same letters of the alphabet are used to identify human and animal red cell antigens, they are species specific. For example antigen A of the dog is not the same as the A antigens of humans, horses, or cats.

Domestic cats have only one known blood group system, which consists of three blood types, A, B, and AB, defined by specific carbohydrates on the red cell membrane.[1] Most cats are type A, but certain breeds have a higher prevalence of type B group; type AB is rare, and inherited as a separate allele. Cats have naturally occurring antibodies to the antigens that they lack, and acute severe reactions have been documented on the first exposure to the foreign antigen. An in-house kit is now available for typing cats, and crossmatching is used routinely.

Dogs have 10 to 12 blood group systems, but most have not been well characterized biochemically. Most of the research on canine blood groups was done more than 40 years ago by Swisher and Young.[10] The various antigens vary in immunogenicity and prevalence. The most significant one is known as dog erythrocyte antigen (DEA) 1.1, which is present in 40% to 50% of dogs.[3] Although naturally occurring antibodies against this antigen have not been recognized, antibodies readily form when a negative dog receives positive red cells. A second positive transfusion is likely to result in an acute hemolytic reaction in the negative dog. Although naturally occurring antibodies have been identified at low titers for a few of the other antigens, they are of minimal clinical relevance, at least for the first transfusion.[3] Typing reagents are available for only six of the canine red cell antigens, and in-house typing is limited to DEA 1.1. Veterinarians in clinical practice may use reference labs to type their donors and, unless immediate typing of recipients is available, many use only DEA 1.1–negative donors. Crossmatching is used to detect any other acquired antibodies in dogs needing subsequent transfusions.

In large animals such as horses, cattle, sheep, goats, and pigs, blood groups have been studied extensively. This information has been used primarily in basic genetics for breeding and identification purposes, rather than for transfusions. Blood groups of cattle appear to be the most complex, with over 80 blood groups and more than 1000 alleles in the B group alone.[6] Before the advent of DNA evaluation, blood typing was used extensively for parentage testing because artificial insemination is commonly used and the sire may be many miles away. Transfusions are used clinically, especially in horses, but typing is available only in reference labs. Horses are sometimes typed and those that are negative for the most antigenic A and Q phenotypes used as donors. South American camelids have become popular as pets and farm animals in the past two decades, but little research on their blood groups has been done; despite that, transfusions of fresh-frozen plasma (FFP) or plasma are frequently used for failure of passive transfer (FPT) in newborns (crias), and red blood cell transfusions are commonly used in llamas and alpacas with anemia.

Transfusions are sometimes given to pet birds or endangered species such as eagles. Historically, blood from species such as chickens or pigeons was used, but it was later shown that red cell survival was poor across avian species.

Hemolytic disease of the newborn (HDN) occurs in domestic animals, most commonly in mules, horses, and cats.[2] The human placenta allows transfer of alloantibodies to the fetus. Because the placental wall in most domestic species is thicker than that in humans, maternal antibodies do not cross the placenta into animal fetuses. Instead, the neonatal animal absorbs these antibodies through colostrum in the first day of life. Even with their first pregnancy, cats with blood type B secrete strong anti-A antibodies in the colostrum. This causes HDN in kittens with A phenotype. Maternal antibodies in horses may develop from exposure to fetal red cells during pregnancy. Foals of subsequent pregnancies can be affected through nursing. The prevalence of HDN is especially high in neonate horses (1%) and mules (10%), the result of a horse/donkey mating.[2] Dogs have been sensitized by transfusion and cattle by vaccines of blood origin. In all of these species, offspring are normal at birth, and develop hemolysis in hours to days after nursing. Maternal antibodies can be detected before parturition, and colostrum withheld from neonates positive for the antigen in question.

Withholding colostrum can protect against HDN, but all domestic animals depend on colostrum also for early protection against infectious diseases. Puppies and kittens receive 5% to 10% of maternal IgG transplacentally. In foals, calves, and crias virtually no in utero transfer of maternal IgG occurs. Any newborn animal deprived of colostrum, either by intent or through failure to nurse, requires supplementation with oral colostrum, or parenteral serum or plasma free of antibodies against their red cell antigens.

Blood components are now routinely prepared in commercial animal blood banks, university hospitals, and large veterinary practices. Greyhounds make excellent canine blood donors because of their size, gentle disposition, high hematocrit (range: 55% to 65%), high prevalence of DEA 1.1–negative type, and ease of blood collection because of the large size of their jugular veins. Blood collection in dogs and large animals is done under manual restraint, whereas most cats need to be heavily sedated or anesthetized. All donors undergo physical examination and routine lab work; they are also screened for the most common transmissible infectious diseases and are blood typed.

Nowadays the following canine blood components are prepared and stored: whole (fresh) blood (WFB), packed red blood cells (pRBCs), FFP, cryoprecipitate (CRYO), cryoprecipitate-poor plasma (cryopoor), plasma, platelet-rich plasma (PRP), and platelet concentrates.[7,9] Some blood banks also prepare pRBCs and FFP from cats; camelid and equine components are also available through some commercial and university blood banks. The preparation of components allows for transfusion of the specific blood product (or products) for the patient's needs and maximizes the number of products available without the need to increase the donor pool. Moreover, with the use of additive solutions, canine pRBCs and whole blood (WB) can be stored for longer periods (5 weeks).[4,8] In 1998, the Food and Drug Administration approved a hemoglobin-based oxygen carrying solution for use in dogs with anemia (Oxyglobin, Biopure Corporation, Boston, Mass.); this product is widely used by veterinary practitioners for the treatment of dogs with acute anemia, because it is readily available, does not require specific storage conditions, and has a long shelf-life. Although not yet

approved in this species, Oxyglobin is also used in cats with anemia, but it may cause systemic and pulmonary hypertension if given rapidly.

In dogs, pRBCs, WFB, and WB are used primarily in patients with acute anemia (e.g., blood loss, hemolysis), whereas in cats red blood cell–containing components are used for patients with chronic anemias (e.g., chronic renal failure, bone marrow disorders).[4,5,8] In dogs, CRYO is used mainly in the treatment or prevention of bleeding in patients with von Willebrand's disease, although a small number of dogs with hemophilia A also benefit from this product; CRYO is rarely used as a source of fibrinogen in dogs. Cryopoor plasma, FFP, and plasma are used mainly in dogs with rodenticide toxicity due to vitamin K antagonists, a common problem in veterinary practices; dogs with pancreatitis, liver disease, disseminated intravascular coagulation, antithrombin deficiency due to protein-losing nephropathy or enteropathy, and hypoalbuminemia also receive these plasma products. In cats, FFP and plasma are used primarily for liver disease.[5] As discussed earlier, FFP and plasma are frequently used in llamas and alpacas for FPT. Because platelet products are difficult to obtain and store in animals, platelet transfusions are rarely used.

REFERENCES

1. Auer L, Bell K: The AB blood group system in cats. Anim Genet 12:287, 1981.
2. Becht JL: Neonatal isoerythrolysis in the foal. Part 1. Background blood group antigens and pathogenesis. Compend Cont Educ Pract Vet 5:591, 1983.
3. Bull RW, Vriesendorp HM, Cech R, et al: Joint report of the 3rd international workshop on canine immunogenetics. Transplantation 43:154, 1987.
4. Callan MB, Oakley DA, Shofer FS, Giger U: Canine red blood cell transfusion practice. J Am Anim Hosp Assoc 32:303, 1996.
5. Castellanos I, Gray TL, Couto CG: Clinical use of blood products in cats: A retrospective study (1997-2000). J Vet Intern Med 18(4):529-532, 2004.
6. Cotter SM: Comparative Transfusion Medicine. San Diego, Academic Press, 1991.
7. Feldman BF, Zinkl JG, Jain NC: Schalm's Veterinary Hematology, 5th ed. Lippincott Williams & Wilkins, Philadelphia, 2000.
8. Kerl ME, Hohenhaus AE: Packed red blood cell transfusions in dogs: 131 cases (1989). J Am Vet Med Assoc 202:1495, 1993.
9. Kristensen AT, Feldman BF: Canine and Feline Transfusion Medicine (Veterinary Clinics of North America, Small Animal Practice). Philadelphia, WB Saunders, 1995.
10. Swisher SN, Young LE: The blood group systems of dogs. Physiol Rev 41:495, 1961.

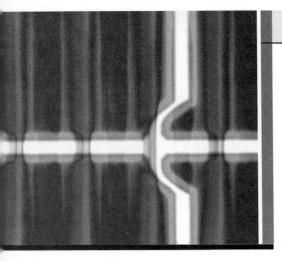

The HLA System

Brian Susskind

LEARNING OBJECTIVES

After reading and studying this chapter the student should be able to:

1. Define MHC and briefly describe the history of the HLA system.
2. Describe the phenomenon of MHC restriction.
3. Briefly describe the physiologic process that takes place when an individual is exposed to a foreign antigen.
4. Discuss the functional differences between MHC (HLA) class I and class II molecules.
5. Define adaptive and innate immunity.
6. Briefly describe the molecular structure of MHC (HLA) class I and class II molecules.
7. Describe how HLA antigens are inherited.
8. Given maternal and paternal haplotypes, determine the possible genotypes of offspring.
9. Explain linkage disequilibrium.
10. Describe both serologic and molecular techniques used to define HLA antigens.
11. Briefly describe the historical development of HLA nomenclatures.
12. Define private and public epitopes.
13. Describe the principle and applications of the complement-dependent cytotoxicity (CDC) test.
14. Discuss the advantages and disadvantages of the CDC procedures versus molecular techniques.
15. Discuss how PRA results are used in clinical decision making.
16. Describe the clinical significance of HLA crossmatch procedures.
17. Describe three methods for purification of B lymphocytes.
18. Discuss briefly three clinical applications of HLA testing.
19. List two HLA-disease associations.
20. Describe the two main theories regarding the etiology of transfusion-related acute lung injury (TRALI).

DISCOVERY OF THE HLA SYSTEM

Over 50 years after the discovery of the ABO blood group system on red blood cells by Karl Landsteiner in 1901, the first human leukocyte antigen (HLA) system was described by Dausset.[1,2] In his 1954 report, Dausset noted **leukoagglutinins** in the sera of **neutropenic** patients who had received many blood transfusions. These leukoagglutinins were alloantibodies produced after exposure to leukocyte antigens foreign to the recipient and were capable of agglutinating white blood cells of other individuals.[2-4] Similar findings were observed in the sera of pregnant women in whom the fetus served as the source of foreign HLA antigens.[5,6]

Leukoagglutinins: Antibodies to antigens on the surface of white cells that can be identified by their ability to agglutinate antigen-positive cells.

Neutropenia: A decrease in the number of circulating neutrophils in the peripheral blood.

CHAPTER SEVEN

The HLA system is the human homolog of major histocompatibility complex (MHC) genes present in all vertebrates and many invertebrates. The MHC was first discovered in mice by Peter Gorer and George Snell, who showed it to be the major barrier to tissue transplantation between different strains of murine species, and dubbed it H-2.[7-9] That HLA is the human homolog of murine H-2 was shown by the observations of Friedman and colleagues in the 1960s, which implied the association between leukoagglutinating antibodies and tissue transplantation.[10] In their studies of skin graft recipients, these investigators noted accelerated skin graft rejection in recipients who were preimmunized with white blood cells from the prospective donor, and family studies showed that the antigens were genetically determined.

As we will see, the name "HLA" is somewhat of a misnomer, because the antigens are more widespread than leukocytes. Indeed, certain HLA antigens are found on nearly every type of cell in the human body. Fortunately, HLA antigens are not expressed or are poorly expressed (**Bg antigens,** including Bg^a [HLA-B7], Bg^b [HLA-B17], and Bg^c [HLA-A28]) on red blood cells.[11]

FUNCTIONS OF MHC GENE PRODUCTS

The role of the MHC remained enigmatic for several decades after its discovery. Why would a gene complex be selected to become the predominant barrier to allografting when, evolutionarily, tissue transplantation was not a natural event? No selective pressure should exist to cause one set of genes to preferentially function in this capacity over the thousands of others in the genome. The enigma began to be resolved in the 1970s by the discoveries of Rolf Zinkernagel and Peter Doherty, who demonstrated that normally T cells only recognize foreign antigens as a complex consisting of an antigen-derived peptide and an MHC molecule.[12-14] Furthermore, under natural conditions the MHC molecules must be the same set of MHC molecules as expressed by the T cells themselves. This phenomenon is referred to as **MHC restriction.**

The landmark discovery of Zinkernagel and Doherty, for which they were awarded a Nobel Prize, led to the realization that the MHC of vertebrate species plays a central role in the processes of recognition and elimination of foreign antigens, and in self vs. non-self discrimination. These processes begin in the thymus during fetal development (and continue beyond birth), where T cells are "educated."[15,16] The mature T cells permitted to leave the thymus and populate the peripheral lymphoid tissue are only those which possess a T-cell receptor (TCR) restricted to recognizing antigens presented in association with "self" MHC class I or class II molecules, but which are not overly reactive to self HLA bearing self-peptides (which could result in autoimmunity).[17-21]

In the periphery, when an individual is exposed to a foreign antigen, the potential pathogen is first engulfed by an antigen-presenting cell (APC), usually a macrophage or dendritic cell. The APC digests the foreign material in a manner such that peptides from it become displayed on the cell surface (antigen process-

Bg antigens: HLA antigens present on red cells that may cause weak and variable reactions with sera containing the corresponding antibody. These antibodies may interfere with the interpretation of pretransfusion antibody detection and identification and may be present as contaminating antibodies in commercial antisera.

MHC restriction: T cells respond to antigens presented in association with the same set of MHC molecules as expressed by the T cells themselves.

ing) in association with the MHC class I or class II molecules (see The Genetics and Biochemistry of the HLA Complex, below). MHC class I molecules are involved in the processing and presentation of intracellular antigens (e.g., viral peptides and endogenous proteins), whereas exogenous antigens, taken into the APC by phagocytosis or pinocytosis and processed in lysosomes and endosomes, are presented in association with MHC class II molecules.

There are important functional differences between MHC class I and II molecules. The CD8 T-cell subset is restricted to recognition of antigenic peptides in association with HLA class I. Because HLA class I is found on virtually every nucleated cell in the body, CD8 cytotoxic T cells play an important role in viral immunity. The CD4 T-cell subset recognizes those antigens that are associated with HLA class II molecules, and, once activated, releases **lymphokines,** which stimulate B-cell expansion, proliferation, and antibody production, or help activate CD8 T cells. Because the CD4 T-cell subset, which recognizes antigen in the context of MHC class II, is the major regulator of the **adaptive immune response** (and also influences **innate immunity** to a considerable extent), the fact that MHC class II expression is normally restricted to APCs probably represents a form of immunologic regulation in itself.

Thus the primary immunologic function of MHC molecules is to bind and "present" antigenic peptides on the surfaces of cells for recognition (binding) by the antigen-specific TCRs of lymphocytes. In light of these findings, it seemed that the enigma of why MHC was the primary immunologic barrier to allografting might be that T cells are constantly surveying the MHC molecules expressed on the surface of cells in the organism.

Genetics and Biochemistry of the HLA Complex

Human leukocyte antigen molecules are encoded by a cluster of genes on the short arm of chromosome six (Fig. 7-1).[22-25] The complex is divided into subregions that code for biochemically related proteins. **Class I HLA molecules** consist of a 45 kd alpha chain glycoprotein that is noncovalently bound to beta 2-microglobulin (Fig. 7-2). Only the alpha chain is encoded by MHC genes and is polymorphic. The beta 2-microglobulin subunit is encoded by a conserved (nonpolymorphic) gene outside of the HLA complex (on chromosome 15). The majority of expressed class I alpha chain genes are located in the HLA-A, HLA-B, HLA-C subregions, and their products, the class I protein molecules, are found on virtually all nucleated cells in the body. **HLA class II molecules** are dimers composed of a 32 kd alpha chain and a 28 kd beta chain (Fig. 7-3). The expressed class II HLA genes are located in the DR, DP, and DQ subregions, and the HLA-DR, HLA-DQ, and HLA-DP molecules are formed between alpha and beta polypeptides encoded within its respective subregion. Class II molecules are expressed primarily on cells such as macrophages, dendritic cells, and B cells, which have the capacity to present antigens to CD4+ ("helper") T cells; CD8+ T cells (e.g., cytolytic T cells) recognize antigenic peptides in combination with HLA class I molecules. Class I and class II genes are highly **polymorphic,** and the ability of HLA molecules to bind a peptide antigen varies among HLA molecules. This factor is believed to underlie one of the mechanisms by which certain HLA alleles render an individual more susceptible to a disease.

As also depicted in Fig. 7-1, the human MHC contains other class I and class II genes, as well as so-called **class III** genes that are not directly involved in clinical

Lymphokines: Belong to the broader class of substances known as cytokines. Cytokines are low molecular weight proteins that participate in the regulation of the immune response. Other cytokines include interferons, interleukins, and monokines. Lymphokines are also discussed in Chapter 2.

Adaptive immune response: Immune system mechanisms that recognize antigens as non-self, specifically respond to the antigens, and respond faster and more vigorously on subsequent exposure to the antigen. Prototypic examples are antibody- and T-cell–mediated immune reactions.

Innate immunity: Inborn immune system mechanisms that confer basic resistance to invasion by bacteria, fungi, viruses, and so on.

Class I genes: In humans these genes encode for the production of the heavy chains of the HLA-A, HLA-B, and HLA-C molecules, as well as the nonclassical molecules.

Class II genes: Genes that encode the production of the α and β polypeptides of the class II molecules (DM, DO, DP, DQ, and DR).

Polymorphic: Pertaining to the existence of two or more phenotypes in the population.

Class III genes: Alleles of the MHC that produce a number of functionally diverse molecules.

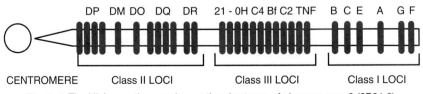

Fig. 7-1 The HLA genetic complex on the short arm of chromosome 6 (6P21.3).

histocompatibility testing. Products of the class I HLA-E, HLA-F, HLA-G genes appear to have functions related to materno-fetal tolerance and tumor immuno-surveillance.[26,27] Class II genes, HLA-DM and HLA-DO, appear to modulate the processing and presentation of peptides, which are ultimately bound and expressed on the surface of APCs in the context of DR, DP, and DQ. Class III genes encode complement components and other molecules not specifically involved in immune recognition (e.g., C2, C4 and factor B, tumor necrosis factor, 21-hydroxy-lase).[22,24,26-30] Additional genes encoded within the HLA complex on the short

Class I

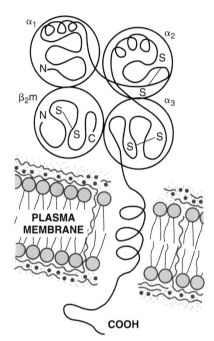

Fig. 7-2 Class I antigen.

Class II

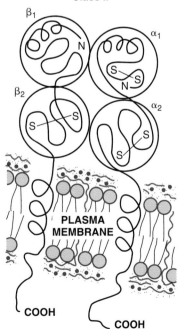

Fig. 7-3 Class II antigen.

arm of chromosome 6 (6p21.3) not depicted in Fig. 7-1 encode other proteins that also play roles in the mechanics of antigen processing and presentation, including, heat shock proteins, peptide transporters, and proteasomes.

HLA Inheritance

The loci of all three genetic regions of the MHC are within 4000 kilobases of each other on chromosome 6, and the MHC is usually inherited en bloc as a complete **haplotype** rather than as individual alleles, unless a recombination or crossing-over event has occurred.[31,32] Because normal individuals inherit one set of chromosomes from each biologic parent, each parent contributes a haplotype, and two haplotypes constitute a genotype. Fig. 7-4 illustrates this concept. HLA genes are codominantly expressed, that is, heterozygous individuals express the alleles of both loci. In solid organ transplantation, when both alleles for the A, B, and DR antigens are matched, it is termed a six-antigen match. (The reader can refer to Chapter 1 for a more complete discussion of patterns of inheritance.)

With the MHC inherited en bloc, certain alleles tend to be inherited together. This phenomenon is referred to as **linkage disequilibrium** and is characterized by the occurrence of linked alleles in a haplotype more often than would be expected by chance alone based on gene frequency.[25,33,34] For example, there is a linkage dis-

Haplotype: The inheritance of Rh antigens is another example of the inheritance of haplotypes (closely linked antigens as a unit). Refer to Chapter 6 for a discussion of the genetics of the Rh system.

Linkage disequilibrium: The occurrence of a haplotype in the population more frequently than would be expected based on probability.

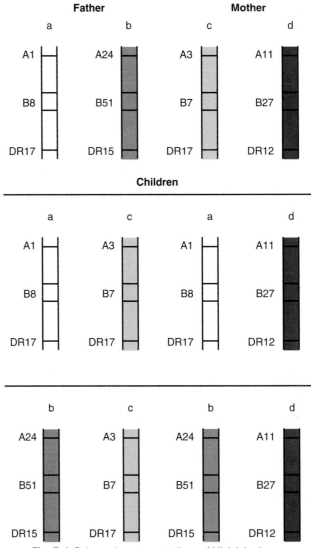

Fig. 7-4 Schematic representations of HLA inheritance.

TABLE 7-1 Example of Linkage Disequilibrium between HLA-A1 and HLA-B8

HLA Antigen	Gene Frequency	Expected Haplotype	Observed Haplotype Frequency
A1	0.15	1.5%	7%-8%
B8	0.10		

HLA, Human leukocyte antigen.

equilibrium between HLA-A1 and HLA-B8 in Caucasians (Table 7-1). The gene frequencies of HLA-A1 and HLA-B8 are 0.15 and 0.10, respectively. Therefore 1.5% (0.15 × 0.10) of all Caucasians should possess both HLA-A1 and HLA-B8. The actual frequency is, however, 7% to 8%. Linkage disequilibrium also exists with various combinations of A, B, and DR loci among defined ethnic populations.[25,35-37]

Nomenclature
Serologic

After their discovery, the methods and principles used for defining HLA antigens were very similar to those used for red cell antigen typing. Patient sera were screened for HLA antibodies, and compatibility between donor cells and recipient sera was established through crossmatching using the same procedure. Terasaki and McClelland introduced the microlymphocytotoxicity test in 1964 as a means to define HLA specificity more clearly.[38] This **complement-dependent cytotoxicity (CDC) test** (see The Complement-Dependent Cytotoxicity Test, later in this chapter) soon replaced the less reliable and more reagent-intensive leukoagglutination test, and became the standard HLA testing technique. Since 1964, 13 international workshops have been held by scientists to exchange information, as well as cell panels and antibodies. This collaborative effort has led to reagent standardization and the development of a common World Health Organization (WHO) approved nomenclature.[39,40]

The "classical" HLA class I and II antigens have been defined by serologic, cellular, or molecular techniques, and are assigned to one of the following series: class I: HLA-A, HLA-B, HLA-C; class II: HLA-DP, HLA-DQ, or HLA-DR. The current serologic classification of HLA antigens is outlined in Table 7-2. With this system, serologically defined antigens are designated with the HLA locus from which they are derived followed by a number that connotes the chronologic order in which they were defined (e.g., HLA-A2 and HLA-B7). From Table 7-2 it is obvious that the numbers for the HLA-A and HLA-B antigens are not in sequence. The numbers for HLA-A and HLA-B were assigned before these two separate loci were recognized.

It used to be that newly defined serologic HLA antigens were preceded by a "w" for "workshop" to indicate their provisional status, until confirmed and formally accepted by the WHO Terminology Committee, when the "w" was dropped (e.g., Aw74). With the advent of molecular HLA typing, the "workshop" designation is no longer required. C-locus encoded antigens are still written with the "w," however, so that these antigens will not be confused with complement proteins (e.g., Cw1 is an HLA antigen whereas C1 is the first component of the complement cascade).

Serologic nomenclature categorizes antigen families as defined by antibody reaction patterns. Many antigens in the HLA system share common antigenic determinants or epitopes. As serologic typing reagents and methods improved, it became possible to more narrowly define or split of some of the originally described antigens. For example, HLA-A25, HLA-A26, HLA-A34, and HLA-A66 are splits of an antigen initially defined as HLA-A10. A common epitope, A10, is present on all four antigen molecules, but other specific epitopes define them as relatively unique molecules. Thus antigenic determinants can be defined as either

Complement-dependent cytotoxicity (CDC) test: Laboratory procedures that use complement fixation and resultant cell lysis as an end point.

Splits/subtypes: HLA antigens tend to be serologically crossreactive but may have additional epitopes that more narrowly define them as split from the broad antigen. Subtypes are serologically definable alleles.

TABLE 7-2 Serologic HLA Antigens

CLASS I				CLASS II	
HLA Ag	Splits and Subtypes†	HLA Ag	Splits and Subtypes	HLA Ag	Splits and Subtypes
A1		B5	B51, B52, B5102, B5103	DR1	DR103
A2	A203, A210	B7	B703	DR2	DR15, DR16
A3		B8		DR3*	DR17, DR18
A9	A23, A24, A2403	B12	B44, B45	DR4	
A10	A25, A26, A34, A66	B13		DR5	DR11, DR12
A11		B14*	B64, B65	DR6	DR13, DR14, DR1403, DR1404
A19	A29, A30, A31, A32, A33, A74	B15*	B62, B63, B75, B76, B77	DR7	
A28	A68, A69	B16	B38, B39, B3901, B3902	DR8	
A36		B17	B57, B58	DR9	
A43		B18		DR10	
		B21	B49, B50, B4005		
Cw1		B22	B54, B55, B56	DQ1	DQ5, DQ6
Cw2		B27	B2708	DQ2	
Cw3*	Cw9, Cw10	B35		DQ3*	DQ7, DQ8, DQ9
Cw4		B37		DQ4	
Cw5		B40*	B60, B61		
Cw6		B41			
Cw7		B42			
Cw8		B46			
		B47,			
		B48, B53, B59, B67			
		B70, B73, B78, B81	B71, B72		

*Molecular nomenclature uses the broad antigen for the allele family (see Table 7-4).
†Subtypes are serologically definable alleles.
HLA, Human leukocyte antigen.

Private epitopes: Antigenic determinants that are detectable on one or a few HLA molecule variants.

Public epitopes: Antigenic determinants that are produced by more than one gene.

Cross-reactive epitope groups (CREGs): Groups of antigens based on their common reactivity with antibodies to public epitopes.

private or public epitopes. **Private epitopes** occur in only one single or a limited number of HLA molecules, and antisera defining these epitopes have sometimes led to the elucidation of individual gene products or subtypes (e.g., A210, A2403, B2708, B5103). In contrast, **public epitopes** are common to more than one gene product, and these shared determinants can be distributed over a broader range of antigens. Bw4 and Bw6 are examples of widely distributed public epitopes. Either determinant can be found on nearly all B-locus gene products, and a few A locus antigens as well.[23] Antibodies to the public epitopes have been used to categorize HLA gene products into cross-reactive epitope groups, or CREGs (Table 7-3). Antibodies to class I antigens often have specificity for these shared epitopes and can exhibit limited or extensive cross-reactivity.[41-46]

Molecular

With the advent of molecular HLA typing in the 1980s, it became possible to define HLA antigens at the DNA level, that is, as alleles of HLA loci that differ in the proteins they encode but that, depending on how many amino acid differences there

TABLE 7-3 Cross-Reactive Epitope Groups of HLA Class I Antigens	
CREG	Broad and Splits of Antigens
A1C	A1, 3, 11, 19 (29, 30, 31,), 36, 80
A2	A2, 9 (23, 24), 28 (68, 69), B17 (57, 58)
A10C	A10 (25, 26, 34, 66), 32, 33, 43, 74
B5C	B5 (51, 52.) 18, 35, 53
B5C2	B5 (51, 52), 15 (62, 63, 71, 72, 75, 76, 77), 17, (57, 58), 21 (49, 50), 35, 53, 73,78
B7C	B7, 8, 13, 27, 40 (60, 61), 41, 42, 47, 48, 54, 55, 56, 81
B8C	B8, 18, 38, 39, 64, 65
B12C	B12 (44, 45), 13, 37, 41, 47, 21 (49, 50), 40 (60, 61)
BW4	A23, 24, 25, 32, B13, 27, 37, 38, 44, 47, 49, 51, 52, 53, 57, 58, 59, 63, 77
BW6	B7, 8, 18, 35, 39, 41, 42, 45, 46, 48, 50, 54, 55, 56, 60, 61, 62, 64, 65, 67, 71, 72, 73, 75, 76

CREG, Cross-reactive epitope group.

were among them, may or may not differ in serologic reactivity. A new form of nomenclature based on HLA specificities defined by molecular techniques was implemented in 1987.[47] HLA alleles are designated with the letter indicating the locus, an asterisk, a two-digit Arabic number that defines the allele family, followed by a two-digit number for the allele. For example, for HLA-A1, there are at least nine genes, the designated alleles of which are A*0101, A*0102, A*0103 . . . A*0109. For most specificities, the allele family corresponds to the serologic specificity of a HLA subtype or "split" (e.g., B*4402, B*4501), although in several cases the numerals of the broad antigen are used (e.g., B*1401, B*1402). Although there is a general correlation between serologically defined HLA antigens and alleles whose DNA sequences are known, a one-to-one correlation between serotype and genotype does not necessarily exist (e.g., the serologic equivalent of DRB1*1415 is DR8). Furthermore, not all of the members of an allele family may be serologically defined (e.g., A*0106).[48]

In 1990 a fifth digit was added to permit the distinction of sequences differing only by noncoding nucleotide substitutions; that is, the gene products would be synonymous at the level of amino acid sequence (e.g., A*01011 and A*01012).[49] In 2002, it became necessary to introduce an extra digit between the current fourth and fifth digit, to allow for up to 99 synonymous variants of each allele (e.g., A*010101 and A*010102). Furthermore, seventh and eighth digits describing variation in introns or 5′ or 3′ regions of the gene were added in 2002, expanding the full name of some alleles to eight digits.[39] Table 7-4 lists some current examples of HLA genetic nomenclature.

CLINICAL HLA TESTING

The three major categories of clinical HLA testing are HLA phenotyping (also called tissue typing), HLA panel-reactive antibody (PRA) testing, and HLA cross-matching. HLA phenotyping is performed because the greater the degree of HLA compatibility between the transplant recipient and donor, the better the clinical outcome (Fig. 7-5). This is especially true for bone marrow transplants, where each HLA mismatch increases the risk of graft-versus-host disease. HLA typing also may be indicated to assist in making diagnoses of some diseases because individuals with particular HLA antigens have greater incidences of certain disorders, for example, **ankylosing spondylitis** and **Reiter syndrome** with B27, or **narcolepsy** with DR2 (the DR15 split of DR2, and DQ6, which is in strong linkage disequilibrium).[50-52] Sensitization to foreign HLA antigens due to blood or platelet

Ankylosing spondylitis: An inflammatory disorder of unknown etiology that primarily affects the axial skeleton, resulting in the loss of spine flexibility.

Reiter syndrome: A syndrome which in its full-blown picture consists of urethritis, arthritis, and conjunctivitis. Urethritis usually occurs first. There are countless clinical symptoms, but the clinical picture is dominated by polyarthritis. There is pain, swelling, redness, and heat in the joints.

Narcolepsy: Intermittent attacks of sleepiness during the daytime.

TABLE 7-4 Selected Examples of Molecular HLA Nomenclature

HLA Ag Serologic Equivalent	Representative Alleles
A2	A*0201
A210	A*0210
B44	B*4402
B64	B*1401
B65	B*1402
None	Cw*140201
	Cw*150202
	Cw*1601
	Cw*171
	Cw*1801
DR1	DRB1*0101
DR103	DRB1*0103
DR17	DQB1*0301, DQB1*0304
DQ2	DQB1*0201
DQ9	DBB1*0303
DR51	DRB5*010101, DRB5*0202
DR52	DRB3*0102, DRB3*0202, DRB3*0302
DR53	DRB4*0102

HLA, Human leukocyte antigen.

HLA-A+B+DR Mismatches
First Cadaver Kidney Transplants 1985-2002

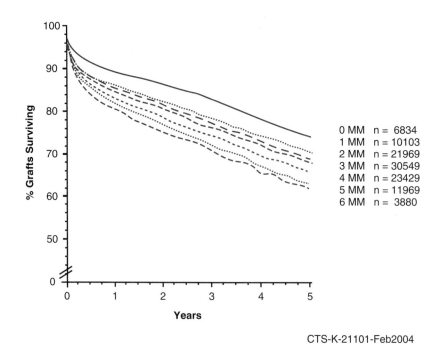

CTS-K-21101-Feb2004

Fig. 7-5 Impact of HLA matching on kidney graft survival. (Collaborative Transplant Study, www.ctstransplant.org/ February 2004.)

transfusion, pregnancy, or previous transplant can cause patients to form antibodies to foreign HLA molecules (hence the reason HLA molecules are often referred to as "HLA antigens"). Presence of anti-HLA antibodies in a patient could cause rejection of an allogeneic organ, tissue, or progenitor cell transplant, or cause a patient to become refractory to platelet transfusions. To determine whether the recipient has previously made antibodies reactive against foreign HLA antigens, HLA antibody screening is performed using panels of cells previously HLA phenotyped. When a donor is ultimately identified for a transplant patient, a donor-specific HLA crossmatch is performed.[53-55]

The Complement-Dependent Cytotoxicity Test

HLA phenotyping, PRA, and crossmatching can all be performed by serologic methodologies. The principles of HLA serologic testing are very similar to those used for red cell testing. For HLA antigen phenotyping ("tissue typing") by the complement-dependent microlymphocytotoxicity (CDC) test, known antisera are used to identify HLA antigens on the lymphocyte surface. Using an analogous procedure, patient sera can be assessed for panel-reactive antibodies (PRAs) by screening against a set of HLA-phenotyped lymphocytes. Also by CDC testing, compatibility between an individual potential donor and the patient can be established through crossmatching of donor cells with patient sera.

Typically, CDC testing is performed in 60- to 72-well microtiter trays, the wells of which can hold approximately 10 μL. The tray wells contain 1 to 2 μL of antisera overlaid with mineral oil to prevent evaporation during the various incubation stages. Trays can be stored at −70° C and thawed at room temperature before use. In this procedure, 1 μL of cells is added to each well and the tray is incubated at room temperature for 30 minutes. After incubation, 5 μL of rabbit serum is added as a source of complement. If antibody were bound to the lymphocyte membrane, complement would be activated, resulting in membrane injury (Fig. 7-6).[38] The degree of injury can then be observed microscopically by the uptake of a vital dye, such as eosin Y or trypan blue, by the injured cells. Wells are usually read under an inverted phase contrast microscope; uninjured cells appear refractile and small, and dead cells appear large, flatter, and darker. The percentage killed is graded from 1 to 8, with 1 representing 0% to 10% decrease in cell viability of the test wells compared to a negative serum control, and 8 representing a

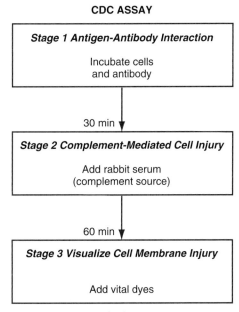

CDC ASSAY

Stage 1 Antigen-Antibody Interaction

Incubate cells
and antibody

30 min

Stage 2 Complement-Mediated Cell Injury

Add rabbit serum
(complement source)

60 min

Stage 3 Visualize Cell Membrane Injury

Add vital dyes

Fig. 7-6 CDC procedure.

TABLE 7-5 CDC Test Recording Results

1 =	0%-10% cell death	Negative
2 =	11%-20% cell death	Negative
4 =	21%-50% cell death	Doubtful or weak positive
6 =	51%-80% cell death	Positive
8 =	81%-100% cell death	Positive
0 =	Well is unreadable	

CDC, Complement-dependent cytotoxicity.

Antiglobulin testing: Refer to Chapter 2 for a discussion of the theory and application of antiglobulin testing.

strong positive reaction with virtually all dead cells (Table 7-5). When at least 50% cell death is noted, the cells tested possess the HLA antigen.

The CDC assay can be enhanced by incorporating an **antiglobulin** reagent into the assay.[56,57] This assay is more sensitive than the standard CDC assay but should not be used for routine HLA typing. It should be reserved for those situations requiring the detection of low levels of HLA antibodies, such as crossmatch testing performed for organ transplantation.[58]

Peripheral blood lymphocytes (PBLs) are the most readily available source of cells to use for clinical HLA testing, although lymphocytes harvested from other tissues can be used, such as lymph node or spleen. Whole blood (or a single-cell suspension prepared from lymph nodes or spleen) is layered over Ficoll-Hypaque, a high molecular weight substance that induces rouleaux formation. Ficoll-Hypaque is more dense than lymphocytes, monocytes, and platelets but less dense than red cells and granulocytes. On centrifugation, the red cells and granulocytes pass through the gradient and form a pellet at the bottom of the tube. Platelets remain in the supernatant while T and B lymphocytes and monocytes remain at the plasma-gradient interface. The T and B lymphocytes are harvested from this interface and washed, and the cell concentration is adjusted to 1 to 2×10^6 cells/mL (Fig. 7-7). T and B lymphocyte viability should be at least 90% to be used in the CDC test. Cells then can be used immediately for testing, or can be frozen in dimethyl sulfoxide (DMSO) and saved for subsequent testing.

Whereas purified suspensions of T and B lymphocytes are used in the microlymphocytotoxicity tests for detection of HLA class I antigens or antibodies (HLA-A, HLA-B, and HLA-C), CDC-based phenotyping, PRA analysis, or crossmatching for class II antigens (HLA-DR and HLA-DQ) requires a purified suspension of B lymphocytes. Historically, this B cell suspension was prepared using nylon wool separation, based on the observation that B lymphocytes preferentially adhere to nylon wool and T lymphocytes do not. The B lymphocytes can then be

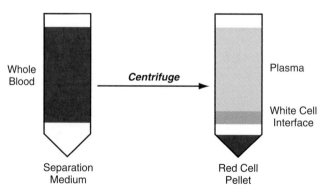

Fig. 7-7 Lymphocyte separation.

eluted from nylon wool. More contemporary methods of preparing purified B-cell suspensions include (1) differential lysis of non-B cells with monoclonal antibodies and complement, (2) positive B-cell selection using magnetic beads coated with a B-cell–specific antibody, and (3) positive B-cell selection using Rosetting techniques. The purified suspension of B lymphocytes can be tested with antisera of known anti-HLA class II specificity using the CDC assay for HLA class II phenotyping of the patient, in a B-cell panel to screen for the presence of anti-HLA class II specific antibodies in the patient's serum, or in a crossmatch to assess whether a patient has donor-specific HLA class II antibody.

Historically and to this day, the majority of tissue-typing laboratories perform HLA typing, crossmatching, and antibody screening by variations on the CDC assay. Recently, alternative approaches to these tests have been described, and include DNA-based methods for HLA phenotyping and flow cytometry, and enzyme-linked immunosorbent assay (ELISA)–based methods for PRA and crossmatch testing. Brief descriptions of the classic, serologic tests and more contemporary forms of HLA phenotyping, PRA and crossmatching, are given here.

HLA Phenotyping

HLA specificities defined by serotyping are the antigenic determinants, formed by clusters of amino acids on the HLA molecule, that are detectable by the specific antibodies. Target cells from either the patient or donor are mixed with various antisera, representing specificities of the known HLA antigens, and complement. The most common source of antisera containing anti-HLA antibodies is the serum of multiparous women who have formed these antibodies in response to pregnancy. Alternative sources include sera from transplant or transfusion recipients, or monoclonal antibodies.[59-63] As previously described, an HLA antigen is identified as being present on the cell surface because a specific anti-HLA antibody binds to the target cell and fixes complement, thereby leading to cell death, which is interpreted as a positive reaction.

More precise assessment of the role of HLA in organ transplantation and disease states is made possible by molecular tissue typing because HLA alleles that are either difficult to identify or not detected by serologic methods can be recognized by molecular methods. Molecular biology techniques now allow identification of HLA differences at the level of single nucleotide variations. This level of resolution is critical especially for hematopoietic progenitor cell (HPC) transplants, in order to minimize the risks of graft-versus-host disease (GVHD) and for successful engraftment.[64,65] Other advantages of molecular HLA typing technologies are that the reagents needed to perform the tests are defined oligonucleotides that are highly specific and synthesizeable, allowing quantitative and qualitative consistency, and also molecular HLA typing may be conveniently performed with small quantities of cells from any number of sources (not just peripheral blood T [class I] or B [class I and class II] cells), for example, whole blood, buccal swabs, and hair follicles.

The methods being employed for molecular HLA typing in most laboratories utilize the polymerase chain reaction (PCR) technique, a method for the amplification of specific DNA sequences. DNA isolated from donor or recipient leukocytes is mixed with Taq (a DNA polymerase) and oligonucleotide primers that are complementary for specific nucleotide sequences contained within the HLA coding regions. The amplified DNA is analyzed to identify the HLA antigens or alleles encoded by the patient's genomic DNA by a variety of methods, including restriction fragment length polymorphism (RFLP) analysis; DNA hybridization techniques with sequence-specific oligonucleotide probes (SSOPs); sequence-specific primers (SSPs), which will cause the HLA allele(s) with complementary matching nucleotide sequences to be selectively replicated by Taq polymerase; and direct nucleotide sequencing on a gene analyzer. Detailed description of these methodologies is beyond the scope of this chapter, so the reader is referred to the bibliography.[66-70] An experienced serology technician, after a moderate amount of training in molecular biology techniques, can obtain highly accurate results by any of these methods.

As predicted in the previous edition of this textbook, as molecular HLA typing has become more readily available, these procedures have replaced some of the conventional serologic and cellular techniques routinely used in the HLA laboratory. With the exception of serology, which is still advantageous in some situations (e.g., when expediency is a high priority, or low start-up cost), molecular HLA typing methods have largely replaced other HLA typing techniques, such as the mixed lymphocyte culture (MLC) test, the primed lymphocyte test (PLT), and isoelectric focusing (IEF). In general, MLC, PLT, and IEF are more laborious, complex, and expensive than molecular HLA typing, as well as less accurate and precise. However, they still have application in clinical and research HLA laboratories.

The MLC and PLT tests, used to determine class II compatibility between donor and recipient, were originally developed because HLA class II antigens are difficult to define serologically. With these tests, donor and recipient lymphocytes that differ by one or more gene product stimulate each other and undergo cellular activation and blast transformation. This activity can be measured by the incorporation of a radioactive DNA precursor that is then synthesized into new DNA. MLC and PLT results are rarely used nowadays to select kidney and bone marrow donors for intended recipients, but are still in use for posttransplantation monitoring (e.g., of donor-specific hyporesponsiveness).[71,72]

IEF is a method that was developed in order to subtype the serologically defined HLA class I and II antigens. The IEF technique uses a special type of gel to establish the proteins' isoelectric points, which are determined by the amino acid composition. With the IEF technique, lymphocytes are treated with a detergent and the HLA antigens are solubilized with special detergents. The solubilized antigens are then radiolabeled, followed by immunoprecipitation with an antibody reactive to the broader class of antigens. The radiolabeled, immunoprecipitated molecules are subsequently subjected to IEF gel electrophoresis, and the dried gels are exposed to x-ray film. Readings made from the autoradiographs characterize the specific subtypes' isoelectric points.[73]

Panel-Reactive Antibodies

Some patients are sensitized against HLA antigens and have formed antibodies, induced through pregnancy, transfusion, or transplantation. Presence of antibodies in patients could result in rejection of the transplanted organs, tissues, or cells.[53] The principle of PRA testing is that lymphocytes of known HLA phenotype are incubated with patient's serum and rabbit complement. If the serum contains antibodies that are able to bind specifically to HLA antigens on the surface of the lymphocytes, complement-mediated cell death will occur.

Alternatives to cell-based, serologic HLA antibody screening techniques have been developed in recent years. The ELISA PRA assay uses soluble HLA antigens captured onto wells of an ELISA plate. Patient sera are added to the wells, and if HLA antibodies are present, they bind to the antigens captured in the wells. The bound antibodies are detected using a horseradish peroxidase-conjugated anti–human IgG antibody and a substrate converted to a colored product by the enzyme. Absorbance is read using an ELISA plate reader, and assay results are analyzed by computer. A second alternative technique employs flow cytometry technology and latex beads coated with purified HLA class I or class II antigens. The bound antibodies are detected using a fluorochrome-conjugated anti–human IgG antibody, and bound fluorescence is read using a flow cytometer or a similar microfluidics system (e.g., Luminex). ELISA and flow PRA bead-based antibody screening is an attractive alternative to serologic methods because neither method require the use of viable target cells or complement, both are designed to detect only antibodies to HLA antigens (eliminating false-positive reaction due to, for example, autoreactive antibodies present in some forms of end-stage renal disease such as lupus nephritis), and both provide an objective readout.

Regardless of method, the serum is typically screened against a panel size of 30 to 60. PRA is calculated as the percentage of the panel that reacts positive to a patient's serum.

$$PRA = (Positive\ reactions/Number\ in\ panel) \times 100$$

By determining the percentage of the panel that antibodies in the serum recognize (% PRA), information that is useful in determining how long a potential transplant patient might have to wait for a suitable donor, or whether a bleeding-disorder patient should receive single-donor vs. pooled platelet. Finding compatible donors is significantly longer for high-PRA patients. Furthermore, highly sensitized transplant recipients are at higher risk of acute and chronic rejection, and may require more intensive immunosuppression.[53,74] The second important part of the PRA screening is determination of the specificities of the HLA antibodies in a patient's sera, by analysis of the reaction pattern. Knowing the antigen specificity of the antibody is relevant in predicting donor-recipient incompatibility in final crossmatch, or in identifying an appropriate, HLA-matched apheresis donor for a highly alloimmunized patient with a bleeding disorder. Both the PRA and the repertoire of anti-HLA antibody specificities can change over time as a result of alloimmunization events or due to naturally occurring epitope spreading.

Crossmatching

The crossmatch procedure is the most important clinical HLA test performed for solid organ transplantation.[75] HLA crossmatching tests a recipient's serum against prospective donor cells to determine whether donor-specific HLA antibodies are present. A negative crossmatch means that there is minimal risk of early acute rejection or graft loss. Crossmatching should also be performed for progenitor transplant recipients whenever the patient has been allosensitized and has made anti-HLA antibody, as demonstrated by PRA.

CDC crossmatch methods suffer the same technical disadvantages of CDC tissue typing and PRA analysis: requiring viable target cells, variable sensitivity of target cells to complement, detection of antibodies against donor HLA and/or non-HLA antigens, a subjective scoring system, and lack of standardization. Alternative approaches to crossmatch testing have been described based on flow cytometry and ELISA. Flow cytometry crossmatching is more sensitive than CDC detection of antidonor antibodies, is complement independent, facilitates the distinction between anti-HLA class I and anti-HLA class II reactivity (T vs. B cell), can employ gating techniques to eliminate nonviable cells, is faster to perform on an individual basis, has an objective readout based on fluorescence intensity units, and has a better clinical correlation for highly allosensitized individuals and regrafts.[76-86] ELISA crossmatch methods, in which solubilized donor HLA antigens are prepared from leukocytes or platelets and captured onto wells of microtiter plates, have also been described.[87-89] Like flow cytometry, ELISA-based crossmatch methods are an attractive alternative to CDC crossmatch methods because they provide increased objectivity in the detection of antidonor Ab and can be more easily standardized and automated. Advantages of the ELISA-based crossmatch assay over CDC-based and flow cytometry–based techniques are that the ELISA methodology does not require the use of viable target cells and is inherently designed to detect only Abs to HLA antigens. Despite the theoretic advantages of ELISA, flow cytometry remains the most popular alternative to the CDC crossmatching, primarily because of its greater sensitivity, because it is faster to perform, and because ELISA requires a greater amount of donor material in order to prepare an adequate amount of solubilized donor HLA antigens. Furthermore, with the advent of solid-phase methods for accurate assessment of the presence of anti-HLA antibody specificities in patient sera, the false-positive aspect of flow crossmatching, that is, that the antibodies detected may be to non-HLA antigens, is less problematic because in clinical HLA testing, as with most high-complexity clinical testing, the results of any one test are not used as the sole means for patient management decisions.

CLINICAL APPLICATIONS OF HLA TESTING
Solid Organ Transplantation

The rapid growth noted over the past 30 years in histocompatibility testing has been paralleled by major advances in the field of tissue and organ transplantation. Class I and II proteins elicit strong cellular and antibody responses as alloantigens. HLA tissue typing, antibody screening (PRA), and donor-specific crossmatching are vital tests for minimizing the likelihood of **hyperacute rejection** or accelerated graft rejection due to anti-HLA antibodies. Although the primary clinical application of HLA testing is in transplantation, other applications include the selection of platelets for alloimmunized thrombocytopenic patients, genetic marker analysis in disputed parentage cases, and risk factor determination for susceptibility to disease.

For many patients, solid organ transplantation is the ideal therapy for the treatment of human diseases that lead to organ system failure. However, allogeneic transplantation of foreign tissue can induce a cellular and humoral response that often leads to graft rejection. The severity of rejection can often be reduced by selecting HLA-matched organs for the intended recipient because the HLA system antigens serve as a transplantation barrier.[90-92] For most solid organ transplants such as kidney and heart, both donor and recipient are tested for HLA-A, HLA-B, and HLA-DR antigens. HLA compatibility influences graft outcome to different degrees in various types of patients.[93,94] During the early posttransplant period, HLA-DR mismatches have a stronger influence on graft survival than HLA-A and HLA-B mismatches. The influence of the three loci is additive so that the survival rate difference between transplants with zero or six mismatches for HLA-A, HLA-B, HLA-DR is approximately 15% at 5 years (see Fig. 7-5). To obtain optimal long-term survival, all three loci must be considered in the donor-recipient matching procedure. Because of the significantly higher graft survival rate of transplants performed when the patient and donor share all six HLA-A, HLA-B, and HLA-DR antigens, or when there are zero antigen mismatches at these loci, kidney transplants between such donor-recipient pairs are given preferential treatment in the United States and Europe.[90,95,96]

The crucial histocompatibility tests for most solid organ transplantation are ABO and the HLA crossmatch between donor cells and recipient sera. A and B blood group antigens are present on vascular endothelium, and the ABO isoagglutinins that all normal individuals possess to those antigens can cause hyperacute rejection. Therefore the same rules that govern the selection of blood for transfusion apply to the selection of solid organ (e.g., renal and heart) transplants.[97,98] Results of HLA crossmatch procedures are also important, especially for renal transplants. A strong correlation exists between acute forms of rejection (hyperacute, accelerated acute, and acute) and the presence of serum antibody directed against donor HLA antigens. As described earlier, the HLA crossmatch procedure can be performed using a CDC test (preferably by antiglobulin method), by flow cytometer, or by ELISA.[76-86,87-89] Oftentimes for urgent, life-saving transplant such as heart and lung transplants, not enough time is available for HLA matching or crossmatching, and the decision of whether to perform the transplant is based on the HLA antibody screen. As long as the patient is negative for preformed anti-

Hyperacute rejection: Rapid and extensive graft rejection associated with preformed HLA or ABO antibodies.

bodies against donor antigens in PRA screening, the organ can be successfully transplanted.[99-103] Posttransplant, regardless of the results of HLA matching and crossmatching, graft rejection must be controlled continuously with immunosuppressive therapy (except with transplants between identical twins). A variety of drugs can be given to decrease the humoral and the cellular immune responses (e.g., cyclosporin, FK506, rapamycin, antilymphocyte globulin). However, these agents have serious side effects, including nephrotoxicity and enhanced risk of infections.

Bone Marrow Transplantation

Bone marrow transplantation is used to treat patients with various hematologic disorders. These include aplastic anemia, various leukemias, severe combined immunodeficiency syndromes, inherited enzyme deficiencies, and hemoglobinopathies. Bone marrow transplant recipients have different types of problems than solid organ transplant recipients because the immune system of the bone marrow transplant recipient must be totally ablated before receiving an allogeneic marrow. This puts the recipient at risk for opportunistic infections. In addition, the allogeneic bone marrow graft is populated with immunologically competent lymphocytes, and these donor lymphocytes can recognize and respond to the HLA antigens in the recipient, resulting in GVHD. Because graft rejection and GVHD are more severe with mismatched HLA antigens, HLA-A, HLA-B, HLA-C, and HLA-DR matching of donor and recipient is important.[64,104-106]

Before 1980, bone marrow transplants were performed only between HLA-identical siblings. This restricted the number of transplants because less than 30% of individuals eligible for transplantation have an HLA-identical sibling. As an alternative, transplants have been successfully performed using HLA-mismatched family donors and HLA-matched unrelated donors. A concerted effort has been made by the National Bone Marrow Donor Program to generate millions of volunteer marrow donors who are willing to donate marrow to support the population of patients who lack HLA-identical siblings.[107-109]

Umbilical cord blood has emerged as an alternative source of hematopoietic stem cells for transplantation.[110-112] Compared to unrelated bone marrow, a lower incidence and severity of GVHD occurs, allowing for more tolerance of HLA mismatches. Because of the importance of graft cell dose, the majority of recipients are children. Compared to bone marrow transplantation, however, engraftment failure rates are higher, and time to engraftment is slower. A mitigating consideration is the fact that because cord blood units can be cryopreserved and banked, they are available more rapidly than unrelated donor bone marrow grafts when a patient urgently requires transplantation.[111]

An important difference between solid organ and bone marrow transplant recipients is that the ABO antigens do not serve as a transplantation barrier for marrow recipients. During the course of the transplant, the recipient's bone marrow hematopoietic stem cells and immune system are ablated and then reconstituted with the donor's. This, however, can cause special problems in the blood bank related to transfusion support and the selection of blood components during the course of engraftment. For example, in a group O patient who has received a group A bone marrow transplant, there may be a time during the engraftment period when the patient continues to produce ABO isoagglutinins anti-A, anti-B, and anti-A,B. In this situation, red cells selected for transfusion should be group O until anti-A and anti-A,B are no longer detected. Components containing significant amounts of plasma, such as platelets and fresh-frozen plasma (FFP), must be compatible with recipient and donor blood groups. In this case, group A platelets and FFP should be selected for transfusion after transplantation.

For an extensive discussion of hematopoietic stem cell transplantation refer to Chapter 19.

Platelet Transfusion

The use of platelet transfusions has increased dramatically with the advent of bone marrow transplantation and more aggressive chemotherapy regimens for patients with malignancies. Patients who receive multiple platelet transfusions are at risk for alloimmunization to the class I antigens expressed on the platelet surface, resulting in refractoriness to random donor platelets. Refractoriness is manifested by a failure to note an expected rise in the patient's platelet count after infusion of an adequate number of platelets. This refractory state can be caused by HLA antibodies produced in response to exposure to HLA antigens on the platelet surface, on the surface of lymphocytes contaminating both red cell and platelet products, and soluble HLA antigens in plasma products.[113]

For refractory patients, transfusion of single-donor platelets from HLA-matched apheresis donors has been shown to have definite benefits with HLA-A and HLA-B matched platelets, resulting in better posttransfusion platelet counts. (Platelets do not express HLA-Cw or HLA-class II antigens.) Selection of donors, however, is not limited to HLA-matched individuals, and can be extended to donors whose HLA phenotype contains antigens that fall within the same CREG as the patient's HLA determinants. Furthermore, by careful PRA and antibody specificity analysis, especially using the newer solid-phase assay available in ELISA, flow cytometry, and Luminex formats, avoidance of "nonpermissible" antigens against which the patient has preexisting antibodies is possible. These options allow for a larger donor base, but carry the risk that the patient will ultimately make antibodies to the selected mismatches. This risk can be managed by the use of single-donor platelets, apheresis platelets, and leukoreduction.

Providing HLA-matched platelets does not ensure good platelet survival because alloimmunization is not limited to the HLA antigens and can also include platelet-specific antigens (e.g., HPA-1).[114,115] Other causes for failure to achieve the expected rise in the platelet count that are nonimmune in origin can include fever, sepsis, hypersplenism, and disseminated intravascular coagulopathy.

Paternity Testing

The high degree of polymorphism characteristic of the HLA genetic complex provides a tool for resolving disputed parentage cases. By using HLA-A and HLA-B typings alone, 93% of falsely accused males can be excluded. HLA typing in combination with red cell antigen testing increases the exclusion rate to 95%. Exclusion rates can increase to over 99% when other polymorphic non-HLA genetic markers are used, including red cell enzymes and serum proteins.[116,117] Nowadays, however, most paternity testing laboratories in the United States use molecular techniques that center on short tandem repeats (STRs), and therefore HLA typing per se is not as widely used for paternity testing as it used to be.[118,119]

HLA-Disease Associations

Because immune activation is a direct result of the interaction between HLA molecules, foreign antigens, and T cells, polymorphisms in HLA molecules can confer differential disease susceptibility. Numerous studies over the past 35 years have documented associations between HLA types and disease susceptibility.[50-52] Due to recent advancements in molecular biology, the basis of HLA and disease association is being clarified at the genetic and structural levels.

The "relative risk" (RR) that an individual with the disease-associated HLA antigen has of developing the disease compared to an individual who lacks the antigen is estimated using a 2×2 contingency table. Statistical significance is tested by chi-square analysis. An illustration with data for a hypothetical study of Reiter's syndrome is given in Table 7-6. The relative risk in this example shows that individuals who are HLA-B27 positive are 45 times more likely to develop the disease than are individuals negative for the antigen. This association is very sensitive:

TABLE 7-6 Analysis for Association between Reiter Syndrome and HLA-B27

			B27 Positive	B27 Negative	
Reiter syndrome	Positive	a =	50	10	= b
	Negative	c =	1000	9000	= d

Relative risk (RR) = ad/bc
  a = Patients with the disease with B27
  b = Patients with the disease without B27
  c = Individual without the disease with B27
  d = Individual without the disease without B27
RR = 45
  $x^2 = 342$; $p < 0.001$

83% of those patients with Reiter syndrome possess the HLA-B27 antigen, and 99.9% of individuals who do not possess B27 do not have the syndrome (negative predictive value).

Several of the more than 70 diseases having a significant association with a particular HLA gene marker are listed in Table 7-7. Diseases with HLA associations affect a wide variety of organ systems. There are, however, several prominent characteristics in common: the diseases are not among the more commonly encountered, a large majority have an immunologic basis, autoimmune pathogenesis is a feature of many, and none are inherited in accordance with classical mendelian genetics.

For many diseases, HLA typing is of limited diagnostic value because the association is not absolute, and a large majority of individuals with the specific HLA type do not develop the disease. For the example shown in Table 7-6, the positive predictive value of the test is only approximately 5% (50 of 1050 individuals with HLA-B27 antigen having Reiter syndrome). The strength of an HLA-disease association depends on several factors. Disease heterogeneity is one, since there are different clinical forms of many diseases, and an HLA association may apply to only one syndrome. For example, of the two major forms of psoriasis (vulgaris and pustularis), only psoriasis vulgaris is HLA associated. In diabetes, **type I (IDDM)** has a positive HLA association whereas type II is not controlled by HLA-linked genes. Another factor relevant to establishing a link between disease and HLA is that in

Type I (insulin-dependent) diabetes mellitus (IDDM): A form of early-onset hyperglycemia resulting from pancreatic hypofunction.

TABLE 7-7 Selected Examples of HLA-Disease Associations

Disease	HLA Allele	RR
Crohn's disease	A3 or B7	8-40
Idopathic hemochromatosis	A3 or B7	3-7
Myasthenia gravis	B8	3-4
Ankylosing spondylitis	B27	136-181
Reiter syndrome	B27	45-51
Psoriasis vulgaris	C6	7-9
Narcolepsy	DR2	130-350
Goodpasture syndrome	DR2	12-16
Multiple sclerosis	DR2	3-5
Celiac disease	DR3 or DR7	8-12
IDDM	DR3 or DR4	3-6
IDDM	Heterozygous for DR3/DR4	14
Graves' disease	DR3	3-5
Pemphigus vulgaris	DR4	7-17
Rheumatoid arthritis	DR4	3-7

most cases the full etiology of HLA-associated diseases is not known. In IDDM only 20% of HLA-identical siblings and 50% of monozygotic twins develop the disease. The implication of these observations is that the presence of susceptibility HLA molecule alone is not sufficient, and that development of HLA-associated diseases is polygenic and involves unknown environmental factors.

Although many probable mechanisms have been proposed to explain the association of HLA antigens and disease, available evidence supports three mechanisms.[50-52] First, certain HLA alleles are in linkage disequilibrium with the disease susceptibility genes. A case in point is **congenital adrenal hyperplasia.** A defect in adrenal 21-hydroxylase causes the disease, and the gene for this enzyme has been mapped to the class III region of the HLA complex. Linkage disequilibrium between defects in the gene encoding this enzyme and B14, B22, B47, B51, and B60 is the reason for this disease association. **Idiopathic hemochromatosis** and narcolepsy, which also have no apparent immunologic basis, likewise appear to be associated with genes on chromosome 6 that are in strong linkage disequilibrium with the related HLA genes, as discerned by family inheritance studies.

The second mechanism is related to the MHC's control of the immune response. HLA may control disease susceptibility due to differences in the binding of antigenic peptides to different HLA molecules. Since an antigenic peptide may be presented to a T cell exclusively by a particular HLA allele, specific disease-inducing epitopes may bind to the HLA molecules associated with that disease. This could explain the immune response to gluten that is associated with DR3 and DR7 in celiac disease. Similarly, particular HLA molecules may be better able to bind an autoantigen and present it to T cells, for example, peptides derived from the thyroid-stimulating hormone receptor in Grave's disease, acetylcholine receptors in myasthenia gravis, and type IV collagen in Goodpasture syndrome. HLA molecules may also control the immune response via their known influence on the development of T-cell receptor specificities. Normally T cells expressing a receptor that recognizes self-antigens presented on self-HLA molecules are deleted in the thymus as they undergo differentiation. Some HLA alleles may be permissive for the development of T cells with autoimmune potential, and failure to eliminate those autoreactive T cells may predispose the individual to disease if presentation of self or self-like antigens occurs in the periphery (e.g., antigenic mimicry). Alternatively, since HLA molecules also play a role in the positive selection of T-cell receptor specificities during thymic education, the consequence of a susceptible HLA haplotype could be failure to develop T cells specific for an immune-inducing epitope of a particular pathogen. Because of a "hole in the T-cell repertoire," the patient is unable to mount an immune response, allowing the etiologic agent to produce a chronic disease.

The third mechanism is related to the HLA antigen structure. HLA antigens have been shown to be antigenically similar to certain bacteria and viruses, which may result in an altered response to the antigen. This "molecular mimicry" theory holds that the disease-associated HLA molecule shares epitopes with the etiologic agent for the disease. Immune response to pathogens that share molecular structure with self-antigens can lead to autoimmune disease (e.g., streptococcal M-associated antigens in rheumatic fever). Therefore cross-reaction between a pathogen and host HLA could be the basis of an HLA-disease association. An alternative hypothesis for the molecular mimicry theory is that because of "self-tolerance," an etiologic agent that mimics a self antigen would not be recognized as foreign.

Transfusion-Related Acute Lung Injury

Transfusion-related acute lung injury (TRALI), a poorly understood but life-threatening complication of blood transfusion, is estimated to occur at a frequency of 1 per 1000 to 1 per 5000 transfusions, with a fatality rate of approximately 10%.[120,121] There are two major theories on the pathogenesis of TRALI: that TRALI is mediated by

Congenital adrenal hyperplasia: Defects associated with the blockage of one or more enzymes necessary for the production of cortisol and resulting in decreased plasma cortisol, increased ACTH, and hyperplasia of the adrenal cortex.

Idiopathic hemochromatosis: The infiltration of iron into the tissues.

antibodies or that it is caused by factors related to the aging of stored blood products. Publications promoting the antibody-mediated theory implicate HLA class I, class II antibodies and neutrophil-specific antibodies, primarily.[120,122-128]

Although a specific diagnostic test does not exist for TRALI, laboratory confirmation of the clinical diagnosis is important. Methods of HLA and neutrophil antibody detection can be performed in suspected TRALI cases. Some have suggested that donors from multiparous women should be screened first. If no antibody is found among multiparous donors, donors of other products the patient received should be tested. Finally, if no antibody is identified among any of the donors tested, the patient should be screened for the presence of HLA and/or granulocyte antibodies. If antibody is found in either the donor or the patient, concordance should be looked for by crossmatch testing between the donor and the recipient and/or HLA phenotyping to prove the presence of the antigen. If concordance is found, this is strongly suggestive of a diagnosis of TRALI. If no antibody is found, including HLA class II antibodies, or no concordance, this does not entirely rule out a diagnosis of TRALI. In up to 15% of TRALI cases reported, no antibody has been identified in either the patient or donor.[121,128,129]

CHAPTER SUMMARY

1. The major histocompatibility complex (MHC) refers to a cluster of genes that are involved in graft rejection and the immune response. In the human, this system is called HLA. Analog MHC systems have been found in all mammals studied so far.

2. The HLA antigens play an important role in the immune system's ability to distinguish self from non-self, and are required for antigen processing and presentation.

3. There are two main classes of HLA genes: class I (including HLA-A, HLA-B, and HLA-C) and class II (e.g., HLA-DR, HLA-DP, and HLA-DQ). A third class (class III) encodes complement components and other molecules not specifically involved in immune recognition. Each gene has a distinct position (or locus) on chromosome 6.

4. This entire area is highly polymorphic, meaning that there are a large number of different genes between different individuals at the same genetic locus. Different forms of genes that occupy the same locus are said to be alleles of each other. It is highly unlikely that two unrelated persons have the same HLA type.

5. Serologic nomenclature categorizes antigen families as defined by antibody reaction patterns. Many antigens in the HLA system share common antigenic determinants or epitopes. These antigenic determinants can also be defined as either private or public epitopes.

6. Nomenclature for HLA antigens assigned by DNA typing consists of the locus (e.g., HLA-DRB1), followed by an asterisk, two arabic digits for the corresponding serologic specificity, and two digits for the specific sequence.

7. For HLA antigen phenotyping ("tissue typing") by the complement-dependent microlymphocytotoxicity (CDC) test, known antisera are used to identify HLA antigens on the lymphocyte surface. Using this same procedure, patient sera can be assessed for panel-reactive antibodies (PRAs) by screening against a panel of HLA-phenotyped lymphocytes, and compatibility between an individual potential donor and the patient can be established through crossmatching of donor cells with patient sera.

8. State-of-the-art histocompatibility testing takes advantage of advances in molecular and ELISA testing methodology to replace conventional serologic testing with methods that are more sensitive and precise, as well as standardizable and automatable.

9. The HLA crossmatch assay is the most important clinical HLA test result for most solid organ transplants. It is used to determine whether a transplant patient has detectable antidonor HLA antibodies. Avoiding antidonor HLA antibodies when selecting donor-recipient pairings results in low likelihood of early acute rejection and graft loss.

10. By molecular tissue typing techniques, HLA antigens that are either difficult to identify or are not detected by serologic methods (e.g., alleles) can be recognized. Reagents needed to perform the tests are readily available from several commercial sources, qualitatively and quantitatively consistent from batch to batch, and highly specific. Molecular HLA typing may be performed with small quantities of cells, including those that are nonviable.

11. The primary stimuli for HLA alloimmunization are transfusion (contaminating leukocytes from blood and blood components), transplantation, and pregnancy.

12. Clinical HLA testing primarily serves the needs of solid organ and progenitor cell transplant programs, transfusion medicine, and disease association studies.

13. Both HLA class I and class II alloantigens can induce transplant immunity at humoral (antibody) and cellular (T lymphocyte) immune levels.

14. Advances in organ transplantation have been accompanied by advances in HLA testing and typing techniques. These, along with improved patient management regimens, allow for the selection of the best possible grafts for patients.

15. Individuals with particular HLA types have a greater incidence of certain diseases. HLA typing may assist in making diagnoses of some of these diseases if the particular HLA antigen carries a high enough relative risk for the disorder (e.g., ankylosing spondylitis, narcolepsy).

16. The functional association between HLA alleles and disease is coming to be understood in molecular terms, and critical sites within "susceptibility" alleles of HLA molecules have been identified in several diseases. This information is important for identifying individuals at risk and devising new strategies for prevention or therapy.

17. HLA testing has improved the selection of platelets for refractory patients by providing matched and selectively mismatched components for transfusion.

REFERENCES

1. Dausset H: Leukoagglutinins. IV. Leukoagglutinins and blood transfusion. Vox Sang 4:190, 1954.
2. Dausset H: Iso-leuco-anti-corps. Acta Haematol 20:156-166, 1958.
3. Brittingham TE, Chaplin H: Febrile transfusion reactions caused by sensitivity to donor leukocytes and platelets. JAMA 165:819, 1957.
4. Payne R: The association of febrile transfusion reactions with leukoagglutinins. Vox Sang 2:233, 1957.
5. Payne R, Rolfs MR: Fetomaternal leukocyte incompatibility. J Clin Invest 37:1756-1763, 1958.
6. van Rood JJ, Eernisse JG, vanLeeuwen A: Leukocyte antibodies in the sera of pregnant women. Nature 181:1735, 1958.
7. Gorer PA: The antigenic basis of tumour transplantation. J Pathol Bacteriol 231-252, 1938.
8. Gorer PA, Snell GD, Amiel JL: The genetic and antigenic basis for tumor transplantation. J Pathol Bacteriol 691-697, 1937.
9. Snell GD, Higgins GF: Alleles at the histocompatibility-2 locus in the mouse as determined by tumor transplantation. Genetics 306-310, 1951.
10. Friedman EA, Retan JW, Marshall DC: Accelerated skin graft rejection in humans preimmunized with homologous peripheral leukocytes. J Clin Invest 40:2162-2170, 1961.
11. Daar AS, Fuggle SV, Fabre JW, et al: The detailed distribution of HLA-A, B, C antigens in normal human organs. Transplantation 38:287-292, 1984.
12. Doherty PC, Zinkernagel RM: Restriction of in vitro T cell–mediated cytotoxicity in lymphocytic choriomeningitis within a syngeneic or semiallogeneic system. J Exp Med 141:502-507, 1975.
13. Zinkernagel RM, Doherty PC: Immunological surveillance against altered self components by sensitised T lymphocytes in lymphocytic choriomeningitis. Nature 25:547-548, 1974.
14. Zinkernagel RM, Doherty PC: Restriction of in vitro T cell–mediated cytotoxicity in lymphocytic choriomeningitis within a syngeneic or semiallogeneic system. Nature 25:701-702, 1974.
15. Rothenberg EV: Stepwise specification of lymphocyte developmental lineages. Curr Opin Genet Dev 10:370-379, 2000.
16. Rothenberg EV: The development of functionally responsive T cells. Adv Immunol 51:85-214, 1992.
17. Baldwin KK, Trenchak BP, Altman JD, Davis MM: Negative selection of T cells occurs throughout thymic development. J Immunol 163:689-698, 1999.
18. Denis F, Rheaume E, Aouad SM, et al: The role of caspases in T cell development and the control of immune responses. Cell Mol Life Sci 54:1005-1019, 1998.
19. Poulin JF, Viswanathan MN, Harris JM, et al: Direct evidence for thymic function in adult humans. J Exp Med 190:479-486, 1999.
20. Ridgway WM, Fathman CG: The association of MHC with autoimmune diseases: Understanding the pathogenesis of autoimmune diabetes. Clin Immunol Immunopathol 86:3-10, 1998.
21. Savage PA, Davis MM: A kinetic window constricts the T cell receptor repertoire in the thymus. Immunity 14:243-252, 2001.
22. Rhodes DA, Trowsdale J: Genetics and molecular genetics of the MHC. Rev Immunogenet 1:21-31, 1999.
23. Natarajan K, Li H, Mariuzza RA, Margulies DH: MHC class I molecules, structure and function. Rev Immunogenet 1:32-46, 1999.
24. Little AM, Parham P: Polymorphism and evolution of HLA class I and II genes and molecules. Rev Immunogenet 1:105-123, 1999.
25. Beck S, Trowsdale J: The human major histocompatibility complex: Lessons from the DNA sequence. Annu Rev Genomics Hum Genet 1:117-137, 2000.
26. Le Bouteiller P, Blaschitz A: The functionality of HLA-G is emerging. Immunol Rev 167:233-244, 1999.
27. Weetman AP: The immunology of pregnancy. Thyroid 9:643-646, 1999.
28. Gadola SD, Moins-Teisserenc HT, Trowsdale J, et al: TAP deficiency syndrome. Clin Exp Immunol 121:173-178, 2000.
29. Hutchinson IV, Pravica V, Hajeer A, Sinnott PJ: Identification of high and low responders to allografts. Rev Immunogenet 1:323-333, 1999.
30. Crawford K, Alper CA: Genetics of the complement system. Rev Immunogenet 2:323-338, 2000.
31. Hiller C, Bischoff M, Schmidt A, Bender K: Analysis of the HLA-ABC linkage disequilibrium: Decreasing strength of gametic association with increasing map distance. Hum Genet 41:301-312, 1978.
32. Bender K, Bissbort S, Hiller C, et al: On regional mapping of human chromosome 6. Review and own findings. Acta Anthropogenet 7:85-105, 1983.

33. Bell JI, Todd JA: HLA class II sequences infer mechanisms for major histocompatibility complex–associated disease susceptibility. Mol Biol Med 6:43-53, 1989.

34. Koller BH, Geraghty DE, DeMars R, et al: Chromosomal organization of the human major histocompatibility complex class I gene family. J Exp Med 169:469-480, 1989.

35. Hiller C, Bischoff M, Schmidt A, Bender K: Analysis of the HLA-ABC linkage disequilibrium: Decreasing strength of gametic association with increasing map distance. Hum Genet 41:301-312, 1978.

36. Degos L, Dausset J: Human migrations and linkage disequilibrium of HL-A system. Immunogenetics 3:195, 1975.

37. Tomlinson IP, Bodmer WF: The HLA system and the analysis of multifactorial genetic disease. Trends Genet 11:493-498, 1995.

38. Terasaki PI, McClalland JD: Microdroplet assay of human serum cytotoxins. Nature 204:2469-2475, 1964.

39. Marsh SGE, Albert ED, Bodmer WF, et al: Nomenclature for factors of the HLA system, 2002. Hum Immunol 63: 1213-1268, 2002.

40. Marsh SGE: HLA nomenclature and the IMGT/HLA sequence database. Novartis Foundation Symposium 254:165-173, 2003.

41. Konoeda Y, Terasaki PI, Wakisaka A, et al: Public determinants of HLA indicated by pregnancy antibodies. Transplantation 41:253-259, 1986.

42. Rodey GE, Neylan JF, Whelchel JD, et al: Epitope specificity of HLA class I alloantibodies. I. Frequency analysis of antibodies to private versus public specificities in potential transplant recipients. Hum Immunol 39:272-280, 1994.

43. Rodey GE, Fuller TC: Public epitopes and the antigenic structure of the HLA molecules. Crit Rev Immunol 7: 229-267, 1987.

44. Duquesnoy RJ, Howe J, Takemoto S: HLA matchmaker: A molecularly based algorithm for histocompatibility determination. IV. An alternative strategy to increase the number of compatible donors for highly sensitized patients. Transplantation 75:889-897, 2003.

45. Takemoto SK: HLA amino acid residue matching. Clin Transpl 397-425, 1996.

46. McKenna RM, Takemoto SK: Improving HLA matching for kidney transplantation by use of CREGs. Lancet 355: 1842-1843, 2000.

47. Dupont B: Nomenclature for factors of the HLA system, 1987. Decisions of the Nomenclature Committee on Leukocyte Antigens, which met in New York on November 21-23, 1987. Hum Immunol 26:3-14, 1989.

48. Marsh SGE, Albert ED, Bodmer WF, et al: Nomenclature for factors of the HLA system, 2002. Tissue Antigens 60:407-464, 2002.

49. Bodmer JG, Marsh SG, Albert ED, et al: Nomenclature for factors of the HLA system, 1990. Hum Immunol 31:186-194, 1991.

50. Abrahamova J, Majsky A: HLA system and some neoplastic diseases. Acta Univ Carol [Med Monogr] (Praha) 123:1-80, 1988.

51. Charron D: HLA class II disease associations: Molecular basis. J Autoimmun (5 Suppl A):45-53, 1992.

52. Nepom GT, Erlich H: MHC class-II molecules and autoimmunity. Annu Rev Immunol 9:493-525, 1991.

53. Gebel HM, Bray RA: Sensitization and sensitivity: Defining the unsensitized patient. Transplantation 69:1370-1374, 2000.

54. Gebel HM, Bray RA, Ruth JA, et al: Flow PRA to detect clinically relevant HLA antibodies. Transplant Proc 33:477, 2001.

55. Kerman RH, Susskind B, Slaton J, et al: Improved graft survival in 100 retransplant recipients following AHG-negative crossmatching. Transplant Proc 29:1451-1453, 1997.

56. Johnson AH, Rossen RD, Butler WT: Detection of alloantibodies using a sensitive antiglobulin microcytotoxicity test: Identification of low levels of pre-formed antibodies in accelerated allograft rejection. Tissue Antigens 2:215-226, 1972.

57. Fuller TC, Phelan D, Gebel HM, Rodey GE: Antigenic specificity of antibody reactive in the antiglobulin-augmented lymphocytotoxicity test. Transplantation 34: 24-29, 1982.

58. Fuller TC, Fuller AA, Golden M, Rodey GE: HLA alloantibodies and the mechanism of the antiglobulin-augmented lymphocytotoxicity procedure. Hum Immunol 56:94-105, 1997.

59. Fuller AA, Rodey GE, Parham P, Fuller TC: Epitope map of the HLA-B7 CREG using affinity-purified human alloantibody probes. Hum Immunol 28:306-325, 1990.

60. Fuller AA, Trevithick JE, Rodey GE, et al: Topographic map of the HLA-A2 CREG epitopes using human alloantibody probes. Hum Immunol 28:284-305, 1990.

61. Mulder A, Kardol M, Blom J, et al: A human monoclonal antibody, produced following in vitro immunization, recognizing an epitope shared by HLA-A2 subtypes and HLA-A28. Tissue Antigens 42:27-34, 1993.

62. Mulder A, Kardol M, Blom J, et al: Characterization of two human monoclonal antibodies reactive with HLA-B12 and HLA-B60, respectively, raised by in vitro secondary immunization of peripheral blood lymphocytes. Hum Immunol 36:186-192, 1993.

63. Mulder A, Kardol MJ, Uit het Broek CM, et al: A human monoclonal antibody against HLA-Cw1 and a human monoclonal antibody against an HLA-A locus determinant derived from a single uniparous female. Tissue Antigens 52:393-396, 1998.

64. Hansen JA, Yamamoto K, Petersdorf E, Sasazuki T: The role of HLA matching in hematopoietic cell transplantation. Rev Immunogenet 1:359-373, 1999.

65. Petersdorf EW, Anasetti C, Martin PJ, Hansen JA: Tissue typing in support of unrelated hematopoietic cell transplantation. Tissue Antigens 61:1-11, 2003.

66. Middleton D: History of DNA typing for the human MHC. Rev Immunogenet 1:135-156, 1999.

67. Welsh K, Bunce M: Molecular typing for the MHC with PCR-SSP. Rev Immunogenet 1:157-176, 1999.

68. Cao K, Chopek M, Fernandez-Vina MA: High and intermediate resolution DNA typing systems for class I HLA-A, B, C genes by hybridization with sequence-specific oligonucleotide probes (SSOP). Rev Immunogenet 1:177-208, 1999.

69. Arguello JR, Madrigal JA: HLA typing by Reference Strand Mediated Conformation Analysis (RSCA). Rev Immunogenet 1:209-219, 1999.

70. Guo Z, Hood L, Petersdorf EW: Oligonucleotide arrays for high resolution HLA typing. Rev Immunogenet 1:220-230, 1999.

71. Kerman RH, Susskind B, Katz SM, et al: Postrenal transplant MLR hypo-responders have fewer rejections and better graft survival than MLR hyper-responders. Transplant Proc 29:1410-1411, 1997.

72. Reinsmoen NL: Cellular methods used to evaluate the immune response in transplantation. Tissue Antigens 59: 241-250, 2002.

73. Yang SY, Morishima Y, Collins NH: Comparison of one-dimensional IEF patterns serologically detectable HLA-A and B allotypes. Immunogenetics 19:217-231, 1984.

74. Kerman RH, Orosz CG, Lorber MI: Clinical relevance of anti-HLA antibodies pre and post transplant. Am J Med Sci 313:275-288, 1997.

75. Cook DJ, Fettouh HI, Gjertson DW, Cecka JM: Flow cytometry crossmatching (FCXM) in the UNOS Kidney Transplant Registry. Clin Transpl 413-419, 1998.

76. Lobashevsky AL, Senkbeil RW, Shoaf JL, et al: The number of amino acid residues mismatches correlates with flow cytometry crossmatching results in high PRA renal patients. Hum Immunol 63:364-374, 2002.

77. Bray RA: Flow cytometry in human leukocyte antigen testing. Semin Hematol 38:194-200, 2001.

78. Cho YW, Cecka JM: Crossmatch tests—an analysis of UNOS data from 1991-2000. Clin Transpl 237-246, 2001.

79. Dilioglou S, Cruse JM, Lewis RE: High panel reactive antibody against cross-reactive group antigens as a contraindication to renal allotransplantation. Exp Mol Pathol 71:73-78, 2001.

80. O'Rourke RW, Osorio RW, Freise CE, et al: Flow cytometry crossmatching as a predictor of acute rejection in sensitized recipients of cadaveric renal transplants. Clin Transplant 14:167-173, 2000.

81. Aziz S, Hassantash SA, Nelson K, et al: The clinical significance of flow cytometry crossmatching in heart transplantation. J Heart Lung Transplant 17:686-692, 1998.

82. Bittencourt MC, Rebibou JM, Saint-Hillier Y, et al: Impaired renal graft survival after a positive B-cell flow-cytometry crossmatch. Nephrol Dial Transplant 13:2059-2064, 1998.

83. Bryan CF, Baier KA, Nelson PW, et al: Long-term graft survival is improved in cadaveric renal retransplantation by flow cytometric crossmatching. Transplantation 66: 1827-1832, 1998.

84. Brando B, Sommaruga E: Flow cytometry cross-match. Eur J Histochem 40:53-62, 1996.

85. Bray RA: Flow cytometry crossmatching for solid organ transplantation. Methods Cell Biol 41:103-119, 1994.

86. Berteli AJ, Daniel V, Pomer S, Opelz G: Clinical relevance of pretransplant flow cytometric crossmatches with T and B lymphocytes in kidney transplantation. Transplant Proc 22:1895-1896, 1990.

87. Buelow R, Chiang TR, Monteiro F, et al: Soluble HLA antigens and ELISA—a new technology for crossmatch testing. Transplantation 60:1594-1599, 1995.

88. Hennessy PK, Adams PW, Inlow JC, et al: Comparison of sensitivity, reproducibility, and test agreement between Amos-modified, AHG, ELISA, and flow cytometry crossmatch methodologies. Hum Immunol 55(Suppl 1):85, 1997.

89. Susskind B, Kerman RH, Nelson R, et al: Comparison between enzyme-linked immunosorbent assay and cytotoxic cross-match procedures for detecting IgG anti-donor antibodies. Transplantation 66:1823-1826, 1998.

90. Takemoto SK, Terasaki PI, Gjertson DW, Cecka JM: Twelve years' experience with national sharing of HLA-matched cadaveric kidneys for transplantation. N Engl J Med 343:1078-1084, 2000.

91. Terasaki PI: The HLA-matching effect in different cohorts of kidney transplant recipients. Clin Transpl 497-514, 2000.

92. Hata Y, Cecka JM, Takemoto S, et al: Effects of changes in the criteria for nationally shared kidney transplants for HLA-matched patients. Transplantation 65:208-212, 1998.

93. Gjertson DW: A multi-factor analysis of kidney regraft outcomes. Clin Transpl 335-349, 2002.

94. Hata Y, Ozawa M, Takemoto SK, Cecka JM: HLA matching. Clin Transpl 381-396, 1996.

95. Danovitch GM, Cecka JM: Allocation of deceased donor kidneys: Past, present, and future. Am J Kidney Dis 42: 882-890, 2003.

96. Opelz G: HLA compatibility and kidney grafts from unrelated live donors. Collaborative Transplant Study. Transplant Proc 30:704-705, 1998.

97. Eastlund T: The histo-blood group ABO system and tissue transplantation. Transfusion 38:975-988, 1998.

98. Benjamin RJ, McGurk S, Ralston MS, et al: ABO incompatibility as an adverse risk factor for survival after allogeneic bone marrow transplantation. Transfusion 39: 179-187, 1999.

99. Tambur AR, Bray RA, Takemoto SK, et al: Flow cytometric detection of HLA-specific antibodies as a predictor of heart allograft rejection. Transplantation 70:1055-1059, 2000.

100. Bishay ES, Cook DJ, Starling RC, et al: The clinical significance of flow cytometry crossmatching in heart transplantation. Eur J Cardiothorac Surg 17:362-369, 2000.

101. Bishay ES, Cook DJ, El FH, et al: The impact of HLA sensitization and donor cause of death in heart transplantation. Transplantation 70:220-222, 2000.

102. Burgess BO, Palmer S, Russell SD, et al: Impact of plasmapheresis/IVIg therapies on antibody levels and graft outcome in heart and lung recipients. Hum Immunol 64:S110, 2003.

103. Lau CL, Palmer SM, Posther KE, et al: Influence of panel-reactive antibodies on posttransplant outcomes in lung transplant recipients. Ann Thorac Surg 69:1520, 2000.

104. Tiercy JM, Villard J, Roosnek E: Selection of unrelated bone marrow donors by serology, molecular typing and cellular assays. Transplant Immunol 10:215-221, 2002.

105. Petersdorf E, Anasetti C, Servida P, et al: Effect of HLA matching on outcome of related and unrelated donor transplantation therapy for chronic myelogenous leukemia. Hematol Oncol Clin North Am 12:107-121, 1998.

106. Petersdorf E, Anasetti C, Martin PJ, et al: Genomics of unrelated-donor hematopoietic cell transplantation. Curr Opin Immunol 13:582-589, 2001.

107. Hurley CK, Wade JA, Oudshoorn M, et al: A special report: Histocompatibility testing guidelines for hematopoietic stem cell transplantation using volunteer donors. Tissue Antigens 53:394-406, 1999.

108. Hurley CK, Setterholm M, Lau M, et al: Hematopoietic stem cell donor registry strategies for assigning search determinants and matching relationships. Bone Marrow Transplant 33:443-450, 2004.

109. Hurley CK: HLA diversity: Detection and impact on unrelated hematopoietic stem cell donor characterization and selection. Int J Hematol 76(Suppl 2):152-154, 2002.

110. Cohena Y, Nagler A: Hematopoietic stem-cell transplantation using umbilical-cord blood. Leuk Lymphoma 44:1287-1299, 2003.

111. Grewal SS, Barker JN, Davies SM, Wagner JE: Unrelated donor hematopoietic cell transplantation: Marrow or umbilical cord blood? Blood 101:4233-4244, 2003.

112. Barker JN, Krepski TP, DeFor TE, et al: Searching for unrelated donor hematopoietic stem cells: Availability and speed of umbilical cord blood versus bone marrow. Biol Blood Marrow Transplant 8:257-260, 2002.

113. Rodey GE: Prevention of alloimmunization in thrombo-cytopenic patients. In Smith DM (ed): Platelets. Arlington, VA, American Association of Blood Banks, 1988.

114. Uhrynowska M, Zupanska B: Platelet-specific antibodies in transfused patients. Eur J Haematol 56:248-251, 1996.

115. Schiffer CA: Management of patients refractory to platelet transfusion: An evaluation of methods of donor selection. Progr Hematol 15:91, 1987.

116. Walker RH, Pohl BA: Paternity testing with an absent mother. The probability of exclusion of red cell surface antigen, Gm, Hp, and HLA systems in North American whites and blacks. Transfusion 29:31-35, 1989.

117. Walker RH, Meyers MA, Phillips LM: The probability of exclusion of the HLA-A,B system in North American whites and blacks in parentage tests. Transfusion 27:75-79, 1987.

118. Henke L, Fimmers R, Josephi E, et al: Usefulness of conventional blood groups, DNA-minisatellites, and short tandem repeat polymorphisms in paternity testing: A comparison. Forensic Sci Int 103:133-142, 1999.

119. Thomson JA, Pilotti V, Stevens P, et al: Validation of short tandem repeat analysis for the investigation of cases of disputed paternity. Forensic Sci Int 100:1-16, 1999.

120. Popovsky MA, Moore SB: Diagnostic and pathogenetic considerations in transfusion-related acute lung injury. Transfusion 25:573-577, 1985.

121. Silliman CC, Boshkov LK, Mehdizadehkashi Z, et al: Transfusion-related acute lung injury: Epidemiology and a prospective analysis of etiologic factors. Blood 101:454-462, 2003.

122. Bux J, Becker F, Seeger W, et al: Transfusion-related acute lung injury due to HLA-A2–specific antibodies in recipient and NB1-specific antibodies in donor blood. Br J Haematol 93:707-713, 1996.

123. Bux J: Molecular nature of granulocyte antigens. Transfus Clin Biol 8:242-247, 2001.

124. Davoren A, Curtis BR, Shulman IA, et al: TRALI due to granulocyte-agglutinating human neutrophil antigen-3a (5b) alloantibodies in donor plasma: A report of 2 fatalities. Transfusion 43:641, 2003.

125. Eastlund DT, McGrath PC, Burkart P: Platelet transfusion reaction associated with interdonor HLA incompatibility. Vox Sang 55:157-160, 1988.

126. Kao GS, Wood IG, Dorfman DM, et al: Investigations into the role of anti-HLA class II antibodies in TRALI. Transfusion 43:185-191, 2003.

127. Kopko PM, Popovsky MA, MacKenzie MR, et al: HLA class II antibodies in transfusion-related acute lung injury. Transfusion 41:1244-1248, 2001.

128. Kopko PM, Marshall CS, MacKenzie MR, et al: Transfusion-related acute lung injury: Report of a clinical look-back investigation. JAMA 287:1968-1971, 2002.

129. Popovsky M, Haley NR: Further characterization of transfusion-related acute lung injury: Demographics, clinical and laboratory features, and morbidity. Immunohematology 16:157-159, 2000.

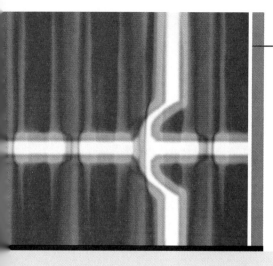

Donation, Preparation, and Storage

The science of immunohematology and the practice of transfusion medicine are dependent on the act of donation. Blood donors represent less than 5% of the population, and it is these unselfish individuals who provide the whole blood product or component(s) that meet the needs of the entire nation. It is therefore essential that we continue to expand and at the same time retain the current donor pool. Donation must be accomplished in such a way that the safety of both the donor and the potential recipient is assured. This is facilitated, in part, by careful donor screening, appropriate record keeping, accurate and sensitive donor testing, efficient component preparation, quality control and quality assurance, continuing education and development, and compliance with established standards of practice.

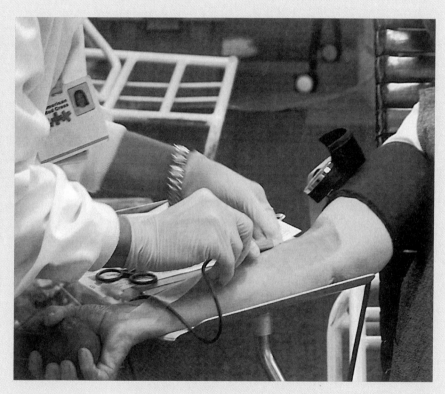

The donated blood can be further processed to produce blood components, which allow for a more efficient utilization of the product and can better meet the transfusion needs of the patient population. Component preparation requires the development of new, safer, and more efficient preparation techniques and careful quality control. Regulatory agencies and voluntary accrediting agencies provide guidelines for practice that serve to ensure the quality and safety of the product.

Once prepared, blood components must be stored at conditions that will maintain viability, sterility, and potency. The length of storage, temperature of storage, and other optimal physical and chemical conditions must be maintained for the shelf life of the product. Continued research results in improved preservation and storage techniques, for example, the development of new plastics for containers and improved anticoagulant/preservative solutions.

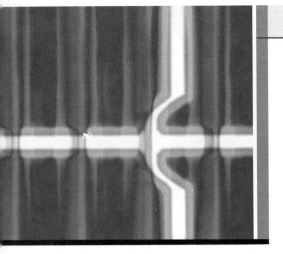

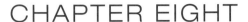

CHAPTER EIGHT

Donor Screening and Blood Collection

Joy L. Fridey and Candace E. Kay

LEARNING OBJECTIVES

After reading and studying this chapter, the student should be able to:

1. Describe the role of the Food and Drug Administration, the American Association of Blood Banks, the College of American Pathologists, and the Joint Commission on Accreditation of Healthcare Organizations in regulating and setting standards for the practice of blood banking and transfusion medicine.
2. Discuss factors that affect blood availability.
3. Describe general approaches for maintaining the safety of the blood supply.
4. Explain the rationale for pre-donation screening.
5. Describe the components of the blood donor screening process.
6. Discuss the major categories of screening questions intended to protect recipients.
7. List approaches to conducting pre-donation screening.
8. Outline major format and design changes in the AABB Uniform Donor History Questionnaire.
9. Determine whether the donor is eligible to donate based on the results of the donor's physical evaluation.
10. Describe the confidential self-exclusion procedure.
11. Discuss the elements of donor consent.
12. List six anticoagulant/preservative/additive solutions that are currently approved for use.
13. Describe several approaches to preparation of the phlebotomy site.
14. List four possible adverse donor reactions, including symptoms and treatment.
15. State specific, current regulations with regard to the retention of donor records.
16. Describe the laboratory testing that must be done on donor blood before release.
17. State the rationale for doing bacterial detection testing on platelet apheresis products and why such testing is not required for a red blood cell product.
18. Describe under what conditions the following tests might be run on donor blood: cytomegalovirus (CMV) screening, special antigen typing, and screening for sickle cell trait.
19. List the 11 items that must be included on the final product label.
20. Define pooling and describe its value in transfusion medicine.
21. Describe the risks and benefits of preoperative whole blood autologous donation.
22. Explain why autologous units should not be crossed over into the general inventory.

23. Describe the benefits and challenges associated with directed donations.
24. Define the term apheresis.
25. Describe how multiple component technology is revolutionizing allogeneic blood collection.
26. Discuss adverse reactions that are unique for apheresis procedures.
27. Define the role that apheresis technology is playing in hematopoietic progenitor cell transplant therapies.

INTRODUCTION: CHALLENGES FOR THE MEDICAL TECHNOLOGIST

Each year in the United States approximately four million patients require transfusions of packed red blood cells, platelets, plasma, or cryoprecipitate. Transfusion is often a life-saving treatment, and is needed across the spectrum of patient care, especially for individuals undergoing surgery, receiving cancer therapy, or recovering from trauma. Because the Food and Drug Administration (FDA) has not yet approved/licensed for human use pharmaceutical products that could perform the oxygenation and hemostatic functions of blood, the blood supply depends almost entirely on voluntary donations by healthy donors or, to a lesser extent, autologous donations by qualified patients.

Two particularly important determinants of feasible and successful transfusion therapy are blood availability and safety. Availability is affected by a complex interplay of factors. The number of annual donations and regulations that affect donor qualification criteria are the most significant. It is estimated that fewer than 5% of potentially eligible individuals donate. Data from the National Blood Data Resources Center (NBDRC) of the American Association of Blood Banks (AABB) demonstrate that transfusion of whole blood between 1999 and 2001 increased by 15%, while collections only increased by 6%. These data also show that the excess of collected vs. transfused units, which was almost 1,200,000 units in 1999, decreased to a startlingly low 205,000 units.[1]

Donor eligibility has been affected by a growing body of standards, regulations, and guidance documents that are intended to diminish not only the risks of known transfusion-transmitted infections, but theoretical ones as well. This has resulted in the deferral of many potential donors and the loss of long-term frequent donors. Increased blood usage, blood type inventory imbalances, and even labor actions or weather patterns—both of which affect the transport of blood—can affect local and national supplies. The net result of these phenomena is that the blood supply in the United States is strained, and chronic, perpetual shortages have become an unfortunate fact of life for blood bankers and patients. Thus, medical technologists are faced with the increasingly difficult challenge of managing unpredictable and sometimes less than optimal hospital inventories.

TABLE 8-1 Per-Unit Risk of Selected Transfusion-Transmissible Viruses

Virus	Risk per Unit
HIV*	1:2,135,000
HCV*	1:1,935,000
HBV	1:205,000
HTLV	1:2,993,000

Source: Dodd RY, Notari EP, Stramer SL: Current prevalence and incidence of infectious disease markers and estimated window period risk in the American Red Cross blood donor population. Transfusion 42:975-979, 2002.
*With nucleic acid testing (NAT).

The good news is that blood safety has improved by orders of magnitude in the past 15 years. In the mid-1980s, direct questioning of donors about risk factors for human immunodeficiency virus (HIV) and hepatitis reduced transfusion transmission of these infections. The implementation of extremely sensitive tests for serologic and/or nucleic acid evidence of HIV types 1 and 2, hepatitis B and C, syphilis, human T-cell lymphotropic viruses types I and II (HTLV-I/II), and West Nile virus nucleic acid testing (NAT) have had a huge and welcome impact on blood safety. Table 8-1 shows the currently estimated per-unit risk for HIV and other viruses. In addition, the AABB and College of American Pathologists (CAP) Standards requiring testing of platelets for evidence of bacterial contamination will reduce the risk of what is currently the major cause of transfusion-associated infection.

This improvement in blood safety has resulted in obvious health benefits, but safety enhancements have also been associated with significant increases in the costs of processing and testing units. These costs are, for the most part, borne by hospitals. Transfusion services have witnessed unprecedented increases in blood expenditures at a time when health care facilities and laboratories are facing major resource challenges. As a result, today's hospital-based medical technologists not only must grapple with managing sometimes scarce supplies, but function within a "do more with less" milieu.

The contributions that medical technologists make to the field of transfusion medicine and blood banking cannot be overstated—neither can their responsibilities. Medical technologists who work in a blood collection facility may be involved in donor screening and blood collection, processing, and testing, and quality programs. Staff employed in transfusion services will likely participate in the management of inventory, some types of processing, compatibility testing, issuing of blood, and quality assurance functions. Regardless of their specific role, medical technologists can enhance their expertise and ability to address challenges by remaining conversant in and informed about all aspects of transfusion medicine and blood banking. The major objective of this chapter is to provide relevant information about blood collection and some aspects of processing.

FACILITIES, REGULATIONS, AND STANDARDS
Blood Banks, Blood Centers, and Transfusion Services: Who Is Who?

The term **blood bank** has been used generically to mean a **blood center,** a hospital-based **transfusion service,** or some combination of these. In this chapter, the use of the words "blood bank" will be avoided (although "blood bankers" will be used in a loose way to refer to those involved in transfusion medicine and blood banking). "Blood centers" will refer to either community or hospital-based collection facilities. "Transfusion service" will refer to the department in a hospital that performs compatibility testing and issues blood. These are somewhat arbitrary designations, in that several community blood centers perform compatibility testing

Blood center (blood bank): A facility that is generally responsible for activities leading to the preparation of suitable blood products for transfusion, including such areas as donor recruitment, phlebotomy, processing, storage, and shipment. Some blood centers have expanded roles, including pretransfusion testing, antigen screening, and reference services.

Transfusion service: A facility traditionally housed in the institution where transfusion takes place, usually a hospital. The role of the blood bank is to provide the necessary testing and support to ensure the appropriate and safe transfusion of blood, blood components, and blood products. Typical roles of the blood bank include pretransfusion testing, antibody identification, product selection, and monitoring of transfusion outcomes.

for hospitals—so-called centralized crossmatching—and some transfusion services may actually process blood collected by a hospital blood center.

Traditionally, blood centers handle donor recruitment, screening, collection of whole blood or apheresis products, serologic and **infectious disease marker (IDM)** testing, preparation of components, storage, and transport. In addition, some community blood centers provide highly specialized services such as **human leukocyte antigen (HLA)** testing, consultation or reference laboratory services for antibody identification problems, crossmatching for out-of-hospital transfusions, educational training for health practitioners and the public, and serve as a general resource on blood-related issues.

The hospital transfusion service is closest to the patient care arena, in that it performs compatibility testing, resolves patient antibody problems, carries out final product preparation (such as pooling of platelet concentrates or thawing of fresh frozen plasma), issues units for transfusion, and investigates transfusion complications or reactions. Transfusion services may also engage in certain types of processing such as irradiation, leukofiltration, and even testing of platelet components for evidence of bacterial detection. Education of health care workers such as medical technologists, pathology residents, and other physicians, including medical staff, is also an activity of some transfusion services. Whether or not a formal training program exists, the transfusion service technologists and medical director should play a role in teaching and reinforcing good transfusion practices to the clinical staff within each institution.

Most hospitals obtain blood from community blood centers, but other models for blood acquisition exist. The gamut of hospital-based collection activities runs from providing solely autologous and/or directed donor services to more complex activities such as component processing and labeling. It is estimated that approximately 10% of all blood in the United States is collected by hospital-based centers.[1] For those centers that engage in collection and processing activities, the medical technologist's responsibilities are much more extensive, not only because of the increased workload, but because regulations pertaining to processing and testing come into play.

Standards, Regulations, and Governing Bodies

Although the major purpose of regulations and standards is to ensure the highest possible level of safety, there are two overarching factors necessary for manufacturing a safe and efficacious blood product: (1) thorough and accurate pre-donation qualification (screening) of blood donors and (2) performing of serologic and IDM testing on all donations, in accordance with test manufacturers' instructions and applicable regulations.

Blood collection and transfusion activities in the United States are monitored and regulated by several entities. Regulatory oversight by the **Food and Drug Administration (FDA)** and state governments is inescapable, whereas accreditation by other agencies such as the **American Association of Blood Banks (AABB)**, the **College of American Pathology (CAP)**, or the **Joint Commission on Accreditation of Healthcare Organizations (JCAHO)** is voluntary. Institutions subscribe voluntarily because of their interest in maintaining and documenting high quality and standards.

All blood collection facilities in the United States are required by the Public Health Service Act to comply with "Current Good Manufacturing Practice for Blood and Blood Components," which is defined in the **Code of Federal Regulations (CFR)**, Title 21, Parts 200-299 and 600-799.[2] These codes, written by the U.S. Congress, are federal laws that are administered by the FDA, which generally conducts inspections of licensed and registered facilities on an annual basis. The goal of these regulations is to enhance the safety, purity, and potency of blood products.

FDA licensure is required if blood will be shipped across state lines; therefore most, if not all, community blood centers are licensed FDA establishments.

Infectious disease marker (IDM) testing: Testing for markers such as antigens, antibodies, or nucleic acid (viral genetic) material present in donated blood to screen for risk of transfusion-transmitted diseases. This testing enhances blood safety but also increases the cost of blood and blood products.

Refer to Chapter 7 for a discussion of the HLA system and implications in blood banking.

Food and Drug Administration (FDA—CBER): A federal agency that promulgates regulations and guidance documents for blood product manufacture and transfusion (refer to www.fda.gov/cber/blood.htm). *CBER,* Center for Biologics Evaluation and Research.

American Association of Blood Banks (AABB): The professional, standard-setting organization for practitioners in the field of transfusion medicine. The AABB provides standards of excellence for transfusion medicine practice and has a voluntary inspection and accreditation program (refer to www.aabb.org).

College of American Pathologists (CAP): A professional organization for clinical pathologists and clinical laboratory scientists. CAP develops standards of practice for clinical laboratories and has a voluntary inspection and accreditation program (refer to www.cap.org/apps/cap.portal).

Joint Commission on Accreditation of Healthcare Organizations (JCAHO): The organization that develops standards for health care delivery and provides a voluntary inspection and accreditation program for hospitals and other health care delivery organizations (refer to www.jcaho.org/).

Code of Federal Regulations (CFR): FDA publication that includes regulations pertaining to, among other things, the manufacture of blood, blood components, and blood products.

Facilities that do not ship across state lines are not required to obtain licensure, but any entity that collects or processes blood must at least be registered. This applies to transfusion services that collect autologous units. Likewise, transfusion services that perform certain types of "manufacturing" such as irradiation, leukofiltration, or component pooling must also register. Transfusion services that only make packed red cells from whole blood units and engage only in compatibility testing and issuing of units do not need to register.

Although some transfusion services are not required by law to have FDA licensure or registration, they are required to report fatalities in transfusion recipients.[2] But even beyond this, the FDA has, in recent years, assumed an oversight role for transfusion services that engage in component manufacturing processes, such as those mentioned previously. If the transfusion service that engages in manufacturing activities does not carry out those processes correctly and loses control of the product (such as issuing it for transfusion), that transfusion service must file a **biological product deviation (BPD)** report with the FDA. Examples of events that would require a BPD report are issuing a pooled platelet product with the wrong expiration time, or a unit for which leukoreduction was ordered but not done.[3]

Most blood centers and many transfusion services are accredited by the American Association of Blood Banks. Such accreditation is voluntary, but is viewed as a means of demonstrating conformance with an internationally recognized standard-setting organization. The AABB establishes minimum standards for blood banks and transfusion services. These standards are published approximately every 18 months in **Standards for Blood Banks and Transfusion Services,** the most current edition of which was published in November 2003.[4] Other AABB publications (such as the Technical Manual,[5] **Circular of Information,**[6] and frequent newsletters) and educational programs provide excellent guidelines and up-to-date information for blood collection practices and the field of transfusion medicine.

Although the combined activities of the FDA and AABB account for most of the regulatory oversight and accreditation, respectively, of blood centers and transfusion services, other agencies inspect for compliance with their own competency, proficiency, and safety criteria. The College of American Pathologists (CAP) inspects and accredits the laboratories of health care facilities, and has a "checklist" exclusively for transfusion services and blood collection programs. Accreditation requires audits every 2 years by assessors who review policies and procedures.[7]

The Joint Commission on Accreditation of Healthcare Organizations (JCAHO) also conducts comprehensive inspections of hospitals every other year. JCAHO has become increasingly interested in transfusion practices. The 2004 Standards require an approach to systematically collect data on processes related to the use, ordering, and administration of blood products. Data must be periodically analyzed and evaluated for undesirable trends. Further, a risk assessment for identifying and decreasing the occurrence of unanticipated adverse events must be conducted proactively.[8]

Blood centers and transfusion services must have written **standard operating procedures (SOPs)** for operational, regulatory, and some administrative activities. These are necessary in order to maintain consistency and ensure conformance with applicable regulations and standards. The actual development of these documents is by no means an easy task, but the **National Committee for Clinical Laboratory Standards (NCCLS)** has developed a standard laboratory procedure format that is recognized by accrediting agencies for its excellence. This format provides a structure for technical procedures that covers all relevant and important aspects.[9] The general requirements of an NCCLS procedure are shown in Box 8-1. The use of SOPs—which should reflect and integrate regulations and standards— is an essential practice for maintaining blood safety and appropriate usage.

Biological product deviation (BPD): A blood product that does not meet good manufacturing standards. A list of BPD codes can be found at www.fda.gov/cber/biodev/bpdrfy02-2.pdf.

Standards for Blood Banks and Transfusion Services (AABB Standards): A publication of the AABB that provides voluntary standards for blood centers and transfusion services. The AABB offers an accreditation program through which institutions can be audited and subsequently accredited to demonstrate conformance with the AABB Standards.

Circular of Information: The Circular of Information for the Use of Human Blood and Blood Components is a publication that provides a review of blood and blood components including composition, indications, contraindications and precautions, instructions for administration, and adverse reactions. The Code of Federal Regulations, Title 21, requires that the Circular be available to medical personnel involved in transfusion processes (refer to www.aabb.org/All_About_Blood/COI/coi0702.pdf).

Standard operating procedures (SOP): An approved set of written procedures that delineate in detail the procedures, policies, and processes performed in a blood center or transfusion service.

National Committee for Clinical Laboratory Standards (NCCLS): A professional organization that develops consensus standards and best practices for clinical laboratory testing (refer to www.nccls.org/).

Box 8-1	NCCLS Format for Laboratory Procedures

Purpose: Briefly state the goal of performing the procedure.

Policy: State the underlying rationale.

Reagents: If applicable, list all reagents that will be used; include those provided by the manufacturer and the facility. Should include directions for preparation and storage and labeling requirements for all reagents.

Equipment: Designate which instrument(s) will be used.

Supplies: List supplies.

Specimen: State the type of specimen, requisite patient preparation, and specific handling conditions.

Special safety precautions: List any that may be appropriate.

Quality control: Briefly describe how this will be assessed.

Procedure: Give a step-by-step, complete description of how the procedure will be performed.

Interpretation/results: State qualitative or quantitative results; provide reference ranges, when applicable; and specify results that warrant referral to a supervisor or medical director.

Calculations: Include equations and examples.

Expected values: Should include expected and/or acceptable quantitative or qualitative results and ranges.

Method limitations: Include interfering substances and linearity limits, and the effect on test results.

Procedure notes: Special comments that pertain to the procedure.

References: Cite texts, literature, regulations, standards, and other documents that serve as basis or logistics for performing the procedure.

Related documents: List other procedures that are related or apply.

Signatures: Section for signature of designated reviewers and those responsible for approval.

Appendices: Applicable documents to illustrate specific steps or items such as forms, labels, tags, or tables.

Source: NCCLS Clinical and Laboratory Technical Procedure Manuals: Approved Guideline, 4th ed. GP2-A4. 22(5), April 2002.

General Policies for Blood Banks and Transfusion Services

Standards of practice are found in the AABB Standards for Blood Banks and Transfusion Services. The framework for this reference is based on the quality management system approach, derived from **International Organization for Standardization (ISO)** elements. Box 8-2 presents an overview of the general policies that apply to all transfusion practices in blood banks and transfusion services. Box 8-3 contains the 10 quality system essentials defined by the AABB in 1997. Many of these general requirements are also requirements of other accrediting agencies, and reflect good laboratory practices and high quality standards.

Standard operating procedures and some policies vary from center to center. Blood collection facilities are permitted to adopt qualification measures that are more stringent than those of governments or accrediting agencies. However, if a blood collection facility wishes to implement screening practices or criteria that appear less rigorous or are different from regulations and standards, they must provide an appropriate rationale supported by data.

International Organization for Standardization (ISO): A nongovernmental organization that promulgates basic quality and safety standards for business and industry (refer to www.iso.org/iso/en/ISOOnline.frontpage).

DONORS AND DONOR SCREENING
Why Donate?

Each year, more than 14 million units of blood and products are collected from about 9 million people who donate at blood centers and mobile blood drives throughout the United States.[1] These people provide for the millions of patients

---

Box 8-2 **General Policies for Blood Banks and Transfusion Services**

I. The blood bank or transfusion service must be under the direction of a qualified licensed physician.
II. Quality management programs should include the following:
  A. A program of quality assessment and improvement to ensure that policies and procedures are properly maintained and executed.
  B. Detailed procedures manuals annually reviewed by the medical director.
  C. Quality control for reagents, equipment, and methods.
  D. Peer-review programs that monitor all categories of transfusion practice, including criteria for evaluating orders, usage, administration policies, and compliance with these criteria.
  E. All tests required by the standards must be performed in an accredited laboratory.
  F. All containers and anticoagulants used for preservation must meet or exceed the FDA criteria.
III. Safety programs should include the following:
  A. Programs to minimize risks to employees, donors, volunteers, and patients.
  B. Procedures for biologic, chemical, and radiation safety and monitoring.
  C. Handling and discarding of blood and blood components in a manner that decreases the potential for exposure to infectious agents.

Box 8-3 **AABB Standards for Blood Banks and Transfusion Services: Quality System Essentials**

Organization: Refers to roles and responsibilities of management, the quality system, and the requirement for development of policies, processes, and procedures.
Resources: Pertains to personnel selection, training, competency assessment, and records.
Equipment: Describes minimum requirements for selection, calibration, maintenance, identification, and control of equipment.
Supplier and customer issues: States expectations regarding suppliers, supplier agreements, and inspection of incoming materials.
Process control: Includes extensive details regarding component collection and production and transfusion-related activities.
Documents and records: Outlines document control and record retention periods.
Deviations, nonconformances, and complications: Presents expectations for follow-up and correction of these occurrences.
Assessments, internal and external: Pertains to expected follow-up of assessment results and monitoring of blood utilization.
Process improvement through corrective and preventive action: Describes specific events and issues that must be addressed. Describes approaches to prevention.
Facilities and safety: General guideline regarding appropriate facility, environmental, and safety conditions.

Source: Fridey JL (chair): Standards for Blood Banks and Transfusion Services, 22nd ed. Bethesda, MD, American Association of Blood Banks, 2003.

---

who are transfused every year in the United States. Who are these donors and why do they donate?

One of the major underpinnings of the safe U.S. blood supply is its volunteer nature. Studies in the 1970s showed that when paid donors were eliminated from the donation pool, the incidence of posttransfusion hepatitis was dramatically reduced.[10,11] Currently, motivations for voluntarily donating are as varied as the type of people who donate. It is likely that the vast majority of individuals do so out of altruism. Some donate for a specific family member or friend (directed, or designated, donations), or because they personally know someone who needed transfusions. A smaller number donate in order to receive a benefit such as a basic health assessment or to receive free laboratory screening such as cholesterol testing. Unfortunately, at least one study has shown that a small but significant number—1.1%—of individuals donate in order to receive free HIV testing.[12]

By definition, volunteerism means that donors are not paid. The FDA also does not permit gifts that are readily convertible into cash to be given to donors. Thus "hot" items—such as sporting event tickets that are likely to be "scalped"—would not be permitted. Neither would savings bonds, certificates of deposit, or other cash alternatives.[13] This regulation exists to decrease the chance that a prospective donor would withhold relevant risk information. However, the FDA does permit small items such as T-shirts, pens, ice cream bars, or sunglasses to be given as tokens of appreciation. Fortunately, most donors simply want to do a good deed, and small take-away gifts are incidental to their demonstration of altruism.

One exception to the no-cash policy exists. Commercial plasma centers that collect plasma for the manufacture of derivatives and pharmaceutical products are permitted to pay donors. This is allowable because the plasma fractionation processes inactivate pathogens. In addition, these companies undergo intense regulatory scrutiny to ensure product integrity and safety.

In the United States, tens of millions of people are eligible to donate blood. Unfortunately, only 3% to 5% of physically capable people do so. That these individuals are the sole source of blood for the entire country says much about their generosity. However, that the entire blood supply depends on this small group of people is disconcerting, and has serious implications for blood availability. Particularly, as regulatory agencies promulgate new deferral criteria and require new tests in the face of real or perceived blood safety threats, the number of donors could be seriously eroded unless new ones step into the supply breach.

Purpose of Pre-donation Screening

The approach to blood safety is multitiered, and is outlined in Box 8-4. A major pillar of safety is donor qualification. One reason for screening donors is to identify health, travel, medications, or infectious disease risks that could expose the recipient to infections or teratogenic substances. The other rationale is to identify medical conditions or health problems that could make donating an unsafe procedure for the donor. Briefly restated, screening is done to protect donors and recipients.

Screening has three possible outcomes for the prospective donor: acceptance, temporary deferral, or permanent deferral. Accepted donors continue on in the donation process. If a donor is temporarily deferred, the reason for and length of the deferral are explained and the donor may be advised to take specific follow-up actions. For example, if the donor's hemoglobin level is seriously low, the donor may be referred to his or her doctor for evaluation. Or, if the hemoglobin is slightly below normal and likely due to dietary factors or menstrual bleeding, iron-containing foods might be suggested. Persons who are not acceptable under any circumstances are permanently deferred. Persons at risk for the transmission of

---

Box 8-4	Mechanisms for Maximizing Blood Safety in the United States

Unpaid, voluntary donor base
Donor education
Pre-donation screening
Pre-donation medical evaluation
Confidential self-exclusion
Postdonation call-back instructions
Infectious disease marker testing

infectious diseases are deferred temporarily or permanently, depending on the nature of the exposure.

The donor screening process has four major components: (1) registration of the donor, at which time demographic information is obtained; (2) presentation of pre-donation educational materials to the donor; (3) a process to solicit information about medical, medication, travel, and social history; and (4) the physical evaluation. After successful completion of these steps, the donor advances to actual phlebotomy.

Registration and Demographic Information

During registration the donor provides identifying and demographic information that is necessary for compliance with regulations pertaining to the ability to trace units, avoid duplication of donor records, and notify the donor about abnormal test results. Demographic information can also be used for recruitment purposes or to mark donation milestones.

Data collected from each prospective donor should include the following:[2,4]

1. **Name**—first, last, and middle initial (not necessarily in that order).
2. **Permanent address;** home and business phone numbers. (E-mail addresses and cell phone numbers are optional but are increasingly valuable communication tools.)
3. **Gender.**
4. **Date of birth and age.** Date of birth is preferable because it can be a second source of permanent identification of the donor.
5. **Date of last donation,** if known by the donor. This information should be easily available to registration personnel so that donors are not accepted before they are eligible. For instance, donors of whole blood are not eligible to donate for 56 days after the previous whole blood donation, except in special circumstances. However, platelet or plasma donors may donate more frequently. For regulatory and operational reasons, it is therefore extremely useful to build future eligibility dates for specific types of donations into registration or other software. Otherwise, a manual system must exist for determining—preferably at the time of registration—whether donors can make their intended component donation on a given day.
6. **Written consent** of the donor to proceed with the donation process.
7. **A unique identifier** such as a social security number, driver's license number, or other unique and permanent number.
8. **Occupation and when the donor must return to work.** This may have relevance for determining when the donor can safely continue performing his or her usual duties. Each blood center should consider those occupations for which blood donation may represent a risk, keeping in mind that the plasma volume removed during whole blood donation returns to normal levels within 24 hours, but the red cell mass and hemoglobin levels may not return to the pre-donation levels for up to several weeks or months.
9. **Race or ethnicity.** This can be useful in selecting appropriate donors to screen for specific antigen-negative products or research protocols that require the race or ethnicity of the donor to be documented.

Before the next steps, the donation process should be clearly explained to the donor, especially if an individual is a first-time donor or the center has changed any of its major screening or collection procedures. The mechanics and purpose of the educational materials, the interviewing process, medical evaluation, other associated activities, and expected length of the donor's visit should be reviewed. This latter information is of particular importance, as donors, like all of us, are juggling increasingly busy lives and schedules. A donor planning to give whole blood can expect the actual phlebotomy to take 10 to 15 minutes, but the entire process takes up to an hour. Plasmapheresis may take 1 to 1.5 hours, and plateletpheresis from 1 to 2 hours.

Presentation of Educational Materials

Immediately before or after registration, donors are required to read information about blood donation and risk factors for infectious diseases. The concept of providing donors with such prescreening educational materials was conceived by the AABB in 1984,[14] and the FDA has required it since 1990.[15] The intention is to educate donors about HIV and acquired immunodeficiency syndrome (AIDS), and prompt donor self-deferral or at least questioning of blood center staff by donors to whom such information might apply. These educational materials, usually presented in a brochure or laminated form, have played an increasingly significant role in familiarizing donors with the donation process and deferrable risks.

In 2000, the AABB convened a multiorganizational **task force** to address a number of donor screening issues, including the content of prescreening educational materials. The task force reviewed materials from more than 20 blood centers and found considerable variation. As a result, the task force designed new educational materials, and recommended that the FDA require their use in all collection facilities. The revised document emphasizes the importance of accuracy and honesty in responding to screening questions, defines the term "sexual contact" (since well over a dozen screening questions ask about sex-related exposures), more clearly explains HIV and AIDS information, and details the donation process.[16] A version of the educational materials is shown in Fig. 8-1.

Task force: A small group of individuals usually selected for their expertise who gather to solve a focused problem.

Mechanics of Screening

The screening process should involve the participation of trained staff and should be done in a setting that offers privacy and confidentiality. The actual screening mechanism varies from center to center. In many collection facilities the donor reads and responds in writing to the questions, and is offered an opportunity to ask for clarification if he or she does not understand a particular item. In this approach, no questions are verbally repeated by staff. Elsewhere, donors review and answer the questions, and either all or some of the items—especially HIV risk questions—are verbally repeated by blood center staff. This latter approach is based on an FDA guidance document that is interpreted by many blood centers as requiring all HIV risk questions to be asked verbally.[17] The AABB task force to redesign the donor screening materials has developed a simplified screening instrument (discussed later) that is intended to be fully donor self-administered.

In the late 1990s several companies developed software for computer-assisted screening (CAS). The donor listens to and/or reads questions that appear on a computer screen, and responses are recorded by the donor or staff, either by use of a touch screen or keyboard.[18,19] Responses that could lead to a deferral are flagged, and follow-up questioning is done by staff. Both of these systems offer the distinct safety advantages of having audio and visual components, standardizing screening, ensuring that no questions are skipped, enabling the use of hierarchic deferral algorithms, being easily modifiable when questions are added or eliminated, and having multiple language applications. These systems have already been approved by the FDA for use in blood collection facilities, and within the next few years will eliminate manual screening systems in most centers.

The contents of the current screening instrument derive predominantly from FDA regulations, guidance documents, and memoranda; the AABB is the source of a few questions. In the early 1990s, the Blood Centers of California, an organization of not-for-profit blood centers, made significant revisions to the wording and organization of the questions; the goal was to standardize donor screening in California and produce a more logical screening tool. This document was

Blood Donor Educational Materials

MAKING YOUR BLOOD DONATION SAFE

Thank you for coming in today! This information sheet explains how **YOU** can help us make the donation process safe for yourself and patients who might receive your blood. **PLEASE READ THIS INFORMATION** *BEFORE* **YOU DONATE! If you have any questions now or anytime during the screening process, please ask blood center staff.**

ACCURACY AND HONESTY ARE ESSENTIAL!

Your **complete honesty** in answering all questions is very important for the safety of patients who receive your blood. **All information you provide is confidential.**

DONATION PROCESS

To determine if you are eligible to donate we will:
–Ask questions about health, travel, and medicines
–Ask questions to see if you might be at risk for hepatitis, HIV, or AIDS
–Take your blood pressure, temperature, and pulse
–Take a small blood sample to make sure you are not anemic

If you are able to donate we will:
–Cleanse your arm with an antiseptic. **(If you are allergic to Iodine, please tell us!)**
–Use a new, sterile, disposable needle to collect your blood

DONOR ELIGIBILITY – SPECIFIC INFORMATION

Why we ask questions about sexual contact:
Sexual contact may cause contagious diseases like HIV to get into the bloodstream and be spread through transfusions to someone else.
Definition of "sexual contact":
The words "have sexual contact with" and "sex" are used in some of the questions we will ask you, and apply to *any* of the activities below, whether or not a condom or other protection was used:
1. Vaginal sex (contact between penis and vagina)
2. Oral sex (mouth or tongue on someone's vagina, penis, or anus)
3. Anal sex (contact between penis and anus)

HIV/AIDS RISK BEHAVIORS AND SYMPTOMS

AIDS is caused by HIV. HIV is spread mainly through sexual contact with an infected person OR by sharing needles or syringes used for injecting drugs.

DO NOT DONATE IF YOU:

–Have AIDS or have ever had a positive HIV test
–Have ever used needles to take drugs, steroids, or anything not prescribed by your doctor
–Are a male who has had sexual contact with another male, even once, since 1977
–Have ever taken money, drugs, or other payment for sex since 1977
–Have had sexual contact in the past 12 months with anyone described above
–Have had syphilis or gonorrhea in the past 12 months
–In the last 12 months have been in juvenile detention, lockup, jail, or prison for more than 72 hours
–Have any of the following conditions that can be signs or symptoms of HIV/AIDS:
  • Unexplained weight loss or night sweats
  • Blue or purple spots in your mouth or skin
  • Swollen lymph nodes for more than 1 month
  • White spots or unusual sores in your mouth
  • Cough that won't go away or shortness of breath
  • Diarrhea that won't go away
  • Fever of more than 100.5° F for more than 10 days

Remember that you *CAN* give HIV to someone else through blood transfusions even if you feel well and have a negative HIV test. This is because tests cannot detect infections for a period of time after a person is exposed to HIV. **If you think you may be at risk for HIV/AIDS or want an HIV/AIDS test, please ask for information about other testing facilities.** *PLEASE DO NOT DONATE TO GET AN HIV TEST!*

Travel to or birth in other countries
Blood donor tests may not be available for some contagious diseases that are found only in certain countries. If you were born in, have lived in, or visited certain countries, you may not be eligible to donate.

What happens after your donation
To protect patients, your blood is tested for hepatitis B and C, HIV, certain other viruses, and syphilis. If your blood tests positive it will not be given to a patient. You will be notified about test results that may disqualify you from donating in the future. **Please do not donate to get tested for HIV, hepatitis, or any other infections!**

Thank you for donating blood today!
(Donor Center Name)
(Telephone Number)

Fig. 8-1 AABB blood donor predonation educational materials.

submitted to the AABB for review, and the AABB subsequently obtained FDA "approval" for the wording, organization, and format changes. The questionnaire was adopted as the official AABB screening instrument, to be used in a standardized way by collection facilities in the United States, and became known as the "Uniform Donor History Questionnaire."[20,21] Answers to the medical history questions are clues to the overall suitability of the potential donor and must be performed in a careful and well-considered manner.

Categories of Questions
Questions to Protect Donors

The goal of most questions for maintaining donor safety is to identify health conditions that would render donation unsafe. Thus, questions about general health on the day of donation, recent pregnancy, heart ailments, and lung ailments are asked. Pregnancy, although in and of itself not a contraindication, especially for autologous donations, has a 6-week deferral, the origin of which dates back many decades. There are actually no data to support a deferral of this length for someone who has been pregnant, but an informal, unpublished 2001 survey of several obstetricians revealed a general unease about allowing donations from someone who has undergone the dramatic physiologic changes that characterize pregnancy.[22] The rationale for deferring donors with certain heart and lung conditions revolves around concerns that rapidly removing approximately 500 mL of whole blood could affect oxygenation and thus cardiac and pulmonary function.

Questions about a history of cancer are not necessarily meant to protect the donor, but are asked because of concerns that transfusing blood from such a donor could somehow put the recipient at risk. There currently are no data to support this thinking, although there is a general consensus that it is not a good idea to collect and transfuse blood from someone who has had certain types of malignancies. In our experience, a history of lymphohematologic malignancies, that is, lymphomas or leukemias, is the basis for permanent deferral. Some blood centers do, however, allow donors who are considered cured or in remission from some types of solid tumors—breast, colon, or prostate, for example—to donate after a specified period of time. This is a somewhat controversial area, and it would not be unexpected if the FDA were eventually to establish deferral criteria. For the most part, at this point in time, decisions about whether to accept such donors is made by the blood center medical staff, and practices are not standardized in the United States.

Questions to Protect Recipients
Infectious Diseases

The vast majority of screening questions are intended to determine if a donor has risk factors for exposure to an increasing number of proven or potentially transfusion-transmissible diseases. In an ideal world, laboratory assays or the availability of FDA-approved pathogen inactivation systems would obviate the need for pre-donation screening. Assays are now performed for HIV-1 and HIV-2 (HIV-1/2), hepatitis C virus (HCV), hepatitis B virus (HBV), human T-cell lymphotropic viruses types I and II (HTLV-I/II), syphilis, and West Nile virus (WNV).[4] However, tests are either not available or easily adaptable to large-scale screening for a host of pathogens such as HIV group O, malaria, *Babesia microti* (the causative agent of babesiosis), *Trypanosoma cruzi* (Chagas' disease), leishmaniasis, sudden acute respiratory syndrome (SARS), or the prions that cause Creutzfeldt-Jakob disease (CJD) or variant Creutzfeldt-Jakob disease (vCJD—the human version of bovine spongiform encephalopathy, otherwise known as "mad cow disease"). Thus the Uniform Donor History Questionnaire (UDHQ) has become a major mechanism by which donors are screened for many diseases.[5]

Travel-Related Questions

Questions designed to identify potentially infected donors fall into two major categories: travel-related risk, and risk of exposure through contact with pathogen-containing blood or other body fluids of humans or insects. International travel and rapidly changing global population demographics have increased the possibility that pathogens can be spread transcontinentally or across oceans within a matter of days, weeks, or months. Not surprisingly, the number of travel-related deferrals and questions has also quickly risen. An example is the 2003 FDA Guidance requiring

TABLE 8-2 Deferrals for Geography- or Travel-Associated Infectious Disease Risks

Country or Region	Infectious Agent	Deferral Period
Numerous global regions[1]	Malaria	Varies with length of time spent there[2]
Cameroon, Central African Republic, Chad, Congo, Equatorial Guinea, Gabon, Niger, Nigeria[3]	HIV, group O	Permanent if transfused or lived in or had sexual contact with someone from any of these countries
Europe[4]	vCJD	Permanent if there 5 years or more, cumulative since 1980
United Kingdom[4]	vCJD	Permanent if 3 months or more, cumulative from 1980 to 1996
Iraq[5]	Leishmania	12 months from departure date
Numerous global regions[6]	Sudden acute respiratory syndrome (SARS)	14 days after return to United States

[1] Health Information for International Travel. Atlanta, 2003–2004, US Department of Health and Human Services, Centers for Disease Control and Prevention.

[2] Interim Standards for Blood Banks and Transfusion Services, 22nd ed. Association Bulletin 04-02. Bethesda, MD, Jan 2004, American Association of Blood Banks.

[3] Interim Recommendations for Deferral of Donors at Increased Risk for HIV Group O Infection. FDA Memorandum. December 1996.

[4] Revised Preventive Measures to Reduce the Risk of Transmission of Creutzfeldt-Jakob Disease (CJD) and Variant Creutzfeldt-Jakob Disease (vCJD) by Blood and Blood Products. FDA Guidance for Industry. January 2002.

[5] Deferral for Risk of Leishmaniasis Exposure. Association Bulletin 03-14. Bethesda, MD, October 2003, American Association of Blood Banks.

[6] Revised Recommendations for the Assessment of Donor Suitability and Blood Product Safety in Cases of Suspected Severe Acute Respiratory Syndrome (SARS) or Exposure to SARS. FDA Guidance for Industry. September 2003.

the addition of three SARS-related questions to the UDHQ.[23] Table 8-2 lists regions that are endemic for certain infections and the reason for donor deferrals.

Deferrals for Exposures to Infectious Materials

Exposure to hepatitis, HIV, HTLV, and many other infectious agents occurs through sexual contact or other types of contact with infected body fluids, especially blood. Thus many of the screening questions ask specifically about such exposures. Persons with HIV, AIDS, HBV, HCV, and HTLV are permanently deferred. Affirmative responses to questions about sporadic, familial, or iatrogenically acquired CJD result in permanent deferral, as do "yes" answers to items that ask about babesiosis or Chagas' disease. Injection of nonprescribed drugs, especially so-called street drugs, male-with-male sex since 1977, and treatment with clotting factors will also bring about permanent deferral. Examples of permanent deferrals are listed in Box 8-5.

Responses to other questions about possible or actual exposures to blood-borne pathogens may result in temporary deferrals ranging from several months to years. One-year deferrals would include occupational or other exposures to blood or body fluids; sexual contact with an HIV- or HBV-infected person; a history of syphilis or gonorrhea; and some types of tattoos and body piercing. Box 8-6 pro-

Box 8-5	Examples of Permanent (Indefinite) Deferrals for Individuals with Infections, Infectious Disease Exposure Risk, or Certain Laboratory Results

INFECTION OR EXPOSURE RISK

History or diagnosis of HIV/AIDS

Viral hepatitis after 11th birthday

Confirmed positive HbsAg assay

Repeatedly reactive for HbcAb more than once

History of or positive tests for HTLV, HCV, or HIV

Donated only unit of blood associated with transmission of hepatitis, HIV, or HTLV

Male-to-male sex since 1977

History of babesiosis or Chagas' disease

History or physical evidence of injection drug use

Use of a needle to administer nonprescription drugs

CJD or CJD risk; vCJD or vCJD risk

---

vides examples of 1-year deferrals. Three relatively recent novel deferrals—based on new donor questions—relate to smallpox vaccination, West Nile virus, and leishmaniasis. Specific deferral periods for these, especially smallpox, are based on somewhat complicated algorithms.[24-26]

Medication Deferrals

Ingestion of aspirin or aspirin-containing products has for many years resulted in temporary deferral for donors of apheresis platelets or some whole blood–derived platelet concentrates, due to the inhibitory effect on platelet function. However, within the past decade a whole new medication deferral category—and accompanying questions—has been added to the screening process: medications with the potential for producing teratogenicity in embryos or fetuses. For example, donors taking medications such as finasteride or dutasteride for prostatic hypertrophy are deferred for specified time periods. Certain psoriasis or acne medications such as Tegison and Acitretin result in permanent and 3-year deferrals, respectively.

Many of the major deferral categories that use questions for identifying donor risks are discussed earlier in this chapter. For further detail and a complete listing of deferral criteria and time frames, the reader is referred to the AABB Standards and Technical Manual.[4,5]

Box 8-6	Examples of 12-Month Deferrals for Exposures or Possible Exposures to Infectious Agents

EXPOSURE TYPE

Blood or blood component transfusion

Tissue or human-derived transplants

Mucous membrane blood exposure

Penetration of skin with nonsterile instruments or equipment (e.g., occupational needle stick, certain types of tattoos)

Sexual contact with persons infected with HBV, HIV (or having HIV risk factors), or symptomatic viral hepatitis

Incarceration for more than 72 consecutive hours

History of syphilis or gonorrhea (or completion of treatment in absence of negative tests)

Sources: Fridey JL (chair): Standards for Blood Banks and Transfusion Services, 22nd ed. Bethesda, MD, American Association of Blood Banks, 2003; Revised Recommendations for the Prevention of Human Immunodeficiency Virus Transmission by Blood and Blood Products. FDA Memorandum. April 23, 1992.

Uniform Donor History Questionnaire (UDHQ): A recently revised questionnaire for the screening of donors of blood and blood components. The questionnaire has been accepted by the FDA (refer to the FDA guidance at www.iso.org/iso/en/ISOOnline.frontpage).

The Uniform Donor History Questionnaire: Taming a Wild Beast

Although it is now possible to test for many blood-borne diseases, there has been a significant reliance on pre-donation screening for infections for which tests are not available. It is highly likely that for the foreseeable future the identification of potentially unsafe donors will be accomplished, in concert with available laboratory testing, through written or computer-assisted screening. It is unlikely that serologic or nucleic acid testing will become the sole means of weeding out unsafe donors. In short, pre-donation screening is here to stay.

The addition of numerous new questions to the **Uniform Donor History Questionnaire (UDHQ)** in the past decade has probably brought about an incremental improvement in blood safety. However, two observations can be made. First, the inclusion of new questions by ever-cautious regulatory agencies has caused a significant loss of donors. This has resulted in appeals to the FDA to balance the risk of adding a new deferral category and question with the possible impact on the blood supply. Second, the history questionnaire itself has taken on gargantuan proportions. Anyone who has donated blood in the past 10 years cannot help but notice the number of questions—approaching 50—and the size and complexity of many of them.

It is indisputable that in the 1970s, 1980s, and even the early 1990s, pre-donation screening played an important role in reducing transfusion-transmitted hepatitis and HIV—especially in the absence of laboratory assays. However, the current enormity and complexity of the UDHQ has raised concerns about its true effectiveness in preventing infectious transmissions. Do donors really understand many of these questions? Do they read them? Is the length and complexity discouraging prospective donors? Have the questions, particularly those added since 1992, been evaluated for comprehension? (The answer to this last question, until recently, was "no.")

As a result of these and many other issues, in 2000 the FDA asked the AABB to assemble a task force to redesign the donor screening materials, making them more understandable and user-friendly. Another goal was to develop an abbreviated questionnaire for frequent donors—and to define "frequent." The simplification process (which did not include an option to eliminate FDA-derived questions) involved the development of a methodology for evaluating questions for comprehensibility. This methodology incorporated the use of focus groups and cognitive testing to evaluate whether individuals representative of typical donors could understand the intent and content of each question. The questionnaire was entirely reworked using state-of-the-art survey design principles.

Feedback from the focus groups and laboratory-based cognitive testing indicated that the questions were too long, contained too many items, and used too much medical jargon. To solve this, many questions were broken up into "sound bites," each of which could receive more attention than a question containing multiple items. When possible, medical jargon was replaced by lay terminology. In addition, the task force received input that the placement of questions required donors to engage in mental "time travel"—because so many questions involve specific time frames. In anticipation of additional deferrable medications being added, it was decided that certain medications should be removed from the questionnaire and placed in a concise companion document that the donor would read.

The end product, developed over a 3-year period, was a document that placed shorter, more concise questions in chronologically ordered time frames. The full-length questionnaire, intended for use by first-time or infrequent donors, has conceptually been approved by the FDA, and appears in Fig. 8-2. It is hoped that by the time this textbook has been published, the FDA will have published a guidance document formally endorsing the revised version. The fate of the proposed abbreviated version has, at this writing, not yet been determined.

The redesign of the UDHQ represents the most far-reaching attempt to develop a pre-donation screening tool that is based on sound survey development, and will result in improved donor comprehension and, optimally, a safer blood supply.

Pre-donation Physical Evaluation

Donors who meet the pre-donation screening qualifications undergo a focused physical evaluation. This is not intended to be a full-fledged medical examination, but is done to identify any obvious medical conditions or abnormalities.

General Appearance of Donor

The physical examination begins by observing the prospective donor's general appearance. The interviewer decides if the donor appears to be in good health, is alert, has no evidence of intoxication or drug-induced mental impairment, has no obvious symptoms of an infection, and appears cognitively capable of giving

	Yes	No	
Are you			
1. Feeling healthy and well today?	❏	❏	
2. Currently taking an antibiotic?	❏	❏	
3. Currently taking any other medication for an infection?	❏	❏	
Please read the Medication Deferral List.			
4. Are you now taking or have you ever taken any medications on the Medication Deferral List?	❏	❏	
5. Have you read the educational materials and had your questions answered?	❏	❏	
In the past **48 hours**	❏	❏	
6. Have you taken aspirin or anything that has aspirin in it?			
In the past **week**			
7. Have you had a headache and fever at the same time?	❏	❏	
In the past **6 weeks**			
8. Female donors: Have you been pregnant or are you pregnant now? (Males: check "I am male.")	❏	❏	❏ I am male
In the past **8 weeks** have you			
9. Donated blood, platelets, or plasma?	❏	❏	
10. Had any vaccinations or other shots?	❏	❏	
11. Had contact with someone who had a smallpox vaccination?	❏	❏	
In the past **16 weeks**			
12. Have you donated a double unit of red cells using an apheresis machine?	❏	❏	
In the past **12 months** have you			
13. Had a blood transfusion?	❏	❏	
14. Had a transplant such as organ, tissue, or bone marrow?	❏	❏	
15. Had a graft such as bone or skin?	❏	❏	
16. Come into contact with someone else's blood?	❏	❏	
17. Had an accidental needle-stick?	❏	❏	
18. Had sexual contact with anyone who has HIV/AIDS or has had a positive test for the HIV/AIDS virus?	❏	❏	
19. Had sexual contact with a prostitute or anyone else who takes money or drugs or other payment for sex?	❏	❏	
20. Had sexual contact with anyone who has ever used needles to take drugs or steroids, or anything *not* prescribed by their doctor?	❏	❏	
21. Had sexual contact with anyone who has hemophilia or has used clotting factor concentrates?	❏	❏	
22. Female donors: Had sexual contact with a male who has ever had sexual contact with another male? (Males: check "I am male")	❏	❏	❏ I am male

Fig. 8-2 AABB full-length donor history questionnaire.

Continued

	Yes	No
23. Had sexual contact with a person who has hepatitis?	☐	☐
24. Lived with a person who has hepatitis?	☐	☐
25. Had a tattoo?	☐	☐
26. Had ear or body piercing?	☐	☐
27. Had or been treated for syphilis or gonorrhea?	☐	☐
28. Been in juvenile detention, lockup, jail, or prison for more than 72 hours?	☐	☐
In the past **three years** have you,		
29. Been outside the United States or Canada?	☐	☐
From **1980 through 1996,**		
30. Did you spend time that adds up to three (3) months or more in the United Kingdom? (Review list of countries in the UK)	☐	☐
31. Were you a member of the U.S. military, a civilian military employee, or a dependent of a member of the U.S. military?	☐	☐
From **1980 to present**, did you		
32. Spend time that adds up to five (5) years or more in Europe? (Review list of countries in Europe.)	☐	☐
33. Receive a blood transfusion in the United Kingdom? (Review list of countries in the UK.)	☐	☐
From **1977 to the present**, have you		
34. Received money, drugs, or other payment for sex?	☐	☐
35. Male donors: Had sexual contact with another male, even once? (Females: check "I am female")	☐	☐	☐ I am female
Have you **EVER**		
36. Had a positive test for the HIV/AIDS virus?	☐	☐
37. Used needles to take drugs, steroids, or anything *not* prescribed by your doctor?	☐	☐
38. Used clotting factor concentrates?	☐	☐
39. Had hepatitis?	☐	☐
40. Had malaria?	☐	☐
41. Had Chagas' disease?	☐	☐
42. Had babesiosis?	☐	☐
43. Received a dura mater (or brain covering) graft?	☐	☐
44. Had any type of cancer, including leukemia?	☐	☐
45. Had any problems with your heart or lungs?	☐	☐
46. Had a bleeding condition or a blood disease?	☐	☐
47. Had sexual contact with anyone who was born in or lived in Africa?	☐	☐
48. Been in Africa?	☐	☐
49. Have any of your relatives had Creutzfeldt-Jakob disease?	☐	☐

Fig. 8-2, cont'd AABB full-length donor history questionnaire.

consent. There is an element of subjectivity in this part of the screening, but trained and experienced staff may be able to detect problems that could affect the donor or recipient if the donation were allowed to proceed.

Determination of Hemoglobin Level

It is important to determine that the prospective donor's hemoglobin level is high enough to support the safe removal of 405 to 550 mL of blood. (The amount of whole blood collected from a donor depends on whether a 450 or 500 mL bag is used.) Samples for determining the prospective donor's hemoglobin (or hematocrit) may be obtained from a peripheral vein or finger stick. The AABB Standards no longer permit using the earlobe as a sample source.[4] The AABB Standards requires that the hemoglobin level for whole blood donation be equal to or greater than 12.5 g/dL (125 g/L) and the hematocrit be equal to or greater than 38%.

Donors whose hemoglobin levels are below acceptable levels are deferred until the hemoglobin standard is met; the actual deferral period is at the discretion of the medical director, or a policy established by the collection facility based on medical input. The donor may be counseled to increase consumption of foods rich in iron if there is no apparent serious underlying medical condition that could be contributing to the low hemoglobin or hematocrit. The minimal hemoglobin or hematocrit leading to the referral of the donor to his or her doctor should be determined by the medical director. Recommending that iron supplements be used is also best done in consultation with the blood center physician.

The hemoglobin or hematocrit could be tested in several ways: (1) use of a spun hematocrit; (2) use of a hematology analyzer, either handheld or countertop; or (3) the use of **copper sulfate ($CuSO_4$)** solution. Although most medical laboratory personnel are familiar with the first two methods, the $CuSO_4$ method may be unfamiliar to those who have not worked in a blood center.

The $CuSO_4$ method is widely used in blood centers because it is a rapid and fairly reliable means of determining that the donor's hemoglobin meets the minimal 12.5 mg/dL level. It is based on the principle that the specific gravity of blood correlates with the hemoglobin level. When a drop of blood having a hemoglobin greater than the minimal level is dropped into a tube of $CuSO_4$ solution with a specific gravity of 1.054, the drop of blood will sink to the bottom. If the donor's hemoglobin is marginal and the specific gravity of the donor's blood drop is the same as that of the $CuSO_4$ solution, the drop may slowly sink. If the hemoglobin is lower than required, the drop of blood may float on the top of the solution, or may fall through it only very slowly. If the drop floats on the top of the solution or takes 15 seconds or longer to reach the bottom, the hemoglobin is too low and the donor should be deferred (Fig. 8-3).

Several comments about the use of $CuSO_4$ solutions are warranted. First, the specific gravity of $CuSO_4$ can change if the container is left uncovered and evaporation occurs. As a result, the specific gravity of the $CuSO_4$ may increase so that a blood drop from a donor with a normal hemoglobin may fall slowly enough—or not at all—resulting in an inappropriate deferral. Therefore the $CuSO_4$ solution should be covered unless in use. Second, it is the experience of these authors that it is becoming increasingly difficult to dispose of used $CuSO_4$ solutions, because they represent a biologic hazard to chemical waste disposal companies. It is likely that blood centers will eventually have to abandon the use of this approach to hemoglobin testing, and turn to automated systems or a spun hematocrit to evaluate iron or red cell levels, respectively.

$CuSO_4$ method: Donor hemoglobin screening can be accomplished by using $CuSO_4$ solutions. The test is based on the relative specific gravity of the solution and the blood. Blood will either float on the surface or sink to the bottom of the $CuSO_4$ solution depending on the hemoglobin concentration.

 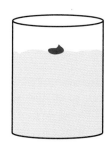 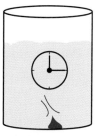 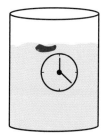

| Blood is first drawn from the finger using a small sterile lancet. A small blood sample is dropped into the $CuSO_4$ solution | The specific gravity of the copper sulfate solution is 1.054 for hemoglobin of 12.5 g/dL. Blood drop floats on top and then... | ...if it falls to the bottom within 15 seconds, there is enough hemoglobin to donate. | If it does not fall, or takes longer than 15 seconds to fall, the hemoglobin level is lower than required to donate. |

Fig. 8-3 Hemoglobin determination using the copper sulfate method.

Pulse

The purpose of taking the donor's pulse is to detect any irregularities of rate or rhythm that could be suggestive of heart disease or other pathologic conditions. The pulse should be between 50 and 100 beats per minute. If the donor engages regularly in physical exercise or is an athlete, a lower pulse may be acceptable; however, this information should be documented on the donor's record. The pulse should be taken for at least 30 seconds, with the option to extend that time to 1 minute if any question or irregularity is noted.[4]

Blood Pressure

Systolic pressure: The period of highest pressure in the arterial system, which corresponds to the time in the heart cycle when the muscle contracts and expels its contents (systole).

Diastolic pressure: The period of lowest pressure in the arterial system, which corresponds to the time in the heart cycle when fibers lengthen and the heart dilates and fills (diastole).

The purpose of evaluating the donor's blood pressure is to avoid drawing blood from a hypotensive or hypertensive individual. A low blood pressure could be a symptom of dehydration or other significant medical condition, unless the donor is an athlete or exercises regularly. In this case, a low-appearing blood pressure may be acceptable, with medical director approval. A donor with a high blood pressure reading that is reliably duplicated is not considered a "well and healthy" donor and should not be accepted that day. The **systolic** pressure should be no higher than 180 mm Hg and the **diastolic** no higher than 100 mm Hg.[4] In evaluating the sounds heard while deflating the blood pressure cuff, the systolic is the first sound while the cuff is being deflated, and the diastolic pressure is marked by the disappearance of heart sounds. Many centers are now using automated blood pressure devices, which have readouts of the systolic and diastolic pressures and eliminate the need for the use of a stethoscope. This removes operator subjectivity, but if such devices are used they should be calibrated on a regular basis.

The pulse and blood pressures are highly variable and may be influenced by a number of factors such as time of day, caffeine ingestion, smoking, intravascular volume, or the donor's state of mind. A donor with an unacceptable blood pressure in the presence of one or more these factors may be asked to sit quietly for several minutes to see if the blood pressure normalizes. Donors who have a history of hypertension but have a normal pressure due to the use of antihypertensive medication are acceptable.

Temperature

An oral temperature above 37.5° C (99.5° F) usually requires that the donor be temporarily deferred.[4] An elevated temperature could be a sign of infection. However, if the donor has smoked, eaten, or consumed hot beverages shortly before evaluation, the temperature could be falsely elevated. The blood center should have a policy for determining the circumstances under which the temperature could be retaken. However, if the donor has not engaged in any activities that could spuriously cause a reading higher than 37.5° C, she or he should be temporarily deferred because of the possible existence of an infection.

Donor Weight

Hypovolemia: Decreased intravascular blood volume.

The acute loss of 15% or more of an individual's blood volume can result in symptoms of **hypovolemia.** The donor's weight in pounds (lb) or kilograms (kg) is the basis for determining blood volume; thus, using a minimum acceptable donor weight is the means by which hypovolemia can be avoided. The AABB standards require that, in order to avoid acute hypovolemic reactions, the maximum whole blood volume that can be removed is 10.5 mL/kg of donor weight; this includes samples for testing as well as the blood in the container.[4] In general, a donor weight of 110 lb or more meets this standard. However, depending on whether a 450 or 500 mL bag is used, the donor's weight may need to be somewhat higher to qualify for the maximal possible volume. A comprehensive discussion, including examples, is provided in a subsequent section.

Venipuncture Site

The antecubital area of the forearm is the preferred site for performing venipuncture. Careful inspection of this area is needed in order to select a suitable vein and to check for skin lesions and evidence of possible injection drug use. If skin lesions, rashes, dermatitis, or evidence of infection is noted, the involved site should not be selected for phlebotomy. Both arms should be evaluated for evidence of possible injection drug use; multiple small scars along the course of a vein or numerous small scars in the forearm are suggestive of intravenous or subcutaneous (i.e., "skin-popping") injection drug use, respectively, and the donor should be permanently deferred. However, it should be kept in mind that frequent blood donors often have scars and pitting in the antecubital area(s), so if the phlebotomist is in doubt about a donor's acceptability, a supervisor or medical director should be consulted.

Confidential Donor (Unit) Self-Exclusion

In some situations, individuals who may not meet health or safety qualification criteria may feel pressured by family members or acquaintances to donate. To prevent the blood from a potentially unsafe donor from being issued for transfusion, the concept of **confidential unit exclusion (CUE)** was conceived and then adopted by U.S. blood centers in the mid-1980s. In this system, the donor was given the opportunity to confidentially indicate that his or her blood might not be safe for transfusion. Thus, a donor who might be at risk for exposure to HIV or hepatitis would be screened and then donate, but somewhere in the process would designate that his or her blood should not be used for transfusion.

> **Confidential unit exclusion (CUE):** The opportunity for a blood donor to indicate in confidence that the donated unit should not be used for transfusion. In such cases, all donor testing is completed and the donor is notified of any abnormal results and offered any necessary consultation.

Although this requirement was eliminated from FDA regulations in April 1992[17] and from the AABB Standards in 1993, the opportunity for donors to privately communicate that their blood should not be transfused is still used in many centers. One approach for CUE is to have the donor place a bar-coded "safe" or "unsafe" sticker on a designated spot on the donor history questionnaire, as seen in Fig. 8-4. Another approach is for the donor to put a label or check mark on a separate form that will then be reviewed by laboratory or other personnel.

The self-exclusion opportunity is given to the donor usually after he or she has successfully completed all phases of the pre-donation screening process, including attentive review of the educational materials. The CUE process should be carefully explained to the donor. To encourage use of the CUE, the donor should be told that his or her answer will be kept confidential. Blood center staff should then discretely turn aside or excuse themselves from the screening room until the donor has completed the procedure. Even though use of a CUE is no longer required, if a blood center employs this process, donors must be informed that if they indicate that their blood should not be used, the unit will undergo infectious disease testing. Further, donors should be told that they *will* be informed of positive test results.[4,17]

Use of the CUE may confer a small measure of added blood safety. In one study, 1446 donors who, for various reasons, were not eligible to donate again, had a 9.8% viral marker discard rate, compared to that blood center's overall viral discard rate of 3.5%.[27] However, of the 2377 donors who had used the CUE and were informed that they were permanently deferred for that reason, 39% requested and, after being further evaluated by a risk factor survey, underwent reinstatement. Feedback provided by many of these reinstated donors indicated that they had misunderstood either the mechanics or appropriate use of the CUE. This latter finding underscores the need to carefully explain the CUE process and its rationale.

Consenting to Donate

If the prospective donor has successfully passed pre-donation screening and the physical evaluation, the final step before donation is to provide written consent to donate. The components of consent include the following:[4,17]

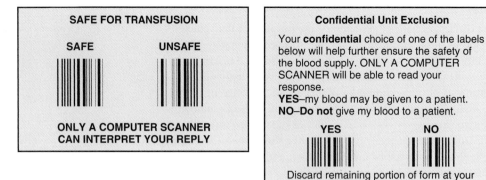

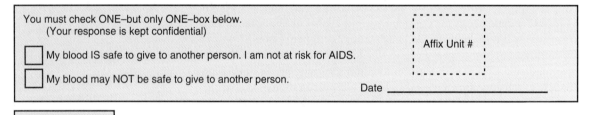

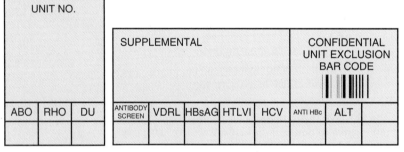

Fig. 8-4 Confidential unit exclusion examples.

1. An explanation of the donation process in terms the donor can understand.
2. An explanation of the significant risks of donation such as syncope, vascular or nerve injury, infection, bruising, hematoma, and in the case of apheresis procedures, citrate-related reactions.
3. A statement that tests will be performed on the donor's blood to reduce the risks of transmitting infectious agents to recipients.

4. A statement that there is a time interval early in infections during which tests for infectious disease may be negative even though disease may be transmitted to the recipient.

5. A statement that if the donor's sample is positive for infectious disease markers, the donor's name will be placed on a confidential deferred donor list.

6. A statement that under some circumstances infectious disease testing may not be done. (Examples include the inadvertent failure of staff to collect specimens for IDM testing, or the occurrence of a failed test run. Donors are informed of this so they do not automatically assume that no notification means they are not infected with HIV or other communicable diseases.)

7. The opportunity to ask questions.

8. The opportunity to give or refuse consent.

9. The actual signature of the donor consenting to the procedure.

In addition to the consent process, the FDA requires that a blood center have a separate mechanism by which the donor reaffirms certain elements that appear in the consent and indicates that he or she understands various recipient safety measures. A suggested statement from the FDA reads as follows:

> I have reviewed and understand the information provided to me regarding the spread of the AIDS virus (HIV) by blood or plasma. If I am potentially at risk for spreading the virus known to cause AIDS, I agree not to donate blood or plasma for transfusion to another person or for further manufacture. I understand that my blood will be tested for antibodies to HIV and other disease markers. If this test indicates that I should no longer donate blood or plasma because of a risk of transmitting the AIDS virus (or other infectious diseases), my name will be entered on a list of permanently deferred donors. I understand that I will be notified of a positive result.

In most states, donors must be at least 17 years old to donate. Put another way, if a donor is 17 or older, consent of a parent or guardian is not required. If an adolescent is not qualified based on age, the adolescent may not give his or her own consent to donate. Consent forms should therefore include a section for the signature of the consenting parent or guardian in this situation.

Pre-donation screening and medical evaluation increase the likelihood that a safe product will be collected for a recipient, and that the donation experience is safe for the "giver." Following completion of the consenting process, the donor will go on to make his or her donation of whole blood or apheresis components.

BLOOD COLLECTION
Selection of Bags, Preservatives, and Anticoagulants

Various types of containers have been used to store blood, including glass bottles that were cleaned and sterilized after use and recycled. Today's containers are flexible plastics especially designed to allow for maximal product stability, cell viability, and sterility. All containers used for the donor phlebotomy are sterile and are intended to be used only once. Blood collection sets consist of a primary bag, satellite bags that are either empty or have additional solutions, and a long plastic tubing line ending with a 16- or 17-gauge needle. The entire collection set is interconnected by tubing lines and is considered a closed system. The only time the entire assembly is open to the environment is when the needle is uncapped and the venipuncture is performed. At the end of the collection, the tubing near the needle is clamped off, the needle is removed from the donor's arm, and the tubing near the needle end is heat-sealed so that the needle may be removed from the blood collection set and discarded. In this way the system retains the integrity required for a closed system.

All containers and anticoagulants used for the preservation and storage of blood and its components must meet or exceed FDA criteria. Today there are a total of six approved anticoagulant/preservative or anticoagulant/preservative/additive solutions that may be used.

All whole blood is collected in clear plastic, pyrogen-free containers that contain an anticoagulant/preservative solution identified as CPD, CP2D, or CPDA-1. Each of these solutions contains sodium citrate, citric acid, dextrose, and monobasic sodium phosphate in established concentrations. The amount of dextrose in each formula varies slightly, and the CPDA-1 contains the extra ingredient of adenine. The citrate compounds prevent coagulation by chelating calcium, and the dextrose provides nourishment for the living red blood cells. Though metabolism is slowed by storage at 1° to 6° C, the cells must have a nutritive source to remain alive. In the CPDA-1, the amino acid adenine is used in the production of the energy molecule adenosine triphosphate (ATP).

CPD and CP2D have an FDA-approved shelf life of 21 days when the product is stored at 1° to 6° C. CPDA-1 has an increased shelf life of 35 days when stored at 1° to 6° C because of the extra nutritional supplement, adenine. Each blood product collected in **CPD, CP2D, and CPDA-1** must have a final hematocrit of 80% or less. In a 450 mL blood collection bag, there is 63 mL of the anticoagulant/preservative solution and a red cell volume of 450 ± 45 mL. This ratio provides the proper proportions of red blood cells to anticoagulant/preservative solution. If a "low-volume" (300 to 404 mL) unit is to be drawn, it is necessary to adjust the amount of anticoagulant/preservative solution in the bag before collection. (See following section on low-volume blood units for more information and a suggested formula.) If a low-volume unit is drawn without adjusting the volume of anticoagulant/preservative solution, that unit must be discarded. The same principle applies to a unit that is "overweight" at a volume of ≥495 mL. In this instance there is too little anticoagulant/preservative to adequately prevent clotting and maintain the viability of the red blood cells. This unit must also be discarded. Currently, 500 ± 50 mL red blood cell collection bags are in use. These bags have 70 mL of anticoagulant/preservative solution.[5,6]

After the blood has been collected into the primary bag with its anticoagulant/preservative solution, an additional solution may be added during the whole blood processing in order to extend the red blood cell product shelf life. The extended shelf life for all red blood cells containing additive solutions is 42 days if blood is stored at 1° to 6° C. This extended shelf life is a critical factor in maintaining an adequate blood supply.

In the blood processing area, the whole blood is centrifuged and excess plasma is removed. This excess plasma is directed into one of the attached empty satellite bags via interconnecting tubing required to maintain the closed system. The bag into which the excess plasma is shunted is then properly labeled, and the connecting tubing heat-sealed and detached from the parent bag. At this time additive solutions may be mixed with the concentrated red blood cells in order to provide additional sources of nutrition, energy production, and cell stabilization. The ingredients of these solutions, in varying combinations approved by the FDA, are dextrose, adenine, monobasic sodium phosphate, mannitol, sodium chloride, sodium citrate, and citric acid. The trade names for these additive solutions are Adsol, Optisol, and Nutricel. The volume of additive solution added to a red blood cell volume of 450 ± 50 mL is 100 mL (for 500 mL collection bags, the volume of additive solutions is about 110 mL). The resulting hematocrit of the red blood cell bag must still be less than or equal to 80% per FDA regulations (usually, the product's hematocrit is approximately 60%). Once the additive solutions have been drained into the parent bag that contains the red blood cells, the tubing of the now-empty additive bag may be heat sealed and detached from the collection set.[5,6]

Unique Product Identification Systems: Control and Tracking

Every blood product is assigned a unique identifier at the time of collection. This identifier is either a number or an alphanumeric combination of letters and

CPD, CP2D, and CPDA-1: Licensed anticoagulant-preservative solutions that can be intended for use for the collection of blood and components for transfusion.

numbers. Whatever type of identification is assigned to a blood product, it must never be removed from the blood product or obscured with other labels or marks. Examples of such identifiers are 03GT123456, R12345, and 123456789. It may happen that a receiving facility's computer system, for example, can only recognize an alphanumeric system but the blood product has a numeric identifier. In such cases, the receiving facility may add its own identifier that must, however, be linked to the original number that is permanently retained on the product bag. There may be a maximum of two product identifiers on a blood product at any one time. At present there is a worldwide effort to adopt a universal identification system for blood products that uses the machine-readable bar-code system. The unique identifier assigned to a unit would be in both letters/numbers and uses the bar-code Universal Product Number (UPN) concept. Many problems with the current labeling programs will be greatly reduced with the use of this international system known as **ISBT 128** labeling. AABB *Standards for Blood Banks and Transfusion Services,* 22nd edition, indicates that blood product labeling should now be in conformance as much as possible with the ISBT 128 directives, although during the transition period the FDA 1985 Uniform Labeling Guidelines are acceptable.[4]

By creating Code 128, the International Society of Blood Transfusion (ISBT) has developed a standardized system for blood labeling and product description (ISBT 128). Bar-coded labels are available for much of the information that is required on each blood product. There is a bar-coded label for the following items: unit ID, expiration date, product type, production site, ABO and Rh type, and type of anticoagulant/preservative/additive solution used. A product modified by irradiation, filtering, or other process has a new product-type bar-coded label that is placed on the unit. In the ISBT 128 system there are currently about 6000 codes for almost any conceivable blood banking product.

The unique blood product identification system is one of the most crucial aspects of transfusion medicine. The unique identifier brings a necessary degree of control over an individual unit of blood that can be processed into multiple components and used by multiple recipients. The tracking of each blood component from the time of collection to transfusion is essential in maintaining a high level of safety in the blood transfusion service.

ISBT 128: An adaptation of a conventional bar-coding system (system 128) used by blood banks throughout the world.

The Phlebotomy

In preparation for venipuncture, the phlebotomist should reidentify the donor using a procedure developed by the blood center. For example, the donor may be asked to state his or her full name and/or other identifying information such as his or her social security number or birth date. The phlebotomist checks the antecubital area of both arms to select the best vein, and the veins may be palpated if the antimicrobial prep has not yet been performed.

Several methods are approved for prephlebotomy preparation of the arm. Because it is impossible to sterilize the arm completely, strict adherence to these methods is necessary to protect the donor and the recipient. Methods approved by the AABB are described in the AABB Technical Manual.[5] It is important to note that the use of green soap is no longer permitted as an alternative scrub solution if a donor is allergic to iodine-based products. Instead, chlorhexidine is an appropriate alternative.[4,28] After the phlebotomy site has been prepared, the donor's arm is not touched again, nor is the vein repalpated before inserting the needle.

During the collection of the product, the anticoagulated bag should be inverted several times to ensure adequate mixing of the anticoagulant with the blood. There must be a method to ascertain when the allowable amount of blood has been removed. This may be done by use of a scale, a trip balance (Fig. 8-5), or a counterweighed balance. Whichever method is used, the method must be calibrated for accuracy each day of use.

Tubing from donor's arm

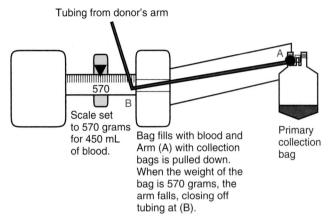

570

Scale set
to 570 grams
for 450 mL
of blood.

Bag fills with blood and
Arm (A) with collection
bags is pulled down.
When the weight of the
bag is 570 grams, the
arm falls, closing off
tubing at (B).

Primary
collection
bag

Fig. 8-5 Gravity scale for monitoring blood donation. The bag fills with blood and the arm **(A)** with the collection bag is pulled down. When the weight of the bag is 570 grams, the arm falls, closing off the tubing at **B.**

Donor Weight as a Function of Collection Container Choice

If a 450 mL bag is used for whole blood collection, the donor must weigh at least 110 lb (50 kg) in order to donate the greatest allowable volume, 495 mL (450 ± 45 mL), in addition to laboratory samples. The total amount of whole blood removed should not be greater than 525 mL. Because a 50 kg (110 lb) person has a blood volume of approximately 3750 mL, the donation of 405 to 495 mL would represent approximately 10% to 13% of the donor's blood volume. If 495 mL of blood were collected and 30 mL taken for testing, the 525 mL removed would total 14% of the donor's blood volume. For this reason, the weight of the donor and amount of blood removed should be carefully monitored, especially if new testing requirements result in the collection of larger volumes of test samples.

The same reasoning applies to the use of 500 mL bags, where the permissible volume collected into the bag is 450 to 550 mL. As noted, the volume needed for test samples must also be included in the calculations. However, in this case, if the maximum volume of blood plus test samples (550 mL and approximately 30 mL, respectively) are removed from a 110 lb person, the total volume would exceed 15% of the donor's blood volume, and the AABB Standard would not be met. (To meet the standard in this situation, the donor would have to weigh 121.5 lb, or 55.2 kg.) Therefore, when collecting a whole blood unit, the bag size, total amount of blood withdrawn, and the donor's weight must all be taken into account in order to avoid acute hypovolemia and meet the AABB Standard. In general, by using the acceptable minimum weight of 110 lb, a safe and appropriate volume can be collected from most donors. However, it is evident that a maximal collection into a 500 mL bag from a donor who just meets a 110 lb weight criterion would result in a collection greater than the allowable amount.

Low-Volume Whole Blood Units

Occasionally it is necessary to remove less blood than the minimal allowable volume of 405 mL. This situation can be encountered when patients who are donating blood for themselves (autologous donation) are small or are children. Low-volume collections are permissible if adjustments are made in the volume of collection bag anticoagulant/preservative, based on the amount of blood that will be collected. Two volumes must be calculated: (1) the volume of blood that can safely be drawn from the donor/patient—a table in the facility's whole blood phlebotomy SOP is a useful tool for this—and (2) the amount of anticoagulant/preservative needed for proper storage conditions, if less than 300 mL is withdrawn.

Of relevance is that the volume of anticoagulant in each phlebotomy bag is the amount required for proper storage of a product containing 450 ± 45 mL, that is, 63 mL. If less than 300 mL of blood is removed from the patient/donor, the volume of anticoagulant must be reduced to provide conditions appropriate for maintaining cell viability during storage. A methodology for making these various calculations follows.

Step 1

Calculate the amount of blood that can be removed, using the donor's weight in the following formula. In pounds:

(Donor weight in pounds ÷ 110 lb) × 450 mL = mL of blood to be withdrawn

In kilograms:

(Donor weight in kilograms ÷ 50 kg) × 450 mL = mL of blood to be withdrawn

Step 2

Determine the correct volume of anticoagulant/preservative that should be in this low-volume unit. The ratio of citrate-phosphate-dextrose (CPD) and citrate-phosphate-dextrose-adenine (CPDA-1) anticoagulant/preservative to blood is 14 mL anticoagulant for each 100 mL of blood. The amount of anticoagulant needed for the specific volume of donor/patient blood is calculated as follows:

Amount blood to be drawn (mL) × (14 mL anticoagulant/100 mL blood) = amount of anticoagulant needed to provide adequate storage conditions using the 14:100 ratio

Step 3

Subtract the number calculated in step 2 from 63 mL, which is the volume of anticoagulant/preservative in a standard 450 mL phlebotomy bag; the resulting number is the amount of solution that must be removed in order to have the correct whole blood:anticoagulant/preservative ratio in the storage bag.

63 mL − volume of anticoagulant needed = mL of anticoagulant to remove from the phlebotomy bag

For example, if whole blood must be drawn into a 450 mL bag from a donor who weighs 70 lb, the calculations would be as follows:

Step 1. (70 lb ÷ 110 lb) × 450 mL = 286.4 mL of blood should be removed from the donor/patient.

Step 2. (286.4 mL blood) × (14 mL anticoagulant/100 mL blood) = 40.1 mL anticoagulant needed.

Step 3. 63.0 mL − 40.1 mL = 22.9 mL of anticoagulant should be removed from the primary bag.

To remove the anticoagulant solution, the bag is placed on a scale, and, based on weight, excess solution is siphoned into a satellite bag until the desired volume of anticoagulant/preservative remains in the primary collection bag. (Note: 1 gram = 1 mL of anticoagulant solution.) Because this process takes place in a closed system, the product retains the original outdate of the anticoagulant/preservative used.

Just before or immediately after the blood has been collected, up to 30 mL of samples for ABO/Rh typing, antibody screening, and infectious disease testing are collected. (In some types of apheresis, samples for laboratory testing are collected from a small satellite pouch just before commencement of apheresis.) Before the whole blood or component leaves the donor's bedside, the identifiers—usually alphanumeric—on the component bag, the segments, the sample tubes, and the donor's record must be rechecked to ensure that all numbers match.

Allogeneic: Refers to the blood or blood products collected from someone other than the intended recipient.

Because **allogeneic** blood donors are considered to represent a healthy population (i.e., generally free of blood-borne diseases), the use of special precautions is not mandated. Gloves must be available for those workers who prefer to use them. However, if the phlebotomist or person doing the physical examination has cuts, scratches, or breaks in the skin, gloves should be worn. At the conclusion of the phlebotomy, the needle must not be recapped but discarded in an approved puncture-proof container for final disposal. Commercially available needle guards are now widely used in order to prevent accidental needle sticks.

The actual donation time for a unit of whole blood is generally 8 to 10 minutes. At the conclusion of phlebotomy, pressure should be applied to the venipuncture site and the donor given written and oral instructions on postphlebotomy care. A sample set of instructions is listed in Fig. 8-6. If the donor has no evidence of developing a reaction, he or she may spend several minutes resting in the chair or proceed to a "canteen" where the donor is encouraged to drink copious amounts of juice, water, or other nondehydrating beverages. Following donation, donors should also be observed for evidence of an impending reaction by appropriately trained staff or volunteers. Some states require that the donor spend at least 15 minutes in the canteen area or chair before leaving the blood drive or center.

A healthy donor's blood volume is approximately 4000 to 5500 mL, or the equivalent of 8 to 11 pints. With adequate fluid replacement, total fluid volume should be restored in less than 72 hours.[29] This process begins in the canteen area, thus the importance of having donors linger a while longer.

1.	After donation, please rest in the donor chair for 10 minutes before getting up. Let one of the staff assist you when you are ready to get up.
2.	Rest in the donor canteen at least 15 minutes. Eat something and drink plenty of water or juice.
3.	Inform a staff member immediately if you have any unexpected reaction, such as lightheadedness, nervousness, queasiness, a flushed look, slight perspiration above the lip, or if the skin is clammy and the color is slightly "off." Staff will ask you how you feel or if you have any questions before you leave.
4.	Drink more fluids than usual in the next 4 hours but avoid alcohol and caffeinated beverages during that period.
5.	Do not smoke for at least 30 minutes after donation.
6.	If there is bleeding from the site where the needle was placed, raise your arm and apply pressure on the bandage until it stops.
7.	If you feel dizzy or faint, lie down or sit down and lower your head between your knees. Call someone to assist you. Do not drive a vehicle if you feel lightheaded or dizzy.
8.	If either bleeding or faintness persists, return to the blood center if possible, or see a physician immediately.
9.	Please contact our blood center if you have any problems related to this donation.
10.	If you become ill in the next 3 to 4 days, contact the blood center with information about your illness. We may want to pull your blood from the shelves so that no patient is adversely affected by your donation. This will, of course, be confidential information shared only with you and the blood center medical staff.

Thank you for your donation.
We hope to see you again soon!

Fig. 8-6 Postdonation instructions.

As an added measure of safety, donors are also instructed to call the blood center if they become ill (especially with an infection) shortly after donation, experience an adverse reaction, or for any reason decide that their blood may not be safe for transfusion. A call-back number should be provided to facilitate this kind of communication. It is not out of the ordinary for donors to forget relevant information during screening, such as recent travel to a malarial area. If the donor subsequently calls and provides information that could affect the safety of the unit, the blood center should have a mechanism for following up this "postdonation information."[4]

Preparation of Segments from the Unit

Blood products are collected and processed in a closed system. This means that no air enters the blood collection bag at the time of collection or during the component processing steps. At the time of phlebotomy, the collection bag tubing that terminates at the needle is allowed to fill with the anticoagulant/preservative solution from the collection bag. One or two drops may fall from the still-capped needle indicating that the line is full of fluid and not air. Once the line is filled, it is clamped off until the venipuncture is done.

As the venipuncture is successfully completed, the clamp is released and the collection proceeds as described previously. At the end of the collection, the line from the donor to the blood bag is again clamped off and the needle is removed from the donor's arm. As the donor applies pressure to the venipuncture site, the needle is heat-sealed from the rest of the tubing. At this time the blood in the tubing line does not contain anticoagulant/preservative solution. In order to mix this fresh blood with the anticoagulant/preservative solution, the tubing must be "stripped" using a special handheld tool or automatic device that pushes the blood from the tubing into the collection bag to mix with the bag solutions. As the stripping device is released, blood refills the tubing. This stripping is done at least three times to ensure good mixing of the collected blood. At some blood centers, it is required that a knot now be made close to the junction of the bag and the tubing.

In both blood centers and transfusion services, it is necessary to perform tests using blood that can be positively associated with the product in the collection bag. To accomplish this, a long piece of tubing that originally was used to interconnect the bags is made into segments or "tails." This tubing line has a number stamped along its length that serves as an identification number for the segments or tails. At the end of each tubing identification number is an "X." The segments or tails are made at each "X" (Fig. 8-7). A heat-sealing device creates a closed band along the tubing at each "X" interval. The heat seal does not sever the tubing, but makes a narrow compressed band that allows each segment to be cut off without opening the blood bag to the air. The last identification number remains attached to the blood bag so that, should any or all of the tails separate from the blood bag, they may be matched up with the correct blood bag.[30]

The blood in the segments is whole blood and so contains both the red blood cells and the plasma. As the unit of blood is allowed to sit in the refrigerator, the blood in the segments separates by gravity into two distinct layers, a compact red blood cell section and a clear plasma layer. Thus it is possible to use one tail to do testing using the red blood cells and the plasma as would be necessary in the crossmatch process. The size of the segments or tails is sufficient to get about 4 to 5 drops of plasma and enough red blood cells to make 3 to 5 mL of a 2% to 5% suspension. This red blood cell suspension may also be used for antigen identification.

Adverse Donor Reactions

Although blood donation is generally considered a safe procedure, it is not without potential complications. Studies have shown that up to 36% of donors may experience an adverse effect, ranging from systemic symptoms of fatigue or vasovagal responses (i.e., lightheadedness or outright syncope), to serious vascular or

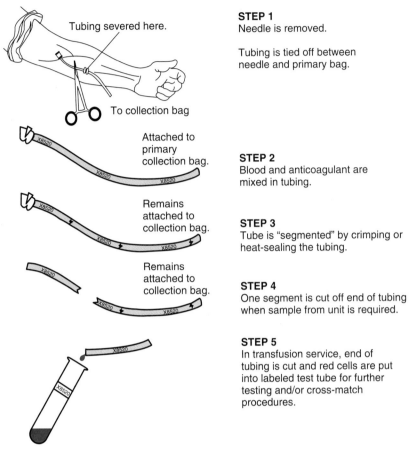

Tubing severed here.

To collection bag

Attached to primary collection bag.

Remains attached to collection bag.

Remains attached to collection bag.

STEP 1
Needle is removed.

Tubing is tied off between needle and primary bag.

STEP 2
Blood and anticoagulant are mixed in tubing.

STEP 3
Tube is "segmented" by crimping or heat-sealing the tubing.

STEP 4
One segment is cut off end of tubing when sample from unit is required.

STEP 5
In transfusion service, end of tubing is cut and red cells are put into labeled test tube for further testing and/or cross-match procedures.

Fig. 8-7 Donor unit segments.

even neurologic injuries.[31,32] In one survey of 1000 donors who were interviewed several weeks after donating, 360 reported one or more adverse reactions: 7.8% of reactions were fatigue, 5.3% were vasovagal in nature, and nausea and vomiting accounted for 1.1%.[31]

Needle injuries can damage blood vessels and include minor ecchymoses (bruises), hematomata, arterial punctures, arteriovenous fistulas caused by arterial punctures, and arterial pseudoaneuryms.[33] Needle-associated nerve injuries have been reported in as many as 1 per 6300 donations,[34] and although the symptoms of shooting pain, burning, or numbness usually resolve spontaneously, their occurrence can be a source of discomfort and concern to the donor.[35,36] Because untoward effects can occur in association with blood donation, phlebotomy staff must be well trained in venipuncture and phlebotomy techniques. They also must be intimately familiar with symptoms of impending reactions, and be able to respond quickly and appropriately. The type of reaction dictates the response. In general, adverse reactions are treated by first suspending or terminating the procedure. If the reaction is minor, the phlebotomist may be able to provide appropriate treatment. However, if the reaction is more severe, it may be necessary to engage the expertise of other staff or the medical director. Some specific reactions are discussed next.

Hematomata and Ecchymoses

One of the more common complications is the development of an ecchymosis or hematomata—subcutaneous, intradermal, or even intramuscular collection of blood—near the venipuncture site. Applying pressure to the area for 5 to 10 minutes helps reduce oozing from the injured vessel wall. The donor should be given instructions on how to care for the arm to prevent further injury. This would include avoidance of lifting or vigorous activity, the application of cold during the first 24 hours, and the circumstances under which the donor should call the center or seek medical care.

Arterial Puncture

Arterial punctures occur when the needle either passes through a vein into an underlying artery, or is inserted directly into an artery. If the needle is pulsating, the blood is redder than usual, or the bag fills up in less than 4 to 5 minutes,[33] it is highly likely that the needle is in an artery. The phlebotomy should be immediately terminated, pressure applied for at least 10 minutes, and a pressure dressing applied. Instructions for aftercare should be similar to those for ecchymoses or hematomata, but the donor should also be told that if evidence of continued bleeding is noticed, the donor should immediately contact his or her physician or go to an urgent care center.

Nerve Injury

Because of the close proximity of nerves to veins, it is also possible that a phlebotomy needle can injure a peripheral nerve. The donor usually describes a sharp, shooting pain. If the donor is in obvious discomfort, the needle should be removed and another vein should be used. The symptoms associated with a nerve injury usually resolve spontaneously, but they may take weeks or months to completely disappear. In most cases, reassuring the donor is an appropriate response. However, if the symptoms persist for a prolonged period of time, the donor should consider consulting a physician. It is worth stating again: The best means of preventing needle injuries is thorough training of phlebotomy staff.

Fainting

Fainting, or syncope, occurs usually as a result of a vasovagal reaction. Symptoms leading up to an actual syncopal episode can include weakness, sweating, lightheadedness, dizziness, or pallor. These symptoms—and the most obvious manifestation, syncope—come about because of a complex interplay of cerebral, brainstem, autonomic nervous system, and even emotional factors such as fear of the sight of blood. Usually the pulse and blood pressure fall. Taken to the extreme, convulsions, or seizures, can also occur.

Treatment for syncope involves lowering the donor's head, raising the donor's feet, loosening constricting clothes, and putting cold compresses on the donor's neck or forehead. It should be noted that many syncopal reactions take place in the canteen, where vasodilation in lower extremity veins can cause gravity-related pooling of blood in the legs. This is the reason that donors should be so carefully observed in the postdonation period, especially in the canteen. Following a syncopal episode, the donor should not be released until the pulse and blood pressure have returned to normal and the donor is feeling well again.

Hyperventilation

Hyperventilation may occur in some donors as a result of anxiety, and could cause a significant drop in CO_2 levels. This can be easily treated by having the donor "rebreathe" into a paper bag. This will increase the CO_2 levels and prevent a more serious reaction such as muscle twitching, tetany, or convulsions. True convulsions are rare, but if they occur, the donor should be protected from injuries and an adequate airway should be maintained.

Nausea and Vomiting

Nausea and vomiting occasionally occur. As in syncope, the factors contributing to this are complex and involve autonomic and central nervous system pathways.

Treatment includes making the donor as comfortable as possible and instructing him or her to breathe slowly. Cold compresses are applied to the donor's forehead and back of neck. Turning the donor's head to the side helps prevent possible aspiration of vomitus.

Cardiac Problems

Serious cardiac problems are extremely rare in a healthy, well-screened blood donor. However, at least 23 deaths associated with donation (whole blood or platelets) have been reported to the FDA since the early 1980s, most of them attributable to cardiovascular disease.[37] If, for any reason, the donor experiences a cardiac or respiratory arrest, cardiopulmonary resuscitation (CPR) should be immediately initiated and emergency medical assistance summoned.

Donors who experience reactions should be provided with as much privacy as possible. Individuals with systemic types of reactions, such as light-headedness, syncope, or convulsions, should not be allowed to leave the collection area until the vital signs have normalized and the donor is feeling well. A blood center should consider having a policy for handling situations in which a donor insists on leaving prematurely. All donor reactions should be noted on the donor's record. This will facilitate donor follow-up and serve as a source of information for future donations. If it is decided that the donor should not donate again, a notation to that effect should also be made.

Donor Records

Blood banks and transfusion services are required to have a system of record keeping, and must have written policies and procedures for donor record storage and retention. Systems must ensure that records are protected from unauthorized alteration or destruction and that they can be retrieved in a reasonable period of time. The system must also ensure the confidentiality of the donor.

Retention of records relating to the donation process, component processing, infectious disease tests, disposition of all donated components, and many other documents must occur for prolonged periods of time or even permanently. FDA regulations and AABB standards specify the length of time that records should be maintained.[2,4]

DONOR PROCESSING: THE LABORATORY

After a red blood cell or platelet apheresis product has been collected at a blood or donor center, it is delivered, under appropriate storage conditions, to a laboratory where the product will be tested. Every single blood product is tested. Only under extraordinary circumstances may a blood product be used before all required testing is completed. One example is a unit donated by a donor who is part of a "dedicated donor" program, whose blood may be transfused before test results are available, provided the donor has undergone testing within the past 30 days and all tests were nonreactive.[38] Repeat donors' records are reviewed before testing to ascertain any previously unacceptable results or notable history. Every time a person donates a blood product, testing must be done on that donor's blood to ensure the safety of that individual blood product.

Testing may be done by the laboratory of a community blood center, by centralized reference centers, or, if the blood is collected by a hospital, in the laboratory—often the clinical pathology department—of that facility. According to AABB Standards and the FDA, all testing must be done in accord with the test manufacturer's instructions. These instructions must be followed exactly, and the specimen for testing must meet the requirements of the manufacturer for acceptability. It is not acceptable, for example, to use the controls from one kit with the reagents from another manufacturer's kit.

Results of testing must be logged or recorded immediately on completion. If testing must be repeated for any reason, the final result must be recorded before interpretation is done. Therefore, initially positive test results must be confirmed by an established protocol, that is, repeated with the same methodology, repeated with a more sensitive or specific method, or confirmed by a definitive test method.

Medically important positive donor test results must be communicated, and documented by the collection facility, to the donor, and any tests requiring Public Health Department notification must be done. Donors are told, before donation during the screening process, that test results for diseases having a potential public health safety concern will be reported, if required by state or other laws. These diseases include HIV, hepatitis, and syphilis, for example.

Donor Testing

All donor testing is done to protect the potential recipients of the blood components. Donor testing evolves as the circumstances within the community change. Testing is accomplished by drawing a series of tubes at the time of the blood unit collection phlebotomy. These tubes are labeled with the same bar-coded unique identification number that is applied to the blood product bag.

The following tests are required at this time:[2,4,5]

1. ABO and Rh typing
2. Antibody screen for unexpected red cell antibodies
3. HbsAg—hepatitis B surface antigen
4. Anti-HBc—antibody to hepatitis B core antigen
5. Anti-HCV—antibody to hepatitis C virus
6. HCV RNA—NAT (nucleic acid amplification test) to detect the RNA of hepatitis C virus
7. Anti–HIV-1/2—antibody to human immunodeficiency virus types 1 and 2
8. HIV-1 RNA—NAT to detect the RNA of HIV-1 virus
9. Anti–HTLV-I/II—antibody to human T-cell lymphotropic virus types 1 and 2
10. Serologic test for syphilis
11. WNV RNA—NAT to detect the RNA of West Nile virus

ABO testing on donor blood products is done using both the **forward** or direct testing of the red blood cells with antisera (anti-A, anti-B, and anti-A,B) and **reverse** typing using the plasma or serum and testing cells that are A_1 or B type.

Rh testing is done on the red blood cells using an anti-D serum. If the test result is reactive (red cells agglutinate with the anti-D serum), the cells are labeled Rh positive. If the test is not reactive (negative) with the anti-D, the cells must be further tested to determine if a **weak D** is present. If further testing demonstrates the presence of weak D, the red blood cells are labeled Rh positive. If further testing confirms the absence of weak D, the cells are labeled Rh negative.

Antibody screening for unexpected red-cell antibodies is done using any of a number of methods (saline, albumin, low ionic strength saline (LISS), polyethylene glycol [PEG]). Unexpected antibodies are the result of transfusion or pregnancy. Blood products found to have unexpected antibodies in the plasma or serum may still be used for transfusion, but the red cells must be washed before use or frozen and then deglycerolized before use.

Viral screen testing for hepatitis (B and C), HIV, and HTLV antibodies is most commonly done using enzyme-linked immunosorbent assay (ELISA or EIA). Testing must be performed according to the manufacturer's instructions, and the control results must be within the manufacturer's specification for the test run to be considered valid. If there is deviation from the manufacturer's instructions, such as an equipment malfunction, error in reagent use, or control deviation, the run is considered invalid. The invalid run must be documented and possible causes determined and documented. All samples processed on such an invalid run must be repeated.

Forward testing (typing): ABO testing that uses reagent antisera (anti-A and anti-B) to identify A and/or B antigens on the red cells. Refer to Chapter 3 for a discussion of the ABO blood group system.

Reverse testing (typing): ABO testing that uses reagent red cells (A1 and B cells) to identify A and/or B antibodies in the serum.

Weak D: An apparently weakened expression of the $Rh_o(D)$ antigen on red cells. For a complete discussion of weak D phenotypes, refer to Chapter 5.

Window period: The period from the time an individual is infected with a disease until it is detectable by laboratory assays.

Additional testing with a different methodology is used to increase the detection sensitivity for both HCV and HIV. Serum is tested for each of these viral diseases using nucleic acid amplification testing (NAT). NAT detects viral RNA and increases the possibility of detecting virus during the serologic **window period** during which antibodies cannot otherwise be detected.

If the screening EIA test is reactive, the serum is again tested—in duplicate. If one or both of the duplicated repeat tests results are reactive, the serum is considered to be "repeatedly reactive." All such units, and all components made from these units, must be discarded. If the duplicated repeat tests are both nonreactive, the test is considered negative and the unit, and all components, may be used.

For repeatedly reactive tests, a confirmatory (or supplemental) test must be done. For HIV, this test is called a "Western blot" assay. If this test is positive using criteria established by the FDA, the donor is considered to be infected with HIV. The donor must be informed of the test results and, in some cases, counseled for follow-up testing and health care. Because of the serious consequences of a positive HIV test, it is critical that the results be as accurate as possible before a final interpretation is made and the donor informed of the results. A comprehensive list of screening tests and companion confirmatory (or supplemental) tests appears in Table 8-3.

For syphilis, a screening test is done. If this test is reactive, a confirmatory test is performed that is specific for the presence of the antibodies to *Treponema pallidum,* the causative agent of syphilis. Many physiologic conditions may cause a false positive in the screening test, for example, pregnancy, autoimmune diseases, or infections. If a confirmatory test is negative, the donor is considered negative for syphilis. However, the FDA requires that the blood product be labeled with both the screening and the confirmatory results.[2] For West Nile virus, NAT is the screening test for detection of viral RNA. If this test is reactive, the donor is deferred (for 28 days from the onset of symptoms or donation) and the unit in question is discarded. The donor is informed of the test result and is asked to have further testing done to confirm the presence of antibody to WNV.[25]

In March 2004, the AABB introduced a new testing requirement for evidence of bacterial contamination of apheresis platelets and platelet concentrates. This testing is done directly on products and not on donor blood samples. The rationale for this new requirement is that bacterial contamination of platelets is the most common transfusion-associated infection risk in the United States today.

Platelet products are stored at room temperature in a volume of glucose-rich plasma that is ideal for platelet survival, but is also ideal for bacterial growth. A common source of contamination is the skin in the donor's antecubital space, where microbial flora abound. The most common contaminants of platelets are the normal skin flora (e.g., *S. epidermidis, P. acnes,* or other *Staphylococcus* coagulase-negative organisms). It is unlikely but nevertheless possible that a donor with occult

TABLE 8-3 Blood Donor Screening and Confirmatory/Supplemental Assays	
Screening Tests	Confirmatory/Supplemental Tests
Syphilis serology: TPPK	Syphilis G EIA
Anti-Hbc EIA	None available
Anti-HCV	Recombinant immunoblot assay (RIBA) HCV 3.0
Anti–HIV-1/HIV-2 EIA	Licensed Anti–HIV-1 Western blot
Anti-HIV-2 EIA	HIV-2 Western blot
Anti–HTLV-1/II	EIA/IFA typing, Western blot, RIPA if applicable
HbsAg EIA	HbsAg confirmatory neutralization
WNV nucleic acid test	None available
HCV/HIV nucleic acid test	None available

bacteremia could pass the screening steps before donation or feel healthy enough to donate. However, if an asymptomatic gram-negative bacteremic donor were to donate, the consequences for the recipient could be dire. This underscores the need for thorough pre-donation screening and careful physical evaluation.

Preventing contamination of platelets is the first line of attack. To this end, the arm scrub is of critical importance. The donor arm venipuncture site must be cleansed with great care using either iodine-based or chlorhexidine scrubs. Repalpation or touching of the venipuncture site is forbidden, even if the phlebotomist uses gloves or gauze as a barrier. This process has been described earlier. A second approach for reducing skin contamination is a diversion of the first few milliliters of blood into a pouch before the blood enters the collection bag. The idea is to reduce or remove any skin fragments and bacteria introduced into the blood during phlebotomy. (This "diverted" blood can also be used for donor viral marker, immunohematologic, or other testing.) Technologies for inactivating pathogens are under development, but at the writing of this chapter are not yet approved by the FDA. Thus, in the absence of approved technologies for pathogen inactivation, it has become necessary to test for bacterial contamination of platelet products.

Testing is done on apheresis platelets by using either of two FDA-approved semiautomated systems. A sample is removed via a sterile connecting device from the apheresis bag 24 hours after collection and is introduced into a culture bottle. The 24-hour waiting period after donation is to allow any contaminants opportunity to grow. The bottle is then monitored (depending on the manufacturer) for either decrease in O_2 levels or increase in CO_2 concentrations. If a positive culture is identified, the source unit is quarantined and further testing and/or donor notification would be done as directed by the collection facility's protocol.

At the writing of this chapter, there are no FDA-approved technologies or assays for bacterial testing of non–leuko-reduced platelet concentrates. Thus concentrates are being tested using alternative approaches. Although these approaches are less sensitive and specific than automated culture systems, they nevertheless represent an improvement in platelet safety. A platelet concentrate can be evaluated using a Gram stain, Wright stain, or acridine orange stain. Swirling is a technique used to evaluate the "normalcy" of platelets by observing the opalescence created by the light shining from the discoid-shaped normal platelets as they move through flowing plasma. As the plasma environment changes in acidity consequent to bacterial growth, the platelets lose their opalescent shimmer. The AABB does not approve of swirling as a routine detection method. Swirling may only be used in emergency situations if the routinely used method cannot be performed.

A simple bacterial detection method that may be used, if validated by the testing site, is a urine dipstick for pH and glucose measurement. Because dipsticks are designed for use with urine or whole blood, it is necessary to establish an interpretive scheme when using the device for testing platelets. The rationale for using dipsticks is that if a product is bacterially contaminated, the pH and glucose levels will decrease.[4,39]

Guarantees of Blood Safety

Today's blood supply is very safe—it is safer than ever before in the history of transfusion medicine. But no laboratory testing or donor history questioning or screening can ever make the supply of human blood products completely safe. Even with the sophisticated assays that are in use, it is possible for an infection to remain undetected if the donor does not yet have serologic (i.e., antibodies) or nucleic acid evidence of infection. This is because all diseases have a "window period" of quiescence or "secrecy" during which a potential donor is asymptomatic, and antigen and/or antibody levels are undetectable. All laboratory tests require threshold levels of antibody or antigen for detection. During the window period, the sensitivity of in vitro testing is not met and therefore it is possible for an infected donor to pass on viable microbes even while still feeling quite healthy.

Although technical errors in testing are extremely rare, they still are possible. Examples may include failure to pipette specimen or deliver reagent. Furthermore, human error in quarantine and release of an infected unit could occur.[40]

One of the fundamental reasons for this permanent condition of uncertainty is obvious. There is no easy, predictive method for anticipating new infectious diseases. The health care industry learned this lesson in the 1980s with the discovery of human immunodeficiency virus, which burst on a totally unprepared world community. Most recently, new blood-borne or potentially blood-borne diseases, such as West Nile virus, have been identified. Malaria was the primary blood-borne parasitic infectious disease of concern for many years, and remains a small but nevertheless possible risk. Now, however, in the early twenty-first century, other parasitic diseases are causing concern within the blood transfusion industry. **Chagas' disease** and **leishmaniasis,** caused by trypanosomes and leishmanial parasites, respectively, have been implicated in causing disease by blood transfusion or tissue transplants. Another infection that is transmitted through tissue is Creutzfeldt-Jakob disease, and it is believed that **variant-CJD** (the human form of bovine spongiform encephalopathy, or "mad cow disease") could be transmitted through transfusion.[41,42] International travel, immigration, and military activity are the primary reasons for the increase in such once rarely seen infections.

Records of Laboratory Testing

The AABB *Standards for Blood Banks and Transfusion Services,* 22nd edition, 2003, contains a comprehensive table of all records that are to be retained by collection facilities, laboratories, and transfusion services. The AABB Standards table includes the retention time for each record type and notes the AABB Standard that applies to each record. In general, 10 years is the maximum *suggested* required time, although applicable state or local laws may supersede AABB-recommended record-retention times. The AABB Standards is referenced to the 21 CFR, 606, and 630. Some records must be permanently retained, such as documentation of notification of significant abnormal laboratory findings, and donor deferral. In general practice, most blood centers and transfusion services keep all donor and blood product records indefinitely.

Laboratories performing tests on blood-product donors must keep records on critical equipment (including computers), reagents, personnel (including training and competency), and test results (both initial and confirmatory). Laboratories must keep records on equipment validation and preventive maintenance schedules, computer validations, reagent accuracy and performance checks, dates of testing, and personnel performing tests. The objective of all record keeping is to create a complete, retrievable, and traceable history of donor testing for each blood product collected. Each donated unit and all its components and any manipulations performed must be traceable from collection until final disposition. The laboratory must establish a total tracking system to meet this FDA requirement.

The FDA requires that laboratory test results be recorded *as they are performed.* The logging of results may be on manual worksheets or in a computer, but it must be immediate. Interpretation of results, however, may be done at a later time. This protocol helps prevent clerical errors and memory lapses.[2]

The federally mandated **Health Insurance Portability and Accountability Act (HIPAA)** requires that confidentiality be maintained and ensured by all persons dealing with health care issues. This includes donor blood products. All laboratories performing donor blood products testing must have a system in place to ensure that test results are not accessible by unauthorized personnel. This is especially important for computerized records. Security passwords and access codes must be implemented and documented by laboratory administration to prevent both record access and alteration.

Chagas' disease: An insect-transmitted parasitic *(Trypanosoma cruzi)* disease that can be transmitted by transfusion.

Leishmaniasis: A parasitic disease spread by the bite of infected sand flies.

Variant Creutzfeldt-Jakob Disease (vCJD): A fatal human neurodegenerative condition transmitted by prions. As with Creutzfeldt-Jakob disease, vCJD is classified as a transmissible spongiform encephalopathy (TSE) because of characteristic spongy degeneration of the brain.

Health Insurance Portability and Accountability Act (HIPAA): Signed into law in 1996, HIPAA was designed to ensure the continuity of health insurance coverage for individuals changing their place of employment. (For additional information on HIPAA, refer to http://dchealth.dc.gov/hipaa/hipaaoverview.shtm).

ADDITIONAL TESTS PERFORMED ON DONOR BLOOD

Additional tests may be performed on donor units. These are not required by the FDA or AABB and are usually done for a specific request or because of the condition of specific recipients. The most common tests are for **cytomegalovirus (CMV),** selected antigens, and sickle cell trait. CMV is a ubiquitous member of the herpes family that can cause flulike symptoms in healthy people, but in most people is asymptomatic and not a significant threat to their well-being. However, the virus can be harbored in all blood components, red blood cells, plasma, and platelets. In people with compromised immune systems due to HIV or chemotherapy for cancers, CMV can be a life-threatening infection that affects multiple organ systems and can cause death. CMV can cause infections in the heart, brain, eyes, and liver. In premature infants, CMV can also be a life-threatening complication. For such persons, a blood product that is CMV negative may be indicated to prevent additional serious health complications. Blood products screened for CMV and found to be negative are labeled "CMV Neg" or "CMV Negative." Screening is usually done by EIA or a latex agglutination test.

All red cells have an array of genetically determined membrane antigens. It is possible to screen cells using antigen-specific sera to determine the antigen typing of a particular donor's red cells. This typing can be very useful in attempts to locate a compatible unit for a recipient with a particular set of plasma **alloantibodies.** If red cells units are antigen typed, a label is placed on the bag (or attached by a tag to the bag) identifying the specific antigens found.

It is possible to screen red cell units for the presence of the **sickle cell trait** and so label the unit. In certain population centers, it is important to do this screening because the structural integrity of red cells in units positive for sickle cell trait may be compromised; this could pose a problem for neonates or those in sickle cell crisis. Under stressful conditions such as **hypoxia** or **acidosis,** the cells from a donor with sickle cell trait may be induced to sickle, causing further problems. Frozen red blood cell products from donors with sickle cell trait do not **deglycerolize** properly and can form a gelatinous mass during the process.

LABELING REQUIREMENTS FOR BLOOD AND BLOOD PRODUCTS
General Requirements

Each product label *must* have the following information before being placed into inventory (i.e., made available for transfusion):
1. Unique identifier—either numeric or alphanumeric
2. Product type (including any modifications from the original product, i.e., irradiation, filtering, etc.)
3. Collecting facility
4. Expiration date (and time if required)
5. Approximate volume
6. Name and volume of anticoagulant/preservative/additive solutions
7. Storage temperature (in degrees Celsius)
8. ABO and Rh type
9. Instructions to transfusionist[6]
10. Phrases "Volunteer Donor" or "Paid Donor" as applicable
11. Component modifying facility—required if product leaves collection facility[2,4]

Fig. 8-8 is an example of a label that would be affixed to an allogeneic red cell unit.

Further label requirements are indicated if the blood product is intended for transfusion. Some blood products are collected for manufacturing of immune globulin G (IgG), or for other uses in reagent manufacturing. Most blood products, however, are collected for transfusion, so the label must also have these additional statements:

Cytomegalovirus (CMV): One of a group of herpes viruses transmitted by viable leukocytes in blood components, which is of special concern when transfusing immuno-compromised recipients.

Alloantibodies: Antibodies against foreign (non-self) red cell or platelet antigens.

Sickle cell trait: A condition that results when an individual is heterozygous for hemoglobin S, that is, inherits one gene for hemoglobin S and one for normal adult hemoglobin (A). Red cells of patients with sickle cell trait can become deformable under certain physiologic conditions, such as hypoxia.

Hypoxia: Insufficient delivery of oxygen to the tissues.

Acidosis: A pathologic condition caused by an increased hydrogen ion concentration and lowered pH.

Deglycerolize: Removal of glycerol (cryoprotective agent) from red cells during the thawing process.

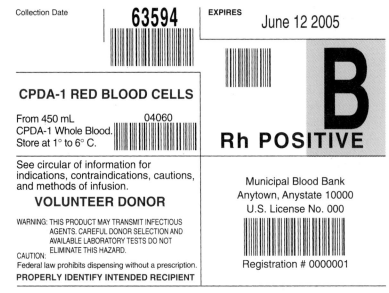

Fig. 8-8 Sample label for red blood cells.

Rx only.

Properly identify intended recipient.

This product may transmit infectious agents.[2,4]

The Code of Federal Regulations, 21 CFR, Part 606.121 specifies the label requirements for all blood products, including the color of the labels, the color of the ink, and the size of the type fonts. Each ABO type must be on a label of a specific color (O is blue, A is yellow, B is pink, and AB is white). Rh types are in black ink on a white ground. Such standardization is an effort to increase safety and reduce error by creating a clear and uniform system that encourages focused attention by all personnel handling the blood products.

Labeling of Autologous Units

Autologous donation: The donation of blood for one's own use.

An **autologous** blood product is one collected from the intended recipient. The labeling of these blood products is the same as for allogeneic (donor) units with the addition of a label that says "For Autologous Use Only." If autologous units are going to be transfused outside the collecting facility, they must be tested for anti–HIV-1/2, anti-HCV, anti–HTLV-I/II, anti-HBc, HCV RNA, HIV RNA, HbsAG, and syphilis. If an autologous unit has a positive result for an infectious disease, a red "BIOHAZARD" label is attached to the unit. Both the AABB Standards and the FDA require notification of the patient and the patient's physician of any positive test results.[2,4,5] Fig. 8-9 is an example of a label that would be affixed to an autologous unit.

Only in "exceptional circumstances" can an autologous unit be used for another patient, but only on a case-by-case basis, only if the infectious disease markers are negative, and only if the medical director approves such an action. Such a **crossed over** unit must have a label indicating "autologous donor."[4]

Crossed over: The process of placing unused autologous units into the homologous blood supply.

Pooled products: Pooling of multiple units of components (e.g., platelets or cryoprecipitate) into one bag for ease of transfusion.

Pooled Products

The two most commonly pooled blood products are cryoprecipitate and platelet concentrates. In each instance these individual products contain very small concentrations of the desired material, cryoprecipitate or platelets. Pooling allows full utilization of a valuable resource and permits customization to patient needs. Cryoprecipitate (informally abbreviated "cryo") contains ≥80 IU of factor VIII (AHF), greater than 150 mg of fibrinogen, and most of factor XIII from the original plasma. Individual cryo units have a volume of about 10 mL.[5] Platelet con-

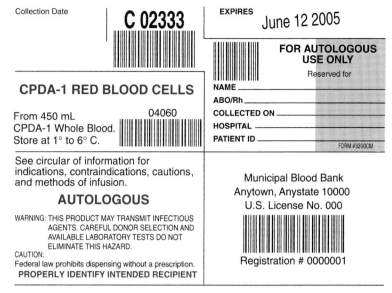

Fig. 8-9 Sample label for autologous red cells.

centrates, by AABB Standards, must contain $\geq 5.5 \times 10^{10}$ platelets in at least 90% of the products and be suspended in sufficient plasma for the pH at the end of storage to be ≥ 6.2.[4]

For cryoprecipitate, it is usual to pool about 10 units for a normal adult recipient. Normal saline is used to rinse each bag and resuspend the cryoprecipitate. It is customary to pool units of the same blood type, but the Rh type need not be identical to that of the recipient. Once the individual units are pooled, the new pool unit must be labeled with a unique identifying number that can be linked to each individual unit used in making the pool. If a manual system is in place, each unit contributing to the pool must be listed against the newly pooled unit identifier. An ideal and appropriate computerized system would have a component manufacturing function that allows multiple units to be pooled and a new identifier and final volume created for the pooled unit. The system used must allow for tracking of the pooled product back to its individual components. The pooled unit is labeled according to the same criteria applied to whole blood. It must have a product type, a new unit numeric/alphanumeric identifier, a new expiration date and time, a new volume, the number of units pooled, the collecting and processing facilities, and volunteer/paid donor.

It is possible to make cryoprecipitate AHF during the initial processing of freshly drawn whole blood. In this situation the pooled cryo is made, assigned a new identifier and volume, given an expiration date of 12 months, and frozen at $-18°$ C. When this single-unit cryo is thawed, the new expiration time for a unit thawed but not pooled in an open system is 6 hours. If individual units of cryo are thawed and then pooled in an open system, the expiration time is 4 hours. If cryoprecipitate is pooled using sterile connecting devices, the post-thaw expiration time is 6 hours.[4,5]

In pooling platelet concentrates, a similar process takes place. Each concentrate is made from a separate unit of whole blood, and must be labeled with the product type, blood type (ABO and Rh), volume, expiration date, and all other information as would be required for a whole blood unit. Generally, an adult requires 6 to 8 platelet concentrates in order to achieve a satisfactory increase in his or her platelet count. The expiration date for platelets pooled in the laboratory is 4 hours, unless the units are pooled using a sterile connecting device; in this case, the expiration date would be that of the first unit that was collected.[4,5]

Labeling as a Final Quality Control Check

Each blood bank or transfusion service must have a system for a final review of all test results and labeling of each blood product. In most blood centers or transfusion services this final check involves two persons who review all requirements for release of a blood product into inventory. When the check is completed, the process is documented on a worksheet or in a computer file as a permanent record of this last review before release to inventory. There should be an SOP to facilitate this review process. If a computer is used to enter data, it should be validated to prevent release of ABO- or Rh-mislabeled products. If any discrepancies are found, they must be resolved before a product is released.[4]

AUTOLOGOUS DONATIONS

An autologous donation is one made by the intended recipient. This is the safest blood because there is no exposure to foreign cellular alloantigens or transfusion-transmissible viral infections (other than any the patient may already have). Thus the patient can avoid the formation of red cell, white cell, or HLA antibodies. In addition, autologous donation increases the likelihood that blood will be available if the patient has a rare blood type or multiple alloantibodies. There are also advantages for blood centers and other patients. Specifically, autologous donation programs can augment the inventory of a blood center and reduce demands on the allogeneic inventory.

There are four broad classifications of autologous procedures: (1) preoperative or predeposit, (2) perioperative hemodilution (acute normovolemic hemodilution [ANH]), (3) intraoperative collection, and (4) postoperative salvage. The type or types of procedures that the patient should undergo in order to avoid or decrease the chance of receiving allogeneic blood should be discussed in advance with the patient, and the risks and benefits of each addressed.

Preoperative (Predeposit) Autologous Donation

Preoperative (predeposit) autologous donation (PAD) can be accomplished either by whole blood phlebotomy or red cell apheresis. Apheresis can usually result in the collection of two red cells units. PAD is most often ordered for use in elective surgeries such as orthopedic procedures, selected gynecologic procedures, and cardiovascular or prostate surgeries. The major justification is the anticipation that at least one unit of blood will be needed intraoperatively or postoperatively. In determining whether a patient should donate preoperatively, the physician should take into account the date of surgery, expected surgical blood loss, the patient's hemoglobin and hematocrit, whether the patient has acceptable peripheral venous access, and the existence of underlying conditions that could be worsened by donating or that would preclude donation.

Date of Surgery

Orders for a patient to donate preoperatively should be timed in such a way that the patient has ample opportunity to do so. Generally, the patient donates one unit per week, as long as the pre-donation hemoglobin and hematocrit stay above the minimum hemoglobin level of 11 g/dL or hematocrit of 33% or greater.[4] Although the minimal allowable time between the last donation and surgery is 72 hours, it is unlikely there will be a meaningful increase in red cell mass this close to surgery—especially if it is the only unit that will be donated. Which type of unit is preferable: one stored in a refrigerator, subject to loss through breakage or other unexpected events, or one stored within its natural environment—the patient's body? Thus blood centers may want to consider whether such a request should be discussed with the ordering physician.

Patient Hemoglobin and Hematocrit

One of the greatest risks associated with preoperative donation is **iatrogenic anemia** or hypovolemia (hypovolemia is less of a problem in red cell apheresis, because intravenous saline is infused during the procedure). As mentioned previously, the minimal

Preoperative (predeposit) autologous donation (PAD): The donation of one or more units of blood by a patient for his or her own use for an anticipated future need such as pending surgery.

Iatrogenic anemia: Anemia resulting from treatment, for example, anemia in newborns resulting from the collection of blood samples for laboratory testing.

acceptable hemoglobin and hematocrit levels are 11 g/dL and 33%, respectively. If these parameters are borderline, removing a unit of autologous blood could render the patient significantly anemic. Further, although **erythropoiesis** can be stimulated by whole blood removal, it generally is not rapid enough to restore the hemoglobin and hematocrit to pre-donation levels, especially if the units are donated less than 3 weeks before surgery.[43] To facilitate erythropoiesis the attending physician may order iron supplements. Administration of erythropoietin to boost the patient's red cell mass is not generally practiced because the patient must be monitored carefully, and use of hematopoietic growth hormones in this setting is not considered cost-effective.

Erythropoiesis: The production of red cells.

Peripheral Venous Access

Occasionally, a patient's veins are so small or inaccessible that successful phlebotomy cannot be performed. Although the attending physician is undoubtedly knowledgeable about many aspects of the patient's health and physical condition, often blood center personnel make the best evaluation regarding the adequacy of venous access. If phlebotomy for whole blood donation is rendered impossible by the patient's anatomy, predeposit autologous donation likely cannot be carried out.

In the order for preoperative autologous donation the physician should specify how many units are needed, and over how long a period of time they should be collected; however, there should be no fewer than 3 days between collections. The collecting center should have an established means of accepting, documenting, and, when appropriate, carrying out attending physician orders for collecting autologous units.

Risks of Autologous Pre-donation

In addition to iatrogenic anemia, the patient could experience the same types of adverse reactions that can occur in allogeneic whole blood or apheresis donations. The risk of bacterial contamination is not eliminated, because inadequate skin preparation or occult bacteremia in the donor are potential sources of bacterial growth or elaboration of endotoxins during storage. In addition, if the unit is inadvertently lost due to breakage or storage problems, the patient may unexpectedly require allogeneic transfusion.

Contraindications for Autologous Donation

Not every patient who will need transfusions should automatically be considered a safe candidate. Preexisting conditions that, in combination with donating a unit of whole blood, could potentially jeopardize the patient's well-being include cardiovascular and pulmonary disease. The collection facility should have SOPs that delineate acceptance criteria, because many patients have underlying medical conditions, some fairly significant. Ultimately, the blood center physician is responsible for establishing acceptance criteria and for determining whether a specific patient should be allowed to undergo whole blood or apheresis red cell collection. The blood center physician can also play an important educational role in the physician and hospital communities regarding the risks and benefits of autologous donation.

Autologous donation should be avoided if the patient has symptomatic coronary artery disease, has congestive heart failure, has had a myocardial infarction within the past 6 months, and/or is on medication for cardiovascular disease. If the patient has pulmonary conditions such as emphysema or chronic obstructive pulmonary disease, the removal of 10% to 15% of the blood volume could affect oxygen uptake and delivery; prudent practice would dictate that other transfusion options be pursued. Uncontrolled hypertension, known cerebrovascular disease including a cerebrovascular accident (stroke) within the previous 6 months, and aortic stenosis are also contraindications for donation.[5]

A final contraindication to autologous donation is the presence or evidence of a bacterial infection. A substantial body of literature about bacterial contamination of blood components exists. Many organisms are capable of growing in blood or components stored at room temperate and even refrigerated at 1° to 6° C. When transfused, bacteria or bacterial endotoxins can produce symptoms ranging from chills and fever to sepsis or even death. Implicated organisms include a broad spectrum such as *Citrobacter, Yersinia, Pseudomonas,* or *Escherichia.*[44-47] If a patient is febrile or reports an infection of the skin, urinary tract, sinuses, gastrointestinal system, pulmonary system, or any other system, that patient should not be permitted to donate. The attending physician should be notified of the deferral and the patient accepted only after the infection has been successfully treated with antibiotics.

General Parameters for Preoperative Autologous Donation

Medical or other qualifying criteria for autologous donation are much less stringent than those for allogeneic donation. The reasons lie in the risk-benefit equation. In the vast majority of circumstances, the indications for autologous donation far outweigh the potential risks of donating. Patients with chronic viral infections or risks associated with nonbacterial infections such as hepatitis or HIV are eligible to donate in many situations. Physical and other parameters such as weight, age, and hemoglobin or hematocrit levels can be substantially different for those patients whose blood will be available only for their own use. These are summarized as follows:[4]

Hemoglobin. $\geq$11 g/dL.

Hematocrit. $\geq$33%.

Age. No upper or lower limit. (Note: Parental or guardian consent must be given for patients under 17 years of age.)

Weight. No minimum weight. If the patient weighs less than 50 kg (110 lb), adjustments in the amount of blood removed must be made before phlebotomy, using the formula presented previously. If less than 300 mL of blood is drawn, the amount of anticoagulant must also be adjusted.

Frequency of donation. Not more often than every 3 days. Not less than 72 hours before scheduled surgery.

Regulatory and Administrative Issues

A facility that collects autologous blood must be registered with the FDA. All activities of the program must conform with Good Manufacturing Practices (cGMPs), and all units tested for certain infectious diseases. Regulations that pertain to staff training, proficiency testing, collection, labeling, storage, documentation, and record keeping also apply.

Although autologous collection programs offer patients, hospitals, and blood centers some significant benefits, such programs are generally more complex, and therefore are more expensive to run. There must be considerable communication with physicians' offices and mechanisms for processing orders. Patients usually require more careful evaluation, and blood center physicians often participate in decisions about patient eligibility. Whereas community-based blood centers—which do not have to deal with third-party payers—can usually count on full reimbursement for collecting and processing autologous units, hospitals may not be able to recover their expenses. However, the availability of autologous units helps meet a patient's transfusion needs in a safer manner, and decreases the hospital's need to purchase allogeneic units from a community blood center.

One additional difficulty associated with autologous programs is that significant wastage of units occurs. In one author's experience, as many as 50% of autologous units were discarded because the units were not needed at time of surgery.[48] In addition to the possibility that some patients may have an unnecessarily and iatrogenically lowered red cell mass going into surgery, the expense associated with this wastage can be considerable. Opportunities abound for educational exchanges between blood bankers and attending physicians, and could improve ordering practices.

Use of Autologous Units for Other Patients

The wastage of autologous units no doubt piques the interest of hospital administrators, who may wonder why such units could not be used for other patients, that is, "crossed over" into the general inventory. In bygone days this practice was permitted if autologous donors underwent the rigorous screening applied to allogeneic donors. However, higher infectious disease marker rates, and concerns that autologous donors might not offer complete medical and social information, prompted the AABB to prohibit crossover. As mentioned previously, only in "exceptional circumstances" can an autologous unit be used for another patient, but only on a case-by-case basis, only if the infectious disease markers are negative, and only if the medical director approves such an action.[4]

Testing and Labeling Requirements for Predeposit Autologous Units

Predeposit autologous blood means units of whole blood collected from the intended recipient in advance of a planned procedure. Blood products that are for autologous use *only* and are not to be shipped do not require infectious disease testing. In practice, however, most blood centers or collection facilities do infectious disease testing on autologous units. If, as mentioned previously, any test is positive, the unit has a "BIOHAZARD" label attached and both the patient and the patient's physician are notified of the test results. If a donor-recipient is to give more than one unit of blood, infectious disease testing need only be done on the first unit collected in each 30-day period. The expiration dates for autologous blood depends on the type of anticoagulant/preservative/additive solution that is in the collection bag.

Autologous blood products are tested for ABO and Rh types and for unexpected antibodies. Historical records should be checked, as with all blood product recipients. Unlike allogeneic units, however, autologous units do not have a blood type label attached. In the usual place for the blood type, a label is affixed that has the patient's name, identification number (medical record or social security number), date of birth, and a space to hand-write the blood type. Fewer errors are likely to occur because the autologous label is so different from an allogeneic label. Other information, such as product type and collection/production facility, is the same as for other blood product labels.[4,5]

Perioperative Procedures

In addition to predeposit autologous donation, three other techniques involve reuse of the patient's own blood. These are employed in the perioperative period and include perioperative hemodilution, intraoperative blood salvage, and postoperative blood salvage. These procedures are discussed in detail in Chapter 14.

DIRECTED DONATIONS

Directed donation, also known as designated donation or patient-specific donation, has been used in transfusion medicine for more than 30 years. Before the HIV epidemic and concerns about blood safety, directed donor blood was used in a different context and for clinically sound reasons. For example, blood from a kidney donor was sometimes transfused into the kidney recipient before renal transplant. Engraftment appeared to be enhanced, and was attributed to an immunosuppressive effect of the transfusion. A common practice for managing alloimmune platelet refractoriness involved—and still involves—the use of **HLA matched** platelets, which are more likely to be found in close relatives. The use of directed donations in other settings was almost unheard of until the 1980s.

As fears of contracting HIV from blood transfusions grew in the early 1980s, patients and their families began to demand the opportunity to select their own donors, rather than accept a unit from the community supply. The belief was that blood from someone known to the patient was safer than that donated by a stranger, and that patients could make better decisions about whose blood was safer. One study, which was done at five large community blood centers, demonstrated that in the early 1990s approximately 2.5% of whole blood units were from directed donors. By 1998, however, directed donations accounted for only 0.9% of donations at these centers.[49] This decrease in use of directed donor blood may be attributed to an overall awareness

Directed donation: The process by which donors designate specific recipients for their donated blood or blood components.

HLA matched: Refer to Chapter 7 for a discussion of the HLA system and blood banking implications.

of increased blood safety and possibly the fact that many community blood centers recover the costs of providing this customized service by charging donors a fee.

Several large studies have shown that the prevalence rate of infectious disease markers is not necessarily lower in directed donors compared to community donors. The study cited previously[49] showed that HbsAg prevalence was greater in directed versus community donors and that HTLV and HBc rates were equivalent. However, the prevalence rates for HIV and HCV were somewhat lower in directed versus community donors. The finding of lower HIV prevalence rates in directed donors was supported by more recent data.[50] However, these more contemporaneous data also show that the prevalence of HBV is 1.6 times greater in directed than community donors and the HCV prevalence is roughly equal in both groups. A study by the American Red Cross comparing prevalence rates of first-time and repeat donors showed that the prevalence of HIV in first-time donors—a category into which many directed donors fall—was twice that of repeat donors, and the prevalence of HCV was more than twice that for repeat donors.[51] Thus, although directed donor HIV rates are lower in some studies, the equivalent or higher risks of other infections suggest that beliefs about better blood safety in directed versus community donors do not derive from data.

Directed donors, who are homologous donors, must meet allogeneic pre-donation and infectious disease qualifying criteria. The only exceptions are that (1) a donor who is part of a "dedicated donor" program for a specific recipient does not have to undergo infectious disease marker testing if testing was done and found to be negative within the previous 30 days,[2] and (2) the donation intervals may be shortened if the donor is evaluated the day of donation by a medical center physician, is deemed healthy to donate, and meets all other qualifying criteria. Directed donors must also review the pre-donation educational materials and consent to donation. Part of this consent should include an acknowledgment by the donor that his or her blood may be given in an emergency to a different recipient, or that the donor's blood may be transfused to another recipient if it is close to expiration or not needed by the intended patient.

Directed donations from certain individuals do present some interesting immunologic problems. If a man donates blood to his wife or sex partner of child-bearing capability, the woman could develop red cell alloantibodies that may increase the risk of fetal hemolytic disease. This kind of donation should be discouraged, but if the parties insist, they should be fully informed of the potential risks and provide written consent.[52]

Graft-versus-host disease (GVHD): The pathologic condition resulting from an immunologic attack by transplanted donor cells against the tissues of the recipient. Refer to Chapter 15 for a discussion of transfusion-associated graft-versus-host disease (TA-GVHD).

Hematopoietic progenitor cells (HPCs): Cells capable of differentiation into all blood cell lineages.

Another risk associated with directed donation from blood relatives, which fortunately is now easily preventable, is **graft–versus–host disease (GVHD).** This severe and often fatal condition is seen most frequently in recipients of allogeneic **hematopoietic progenitor cell (HPC)** or bone marrow transplant recipients. It is caused by an immunologic assault of healthy donor lymphocytes against the skin, gastrointestinal tract, or liver of the recipient. GVHD is also a risk, albeit rare, of transfusion, especially if the donor is a first-degree relative (sibling, parent, or child).[53,54] Such a scenario can be avoided, however, by irradiating the unit with the dose required by AABB Standards.[4] Irradiation confers protection against GVHD by inactivating donor lymphocytes.

In spite of the fact that directed donations may not represent the risk-free transfusion approach that patients may have hoped for, it does offer some definite advantages. It enables recipients and their families to participate in at least one aspect of the patient's care. Special "dedicated donor" programs in which only a few donors support the patient can limit the patient's exposure to allogeneic blood. Directed donations also can improve hospital inventories and decrease dependence on the community donor base. The authors' medical center, in which almost 50% of plateletpheresis units are from directed donors, has increasingly recognized the value of patient-specific donations, for all these reasons.

APHERESIS

The term **apheresis,** also known as **hemapheresis,** derives from the Greco-Latin word aphairesis, "to take away."[55] In the medical context, it refers to a procedure in which whole blood is taken from an individual, a specific portion or portions shunted into a separate receptacle, and the remainder reinfused to the patient or donor. Fig. 8-10 shows a flowchart of the apheresis process.

The ultimate use or disposal of the collected component depends on the indication for conducting apheresis. Hemapheresis is used for collecting blood components intended for transfusion or further processing, to remove cells or a pathologic plasma substance contributing to a patient disease, or for harvesting autologous or allogeneic progenitor cells (HPC) that will used in bone marrow rescue after intensive cancer treatment. Each of these categories will be discussed.

Apheresis/hemapheresis: The process of removing blood from a donor or patient, processing the blood to separate selected elements, and returning the unharvested portion to the donor or patient. Apheresis can be cytapheresis, in which cellular components are harvested, or plasmapheresis, in which plasma is harvested.

Apheresis for Collecting Blood Components

Technological advances in automated cell separators, also known as apheresis instruments, have ushered in a new era in blood collection: the era of multiple component technology. The integration of sophisticated computer software into cell separators and increased automation has broadened the potential array of blood components that can be simultaneously collected. Apheresis can now be used to safely collect up to three full-dose platelet units, two packed red cell units, three units of plasma (so-called "jumbo" plasma), or any combinations thereof, providing the amount and type of component removed meet FDA and AABB safety and product parameters.[2,4,5] For example, a donor who meets certain hematocrit, platelet count, body weight, and other specific eligibility criteria could, in one donation, give two or three platelet units, a plasma unit, and a red cell unit.

Refer to Chapter 17 for a discussion of therapeutic apheresis.

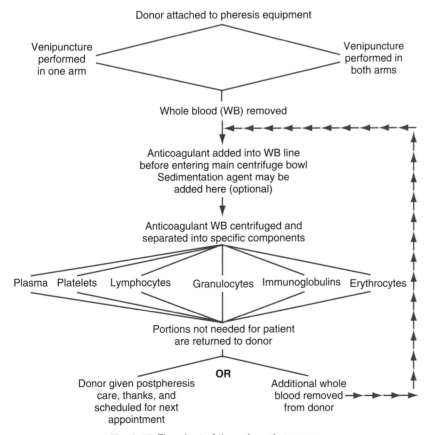

Fig. 8-10 Flowchart of the apheresis process.

In addition to enhancing safety by exposing recipients to fewer allogeneic units, the use of multiple component technology can have a positive impact on component availability, especially during these times of chronic blood shortages. Another benefit is that components are collected in a standardized manner with measurable and consistent product characteristics. Furthermore, using apheresis procedures to collect several components from one donor introduces major efficiencies into the collection process by reducing the costs that would otherwise be incurred by recruiting and testing individual donors of single products.

Many cell separators are highly computerized, employ touch screens for communication between the operator and instrument, have multiple built-in alarm and safety systems, and use preassembled kits that load easily into the machine and can be quickly removed. The instruments record myriad data on each collection, and it is now possible to upload this information into data files or a centralized database.

During the actual apheresis procedure, whole blood is directed into a centrifugation chamber where density gradients separate various portions of the blood, enabling the selective removal of the target component. This component is shunted into its own receptacle, and the remaining portions of the blood returned to the donor or patient, along with a citrate-based anticoagulant (see Fig. 8-10). The blood removal and return cycles involve either continuous or intermittent flow. A typical collection can take anywhere from 30 minutes to 2 hours, depending on the size of the donor and the component types that are programmed into the cell separator.

Complications of Apheresis

Apheresis donors are subject to the same risks that are associated with whole blood donation. Reactions that are unique to apheresis donation include the following:

1. Mechanical hemolysis, exposing the donor to free hemoglobin.
2. Equipment or kit failure resulting in an inability to return blood in the extracorporeal circuit to the donor.
3. Citrate reactions or **citrate toxicity.** Citrate is used as an anticoagulant, and is mixed with the blood being returned to the donor. Because it binds ionized calcium, it can cause symptoms of hypocalcemia. Mild symptoms include perioral paresthesia, or tingling or numbness of the lips. This is easily prevented and treated by educating the donor about citrate-related symptoms and giving the donor oral calcium supplements. If not managed proactively, however, citrate reactions can lead to severe muscle spasms or tetany that could require intravenous calcium administration.

Citrate toxicity: An adverse effect of citrate administration caused by the chelation of calcium and subsequent hypocalcemia.

Plateletpheresis

Probably the most dramatic impact of current apheresis instrumentation is the ability to collect—in one donation event—up to three units of platelets, each of which meets the required $\geq 3 \times 10^{11}$ platelets per unit. (A single apheresis platelet unit is essentially the equivalent of six pooled concentrates.) Most apheresis machines now also perform leukoreduction and, absent procedural complications, the end product has fewer than the 5×10^6 white cells required to meet applicable leukoreduction standards.[4] This almost completely eliminates the need for bedside filtration or filtration by the transfusion service. If the apheresis procedure is hampered by vein performance or technical problems, it may be necessary to perform a white cell count on the product or use a leukoreduction filter in order for the product to meet the leukoreduction specifications. If a transfusion service obtains plateletpheresis units that do not meet leukoreduction standards, the hospital must have some mechanism for performing filtration if ordered by the attending physician.

Donor safety and recipient safety have also been the focus of regulations and standards that govern plateletpheresis. The donor must meet all allogeneic prescreening criteria. The donor should not have taken aspirin or aspirin-containing products within 36 hours of donation, because aspirin and certain other medications can cause irreversible platelet dysfunction.[56]

The donor's preapheresis platelet count must be ≥150,000/μL if apheresis is performed more than once every 4 weeks. If collections are done less frequently, the preapheresis or postapheresis counts from the previous donation may be used as the basis for determining eligibility. If the postprocedure count from the previous donation is less than 150,000/μL, a precount must be done. Individuals who donate platelets may give up to 24 times a year, but not more frequently than once every 2 days in a 7-day period. Plateletpheresis generally lowers the donor's platelet count by 20% to 30%,[57] but the count returns to pre-donation levels within approximately 72 hours of apheresis.

While current apheresis technology offers tremendous promise for improving the blood supply, it has also introduced a new level of regulatory complexity, especially with regard to tracking donor red cell loss. Red cell loss from apheresis donation is usually fairly small. If a platelet donor *only* donates apheresis platelets, the red cell loss—barring unforeseen events—is low enough to allow 24 donations a year. Such information must be recorded and considered in the timing of future platelet donations, but if the donor only donates platelets, this process is fairly straightforward. However, tracking and deferral intervals become much more complicated if an individual also donates whole blood occasionally—or during the platelet collection donates a 200 mL red cell unit.[58-60] If the donor has donated whole blood recently, that donor must be deferred for at least 8 weeks unless the extracorporeal volume of the apheresis instrument is less than 100 mL. If, during plateletpheresis, the donor has also contributed an apheresis red cell unit, that must also be accounted for in the tally. Obviously, this all requires a tracking system, and collections staff must be trained in the use of that system and proactively monitor red cell loss. This information is much easier (and more reliable) to track if computer systems are used. Software specifically designed for this purpose can track apheresis procedure–related red cell loss, upload the information into a central database, and prevent collection from an ineligible donor.

Red Cell Apheresis

Most automated cell separators are now approved by the FDA for collecting two units of red cells. However, depending on the specific system and manufacturer, the qualifying weight and hematocrit usually significantly higher than for whole blood donation. In general, females must weigh at least 130 lb and have a minimum height of 5 feet 1 inch; males should weigh at least 150 lb and measure 5 feet 3 inches. A minimum hematocrit of 40% is required for both genders.[5,58] Intravascular volume is maintained by the simultaneous infusion of intravenous fluids, so that the donor is essentially euvolemic at the conclusion of the collection. However, following a double-unit red cell apheresis, the donor must be deferred for 16 weeks. Red cell loss must be carefully tracked.

The introduction of dual red cell apheresis represents another leap forward in keeping pace with increasing demands on the blood supply. Focused targeting of selected donor populations can significantly improve red cell collections. A preferred donor would be a type O or A male, who donates only occasionally, weighs more than 130 lb, and is willing to spend a few extra minutes in the donation process. Another advantage to automated red cell collection is that the final volume and concentration are standardized and consistent. Finally, as seen in double and triple plateletpheresis collections, the recruitment, screening, and testing costs of producing two apheresis red cell units are half that for two whole blood units.

Granulocytapheresis

Granulocytes are occasionally used to treat sepsis in neonates or adults. Early studies using whole blood, buffy-coat derived granulocytes did not make a convincing case for these products,[61] largely because a therapeutic dose could not be obtained. AABB Standards require that the method used to collect granulocytes for adults must result in a minimum number of 1×10^{10} granulocytes in at least 75% of the apheresis units that are tested.[4] Granulocytapheresis is the best approach for meeting that standard, because it is much more efficient and facilitates the collection of large numbers of cells.

Several factors play a role in the success of granulocyte transfusions in treating sepsis. These factors, based on a meta-analysis of randomized, controlled studies, are the daily dose, which must be at least 1×10^{10} cells, and the absence of recipient alloantibodies to the donor's granulocyte antigens.[62] Even though the dose of 10 billion cells was associated with clinical improvement, daily turnover of granulocytes in an adult is estimated to be 100 billion cells. During serious infections, turnover can be at least 200 billion cells a day.[63] This has led to the practice of improving apheresis yields by administering a sedimenting agent to the donor during collection, or by prestimulating the donor with pharmacologic agents.

The most commonly used sedimenting agent is **hydroxyethyl starch (HES),** a colloid with rouleaux-promoting properties that helps to sediment the red cells.[64] This results in a sharper interface between the white and red cell layers, and allows for better separation of the white cells. However, the body stores HES, sometimes for years, and collection centers should monitor the cumulative dose, the maximum of which must be determined by the medical director.[4] Because HES is a volume expander, its use should be avoided in conditions that could be exacerbated by increased volume; such conditions include but are not limited to hypertension and chronic steroid use. HES can also cause allergic reactions (anaphylaxis) that can be severe and rapid. If signs or symptoms of anaphylaxis occur, the procedure should be terminated and epinephrine administered.

Another approach to increasing a donor's granulocyte count is premedication with steroids such as prednisone or dexamethasone. These medications can usually double the number of circulating granulocytes, but should not be administered to individuals with hypertension, peptic ulcer disease, or diabetes.[5]

Premedication of the donor with growth factors, such as **granulocyte colony stimulating factor (G-CSF),** can mobilize the bone marrow to produce and release dramatic numbers of granulocytes. Studies have shown that, using G-CSF (which is commonly used to mobilize HPCs in allogeneic or autologous stem cell harvests), granulocytapheresis products from a G-CSF–stimulated donor may contain as many as 4.3 to 5.1×10^{10} cells![65,66] However, numerous side effects occur with G-CSF administration, including flulike symptoms, bone pain, and thrombocytopenia. Because G-CSF has not yet been approved by the FDA in this setting, blood centers should consider off-label usage only after getting special FDA approval.

Granulocyte donors must meet all the usual allogeneic criteria. If a donor is going to make serial donations, or donate several times within a short time frame, prudence dictates that the donor's cell counts be closely monitored.

Granulocytes must be transfused within 24 hours, and should not be administered through a microaggregate or leukoreduction filter.

Plasmapheresis

Plasmapheresis is, as the term suggests, the selective removal of plasma from the donor's whole blood during apheresis (only automated methods will be discussed). Plasma may be collected either for transfusion to replace certain clotting factors, or to undergo further manufacturing for pharmaceuticals such as clotting factor concentrates, albumin, immunoglobulins, or vaccines. If the product is intended for transfusion, the donor must meet all allogeneic criteria; usually the plasma is made into fresh frozen or frozen plasma, stored frozen, and thawed before transfusion. If the donor is in a "frequent" plasmapheresis program, that is, donates plasma more than once every 4 weeks, additional medical and laboratory evaluation must take place, including measurement of serum protein levels and serum protein electrophoresis.[2]

Hydroxyethyl starch (HES): A red cell sedimenting agent used in apheresis procedures. HES is also useful as a cryoprotective agent.

Granulocyte colony stimulating factor (G-CSF): Refer to Chapter 19 for a discussion of the use of G-CSF for the mobilization of hematopoietic stem cells.

Therapeutic Apheresis

The term **therapeutic apheresis** is used to describe the removal of pathogenic substances from the circulation, and is usually accomplished with an automated cell separation device. It is intended to ameliorate symptoms of, or, in some instances, treat, a spectrum of diseases. Substances targeted for removal range from large numbers of cells (cytapheresis)—for instance, those seen in blast crisis of acute leukemia—to pathologic antibodies in plasma (plasmapheresis). The concept of removing the "bad" part from blood and replacing it with or leaving only the "good" goes back to fifteenth century and the first recorded transfusion of Pope Innocent VIII. Today's modern medical equipment and apheresis machines simply make the procedure more sophisticated.

As apheresis technologies developed during the late twentieth century, there was great optimism that apheresis could be used to cure a nearly limitless number of diseases. However, in the 1970s and 1980s, its growing popularity, especially for autoimmune diseases, raised concerns about whether it was truly an effective treatment modality for many conditions. Thus, to provide guidance to clinicians, the AABB and other organizations developed usage guidelines based on an exhaustive literature review. The resulting four categories of indications and examples of conditions that fall within specific categories[67,68] are shown in Table 8-4.

The word "plasmapheresis" used in the therapeutic context is somewhat of a misnomer. Although plasma is removed, it must be replaced—but not necessarily with plasma. Usually the replacement fluid is a crystalloid (e.g., saline) or colloid (e.g., albumin), or a combination of these. Only in specific disease entities such as **thrombotic thrombocytopenic purpura (TTP)** should the replacement fluid be plasma. The reasons that plasma replacement should be avoided (unless the patient has TTP) are that a large infusion of plasma increases the chance of exposure to infectious agents and can be associated with severe citrate or allergic reactions. A growing practice for treating TTP involves fluid replacement with plasma from which the cryoprecipitate has been removed, so-called cryosupernatant plasma.[69]

Therapeutic apheresis can have significant complications, not the least of which are those associated with the use of vascular access devices. Citrate, which is given to prevent clotting of the returning blood and replacement fluids, decreases serum calcium levels by binding ionized calcium. Symptoms of citrate toxicity, such as perioral paresthesias or numbness and tingling of the lips, can be mild. However, if not treated (or prevented) by administering oral or intravenous calcium, citrate toxicity can lead to tetany or even cardiac arrhythmias.

In 1983 the estimated fatality rate of therapeutic apheresis was 3 deaths per 10,000 procedures.[70] Although therapeutic apheresis is now much safer due to increased automation, computerization, and lower extracorporeal volumes (especially in continuous flow instruments), close monitoring by physicians and staff is an absolute requirement for identifying and treating adverse effects.

For a more complete discussion of therapeutic apheresis, refer to Chapter 17 in this text.

Apheresis in Hematopoietic Progenitor Cell and Bone Marrow Transplants

Advances in cancer treatment have introduced new roles for apheresis. The major application is in the collection of autologous or allogeneic hematopoietic progenitor cells (HPCs, also loosely called "stem cells") for bone marrow rescue after high-dose chemotherapy. Before apheresis, patients who serve as their own (autologous) donors undergo bone marrow mobilization with growth factors such as G-CSF and/or granulocyte-macrophage colony stimulating factor (GM-CSF). Under the powerful effect of these drugs, the marrow releases millions of HPCs into the bloodstream, from which they are harvested by leukapheresis. The cells are processed to remove excess plasma, cryopreserved, usually with dimethyl sulfoxide

Therapeutic apheresis: Application of apheresis procedures to the treatment of disease. Refer to Chapter 19 for a discussion of therapeutic apheresis.

Thrombotic thrombocytopenic purpura (TTP): A microangiopathic disorder. Refer to Chapter 19 for a discussion of the use of therapeutic apheresis in TTP.

TABLE 8-4 Clinical Indication Categories* for Therapeutic Apheresis and Selected Conditions†

Category I: Evidence supports therapeutic apheresis as standard first choice of therapy or plays a significant adjunctive role in other therapies.

Category II: Efficacy of therapeutic apheresis is generally considered to be appropriate and acceptable.

Category III: Evidence is not adequate to determine efficacy.

Category IV: Available literature shows no support for therapeutic effectiveness.

Condition or Disease	Category	Procedure
Chronic inflammatory demyelinating polyneuropathy	I	Plasmapheresis
Cryoglobulinemia	I	Plasmapheresis
Goodpasture syndrome	I	Plasmapheresis
Guillain-Barré syndrome	I	Plasmapheresis
Hyperviscosity syndrome	I	Plasmapheresis
Leukemia with hyperleukocystosis	I	Leukapheresis
Myasthenia gravis	I	Plasmapheresis
Peripheral HPC for hematopoietic reconstitution	I	Cytapheresis (RBC exchange)
Posttransfusion purpura	I	Plasmapheresis
Symptomatic thrombocytosis	I	Leukapheresis
Thrombotic thrombocytopenic purpura	I	Plasmapheresis
Poisoning or drug overdose	II	Plasmapheresis
Hemolytic uremic syndrome	II	Plasmapheresis
Hyperparasitemia (malaria)	II	Red cell exchange
Rapidly progressive glomerulonephritis	II	Plasmapheresis
Systemic vasculitis (related to rheumatoid arthritis or SLE)	II	Plasmapheresis
ABO-incompatible organ transplant	III	Plasmapheresis
Coagulation factor inhibitors	III	Plasmapheresis
Maternal treatment for HDN	III	Plasmapheresis
Multiple sclerosis	III	Plasmapheresis
AIDS	IV	Plasmapheresis
Amyotrophic lateral sclerosis	IV	Plasmapheresis
Hepatic failure	IV	Plasmapheresis
Lupus nephritis	IV	Plasmapheresis
Psoriasis	IV	Plasmapheresis

*Leitman SF, Ciaverella D, McLeod B, et al: Guidelines for Therapeutic Hemapheresis. AABB Extracorporeal Therapy Committee. 1992, revised 1994, American Association of Blood Banks.
†Brecher ME (ed): Technical Manual, 14th ed. Bethesda, MD, 2002, American Association of Blood Banks.

(DMSO), and stored in a frozen state. After the patient has received intensive cancer therapy—which essentially ablates the bone marrow—the stem cells are thawed and reinfused. Engraftment usually takes place within several weeks. The major clinical indications for stem cell transplants are lymphohematologic malignancies such as lymphomas, leukemia, and multiple myeloma.

Leukapheresis is also performed to collect HPCs from allogeneic donors. The donor, usually a sibling or an HLA-matched, unrelated donor, is prestimulated with growth factors and undergoes apheresis to harvest peripheral blood HPCs. The collection is timed to coincide with the conclusion of the patient's curative chemotherapy, and the HPCs are usually not frozen but infused shortly after collection. Although leukapheresis is the predominant approach to collecting allogeneic HPCs, bone marrow harvests are occasionally done instead. In this situation, apheresis instruments are used to remove red cells from marrow when the donor and patient are an ABO mismatch. This prevents hemolysis of donor red cells by a type O recipient's anti-A, anti-B, or anti-AB.

A third application of apheresis in the hematologic transplant arena is for red cell exchanges, done for ABO minor mismatches. In this situation, the type A, B, or AB recipient undergoes red cell exchange with type O cells. This "converts" the patient to type O, so that as the transplanted HPCs of the type O donor begin producing anti-A, anti-B, or anti-AB, there are so few recipient red cells remaining that hemolysis is avoided.

As HPC transplants have grown increasingly commonplace, so too has the promulgation of standards and regulations. The AABB and Foundation for the Accreditation of Cellular Therapies have both developed standards for HPC therapies.[71,72] These standards establish minimum criteria for most, if not all, activities associated with HPC transplants. The FDA also plans to regulate tissue products, including HPCs.[73] Refer to Chapter 19 of this text for a more complete discussion of HPC collection, processing, storage, and transplantation.

CHAPTER SUMMARY

1. Although blood banks and transfusion services often perform many of the same services, a general definition of each organization shows their differences. A blood bank handles donor recruitment, screening, phlebotomy, serologic testing, preparation of components, and storage and distribution of blood and its products. A hospital transfusion service provides direct transfusion medicine services to the patient.

2. Regulatory oversight of blood centers and transfusion services is done to protect donors and patients. Compliance with regulations is mandatory. Membership in most accrediting agencies is voluntary, but member organizations must comply with all applicable standards. The FDA regulates blood centers with the Code of Federal Regulations, memoranda, guidance documents, and through unannounced inspections, usually on an annual basis. The American Association of Blood Banks provides voluntary inspection and accreditation with biannual inspections, using their Standards for Blood Banks and Transfusion Services as guidelines.

3. Blood donors are not paid for their donations. They donate primarily for altruistic reasons but occasionally for the opportunity to receive basic health screening. A small but significant number of donors apparently donate to receive free HIV testing. Only 3% to 5% of healthy, eligible persons donate in the United States each year.

4. Donor screening before donation has two purposes: to protect the donor and the recipient. The outcome of donor screening is acceptance of the donor, temporary deferral, or permanent deferral.

5. The screening process includes a limited physical evaluation. The donor may be offered the opportunity to confidentially indicate that his or her blood should not be used for transfusion. Potential donors must pass all parts of the screening process before actual phlebotomy takes place.

6. The risks of donation must be explained, and the donor must give written consent.

7. Numerous tests are performed on each donation, regardless of whether the donor is a first-time or a repeat donor. These tests are ABO group, Rh type, antibody screening, HBs antigen, HB core antibody, HCV antibody, HTLV-I/II antibody, HIV-1/2 antibody, syphilis antibodies, WNV, HIV/HCV, and NAT testing. All tests must be negative or as expected before the product is released for transfusion.

8. In addition to the 12 tests always performed on a donor's sample, several other tests are often performed to provide specific blood for selected patients. These can include CMV testing, testing for sickle cell trait, and selected antigen typing.

9. The FDA and the AABB specify specific labeling protocols for blood products. These include proper name of the product; ABO and Rh type (where needed for product); name and address of the facility that collected the blood and/or made the component; the unique number assigned to the donor and the blood product; the expiration date of the product; instructions to the transfusionist; recommended storage temperature; approximate amount of product in the container; the anticoagulant/preservative/additive solution used; and appropriate classification of the donor as volunteer, paid, or autologous.

10. Records of all phases of the donor interview, serologic testing, products made, and final disposition must be stored and available according to the regulations of the FDA, the AABB, and state and local laws. Most facilities retain these records indefinitely.

11. Specialized collections include autologous and directed donations as well as apheresis for collecting blood components, performing therapeutic hemapheresis, and collecting or processing hematopoietic progenitor cells. Apheresis is the process of removing whole blood

from a donor or patient, separating out a specific desired component, and returning the remainder to the donor or patient.

12. An autologous donation is one in which the intended recipient donates his or her own blood or component for future intended transfusion. There are four types of autologous transfusion: preoperative or predeposit, perioperative hemodilution, intraoperative salvage, and postoperative salvage.

13. Patient-directed units are donated for a specific recipient. Infectious disease marker prevalence data show that these units are not necessarily safer than those donated by community donors. However, a directed donor program can serve as a source of whole blood or apheresis components, and decrease reliance on community blood centers. Directed donations from first-degree blood relatives should be irradiated before transfusion to prevent graft-versus-host disease in the recipient.

REFERENCES

1. Shoos-Lipton K: American Association of Blood Banks. National Blood Data Resources Center Survey. Bethesda, MD, American Association of Blood Banks, 2001.

2. Code of Federal Regulations, Title 21. Parts 200-299 and 600-799. Washington, DC, Department of Health and Human Services, Food and Drug Administration, US Government Printing Office, 2003.

3. Biological Product Deviation Reporting for Blood and Plasma Establishments. Food and Drug Administration, Guidance for Industry, August 2001.

4. Fridey JL (ed): Standards for Blood Banks and Transfusion Services, 22nd ed. Bethesda, MD, American Association of Blood Banks, 2003.

5. Brecher ME (ed): Technical Manual, 14th ed. Bethesda, MD, American Association of Blood Banks, 2002.

6. Circular of Information for the Use of Human Blood and Components. Bethesda, MD, American Association of Blood Banks, America's Blood Centers, American Red Cross, 2002.

7. College of American Pathologists Laboratory Accreditation Program. Transfusion Medicine Checklist. December 2003.

8. Comprehensive Accreditation Manual for Hospitals: The Official Handbook. Oakbrook Terrace, IL, Joint Commission on Accreditation of Healthcare Organizations, 2004.

9. NCCLS Clinical Laboratory Technical Procedure Manuals; Approved Guideline, 4th ed. GP2-A4. 22(5), April 2002.

10. Wash JH, Purcell RH, Morrow AG, et al: Post-transfusion hepatitis after open heart operations: Incidence after administration of blood from commercial and volunteer donor populations. JAMA 211:261-265, 1970.

11. Goldfield M, Bill J, Black H, et al: The consequences of administering blood pretested for HbsAg by third generation techniques: A progress report. Am J Med Sci 270:335-342, 1975.

12. Damesyn MA, Glynn SA, Schreiber GB, et al: Behavioral and infectious disease risks in young blood donors: Implications for recruitment. Transfusion 43:1596-1603, 2003.

13. Compliance Policy Guidance for FDA Staff and Industry. Blood Donor Classification Statement, Paid or Volunteer Donor. Chapter 2, Subchapter 230, Section 150. May 7, 2002.

14. Standards for Blood Banks and Transfusion Services, 11th ed. Arlington, American Association of Blood Banks, 1984.

15. Recommendations for the Prevention of HIV Transmission by Blood and Blood Products. FDA Memorandum. February 5, 1990.

16. Final Report of the Task Force to Redesign the Blood Donor Screening Questionnaire. American Association of Blood Banks, March 2002.

17. Revised Recommendations for the Prevention of HIV Transmission by Blood and Blood Products. FDA Memorandum. April 23, 1992.

18. Zuck TF, Cumming PD, Wallace E: Computer-assisted audiovisual health history self-interviewing: Results of the pilot study of the Hoxworth Quality Donor System. Transfusion 41:1469-1474, 2001.

19. Donor-ID Screening System: www.Healthcare-ID.com

20. Uniform Donor History Questionnaire. Association Bulletin #95-5. American Association of Blood Banks, 1995.

21. Uniform Donor History Questionnaire. Association Bulletin #99-10. American Association of Blood Banks, 1999.

22. Fridey JL (chair): AABB Task Force to Redesign the Uniform Donor History Questionnaire. Unpublished data. 2001.

23. Revised Recommendations for the Assessment of Donor Suitability and Blood Product Safety in Cases of Suspected Severe Acute Respiratory Syndrome (SARS) or Exposure to SARS. FDA Guidance for Industry. September 2003.

24. Recommendations for Deferral of Donors and Quarantine and Retrieval of Blood and Blood Products in Recent Recipients of Smallpox Vaccine (Vaccinia Virus) and Certain Contacts of Smallpox Vaccine Recipients. FDA Guidance for Industry. December 2002.

25. Revised Recommendation for the Assessment of Donor Suitability and Blood and Blood Product Safety in Cases of Known or Suspected West Nile Virus Infection. FDA Guidance for Industry. May 2003.

26. Deferral for Risk of Leishmaniasis Exposure. Association Bulletin #03-14. American Association of Blood Banks, 2003.

27. Silvergleid AJ, Pike SL: Confidential unit exclusion: One blood center's experience. Transfusion 39(Suppl):S111-P:28S, 1999.

28. Further Guidance on Methods to Detect Bacterial Contamination of Platelet Components. Association Bulletin #03-12. American Association of Blood Banks, October 2003.

29. Ali AM, McCandy AT, Ali MAM, et al: An approach to determine objectively minimum hemoglobin standards for blood donors. Transfusion 25:286, 1985.

30. Code of Federal Regulations, Title 21. Parts 640.1 and 640.10. Washington, DC, Department of Health and Human Services, Food and Drug Administration, US Government Printing Office, 2003.

31. Newman BH, Pichette S, Pichette D, Dzaka E: Adverse effects in blood donors after whole blood donation: A study of 1000 blood donors interviewed 3 weeks after whole blood donation. Transfusion 43:598-603, 2003.

32. Newman BH: Donor reactions and injuries from whole blood donation. Transfusion Medicine Reviews 11:64-75, 1997.

33. Newman BH: Arterial puncture phlebotomy in whole blood donors. Transfusion 11:1390, 2001.
34. Newman BH, Waxman DA: Blood donation-related neurologic needle injury: Evaluation of 2 years' worth of data from a large blood center. Transfusion 36:213-215, 1996.
35. Horowitz SH: Venipuncture-induced causalgia: Anatomic relations of upper extremity superficial veins and nerves and clinical considerations. Transfusion 40:1036-1040, 2000.
36. Horowitz SH: Peripheral nerve injury and causalgia secondary to routine venipuncture. Neurology 44:962-964, 1994.
37. Epstein J: FDA Blood Products Advisory Committee Meeting. December 2003.
38. Code of Federal Regulations, Title 21. Part 610.4(b). Washington, DC, Department of Health and Human Services, Food and Drug Administration, US Government Printing Office, 2003.
39. Further Guidance in Methods to Detect Bacterial Contamination of Platelet Components. AABB Association Bulletin #03-12, October 1, 2003.
40. Epstein J: Food and Drug Administration, Center for Biologics and Evaluation. CDC Donor Suitability Workshop, Atlanta, 2000.
41. Llewelyn CA, Hewitt PE, Knight RSG, et al: Possible transmission of variant Creutzfeldt-Jakob disease by blood transfusion. Lancet 363(9407):417-421, 2004.
42. Houston F, Foster JD, Chong A, et al: Transmission of BSE by blood transfusion in sheep. J Gen Virol 83:2897-2905, 2002.
43. Toy P, Ahn D, Bacchetti P: When should the first of two autologous donations be made? (abstract) Transfusion 34(Suppl):14S, 1994.
44. Stenhouse MAE, Milner LV: *Yersinia enterocolitica*: A hazard in blood transfusion. Transfusion 22:396, 1982.
45. Sazama K: Bacteria in blood for transfusion: A review. Arch Pathol Lab Med 118:350-365, 1994.
46. Klein HG, Dodd RY, Ness PM, et al: Current status of microbial contamination of blood components: Summary of a conference. Transfusion 37:95-101, 1997.
47. Yomtovian R, Palavecino E: Bacterial contamination of blood products—history and epidemiology. In Brecher M (ed): Bacterial Contamination of Blood Products—History and Epidemiology. Bethesda, MD, American Association of Blood Banks, 2003.
48. Traubert J, Fridey JL: Blood Bank of San Bernardino and Riverside Counties. Unpublished data. 2000.
49. Willams AE, Wu Y, Kleinman SH, et al: The declining use and comparative seroprevalence of directed whole blood donations. S12-030B. AABB 53rd Annual Meeting, November 2000.
50. Schreiber GB: Westat, Inc, and the National Heart, Lung, and Blood Institute Retrovirus Epidemiologic Donor Study. Personal communication, 2002.
51. Dodd RY, Notari EP, Stramer S: Current prevalence and incidence of infectious disease markers and estimated window-period risk in the American Red Cross Donor population. Transfusion 42:975-979, 2002.
52. Kanter MH, Hodge SE: Risk of hemolytic disease of the newborn as a result of directed donations from relatives. Transfusion 29:620, 1989.
53. McMilin KD, Johnson RL: HLA homozygosity and the risk of related-donor transfusion-associated graft-vs-host disease. Transfus Med Rev 7(1):37-41, 1997.
54. Thaler M, Shamiss A, Orgard S, et al: The role of blood from HLA-homozygous donors in fatal transfusion-associated graft-versus-host reaction after open heart surgery. N Engl J Med 321:25-28, 1989.
55. Soukhanov AH (ed): American Heritage Dictionary of the English Language, 3rd ed. Boston, Houghlin Mifflin, 1992.
56. Burch JW, Stanford N, Majerus PW: Inhibition of platelet prostaglandin synthesis in oral aspirin. J Clin Invest 61:314, 1978.
57. Strauss RG, Huestis DW, Wright DG, et al: Cellular depletion by apheresis. J Clin Apheresis 1:158, 1983.
58. Recommendations for Collecting Red Cells by Automated Apheresis Methods. FDA Guidance for Industry. February 13, 2001.
59. Revised Guidelines for the Collection of Platelets Pheresis. FDA Memorandum. October 7, 1988.
60. Donor Deferral Due to Red Cell Loss During Collection of Source Plasma by Automated Plasmapheresis. FDA Memorandum. December 4, 1995.
61. Anderson KC, Ness PM: Scientific Basis of Transfusion Medicine. Philadelphia, WB Saunders, 1994.
62. Vamvakas EC, Pineda AA: Meta-analysis of clinical studies in the efficacy of granulocyte transfusions in the treatment of bacterial sepsis. J Clin Apheresis 11:1-9, 1996.
63. Leitman S: Cytokine Mobilization in Granulocytapheresis Donors: Literature Review. AABB Annual Meeting Compendium, 1997.
64. Mishler JM, Haddock DC, Fortuny IE, et al: Increased efficiency of leukocyte collection by the addition of hyroxyethyl starch to the continuous flow centrifuge. Blood 44:571, 1974.
65. Caspar CB, Seger RA, Burder J, Gmur J: Effective stimulation of donors for granulocyte transfusions with recombinant methionyl granulocyte colony stimulating factor. Blood 81:2866-2871, 1993.
66. Leitman SF, Obitas JM: Optimization of granulocytapheresis mobilization regimens using granulocyte colony stimulating factor and dexamethasone. Blood 88:331a, 1996.
67. Leitman S: Guidelines for Therapeutic Hemapheresis. Bethesda, MD, American Association of Blood Banks, 1992.
68. Owen HG, Brecher ME: Management of the therapeutic apheresis patient. In McLeod BC, Price TH, Drew MJ (eds): Apheresis: Principles and Practice. Bethesda, MD, American Association of Blood Banks, 1997.
69. Owens MR, Sweeney JD, Tahhan RH, et al: Influence of type of exchange fluid on survival in therapeutic apheresis for thrombotic thrombocytopenic purpura. J Clin Apheresis 10:178-182, 1995.
70. Huestis DW: Mortality in therapeutic hemapheresis (letter). Lancet 1:1043, 1983.
71. Standards for Hematopoietic Progenitor Cell and Cellular Product Services, 3rd ed. Bethesda, MD, American Association of Blood Banks, 2002.
72. Standards for Hematopoietic Progenitor Cell Collection, Processing, and Transplantation. Omaha, Foundation for the Accreditation of Cellular Therapy, 2002.
73. Current good tissue practice for manufacturers of human cellular and tissue-based products; inspection and reinforcement. Federal Register 66(50), 2001.

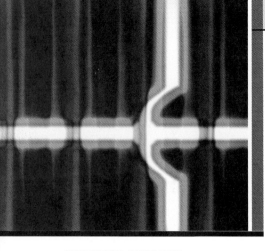

Component Preparation

Dorothy A. Bergeron[*]

LEARNING OBJECTIVES

After reading and studying this chapter, the student should be able to:

1. Describe the benefits of component therapy compared with whole blood administration.

2. Briefly describe the features of a standard triple-pack bag used for blood collection and discuss why these features are important in blood collection, component preparation, storage, testing, and infusion.

3. Describe how sterile connection devices are used in blood component preparation.

4. State the effect of nonsterile entry on the shelf life of blood components stored at 20° to 24° C and at 1° to 6° C.

5. Describe how the theory of differential centrifugation is applied to the preparation of blood components.

6. List four criteria used when calibrating centrifuges for the preparation of blood components.

7. For each of the following blood components, briefly describe the proper name, method(s) of preparation, storage characteristics, shelf life, labeling requirements, composition, approximate volume, quality control standards, and special considerations, if any:

   Whole Blood
   Red Blood Cells
   Red Blood Cells Leukocytes Reduced
   Red Blood Cells Frozen and Red Blood Cells Deglycerolized
   Red Blood Cells Rejuvenated
   Platelets

   Fresh Frozen Plasma and thawed plasma
   Liquid Plasma
   Cryoprecipitated AHF
   Granulocytes
   Platelet Pheresis

8. Describe how fibrin glue is used.

9. List the anticoagulant or anticoagulant/preservative solutions presented in this chapter and include the abbreviation and the shelf life of blood collected in each product.

10. Briefly describe the AABB criteria for determining shelf life for red cell component storage.

11. Discuss the criteria regarding the use of fresh whole blood and describe which clinical situations warrant the use of this product.

12. Discuss record-keeping standards for blood banks and transfusion services.

13. Briefly describe each of the following blood products:

    Normal serum albumin
    Plasma protein fraction
    Factor VIII concentrate
    Factor IX concentrate
    Synthetic volume expanders

14. Briefly describe two types of compounds that are being researched as substitutes for red cell transfusion.

OVERVIEW

Today's physicians ordering transfusion therapy for their patients can select from a wide variety of **components.** The ability to provide transfusion products for each patient's specific needs greatly improves treatment outcomes while it maximizes donor resources. For a transfusion of red cell products alone, the physician may choose from an number of specialized products, including Whole Blood, Red Blood Cells, Red Blood Cells Deglycerolzed, Red Blood Cells Washed, Red Blood Cells Rejuvenated, Red Blood Cells Irradiated, and Red Blood Cells Leukocytes Reduced.

With the exception of the specialized apheresis donation process, a blood donor donates the product known as Whole Blood, from which component preparation begins. The ability to separate various components from Whole Blood is desirable for the following three reasons:

1. Separation of blood into its constituent parts allows for optimal survival of each of those parts. Whole Blood storage conditions are not optimal for all functional components of blood. For example, after 24 hours of storage at 1° to 6° C, Whole Blood has few viable platelets and granulocytes.[1] Stable coagulation factors are well maintained during storage, but heat-labile Factors V and VIII decrease with time and may not be adequate to correct specific deficiencies in patients. The separation of blood into the various components allows storage of each component at the temperature and storage conditions required for maximum in vitro survival.

2. Component preparation allows transfusion of only that specific portion of the blood product that the patient requires. For example, a leukemia patient who requires platelet transfusion to control potential bleeding may not need concomitant red cell transfusion.

3. Transfusing only the specific portion needed avoids the use of unnecessary transfusion, which could be contraindicated in a patient. For example, because of the risk of **hypervolemia,** an elderly anemic patient in congestive heart failure may not easily tolerate the transfusion of 2 units of Whole Blood with its 250 mL of plasma plus red blood cells. The same patient would be better served by transfusion of 2 units of Red Blood Cells with the plasma removed from each unit.

It is important to recognize that when blood is separated into specific components, those components may carry with them the same potential for disease transmission and adverse transfusion reactions as the original unit of whole blood. For example, a unit of Whole Blood that tests positive for hepatitis B surface antigen can pass hepatitis B to recipients of any products made from that unit. To reduce the risk of transfusion-transmitted infection, no blood or components are released for transfusion until all testing is completed and the unit is cleared for safe transfusion. If any of the tests discussed in Chapter 8 are repeatedly positive or have unexpected test results, appropriate products from that donation are quarantined and destroyed.

Component: A product made from the source product, whole blood. Components are broken into two general classes: cellular products and plasma products.

Hypervolemia: Increased blood volume.

*The author would like to recognize the contributions of Judith A. Young to this chapter in the previous edition.

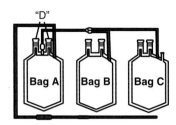

Fig. 9-1 Standard triple-pack collection bag. Bag A is the primary collection bag. Bags B and C are used to hold plasma and platelet products. "D" is the portal that is used to enter the bags either for transfusion of the product or for further processing.

PRINCIPLES OF COMPONENT PREPARATION

Component preparation programs must incorporate the principles of aseptic techniques using sterile, pyrogen-free equipment and solutions.[2] Blood bags used for phlebotomy have integral, sterile extra bags known as **satellite bags** attached to the main collection bag. After 450 ± 45 mL (or 500 ± 50 mL) of donor's blood is collected into the primary phlebotomy bag, which contains the appropriate anticoagulant/preservative, selected components can be transferred into the satellite bags through a closed system of tubing. The original phlebotomy bag may have one, two, or three satellite bags attached. Selection of the bag into which to draw the donor blood is based on anticipated component needs and current inventory. Fig. 9-1 shows a diagram of a standard triple-pack collection bag that allows Red Blood Cells, Platelets, and a plasma product to be made from a single donation in a closed, sterile system.

At times it is desirable to make components or smaller aliquots of a primary bag that has no satellite bags. For example, a request might be made to prepare a 50 mL aliquot of Red Blood Cells for transfusion to a neonatal patient from a unit of Red Blood Cells. If no satellite bags are attached to the red cell unit, it is possible to connect additional satellite bags using one of two methods. One of these methods requires opening the system, and the other maintains the closed sterility of the system. The open system entry involves using one of the portals on the top of the primary bag as the point at which an extra satellite bag is attached. Because this involves possible contamination of components, these products have a significantly shorter shelf life. The second closed separation method allows for the attachment of an additional bag or bags to the original product bag by means of a device known as a **sterile connection device** (or **sterile docking device**). This device allows the tubing from two separate bags to be welded together without losing the sterility of either. Tubing from transfer bags, needles, filters, and collection or pheresis sets may be welded together as long as the diameter and materials of the tubing to be connected are similar. Because each part connected/welded together maintains its internal sterility during this process, the original outdate of each product or bag is maintained. The facility using the device must follow the manufacturer's procedure and maintain the equipment as required. Any variation from the procedure could result in nonsterile connections.

In the preparation of all components, if the sterility of the preparation is compromised or in question, the outdate of the products involved must be changed to a shorter date, depending on the product involved. In general, if a component is stored at 1° to 6° C, the outdate is 24 hours.[2] A break in the seal of a product stored at 20° to 24° C requires that the product be used within 4 hours of the breach.[2]

Differential Centrifugation and Component Preparation

Component preparation and separation are based on the principle that different components of whole blood have different specific gravities. For example, red blood cells represent the heaviest portion of whole blood, with a specific gravity of 1.08 to 1.09, whereas platelets range between 1.03 and 1.04. Using **differential**

Satellite bags: Additional bags attached to the main donor set by sterile tubing. These satellite bags are used for the removal of various blood components, avoiding nonsterile entry of the system.

Sterile connection (docking) device: Instruments capable of heat-welding plastic tubing in a sterile manner, often used when blood components are needed and satellite bags are not available.

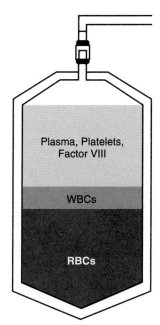

Fig. 9-2 Separation of various components in a unit of whole blood after settling/centrifugation.

centrifugation to spin the donated unit, the components separate into layers in the blood bag, with the heaviest component settling to the bottom. Fig. 9-2 is a diagram of the way individual components separate out in the primary bag after centrifugation. Centrifuges used for this separation are calibrated to deliver the highest product yield in the shortest time at the lowest possible spin. The procedure is designed to cause the least amount of trauma to each product. Fig. 9-3 presents a flowchart of the process. In a unit of whole blood, the centrifuged products settle out in the following layers, starting from the bottom of the bag: red blood cells, white blood cells, and platelet-rich plasma (PRP) (see Step 2, Fig. 9-3). After separating the red blood cells from the PRP, the plasma is centrifuged again for a longer time and at a harder spin, known as a heavy spin. This time the platelets are the heaviest product and they settle to the bottom of the bag (Step 4, Fig. 9-3). The plasma is drawn off into the sterile connected satellite bag with platelets remaining in the first bag (Step 5, Fig. 9-3). Both products are then properly labeled and stored under appropriate conditions until completion of testing and final distribution.

As discussed earlier, it is possible to make some components without either satellite bags or the sterile tubing welder. In this method, the entry portal shown in Fig. 9-1 is opened and a satellite bag added at that portal. Components prepared in this manner are said to be prepared in an "open" system and carry an increased risk of bacterial contamination. Because the seal has been broken, the expiration dates are shortened. As mentioned previously, components stored at 1° to 6° C have a shelf life of no more than 24 hours from the time the system was first opened. The shelf life for components stored at 20° to 24° C is shortened to 4 hours.[2] Products such as washed red blood cells or frozen-deglycerolized red blood cells are examples of products often prepared in an open system.

RED BLOOD CELL COMPONENTS
Whole Blood

Depending on the collection system, a unit of **whole blood** contains 450 ± 45 mL or 500 ± 50 mL of blood plus an **anticoagulant/preservative** solution.[3] The name of the anticoagulant/preservative used during collection is included in the

Differential centrifugation: The separation of components of differing densities by centrifugation. This technique is used for most blood component preparation.

Whole blood: The source product for all blood component production, which consists of red blood cells, white cells, platelets, and plasma collected into an approved anticoagulant/preservative solution.

Anticoagulant/preservative: A solution designed to preserve the viability and function of the collected blood (preservative) and prevent clotting (anticoagulant). Such solutions provide buffering capability and nutrients for cellular metabolism during storage.

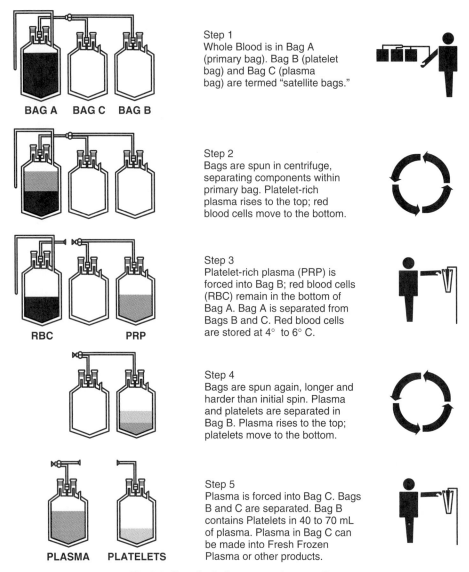

Step 1
Whole Blood is in Bag A (primary bag). Bag B (platelet bag) and Bag C (plasma bag) are termed "satellite bags."

BAG A   BAG C   BAG B

Step 2
Bags are spun in centrifuge, separating components within primary bag. Platelet-rich plasma rises to the top; red blood cells move to the bottom.

Step 3
Platelet-rich plasma (PRP) is forced into Bag B; red blood cells (RBC) remain in the bottom of Bag A. Bag A is separated from Bags B and C. Red blood cells are stored at 4° to 6° C.

RBC   PRP

Step 4
Bags are spun again, longer and harder than initial spin. Plasma and platelets are separated in Bag B. Plasma rises to the top; platelets move to the bottom.

Step 5
Plasma is forced into Bag C. Bags B and C are separated. Bag B contains Platelets in 40 to 70 mL of plasma. Plasma in Bag C can be made into Fresh Frozen Plasma or other products.

PLASMA   PLATELETS

Fig. 9-3 Flowchart of component preparation.

oxygen-carrying capacity: The relative ability of red blood cells to combine with oxygen and release the bound oxygen to tissues.

hypovolemia: Decreased blood volume.

The reader can refer to Chapter 17 for an additional discussion of the use of whole blood versus red blood cells and fresh blood versus stored blood in various clinical settings.

proper name of the product, such as CPDA-1 (citrate-phosphate-dextrose-adenine-1) Whole Blood. The Food and Drug Administration (FDA) must license all anticoagulant/preservative solutions. Table 9-1 provides a list of the currently approved solutions.

Storage temperature must be between 1° and 6° C for the shelf life of whole blood. The determination of the shelf life or expiration date of a whole blood and/or red cell unit is based on the criterion that at least 75% of transfused red blood cells be found in the recipient's circulation 24 hours after transfusion of the product.[1] The shelf life varies with the anticoagulant/preservative used during collection of the blood. Expiration dates are listed in Table 9-1.

Whole Blood has a hematocrit of 30% to 40% and is indicated primarily for those patients who have a symptomatic decrease in **oxygen-carrying capacity** combined with **hypovolemia** of sufficient degree to be associated with shock. In today's transfusion practice, with its emphasis on component therapy, Whole Blood is generally not available. Patients who might have received Whole Blood in the past are now treated with individual components coupled with asanguineous solutions, as needed. The major use of Whole Blood is for autologous transfusion.[1]

TABLE 9-1 Blood Anticoagulant Preservative Solutions Licenses by the FDA

Anticoagulant/Preservative	Abbreviation	Expiration
Acid-citrate-dextrose	ACD	21 days
Citrate phosphate dextrose	CPD	21 days
Citrate phosphate double dextrose	CP2D	21 days
Citrate phosphate dextrose adenine	CPDA-1	35 days
CPD plus additive solution (Fenwal)	AS-1	42 days
CPD plus additive solution (Cutter)	AS-3	42 days
CPD plus additive solution (Terumo)	AS-5	42 days

Fresh Blood

Special requests for fresh Whole Blood may be received on occasion for selected patients such as the neonatal patient. Although justification for **fresh blood** is often difficult, it may be ordered in a belief that fresh blood provides the greatest oxygen-carrying capacity because it has the maximum level of 2,3-diphosphoglycerate (2,3-DPG) and minimal amounts of metabolic waste products such as potassium when compared with older blood. The 2,3-DPG levels are not considered a problem in routine transfusion because the 2,3-DPG levels return to normal within 12 to 24 hours after transfusion.[4] Concerns about 2,3-DPG and potassium levels may be important in the premature neonate and in other patients with impaired cardiac function, hemorrhagic shock, or severe pulmonary disease.[5]

Newborns may be candidates for fresh blood. Newborns have a high percentage of fetal hemoglobin, which does not release oxygen to the tissues as well as adult hemoglobin. Their 2,3-DPG levels may be severely decreased in certain conditions such as respiratory distress syndrome. In addition, the transfused blood represents a large portion of their total blood volume. In these cases, fresh blood, less than 7 days old, with higher levels of 2,3-DPG could be of clinical value in the seriously ill infant.[6] Using the same rationale, an **exchange transfusion** is another procedure in which it is appropriate to use blood less than 7 days old.

Concerns about elevated potassium and hyperkalemia caused by potassium in stored blood are rarely justified.[7] Possible exceptions are patients who are persistently hypotensive, poorly perfused, and acidotic and who require large amounts of blood.[5]

The definitions of fresh blood may vary. In today's blood banks, which perform extensive testing on products before issuing them to ensure blood safety, it is difficult to provide blood available for transfusion earlier than 72 hours after phlebotomy. Blood that falls into the range of 3 to 7 days after phlebotomy is more practical and is readily available for the few special patients who require this product.

Red Blood Cells

Red Blood Cells are prepared by removing most of the plasma from a unit of Whole Blood. Because red blood cells have a higher specific gravity than plasma, the red blood cells move to the lower portion of the collection bag by either gravitational settling or centrifugation. The plasma portion is then removed from the top of the bag into a satellite bag. This plasma portion may be used for further component separation. The separation of plasma from Whole Blood may occur any time during the shelf life of the original unit.[3]

The proper name for the Red Blood Cells includes the anticoagulant/preservative used in the primary bag. For blood donated into a bag containing CPDA-1, the red cell product made is labeled as CPDA-1 Red Blood Cells. All anticoagulant/preservative solutions discussed under Whole Blood are approved for Red Blood Cells. Red Blood Cells should have a final hematocrit that does not exceed 80% and must be stored at 1° to 6° C.[2]

Fresh blood: Whole blood or red blood cells selected for transfusion early (generally less than 7 days) within the storage period in order to minimize the infusion of cellular breakdown products and metabolic waste and to optimize levels of red cell 2,3-DPG and ATP.

Refer to Chapter 17 for an additional discussion of the use of fresh blood in neonatal and massive transfusion.

Exchange transfusion: The repeated withdrawal and transfusion of small amounts of blood.

The reader can refer to Chapter 17 for an additional discussion of transfusion in neonatal and pediatric patients. Chapter 16 provides a more in-depth treatment of transfusion in hemolytic disease of the fetus and newborn.

Red Blood Cells: The blood component prepared by removing most of the residual plasma (200 to 250 mL) from a unit of centrifuged or sedimented whole blood. Red Blood Cells have the same red cell volume and therefore the same oxygen-carrying capacity as Whole Blood but in a significantly reduced volume.

Symptomatic anemia: A decrease in the number of circulating red blood cells, the amount of hemoglobin, or the volume of packed red blood cells per volume of blood. When anemia is severe enough, a patient has some or all of the following symptoms: pallor, weakness, vertigo, headache, sore tongue, drowsiness, malaise, dyspnea, tachycardia, palpitation, angina pectoris, gastrointestinal disturbances, amenorrhea, and slight fever.

If the plasma is removed from the Whole Blood by means of an attached satellite bag or a sterile connection device, the Red Blood Cells have the same shelf life as the original Whole Blood product. However, if the primary collection bag had to be entered and the sterility of the unit was compromised, the shelf life of the Red Blood Cells is 24 hours from the time the primary collection bag was entered.[2]

Red Blood Cells are the preferred product for patients with **symptomatic anemia** because they provide the needed oxygen-carrying capacity without unnecessary volume. Red Blood Cells may also be used for newborn exchange transfusions. (Refer to the discussion of fresh blood.)

Fig. 9-4 shows the standard common label used for Red Blood Cells drawn in CPDA-1 with an explanation of the bar codes found on the label.

Additive Solutions

The shelf life of a unit of Red Blood Cells can be increased to 42 days by using additive solutions. An additive solution (AS) contains dextrose, adenine, sodium chloride, and either monobasic sodium phosphate (AS-3) or mannitol (AS-1 and AS-5). AS-3 also contains sodium citrate and citric acid.[1]

The collection system for additive red blood cells consists of the primary collection and two satellite bags. One of the satellite bags is empty and the other contains the additive solution. To prepare the component, as much plasma as possible is removed from the Whole Blood unit. The plasma is expressed into the empty satellite bag. Once the plasma is removed, the AS is added to the Red Blood Cells.[1] Approximately 100 to 110 mL of AS is added to the red blood cells, with a resultant hematocrit between 55% and 65%.[3]

Red Blood Cells Washed

Red Blood Cells Washed: Red blood cells that have been subjected to serial washing and centrifugation processes in order to remove platelets, plasma, and most of the white blood cells.

Washing Red Blood Cells removes almost all of the plasma, leukocytes, and platelets from the original unit. **Red Blood Cells Washed** can be prepared by using an automated cell washer or by centrifugation. Red blood cells from any in-date unit are mixed with large volumes of physiologic saline. The red cell–saline

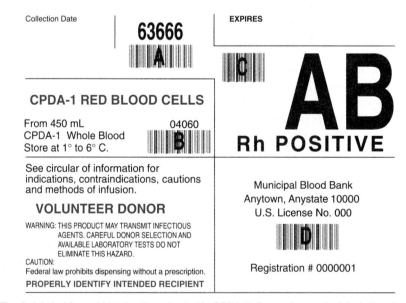

Fig. 9-4 Label for red blood cells collected in CPDA-1. Bar codes on the label allow for accurate computer reading of critical information on the product, confirming the visual inspection of this information. Bar-coded information can include **(A)** unique unit number, **(B)** specific product name, **(C)** ABO/Rh of product, **(D)** facility collecting product. Some facilities use bar codes to check the expiration date and the donor designation (e.g., volunteer, autologous).

mixture is then centrifuged and the supernatant is removed. The procedure removes about 99% of the plasma proteins and up to 20% of the red blood cell mass. Depending on the methodology, washing also removes between 70% and 95% of the leukocytes. Following completion of the washing process, the red blood cells are suspended in 0.85% normal saline. Because the original collection bag must be opened to facilitate the washing process, a washed red blood cell product has a shelf life of 24 hours from the time of entry.[1,2]

The utilization of Red Blood Cells Washed is of particular value in reducing the incidence of **febrile** and **urticarial** reactions in some patients.[8] Red Blood Cells Washed are of special value in patients who have developed antibodies to plasma proteins.[1] The procedure is not recommended for leukocyte reduction when prevention of alloimmunization is desired.[1]

One type of patient who is an excellent candidate for transfusion with Red Blood Cell Washed is the IgA-deficient patient. Although IgA deficiency occurs in approximately 1 in 700 persons,[9] not every IgA-deficient person develops anti-IgA. The patient most at risk for anti-IgA development is the IgA-deficient patient who has been previously transfused or pregnant.[10] The rare patient who does develop anti-IgA can experience severe, potentially fatal **anaphylaxis** when receiving products carrying IgA. Because most people, including blood and platelet donors, carry IgA in their plasma/serum, the patient with anti-IgA has only two choices for transfusion: receive products from another IgA-deficient person or have the IgA-containing plasma removed before transfusion of the products. Because the number of IgA-deficient persons is small, Red Blood Cells Washed become a valuable tool in the transfusion therapy of this patient.[11]

Red Blood Cells Frozen and Red Blood Cells Deglycerolized

Using cryopreservation procedures can extend the shelf life of Red Blood Cells. **Freezing Red Blood Cells** is of primary value when storing units of blood that would likely exceed their expiration date before transfusion could occur if the cells were stored in a liquid form. For example, blood from rare donors or autologous units for a future scheduled surgery may be available in a frozen state for up to 10 years. Freezing red blood cells also allows for stockpiling inventory that may be needed for military activity or natural disaster.[1]

Freezing of red blood cells requires the addition of a **cryoprotective agent** before freezing to prevent cellular damage or hemolysis.[12] To provide maximum protection, an optimal balance between cellular dehydration and intracellular ice crystal formation must be achieved. Although a variety of methods have been used to freeze human red blood cells, the high-glycerol method is the most effective and is the one used by the vast majority of organizations today.[13]

In the high-glycerol method, glycerol is the cryoprotective agent. The final concentration of glycerol is 40% weight of solute per volume of solution (w/v), with approximately 400 mL of 6.2 M glycerol added to the red blood cells. (It is the use of this high concentration of glycerol that gives the procedure its name.) To enhance diffusion of glycerol into the red blood cells, the red blood cells and glycerol are warmed to at least 25° C by using a dry warming chamber for 10 to 15 minutes or by allowing them to sit at room temperature for 1 to 2 hours.[1,14] Because rapid addition of this concentration of glycerol, which is hypertonic to red blood cells, could damage the red blood cells, the process is a two-step method. In the first stage about 100 mL of glycerol is added to red blood cells as they are agitated on a shaker. The shaker is then turned off, allowing for gradual equilibration between the glycerol and the red blood cells. After about 5 to 30 minutes, these glycerolized cells are transported to the freezing bag. The remaining 300 mL of glycerol is added slowly and in a stepwise fashion, with gentle mixing. The glycerolization process should be performed at temperatures between 25° and 32° C, and the process should be completed within 4 hours. The bag containing the

Febrile transfusion reaction: Transfusion reaction associated with a fever in the absence of hemolysis. Most such reactions are due to HLA antibody formation by the recipient or by the presence of cytokines. Refer to Chapter 15 for a discussion of adverse reactions to transfusion.

Urticarial transfusion reaction: An allergic reaction characterized by the development of hives. Refer to Chapter 15 for a discussion of adverse reactions to transfusion.

Anaphylaxis: An allergic reaction to foreign substances that can be associated with fever, redness of the skin, itching, urticaria, dyspnea, chest constriction, cyanosis, irregular pulse, convulsions, hypotension, and death. Anaphylactic reactions to transfusion are discussed in Chapter 15.

Red Blood Cells Frozen: Red blood cells from a Whole Blood donation that are separated and frozen. Freezing allows for extended storage and is especially valuable for rare blood stockpiling.

Cryoprotective agent: A chemical agent, such as glycerol, capable of protecting cells from freeze injury.

glycerolized cells is placed in a protective canister and frozen in a −80° C freezer. The frozen red blood cells are then stored at −65° C or colder for up to 10 years from the date of the original phlebotomy.[1,2]

A Special Collection Bag for Freezing Red Blood Cells

During glycerolization, the red blood cells are transferred from the primary collection bag into a larger bag for glycerolization and freezing. This step introduces an opportunity for bacterial contamination and clerical errors. In the late 1980s, a collection bag was designed specifically to allow collection and freezing of red blood cells in one integrated system. The Department of Defense has adopted this bag for its collections to allow for greater ease and security in preparing frozen red blood cells. The collection system consists of an 800 mL primary collection bag and a set of satellite bags, one of which contains the cryopreservative agent. This setup allows for the addition of the glycerol directly to the primary drawing bag, eliminating the need to enter the primary unit. Collection, rejuvenation, glycerolization, freezing, deglycerolization, and washing can be done in the same bag that was used in the initial collection of the unit.[1,15]

Time Constraints on Freezing of Red Blood Cells

The American Association of Blood Banks (AABB) Standards allow for differences in freezing times depending on the manner in which the cells were originally processed. Red Blood Cells collected in CPD and CPDA-1, without any additive solution, may be frozen within 6 days of collection. Red Blood Cells collected and then processed with an additive solution may be frozen any time before the expiration date. Red Blood Cells that have been **rejuvenated** can be frozen up to 3 days after the expiration date.[1,2] Products frozen must be labeled with the cryoprotective agent used. If the red blood cells were rejuvenated, the solutions used for the rejuvenation must also be listed on the label. A more complete discussion of the rejuvenation process is found later in this chapter.

Thawing/Deglycerolization

The deglycerolization or thawing process is the reverse of the glycerolization or freezing process. The cryoprotective glycerol must be slowly removed and replaced with isotonic solution before transfusing the cells to the patient. The deglycerolizing process can use the same equipment that is used in the process of washing red blood cells, but a longer, more gradual washing is used to allow the red blood cells to gradually equilibrate to their isotonic state.

The deglycerolization process involves three basic steps. The general procedure allows for (1) equilibration of thawed red blood cells with hypertonic solutions, (2) washing with solutions of gradually decreasing hypertonic strength, and (3) resuspension in an isotonic electrolyte solution containing glucose.

In the high-glycerol method, the unit is first allowed to thaw at 37° C or 42° C, depending on whether or not units are frozen using the primary collection bag system. Once thawed, the unit is diluted with 12% sodium chloride, and then washed. The washing process continues using decreasing strengths of sodium chloride until the final deglycerolized red blood cells are suspended in 0.9% NaCl with 0.2% dextrose. The dextrose provides the required nutrition for the red blood cells until transfusion.

Red Blood Cells, Frozen, once thawed and deglycerolized, are stored at 1° to 6° C and have a shelf life of 24 hours (or 2 weeks if a closed system is used) from the time deglycerolization was begun. The deglycerolized red blood cells should have a recovery of 80% or more of the original red blood cells and a viability of at least 70% of the transfused red blood cells 24 hours after transfusion.[2] The proper name of the product includes the original anticoagulant/preservative of the red blood cells and the words Red Blood Cells Deglycerolized. An example of the label for a frozen unit is seen in Fig. 9-5. The label for the same unit after deglycerolization is shown in Fig. 9-6.

Red Blood Cells Rejuvenated: Red blood cells to which agents have been added that are capable of restoring concentrations of ATP and 2,3-DPG in stored red cell products. Adequate levels of ATP are necessary for red blood cell viability, and 2,3-DPG is necessary for satisfactory oxygen delivery to tissues.

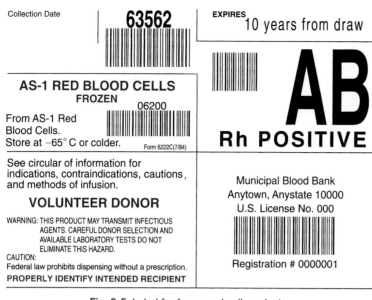

Fig. 9-5 Label for frozen red cell products.

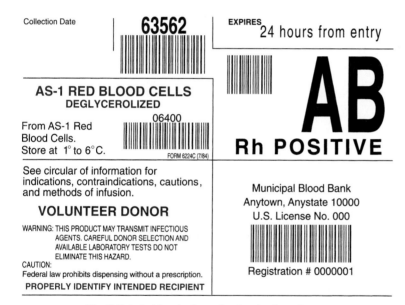

Fig. 9-6 Label for deglycerolized red cell products.

Red Blood Cells Leukocytes Reduced

The presence of leukocytes in red blood cell components has been associated with a variety of adverse effects following transfusions. Among these effects are alloimmunization to foreign **human leukocyte antigens (HLAs),** refractoriness to platelet transfusions, nonhemolytic febrile transfusion reactions (NHFTRs), and disease transmission. Reducing the number of leukocytes in the component can play a role in reducing the incidence of such adverse effects.[16]

The number of leukocytes in a unit of whole blood is about 10^9. A red blood cell product can be labeled **leukoreduced** only if it is prepared by a method that reduces the leukocyte count in the product to less than 5×10^6.[2] Preparation of the product must also retain 85% of the original red blood cells.[1] The number of leukocytes in a unit of whole blood can be reduced by a variety of procedures, including (1) centrifugation, (2) saline washing, (3) freezing and deglycerolizing, (4)

Human leukocyte antigens (HLAs): Glycoprotein antigens found on the surface of all nucleated cells of the body, including most circulating blood cells: lymphocytes, monocytes, granulocytes, and platelets. The HLA system is discussed in detail in Chapter 7.

Leukoreduced (Red Blood Cells Leukocytes Reduced): Red blood cells that have been processed to reduce the number of leukocytes to less than 5×10^6 by means of differential centrifugation, washing, or filtration.

bedside filtration, and (5) prestorage filtration. Each of these methods is discussed here; however, filtration is currently the most effective and frequently used methodology in today's blood bank. Table 9-2 compares and contrasts the various procedures.

Centrifugation for Leukocyte Reduction

One of the earliest methods used to reduce the number of leukocytes is centrifugation. In this method, the unit of blood is centrifuged and the buffy coat layer between the red blood cells and the plasma is drawn off into a satellite bag, along with some of the red blood cells. A variation of this method is to spin the red blood cells in an inverted position so the red blood cells can be drained into the satellite bag, leaving the leukocytes and plasma behind in the primary bag. Although this is a simple, cost-effective technique compared with other methods, the reduction in leukocytes is not sufficient to meet current AABB standards for leukocyte reduction. In addition, up to 20% of red blood cells are lost by this method.[8]

Saline Washing Cells for Leukocyte Reduction

Washing of red blood cells removes leukocytes, platelets, and plasma. A more detailed discussion of the washing process is provided in this chapter. Saline washing was once frequently used, but, with the advent of filtration methods for leukocyte reduction, the popularity of washed red blood cells and the need for washed platelets as a means to prevent febrile reactions and alloimmunization have declined. The primary use of washed products remains the IgA-deficient patient with anti-IgA.

Frozen/Deglycerolized Red Blood Cells for Leukocyte Reduction

The processes associated with freezing and thawing red blood cells also result in a product with a decreased concentration of leukocytes. Deglycerolized red blood cells have a level of leukocyte reduction in the range of 95% to 99% but have a red cell loss of 20%.[17] The use of frozen/deglycerolized red blood cells for leukocyte reduction products is an expensive alternative for leukocyte-reduced cells and in most cases would be inappropriate, the exception being patients who have antibodies to high-incidence or rare antigens. A more complete discussion on frozen/deglycerolized red blood cells is found earlier in this chapter.

TABLE 9-2 Methods For Leukocyte Reduced Red Blood Cells

Method	Percent of WBCs Removed	Percent of RBCs Remaining	Outdate	Advantages	Disadvantages
Centrifugation[8]	70-80	80	Original	Simple	Poor WBC removal; loss of RBCs
Washed Red Cells[8]	70-95	86	24 hours	Removes platelets, plasma	Short OD; labor intensive
Spin cool filtration	82-92	92	Original	Cost effective, good OD	Requires centrifuge
Bedside filtration	99-99.9	90	Original	No special handling	Filters more expensive
Prestorage filtration	99.7-99.9	90	Original	Removes WBC and microaggregates	Filters more expensive Labor intensive; must be done at center within 8 hours of drawing
Frozen/thawed units	95-99	90	24 hours	Patients with antibodies who require rare blood	Expensive; short shelf life

RBC, Red blood cells; OD, Outdate; WBC, white blood cells.

Filtration Methods for Leukocyte Reduction

The most effective and efficient method for reducing the number of leukocytes in a unit is by filtration. Filtration can be done concurrently with transfusion or immediately after collection. Using current techniques, filtration reduces the number of leukocytes by at least 3 logs.[16]

Bedside Filtration Method of Leukocyte Reduction

Leukocyte-reduction filters are used during infusion in place of the standard blood **filter.** This technique allows any unit of red blood cells to be filtered for leukocyte reduction, regardless of the age of the product, and requires no special handling of the unit before transfusion. Leukocyte-reduction bedside filters are available for both red cell and platelet transfusions.

Leukocyte beside filters reduce leukocytes in the product by 99% to 99.9% of the original number but allow greater than 90% of the red blood cells to be transfused.[18,19] Although they are more expensive than the standard blood and platelet filters, the product is effectively leukocyte reduced with ease and convenience. Because filtering is accomplished at the time of transfusion, no products are wasted by having them prepared ahead of time and then not used for the patient.

Prestorage Filtration for Leukocyte Reduction

Another method of leukocyte reduction is the prestorage filtration system. Donor's red blood cells are filtered, within 8 hours of phlebotomy, using a sterile filter. Leukocytes begin to disintegrate quickly when stored at 1° to 6° C. These white cell fragments may be capable of initiating an immune response and carry viral activity.[20,21] In addition, the disintegration of the leukocytes causes release of cellular contents, such as histamine and cytokines, into the component. These products are known to cause nonspecific reactions and alloimmunization in patients. To prevent this fragmentation of leukocytes, it may be desirable to remove white cells before storage. This can be accomplished by using one of two technologies: a sterile connection device or an in-line filter.

Using a sterile connection device, a filter can be connected to a unit of blood before storage and then connected to another sterile bag. The cells can be filtered from the primary drawing bag through the filter into the attached bag, which is labeled as required for leukocyte-reduced products. This product retains the original expiration date of the initial product.[22]

The second technology incorporates a leukocyte filter in the original collection bag. Within the first 8 hours after phlebotomy, the donor's red blood cells are passed through this filter into an attached collection bag. The filtered red blood cells in the bag are leukocyte reduced and retain the original outdate. Leukocyte removal with this system is 96.2% to 99.7%, with greater than 90% of the original red blood cells remaining.[23] The proper name of this product prepared by either method is Red Blood Cells Leukocytes Reduced and includes the name of the anticoagulant/preservative used.

Red Blood Cells Rejuvenated

Red blood cells stored at 1° to 6° C continually lose both 2,3-DPG and adenosine triphosphate (ATP). The level of 2,3-DPG correlates with the ability of the cells to deliver oxygen to the tissues.[4] The viability of the red blood cells correlates with ATP levels. After transfusion, the levels of both 2,3-DPG and ATP return to normal in the patient within 24 hours of transfusion.[4] If necessary, it is possible to restore the levels in vitro before transfusion by the use of "rejuvenation" solutions.[24,25] FDA-licensed rejuvenation solutions contain pyruvate, inosine, adenine, and phosphate.[1]

Rejuvenation requires collection of a unit of Whole Blood in CPD or CPDA-1. Red Blood Cells must then be prepared. Rejuvenation of the Red Blood Cells

All blood and blood components must be administered through a filter. Requirements for blood filtration can be found in Chapter 11.

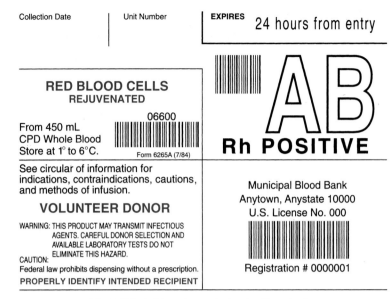

Fig. 9-7 Label for rejuvenated red cell products.

can be done any time between 3 days after collection and 3 days following expiration of the original unit.[1] Rejuvenation of Red Blood Cells within the first 3 days of collection results in elevated levels of 2,3-DPG, which have been shown to interfere with oxygen-carrying capacity of cells following transfusion.[1]

The Red Blood Cells are incubated with the rejuvenating solution at 37° C for 1 hour. Once the Red Blood Cells are rejuvenated, they may be transfused immediately or frozen. If the cells are to be transfused, they must be washed, stored at 1° to 6° C, and transfused within 24 hours of initial entry into the red cell product. If cells are to be frozen, the glycerolization process should begin immediately after removal of the rejuvenation solution. In either case, the washing process is crucial because the presence of inosine is toxic to patients and interferes with the glycerolization process.

Labels on the final rejuvenated product, either Red Blood Cells Washed or Red Blood Cells Deglycerolized must indicate that rejuvenation solution was used. An example of a product label for a red cell product that has been rejuvenated and washed is seen in Fig. 9-7.

Rejuvenation is an expensive process because it involves not only the rejuvenation process itself but the washing of the red blood cells. However, it can be an excellent tool for preserving rare units of blood, maximizing the product's availability in the liquid state, and then rejuvenating it and freezing it for subsequent use.

PLATELETS

Platelets play a significant role in normal hemostasis by repairing breaks in the small blood vessel walls and releasing phospholipid and other release products that are required for in vivo hemostasis. The platelets themselves contain some platelet-bound Factor V and Factor VIII, which are released on transfusion, contributing further to hemostasis. Platelets used for transfusion may come from the routine whole blood donor or may be collected from a single donor using the cytapheresis process. The first section of this discussion on platelets deals with Platelets prepared from Whole Blood donations; Platelets Pheresis are discussed later.

Platelets

Administration of a single unit of Platelets should raise the recipient's platelet count by 5 to 10×10^9/L if the thrombocytopenia is not due to increased platelet

Platelets: Cellular elements separated by differential centrifugation from a single Whole Blood donation (random platelets) and used to treat patients with qualitative and quantitative platelet disorders. Platelets can also be collected by apheresis and are useful for patients requiring HLA-matched products.

destruction.[1] A normal adult dose of Platelets is 4 to 8 units of Platelets prepared from Whole Blood donations.[1] The need for platelet transfusion is determined by the patient's platelet count, the template bleeding time, and the patient's clinical condition.[26] A platelet count of 20 to 50×10^9/L may be well tolerated in a stable patient with uncomplicated hypoproliferative thrombocytopenia, requiring no treatment. On the other hand, a count of 100×10^9/L or higher may be desired before performing surgery or other invasive procedures. In patients undergoing eye surgery or repair of central nervous system structures, baseline platelet counts of 100×10^9/L are desirable since even small amounts of bleeding can have a serious negative impact on patient outcomes.[27] Platelet transfusion effectiveness should be monitored by platelet counts at 1 hour and again at 18 to 24 hours following transfusion, as well as by observing changes in the clinical condition of the patient.

Preparation of Platelets

Preparation of Platelets from random whole blood donors is a two-step process. The first step uses a low-speed centrifugation (light spin) to separate the red blood cells from the plasma. The light spin allows the platelets to remain in the upper (plasma) portion of the collection bag. This plasma product is termed *platelet-rich plasma (PRP)*. Refer to Fig. 9-3, Steps 2 and 3, for a visual representation of this step. The spin time for a light spin must be determined for each centrifuge periodically, using the manufacturer's directions and institutional quality control data.

The PRP is then spun at a higher velocity (hard spin). The hard spin forces platelets to the bottom of the satellite bag. The platelet-poor plasma is expressed into another bag, and the residual platelet pellet is resuspended in a small volume of plasma. This is shown in Steps 4 and 5 of Fig. 9-3. The platelet bag is allowed to rest at room temperature for 1 hour. In general, the platelet component is placed on a rotator to resuspend the platelets, which undergo aggregation during the centrifugation process.[1]

Shelf Life, Quality Control, and Labeling of Platelets

The shelf life of the Platelet product depends on a combination of factors: platelet count, plasma volume, maintenance of the appropriate temperature of storage, continued agitation during storage, the permeability of the plastic used in the storage bag, and the pH.[28] Platelets are extremely sensitive to temperature and pH changes. A decrease in pH below 6.0 causes irreversible changes in the platelet shape, severely affecting their ability to function in vivo.[29] AABB Standards requires suspension of platelets in a volume of plasma that will maintain the pH at 6.2 or higher.[2] The usual volume of plasma is between 40 and 70 mL. Platelets are stored at room temperature with continual agitation for up to 5 days.

Quality control on Platelets involves both a platelet count and measurement of pH. At the end of allowable storage time, the platelet product must have at least 5.5×10^{10}/L platelets per bag with a pH of 6.2 or higher. These values must be seen in 90% of products tested.[2]

Platelets are labeled to indicate the anticoagulant/preservative used in the original collection bag. A sample Platelet label can be found in Fig. 9-8. The proper name for platelets harvested from Whole Blood units is Platelets.

Platelets Pheresis

Platelets may also be collected by cytapheresis methods, which allow for the return of red blood cells and all but 180 to 250 mL of plasma to the donor. The process of collecting only platelets during a cytapheresis process is called plateletpheresis. Platelets Pheresis may be used in any patient who requires platelet transfusion and may be especially effective in patients who have become **refractory** to random donor platelets and therefore require HLA-matched platelet products.[30] Use of HLA-matched or platelet crossmatch-compatible Platelets Pheresis may be of

Refractory: A state of general unresponsiveness to therapy. Patients who do not respond to Platelet transfusion with the expected increase in platelet number are termed refractory.

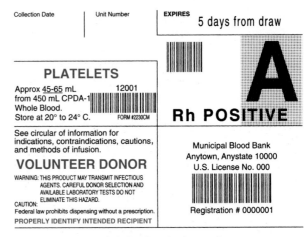

Fig. 9-8 Label for platelet products.

considerable value in these patients. A major benefit of Platelets Pheresis in the multiply transfused recipient is the decrease in exposures to random donors.

Because of the short 5-day life span of platelets in vitro, many collection centers use Platelets and Platelets Pheresis interchangeably to maintain the inventory of this product. Because Platelets Pheresis units contain the equivalent of five to eight random Platelet units, they can be used for any platelet order of this volume or greater.[3] Platelets Pheresis contain platelets suspended in 180 to 250 mL of plasma. They are stored at room temperature (20° to 24° C) with agitation for up 5 days after phlebotomy if they are collected in a closed system. Quality control on the Platelets Pheresis must demonstrate a pH of 6.2 or higher and a platelet count of $3.0 \times 10^{11}/L$ at the end of the allowable storage time in at least 90% of units tested.[2] The proper name for this product is Platelets Pheresis.

Platelets Leukocytes Reduced

The number of leukocytes found in platelet components can be further reduced using filtration. Platelets from whole blood can be labeled Platelets Leukocytes Reduced if the final component contains less than $8.3 \times 10^5/L$ leukocytes. Platelets Pheresis can be labeled Platelets Pheresis Leukocytes Reduced if the final component contains less than $5 \times 10^6/L$ leukocytes.[2]

Platelets Washed

Platelets can also be washed to remove white cells and plasma proteins.[31] Washed platelets are not licensed by the FDA, nor are there AABB standards for this product. Washed platelets are of particular value when working with a true IgA-deficient patient who has developed anti-IgA.

Failure to See the Expected Clinical Response

Expected response from transfusion with Platelets may not be seen in certain clinical conditions. Some patients may actually develop antibodies to platelet antigens or HLA antigens and become refractory to random platelet transfusion, whereas others may have underlying clinical conditions that may shorten platelet survival in vivo.

Platelet survival is shortened in patients with fever, infections, active bleeding, disseminated intravascular coagulation, or splenomegaly.[32] In these clinical conditions, the physician should treat the underlying disease concurrently with platelet therapy. Platelets in these patients should be used only to control active or potential hemorrhage.

Platelet survival: Platelet posttransfusion increments can be affected by excessive destruction or utilization of transfused platelets by both immune and nonimmune mechanisms. Component therapy for patients refractory to platelet transfusion is further discussed in Chapter 14.

PLASMA COMPONENT PREPARATION

The plasma portion of the whole blood donation offers a number of opportunities for component production. Plasma can be obtained following centrifugation of a unit of whole blood or apheresis collection. Approximately 180 to 300 mL of plasma is obtained from a single unit of Whole Blood, depending on the donor hematocrit. Depending on the weight of the donor, between 500 and 800 mL of plasma is obtained from plasmapheresis. The plasma can then be treated to prepare various plasma components. Plasma components are generally used to replace soluble clotting factors in patients for whom no specific coagulation concentrates are available.[3] The time frame in which the plasma components are prepared determines the amount and type of coagulation factors present. A variety of plasma components can be prepared, but we will limit discussion to Fresh Frozen Plasma (FFP) as an example of a component rich in labile coagulation factors and Liquid Plasma as an example of a component deficient in labile coagulation factors. We will then discuss preparation of Cyroprecipitated Antihemophilic Factor (AHF).

Fresh Frozen Plasma

Fresh Frozen Plasma is plasma that is separated from a unit of whole blood and frozen at −18° C or colder. According to the AABB Standards, the freezing must occur within the time frame appropriate for the anticoagulant or collection process.[2] Rapid freezing can occur by placing the plasma in a dry ice–ethanol or dry ice–antifreeze bath, between layers of dry ice, in a blast freezer, or in a mechanical freezer maintained at −65° C or colder. If the plasma is placed in a liquid bath, the AABB Standards require that the bag be protected from chemical alteration. Storage of this product at −18° C or below maintains all coagulation factors for 1 year from the date of phlebotomy. The final product is called "Fresh Frozen Plasma." The label identifies the volume of plasma in the product and the anticoagulant/preservative used. See Fig. 9-9 for an example of labels for FFP.[1,2]

FFP contains plasma proteins plus all coagulation factors, including the labile Factors V and VIII. True clinical need for FFP is relatively limited. Decisions to use the product should be based on replacing all or any of the soluble coagulation factors, the fibrinolytic system factors, or the inhibitors of coagulation such as antithrombin III. FFP should not be used as a general volume expander because safer, less expensive products are readily available, nor should it be used when a more appropriate and specific therapy is available. For example, FFP contains at least 180 mL of donor plasma plus a minimum of 80 IU of Factor VIII; transfusing this product specifically for Factor VIII means giving the patient considerably more volume than may be necessary. Use of specific Factor VIII concentrates with lower volume would be more beneficial to the patient.

The National Institutes of Health published a Consensus Conference report that provided specific guidelines on the appropriate use of FFP.[33] These indications have been updated[34] and are listed in Summary 9-1.

Thawing FFP for Transfusion

FFP is prepared in the transfusion service by thawing the frozen product at 30° to 37° C in a water bath or in an approved microwave thawing device. If thawed in a water bath, the entry ports must be protected so that water cannot contaminate the units. If the product is being transfused for its labile factors, the FFP must be stored at 1° to 6° C and the transfusion must take place no later than 24 hours after thawing the product.[1]

Liquid Plasma

Liquid Plasma is plasma that can be separated from the donor's red blood cells at any time up to 5 days after the expiration of the original product. The product is called Liquid Plasma. Liquid Plasma is stored at 1° to 6° C and can be used up to

Fresh Frozen Plasma: Plasma separated from Whole Blood within 8 hours of donation and frozen at −18° C or below. This process preserves levels of stable and labile coagulation factors for the storage period of 1 year.

Liquid Plasma: The product prepared by the separation of plasma from Whole Blood before the fifth day after expiration. When stored in the frozen state at −18° C, the product can be kept for up to 5 years and is known as Plasma.

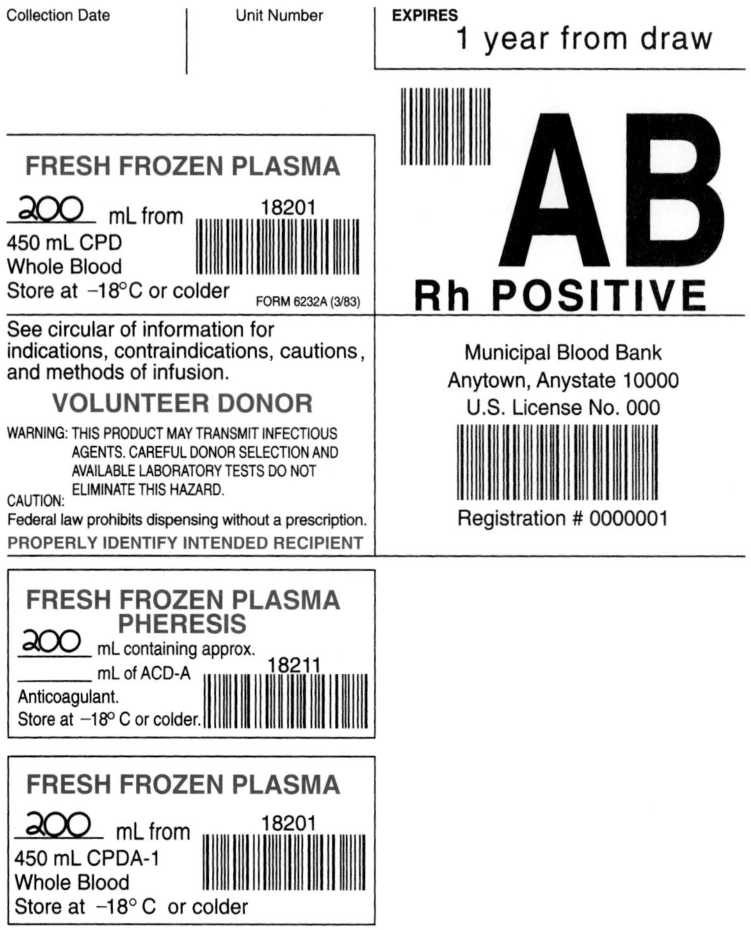

| Collection Date | Unit Number | EXPIRES
1 year from draw |

FRESH FROZEN PLASMA

_200_ mL from   18201
450 mL CPD
Whole Blood
Store at −18°C or colder   FORM 6232A (3/83)

AB
Rh POSITIVE

See circular of information for indications, contraindications, cautions, and methods of infusion.

VOLUNTEER DONOR

WARNING: THIS PRODUCT MAY TRANSMIT INFECTIOUS AGENTS. CAREFUL DONOR SELECTION AND AVAILABLE LABORATORY TESTS DO NOT ELIMINATE THIS HAZARD.

CAUTION:
Federal law prohibits dispensing without a prescription.
PROPERLY IDENTIFY INTENDED RECIPIENT

Municipal Blood Bank
Anytown, Anystate 10000
U.S. License No. 000

Registration # 0000001

FRESH FROZEN PLASMA
PHERESIS
_200_ mL containing approx.
_____ mL of ACD-A   18211
Anticoagulant.
Store at −18° C or colder.

FRESH FROZEN PLASMA
_200_ mL from   18201
450 mL CPDA-1
Whole Blood
Store at −18° C or colder

Fig. 9-9 Label for fresh frozen plasma products.

Summary 9-1

Indications for the Appropriate use of Fresh Frozen Plasma

1. As a replacement for isolated factor deficiencies, unless safer, purified products exist
2. To reverse the effect of sodium warfarin (Coumadin)
3. In the massive transfusion case (greater than one blood volume in several hours)
4. For treatment of thrombocytopenic purpura

---

5 days after the expiration date of the original whole blood product.[2] Liquid Plasma contains all stable coagulation factors, but reduced levels of labile factors. Therefore the product is indicated in patients with reduced levels of the stable coagulation factors.[1,3]

Cryoprecipitated Antihemophilic Factor (Cryoprecipitated AHF or CRYO)

The cold-insoluble precipitate recovered from a controlled thaw of FFP is known as **Cryoprecipitated Antihemophilic Factor** (Cryoprecipitated AHF). Cryoprecipitated AHF can be prepared from a unit of FFP any time within 12 months of collection. The FFP is thawed by placing the unit in a 1° to 6° C cir-

Cryoprecipitated Antihemophilic Factor: The cold-insoluble portion of plasma. The component is rich in Factor VIII:C, von Willebrand factor, Factor XIII, fibrinogen, and fibronectin.

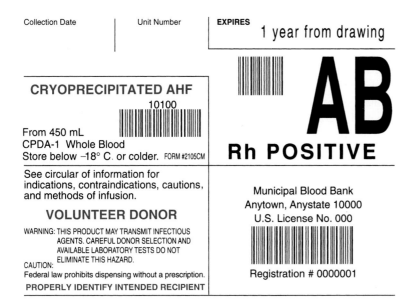

Collection Date	Unit Number	**EXPIRES**

1 year from drawing

CRYOPRECIPITATED AHF
10100

From 450 mL
CPDA-1 Whole Blood
Store below −18° C. or colder. FORM #2105CM

AB

Rh POSITIVE

See circular of information for
indications, contraindications, cautions,
and methods of infusion.

VOLUNTEER DONOR

WARNING: THIS PRODUCT MAY TRANSMIT INFECTIOUS
AGENTS. CAREFUL DONOR SELECTION AND
AVAILABLE LABORATORY TESTS DO NOT
ELIMINATE THIS HAZARD.
CAUTION:
Federal law prohibits dispensing without a prescription.
PROPERLY IDENTIFY INTENDED RECIPIENT

Municipal Blood Bank
Anytown, Anystate 10000
U.S. License No. 000

Registration # 0000001

Fig. 9-10 Label for cryoprecipitate.

culating waterbath or in a refrigerator. The cryoprecipitate can be seen as the white material that remains in the bag after the plasma portion is thawed to slush. The Cryoprecipitated AHF is separated from the plasma as soon as possible to prevent the precipitate from going back into solution. The Cryoprecipitated AHF is suspended in 10 to 15 mL of plasma and frozen within 1 hour and can be stored at −18° C or lower for up to 12 months from the original phlebotomy.[1,2] According to the AABB Standards, the final product must contain Factor VIII levels greater than or equal to 80 IU/bag and fibrinogen levels greater than or equal to 150 mg in all bags tested.[2] Fig. 9-10 provides an example of a cryoprecipitate label. The proper name of this product is Cryoprecipitated AHF, however, it is often abbreviated as Cryo.

Cryoprecipitated AHF is rich in coagulation Factor VIII, both Factor VIII:C (procoagulant activity factor) and Factor VIII:vWF (von Willebrand factor), Factor XIII, and fibrinogen (Factor I). The primary indications for use of Cryoprecipitated AHF include bleeding associated with Factor VIII deficiency, von Willebrand's disease in cases where factor concentrates are not available, and fibrinogen or Factor XIII replacement in patients whose laboratory studies support these specific needs.

Cryoprecipitated AHF is also used in combination with thrombin as a topical agent to stop bleeding when applied directly as **fibrin glue** to a wound or surgical site. This product has been successfully used to control bleeding in cases of removal of urethral stones and in stabilization of auditory ossicles.[35] It is important to recognize that although Cryoprecipitated AHF used in this manner is applied only topically rather than intravenously, the product still carries the same risk of disease transmission as intravenous infusion.

Fibrin glue: The combination of thrombin and cryoprecipitate used topically to arrest surgical bleeding.

Cryoprecipitated AHF is prepared for transfusion or fibrin glue application by thawing the component at 37° C. The thawed component is stored at room temperature (20° to 24° C). It must be transfused within 4 hours if being used for Factor VIII activity.[2]

GRANULOCYTES

Granulocytes are collected by cytapheresis. The product has limited and specific use in transfusion medicine. It contains large numbers of granulocytes, other leukocytes, platelets, and 20 to 50 mL of red blood cells. Each granulocyte product should contain a minimum of 1.0×10^{10}/L granulocytes in 200 to 300 mL of

Granulocytes: Products prepared from a single donor by apheresis techniques. The component contains granulocytes, variable amounts of lymphocytes, platelets, and red blood cells suspended in approximately 250 mL of plasma.

plasma.[2] Once collected, the unit is stored at 20° to 24° C with an expiration date of 24 hours.[2] The proper name of the product is Granulocytes.

Given the volume of plasma and the number of red blood cells in the component, special consideration must be given when selecting Granulocytes for transfusion. The procedure used to prepare Granulocytes generally results in a product that contains more than 2 mL of red blood cells. Therefore ABO-compatible units must be used and a crossmatch is required.[2] Because the donor plasma volume is between 200 and 400 mL, no clinically significant antibodies should be present in the plasma. In an effort to reduce graft-versus-host disease (GVHD), irradiation of the unit before transfusion is recommended.[1] This product is named Granulocytes Irradiated.

Granulocytes are used only in carefully selected patients and are not transfused prophylactically.[1] (Chapter 14 outlines the recipient criteria.) The course of treatment for the patient receiving granulocyte transfusion depends on the clinical progress of the patient. In successful treatment, the patient's fever should drop, the infection should improve, and the absolute granulocyte count should return to at least 500×10^6/L or 500/μL.

IRRADIATION OF BLOOD PRODUCTS

Any component that contains viable lymphocytes can be irradiated. Irradiation limits the availability of these lymphocytes to proliferate, thereby reducing the risk of GVHD in the recipient. (Refer to Chapter 15 for a discussion of GVHD.) Irradiation is recommended for recipients who are severely immunocompromised, such as bone marrow transplant patients, neonates who received intrauterine transfusions and exchange transfusions, and persons who are recipients of designated donations from any blood relative.[1] The AABB Standards for Blood Banks and Transfusion Services requires irradiation of cellular components when the patient is clearly at risk for GVHD, the donor is a blood relative of the recipient, or the donor is HLA compatible with the recipient.[2] Irradiation of the product inactivates the lymphocytes, leaving the platelets, red blood cells, and granulocytes undamaged.[2,36]

Irradiated blood is prepared by exposing the component to a standard source of gamma irradiation. That standard dose is a minimum of 25 Gy (2500 cGy) targeted to the central portions of the component and 15 Gy (1500 cGy) to any other point of the component.[2] Irradiated products must be labeled as such. Because there is some hemolysis, irradiated red blood cells maintain the same expiration date as the original unit or expire 28 days from the date of irradiation, whichever is the earliest date. The expiration dates for platelet or granulocyte products are the same as the original date.[1,2]

QUALITY CONTROL AND QUALITY ASSURANCE

Refer to Chapter 21 for an in-depth discussion of quality control and quality assurance.

The component preparation section of the blood bank must participate in periodic quality control and quality assurance programs, just as is done in all areas of the laboratory. Each product has specific quality control values to be maintained. The FDA and AABB provide specific guidelines and regulations on frequency of testing. The quality control values expected as minimums for all products discussed so far are included in Summary 9-2. The equipment used to prepare the products is also subject to strict quality control requirements and testing. For example, the centrifuges used to spin products for separation must be checked periodically for speed, timer accuracy, and ability to maintain the required temperature during centrifugation. Refrigerators, freezers, and the ambient temperature of the preparation area must be monitored to ensure that appropriate temperatures for the products are maintained at all times during the processing. Devices used for thawing products, as in the preparation of cryoprecipitate, must be quality controlled for the appropriate temperature on each day of use.[2]

Summary 9-2

Summary of Quality Control Requirements for Components

RED BLOOD CELLS

Hematocrit: less than or equal to 80%

Survival: minimum of 75% of red blood cells surviving in patient 24 hours after transfusion

PLATELETS

Platelet count: 5.5×10^{10} or greater in 90% of units tested

pH: 6.2 or greater

PLATELETS PHERESIS

Platelet count: 3.0×10^{11} or greater in 90% of units tested

pH: 6.2 or greater

CRYOPRECIPITATE

Factor VIII content: 80 IU or greater in 100% of units tested

Fibrinogen content: 150 mg or greater in 100% of units tested

GRANULOCYTES

Granulocyte count: 1.0×10^{10} or greater in 75% of units tested

RED BLOOD CELLS LEUKOCYTE REDUCED

Minimum of 85% red blood cells remaining in leukocyte-reduced product

Leukocyte count: less than 5×10^6 in at least 95% of units tested

RED BLOOD CELLS DEGLYCEROLIZED

Mean recovery greater than 80% of red blood cells in original unit

Minimum of 75% of red blood cells surviving in patient 24 hours after transfusion

RECORD KEEPING FOR COMPONENT PREPARATION

In the component preparation area, the record-keeping system of a blood bank must make it possible to trace any unit of blood or component from its source to its final disposition. It must be possible to review all records applying to the specific component and to investigate any adverse reaction a patient might experience following transfusion of any component. Records must be retained as defined by the appropriate accrediting agency or mandated by federal, state, or local agency. Documents and records can be kept in any system that allows for their safekeeping. They must be organized in a way that allows for retention for specific periods of time and easy accessibility for review or retrieval.[1,2]

Refer to Chapter 22 for an in-depth discussion of record-keeping requirements.

OTHER MISCELLANEOUS BLOOD PRODUCTS

In addition to the products prepared routinely by most collection facilities, other products used in transfusion medicine are prepared by large-scale commercial companies. These products use large pools of plasma as the source of the product. Each of the plasma donors who are part of the pool is drawn and tested in accordance with FDA regulations.

Plasma drawing centers are inspected and accredited by the FDA under the regulations set for their industry. In addition, the plasma industry has its own professional organization that monitors its activities. That organization, the **Plasma Protein Therapeutics Association (PPTA)**, has an internal program for certification which provides standards for that industry, just as the AABB provides

Plasma Protein Therapeutics Association: The professional association that develops standards of practice for the plasma industry.

standards for blood banks and transfusion services. This program, called International Quality Plasma Program Certification (IQPPS), involves third-party inspection, adherence to standards, and ongoing reinspection. To qualify, a facility must adhere to additional donor selection and facility standards to include exclusive use of local community donors, drug testing of donors, additional precautions to educate and disqualify high-risk persons, viral marker rate limits, use of a national donor deferral registry, employee training standards, facility maintenance and appearance standards, and standards for laboratory testing. After the initial inspection, follow-up inspections are done on a biannual basis to ensure continued adherence to these standards.[37] These organizations provide the raw material for the miscellaneous products discussed in this section. A significant step in the manufacturing of these products is the ability of the manufacturer to use viral inactivation and purification methods to reduce the risk of the transmission of infectious diseases such as hepatitis B virus, human immunodeficiency virus (HIV), human T-cell lymphotropic virus type I (HTLV-I), hepatitis C virus (HCV), and others. These methods, which include heat treatment and ultraviolet procedures, cannot be used on the fragile cellular products, such as red blood cells or platelets, but cause no damage to plasma. Thus, many of these plasma products carry minimal risk of infectious disease. A brief description of some of these products follows, with a summary of other products in Table 9-3.

TABLE 9-3 Representative Plasma Derivative Products and Major Indications for Use

Product	Indication
Albumin	Restoration of plasma volume subsequent to shock, trauma, surgery, and burns
Alpha$_1$-proteinase inhibitor	Used in the treatment of emphysema caused by a genetic deficiency
Anti-inhibitor coagulation complex	Treatment of bleeding episodes in the presence of Factor VIII inhibitor
Antithrombin III	Treatment of bleeding episodes associated with liver disease, antithrombin III deficiency, and thromboembolism
Cytomegalovirus immune globulin	Passive immunization subsequent to exposure to cytomegalovirus
Factor IX complex	Prophylaxis and treatment of hemophilia B bleeding episodes and other bleeding disorders
Factor XIII	Treatment of bleeding and disorders of wound healing due to Factor XIII deficiency
Fibrinogen	Treatment of hemorrhagic diathesis in hypofibrinogenemia, dysfibrinogenemia, and afibrinogenemia
Fibrinolysin	Dissolution of intravascular clots
Haptoglobin	Supportive therapy in viral hepatitis and pernicious anemia
Hepatitis B immune globulin	Passive immunization subsequent to exposure to hepatitis B
IgM enriched immune globulin	Treatment and prevention of septicemia and septic shock due to toxin liberation in the course of antibiotic treatment
Immune globulin (intravenous and intramuscular)	Treatment of agammaglobulinemia and hypogammaglobulinemia; passive immunization for hepatitis A and measles
Plasma protein-fraction	Restoration of plasma volume subsequent to shock, trauma, surgery, and burns
Rabies immune globulin	Passive immunization subsequent to exposure to rabies
Rh$_0$(D) immune globulin	Treatment and prevention of hemolytic disease of fetus and newborn resulting from Rh incompatibility and incompatible blood transfusions
Rubella immune globulin	Passive immunization subsequent to exposure to German measles
Serum cholinesterase	Treatment of prolonged apnea after administration of succinylcholine chloride
Tetanus immune globulin	Passive immunization subsequent to exposure to tetanus
Vaccinia immune globulin	Passive immunization subsequent to exposure to smallpox
Varicella zoster immune globulin	Passive immunization subsequent to exposure to chickenpox

Clotting Factor Concentrates
Factor VIII Concentrate

Factor VIII concentrate, or antihemophilic Factor (AHF), is a specific treatment for Factor VIII deficiency (hemophilia A) prepared from large donor pools of plasma. The pooled plasma is fractionated, lyophilized, and stored at 1° to 6° C until used. A process of heat treatment reduces the risk of hepatitis, HIV, and other infectious disease transmission. Advances in recombinant-based technology have led to production of recombinant Factor VIII products. These are now the preferred treatment for patients with hemophilia A. The recombinant process further reduces the risk of transmissible disease.[38]

Factor IX Concentrate

Factor IX concentrate (prothrombin complex) is prepared commercially by fractionation of pooled plasma. The final product contains significant levels of Factors II, VII, IX, and X. It is a lyophilized product and is stored at 1° to 6° C. As with Factor VIII, the newer Factor IX concentrates produced by recombinant technology are becoming the preferred method of treatment for patients with Factor IX deficincy.[1,38]

Normal Serum Albumin

Normal serum albumin (NSA) is 96% albumin and 4% globulin plus other proteins. It is a pooled plasma product and is heat treated to inactivate viruses. It is used as a colloid volume expander in patients who are hypovolemic and **hypoproteinemic.** The difference in **oncotic pressure** found in the intravenous or intravascular space when NSA is infused draws the extravascular fluids into the intravascular flow, where it is needed. NSA is supplied as a 5% or a 25% solution. The 5% solution is osmotically and oncotically equivalent to plasma. The 25% solution is markedly hyperoncotic. This makes it of special value in shock patients because it can increase the plasma volume rapidly by drawing the extravascular fluid reserve into the vascular spaces.[1,39]

Hypoproteinemic: Referring to an abnormal decrease in the concentration of protein in the blood.

Oncotic pressure: The pressure exerted by colloids in solution. This pressure affects the balance of fluid in the intravascular and extravascular spaces. Decreases in blood protein (colloid) result in the movement of water out of the vascular compartment and into the extravascular spaces, resulting in edema. Increases in intravascular oncotic pressure (as with the infusion of 25% albumin) results in the movement of water into the vascular compartment.

Plasma Protein Fraction

Plasma protein fraction (PPF) is prepared in a manner similar to normal serum albumin. The major difference between the two products is that PPF does not have as high an albumin content as NSA. The level of albumin in this product is 80% to 85%. It can be stored at room temperature for 3 years or 1° to 6° C for 5 years. It is used as a volume expander in patients who need both volume and protein.[39]

ALTERNATIVES TO HUMAN BLOOD PRODUCTS

The products discussed in this chapter so far are processed from donations of human blood or specific components. There are, in addition, products used in transfusion therapy that are not of human origin. One large group, synthetic volume expanders, has been in wide use for many years, whereas other groups such as recombinant human hematopoietic factors are relatively recent but well-accepted therapy. Current research is under way to produce artificial blood or blood substitutes. We look briefly at each of these alternatives to human source products.

Synthetic Volume Expanders

Volume expanders provide a safe alternative with regard to disease transmission because they can be sterilized and contain no human plasma. When patients require overall volume expansion without concomitant need for the oxygen-carrying capacity of red blood cells or the hemostatic effect of platelets or plasma products, synthetic volume expanders provide a safe and cost-effective alternative. The two major categories of synthetic volume expanders are crystalloid solutions and colloid solutions.

Crystalloid Solutions

The two most commonly used crystalloid solutions are normal saline and Ringer's lactate (or lactated Ringer's solution). Both are isotonic and isosmotic with human plasma. Normal saline contains only sodium ions and chloride ions in concentrations normally found in humans and is the diluent of choice in blood and blood product transfusion.

Ringer's lactate, by comparison, contains potassium, calcium, and lactate in addition to sodium and chloride. The presence of calcium contraindicates this product as a diluent during transfusion of blood. The calcium can overcome the anticoagulant effect of CPDA-1, allowing small clots to develop.[40] Both normal saline and Ringer's lactate expand the plasma volume quickly on a temporary basis. Two thirds of the solution leaves the intravascular space within 24 hours of infusion.

Colloid Solutions

The other group of synthetic volume expanders is the colloid group, which includes dextran, either a high molecular weight dextran (dextran 70) or a low molecular weight product (dextran 40). Dextran should not be used in the infusion set with blood because dextran causes red blood cells to clump in the tubing. Those red blood cells eventually swell and hemolyze as the dextrose and associated water diffuse into the red blood cells from the solution.[40] Samples collected for transfusion service testing that have dextrose in the sample may demonstrate rouleaux formation owing to the clumping effect of the dextrose on the red blood cells.[41] Colloid solutions remain in the intravascular space better than crystalloid solutions. They are especially useful in hemorrhagic shock treatment. Like crystalloid solutions, colloids are sterile and do not transmit infectious disease.

Recombinant Human Hematopoietic Factors

It is possible to prepare synthetically certain human hematopoietic factors for use in selected patients. These products are free from infectious disease transmission.

Recombinant Human Erythropoietin (Hematopoietic Factor)

The first of these products to be put into large-scale clinical use was Recombinant Human Erythropoietin, or r-HuEPO. This product is prepared by recombinant DNA technology to stimulate red cell production in anemic patients with end-stage renal disease.[42] These patients are frequently undergoing renal dialysis and require ongoing transfusion therapy. Use of r-HuEPO stimulates their own marrow to produce enough red blood cells that transfusion of red blood cells may be virtually eliminated.[43] This product has also been approved for the presurgical patient who needs a higher hemoglobin in a short time so that surgery can safely be done.[1]

Although human erythropoietin is not a blood component, it is effective in stimulating red cell production and decreasing the need for transfusion in selected recipients. This hormone is discussed in Chapter 14.

Granulopoietic Factors

Another recombinant hematopoietic factor is one capable of stimulating specific granulocyte factors, or **granulopoietic factors**, such as Recombinant Human Granulocyte Colony Stimulating Factor (rhG-CSF) or Granulocyte-Macrophage Colony Stimulating Factor (rhGM-CSF). These recombinant factors can be engineered to stimulate the production of very specific cells. Only G-CSF and GM-CSF are FDA approved for the management of neutropenia.[1] The potential in recombinant hematopoietic production is exciting as the ultimate in specific therapy for specific patient needs without the risk of disease transmission.

Granulopoietic factors: Naturally occurring glycoproteins that stimulate the development of granulocytes (granulocytopoiesis).

Artificial Blood Substitutes

The development of artificial sources for blood has been a subject of scientific research for many decades. The major advantages being sought are increased safety (no infectious disease transmission), increased availability of the product (no blood shortages or public appeals for donors), stable and rapid oxygen–carrying capacity, and no need to perform compatibility testing or even ABO/Rh typing before transfusion. Work is being done using a variety of different approaches to solving this problem. Those approaches that have made it to clinical trial are discussed here.[44]

The search for a modified hemoglobin product includes looking for a hemoglobin that is not toxic in the patient but remains in the circulation long enough to benefit the patient. Attempts to do this include working to attach the heme molecule to a polymer or, alternatively, encapsulating the hemoglobin to prevent its premature loss from the system.[45] The other direction that this research is taking is using perfluorocarbons as a source of oxygen transport rather than the red blood cells or hemoglobin molecules. This research has yielded a stable emulsion that has potential but has not yet been entirely successful. With the potential seen in recombinant technologies, a recombinant-based hemoglobin product that contains the best features found in both these research focuses may be the best answer at some time in the future. Clearly the advantages of an artificial product make the search well worthwhile.

CHAPTER SUMMARY

1. The practice of separating whole blood into components is desirable because it allows for optimal survival of each product and specific therapy tailored to the patient's unique needs and avoids unnecessary transfusion of products.
2. Although a unit of whole blood is separated into various components, it is important to realize that most products carry the same potential for infectious disease transmission found in the original unit of whole blood.
3. Two essential tools for the sterile separation of components from whole blood are attached satellite bags and sterile connection devices.
4. Components are separated into their individual parts in a unit of whole blood using the specific weight of each component and differential centrifugation.
5. The shelf life of the various products is determined by a number of factors (e.g., survival studies done in vivo) and varies with the type of anticoagulant/preservative used, whether preparation was done in a closed sterile system or an open nonsterile system, and the storage conditions of the product.
6. Each product has specific preparation procedures, storage temperatures, quality control standards, and labeling requirements.
7. Leukocyte-reduced red blood cells are useful in the patient who has experienced febrile reactions to past transfusions. There are several methods for leukocyte reduction: saline washing, filtration, and prestorage filtration.
8. Platelets play an important role in homeostasis and can be made from whole blood within 8 hours of phlebotomy or collected selectively by a process known as plateletpheresis.
9. Certain patients who are immunocompromised may require products that have been irradiated to reduce risk of graft-versus-host disease (GVHD). Products from blood relatives should also be irradiated to decrease this risk to the recipient.
10. Records of procedure manuals, actual product preparation, storage, quality control of products, and storage and final disposition of all products must be maintained for a minimum of 5 years.
11. Other products for transfusion medicine are prepared by commercial plasma companies in large-scale manufacturing. These companies have internal standards established by their own professional organization and are inspected by the FDA.
12. The future of blood component therapy may include the use of synthetic products such as recombinant hematopoietic factors, perfluorochemicals, and hemoglobin substitutes.

REFERENCES

1. Brecher ME (ed): Technical Manual of the American Association of Blood Banks, 14th ed. Bethesda, MD, American Association of Blood Banks, 2002.
2. Standards for Blood Bank and Transfusion Services, 22nd ed. Bethesda, MD, American Association of Blood Banks, 2003.
3. Circular of Information for the Use of Human Blood and Blood Components. Bethesda, MD, American Association of Blood Banks, 2003.
4. Sohmer PR, Dawson RB: The significance of 2,3-DPG in red cell transfusions. Crit Rev Clin Lab Sci 11:107-174, 1979.

5. Simpson MB Jr: Adverse reactions to transfusion therapy: Clinical and laboratory aspects. In Koepke JA (ed): Laboratory Hematology. New York, Churchill-Livingstone, 1984.

6. Delivoria-Papadopoulous M, Martens RJ, Anday EK, et al: Neonatal oxygen transport, the role of exchange transfusion. In Sherwood WS, Cohen A (eds): Transfusion Therapy: The Fetus, Infant, and Child. New York, Masson, 1980.

7. Howland WS: Calcium, potassium and pH changes during massive transfusion. In Musbacker J, Flecher J (eds): Massive Transfusion. Washington, DC, American Association of Blood Banks, 1978.

8. Wenz B: Clinical and laboratory precautions that reduce the adverse reactions, alloimmunization, infectivity and possible immunomodulation associated with homologous transfusion. Transfus Med Rev 4 (Suppl 1):3-7, 1990.

9. Mollison PL, Engelfriet CP, Contreras M: Blood Transfusion in Clinical Medicine, 8th ed. London, Blackwell Scientific, 1987.

10. Vyas GN, Holmdahl L, Perkins HA, et al: Serological specificity of human anti-IgA and its significance in transfusion. Blood 34:573-581, 1969.

11. Mentiove JE, McElligott MC, Aster RH: Febrile transfusion reactions: What blood component should be given next? Vox Sang 42:318-321, 1982.

12. Meryman HT: Cryopreservation of blood and marrow cells: Basic biological and biophysical considerations. In Petz LD, Swisher SN (eds): Clinical Practice of Blood Transfusions. New York, Churchill-Livingstone, 1981.

13. Valeri CR: Frozen preservation of red blood cells. In Simon TL, Dzik WH (eds): Rossi's Principles of Transfusion Medicine. Philadelphia, Lippincott, 2002.

14. Valeri CR: Simplification of the methods of adding and removing glycerol during freezing-preservation of human red blood cells with high or low glycerol methods: Biochemical modification prior to freezing. Transfusion 15:195-218, 1975.

15. Valeri CR, Valeri DA, Anastasi J, et al: Freezing in the primary polyvinylchloride plasic collection bag: A new system for preparing and freezing non-rejuvenated and rejuvenated red blood cells. Transfusion 21:138-141, 1981.

16. Dzik WH: Leukoreduced blood components: Laboratory and clinical aspects. In Simon TL, Dzik WH (eds): Rossi's Principles of Transfusion Medicine. Philadelphia, Lippincott, 2002.

17. O'Neill EM: Red cell transfusions. In Kasporin CA, Rzasa M (eds): Transfusion Therapy: A Practical Approach. Arlington, VA, American Association of Blood Banks, 1991.

18. Sorchia G, Wenz B, Rebulla P, et al: Removal of white cells from red cells by transfusion through a new filter. Transfusion 30:30-33, 1990.

19. Bock M, Wagner M, Knuppel W, et al: Preparation of white cell–depleted blood: Comparison of two bedside filter systems. Transfusion 30:26-29, 1990.

20. Engelfriet CP, Diepenhorst P, Giesson MVD, et al: Removal of leukocytes from whole blood and erythrocyte suspensions by filtration through cotton wool. Vox Sang 28:81-89, 1975.

21. Blajchman MA, Bardossy L, Carmen RA, et al: An animal model of allogenic donor platelet refractoriness: The effect of the time of leukodepletion. Blood 79:1371-1375, 1992.

22. Pietersz RNI, Steneker I, Reesink HW: Prestorage leukocyte depletion of blood products in a closed system. Transfus Med Rev 7:17-24, 1993.

23. Davey R, Sohmer P, Nelson E: Clinical studies of stored leukopoor units prepared with an integral in-line filter (abstract). Transfusion 25:477, 1985.

24. De Venuteo F, Grennemann G, Wilson SM: Rejuvenation of human red cells during liquid storage. Transfusion 14:338, 1974.

25. Moore GL, Faitta ML, Blake B, et al: Storage, rejuvenation, and restorage of human red cells for periods up to 56 days. Transfusion 14:249-252, 1974.

26. Simpson MB: Platelet transfusion in selected clinical situations. In Smith DM, Summers SH (eds): Platelets. Arlington, VA, American Association of Blood Banks, 1988.

27. Simpson MB: Platelet function and transfusion therapy in the surgical patient. In Schiffer CJ (ed): Platelet Physiology and Transfusion. Washington, DC, American Association of Blood Banks, 1978.

28. Slichter SJ: Optimum platelet concentrate preparation and storage. In Garratty G (ed): Current Concepts in Transfusion Therapy. Arlington, VA, American Association of Blood Banks, 1985.

29. Rowley K, Snyder EL: Platelet storage. In Cash JD (ed): Progress in Transfusion Medicine, vol 2. New York, Churchill-Livingstone, 1987.

30. Miyamoto M, Sasahawa S, Ishikawa Y, et al: Leukocyte-poor platelet concentrates at the bedside by filtration through Sepacell-PL. Vox Sang 57:164-167, 1989.

31. Buck SA, Kickler TS, McGuire M, et al: The utility of platelet washing using an automated procedure for severe platelet allergic reactions. Transfusion 27:391-393, 1987.

32. Daly PA, Schiffer CA, Aisner J, et al: Platelet transfusion therapy. JAMA 243:435-438, 1980.

33. NIH Consensus Conference: Fresh frozen plasma: Indications and risk. JAMA 253:551-553, 1985.

34. College of American Pathologists Practice Guidelines Development Task Force: Practice parameter for the use of fresh-frozen plasma, cryoprecipitate, and platelets. JAMA 271:777-781, 1994.

35. Reiss RF, Oz MC: Autologous fibrin glue: Production and clinical use. Transfus Med Rev 10:85-92, 1996.

36. Zimmerman SE: Adverse effects of blood transfusion. In Kasprisin CA, Rzasa M (eds): Transfusion Therapy: A Practical Approach. Arlington, VA, American Association of Blood Banks, 1991.

37. Plasma Protein Therapeutics Association: www.pptaglobal.org/en/qualitysafety_iqpp.cfm

38. Lusher JL: Congenital disorders of clotting proteins and their management. In Simon TL, Dzik WH (eds): Rossi's Principles of Transfusion Medicine. Philadelphia, Lippincott, 2002.

39. Van Akem WG: Preparation of plasma derivatives. In Simon TL, Dzik WH (eds): Rossi's Principles of Transfusion Medicine. Philadelphia, Lippincott, 2002.

40. Ryden SE, Oberman HA: Compatibility of common intravenous solutions with CPD blood. Transfusion 15:250-255, 1975.

41. Mollison PL, Engelfriet CP, Contreras M: Blood Transfusion in Clinical Medicine, 8th ed. London, Blackwell Scientific, 1987.
42. Winearls CG, Oliver DO, Pippard MJ, et al: Effect of human erythropoietin derived from recombinant DNA on the anaemia of patients maintained by chronic haemodialysis. Lancet 2:1175-1178, 1986.
43. Eschbach JW, Egric JC, Downing MR, et al: Correction of the anemia of end stage renal disease with recombinant human erythropoietin: Results of a combined phase I and II clinical trial. N Engl J Med 316:73-78, 1987.
44. Djordjevich L, Miller IF: Synthetic erythrocytes from lipid encapsulated hemoglobin. Exp Hematol 8:584, 1980.
45. Ivankovich L, Djordjevich L, Mayoral J: Synthetic erythrocytes. In Bolin RB, Geyer RP (eds): Advances in Blood Substitutes Research. New York, Alan R Liss, 1983.

FURTHER READING

Anstall HB, Blaylock RC, Craven CM: Managing Hazards in the Transfusion Service. Chicago, ASCP Press, 1993.

Mollison PL, Engelfriet CP, Contreras M: Blood Transfusion in Clinical Medicine, 10th ed. London, Blackwell Scientific, 1997.

Petz LD, Swisher SN (eds): Clinical Practice of Transfusion Medicine, 3rd ed. New York, Churchill-Livingstone, 1996.

Simon TL, Dzik WL (eds): Rossi's Principles of Transfusion Medicine, 3rd ed. Philadelphia, Lippincott Williams & Wilkins, 2002.

Smith DM, Dodd RY (eds): Transfusion-Transmitted Infections. Chicago, ASCP Press, 1991.

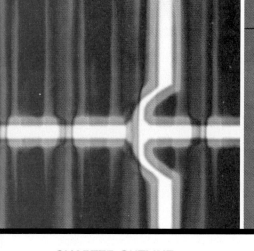

CHAPTER TEN

Blood Component Preservation and Storage

Kay Doyle

LEARNING OBJECTIVES

After reading and studying this chapter, the student will be able to:

1. Discuss the major scientists/clinicians and their contributions in blood preservation and storage.
2. Describe the structure of the RBC and hemoglobin.
3. Explain the functions of hemoglobin, including O_2 and CO_2 transport and the Bohr effect
4. Discuss the production of 2,3-BPG in the RBC Lubering-Rapaport shunt.
5. Explain the role of 2,3-BPG in hemoglobin's delivery of O_2 to the tissues.
6. Describe the oxygen-dissociation curve and list the conditions that cause it to shift to the left or right.
7. Describe the principle of cooperative binding kinetics (cooperativity) in hemoglobin's binding of O_2 and the effect of 2,3-BPG.
8. Discuss the biochemical changes (storage lesion[s]) that occur in stored blood.
9. Compare and contrast the RBC anticoagulant/preservative solutions (ACD, CPD, CP2D, CDPA-1, AS), including historical and/or current applications, chemical ingredients, biochemical changes, and shelf life.
10. Explain the sequence of events in preparing stored RBCs with additive solution.
11. Describe the preparation and shelf life of RBCs with rejuvenation solutions.
12. Discuss the appropriate storage conditions and temperatures for the following blood components:
    Whole Blood
    RBC components (i.e., Red Blood Cells Leukocytes Reduced, Red Blood Cells Washed)
    Plasma components (i.e., Cryoprecipitated AHF)
    Platelet components (i.e., Platelets Pooled, Platelets Pheresis)
    Granulocytes
13. Explain the AABB requirements, including quality control regulations, for refrigeration, freezer, and room temperature storage equipment for blood component products.
14. Discuss the factors that influence stored platelet viability.
15. Describe the storage lesions that occur in stored platelets.
16. Discuss the criteria for visual inspection of blood components.
17. Explain the AABB requirements for blood component shipping (i.e., RBC components, plasma components, Platelets, and Granulocytes).

HISTORICAL PERSPECTIVES OF TRANFUSION

In ancient times, people thought that strength and courage could be transferred to the weak by bathing in or ingesting blood from dying gladiators. By the second to third century, this practice was replaced by bleeding to remove "bad blood." This procedure continued well into the eighteenth century.[1,2]

The year 1492 is often credited with the first human blood transfusion that was given to Pope Innocent VIII who had suffered a stroke the previous year. However, a review of most accounts of this event show that the Pope probably ingested the blood ("given a draught of blood") as was the practice during that time.[1,2]

In the early 1600s, William Harvey discovered the circulatory system in the human body, while the work of Wren, Wilkins, Boyle, and Willis demonstrated that "IV injection of substances was possible."[3] Both of these discoveries opened the way for modern transfusion medicine. The idea of transfusing blood was first described in 1615 by Andreas Libavius, a chemist and physician in Saxony. He wrote of a procedure using male/female silver tubes to connect the arteries of a young man to those of an old man. He believed that "the hot and spirituous blood of the young man will pour into the old one as it were from a fountain of life, and all of his weakness will be dispelled." However, there is no documentation that Libavius ever performed this type of transfusion.[1,2]

Richard Lower first attempted to transfuse dogs by connecting the jugular veins of two animals. However, this failed due to clotting problems. In 1665 at Oxford, he was the first to successfully transfuse blood between two animals using the jugular vein of one dog connected to the cervical artery of another. The literature is full of accounts of attempted transfusions between different types of animals using different devices and methods during this time period.[1,2]

Various people are credited with the first human transfusion. In October 1666, Johann-Daniel Major of Germany is reported to have transfused his professor, who was suffering from paralysis. In June 1667, Jean Baptiste Denis transfused a young boy with a persistent fever. He accomplished this by connecting a lamb's carotid artery to the boy's arm vein to transfuse the blood. The only consequence was that the boy "felt a great heat along his arm."[1] Denis repeated these transfusions on other patients with mixed results. His most famous case involved a 34-year-old patient named Antoine Mauroy, who was transfused in Paris in December 1667 with calf's blood by connecting the animal's femoral artery to the man's arm vein. Mr. Mauroy exhibited pain in the kidney and chest, and about 1 week later, he passed dark, bloody urine, which was described as being "black as soot."[1,2] Greenwalt credits this as the "first incompatible transfusion reaction" ever recorded.[1] In November 1667, Richard Lower and Edmund King transfused Arthur Cona, an "eccentric scholar" from Cambridge, with sheep's blood with no described adverse results.[1] However, because of various adverse reactions in humans following these transfusions, several countries in Europe passed laws prohibiting this practice during this time.[2]

The first transfusion in America and what appears to be the first human-to-human transfusion occurred in 1795, in Philadelphia, Pennsylvania. Philip Syng Physick is credited with performing this procedure on an obstetric patient in an editorial comment by William De Wees in the 1825 edition of the *Philadelphia Journal of the Medical and Physical Sciences.*[4] There is no detailed account to substantiate this comment, and it appears that Dr. Physick performed the procedure only this one time.

With this one exception, human blood transfusions were largely abandoned for 150 years between 1667 and 1817 due to various laws, which forbade them in France, England, and Italy.[1,2] In the early nineteenth century, the English obstetrician, James Blundell, became interested in transfusions to help women who were dying from postpartum bleeding complications. He followed the advice of a University of Edinburgh medical contemporary, Dr. John Leacock, who published his studies in 1817 in which he concluded that species-specific (homologous) blood transfusions were preferred. Detailed accounts describe several human-to-human transfusions that Blundell performed starting in 1818, first using a brass syringe to obtain the donor's blood and then injecting it into the patient's vein.[1-3] He later invented a device known as the "Impellor" which was used until the late 1800s. This device, which was usually attached to the chair the donor was sitting in, had a funnel that collected the donor's blood. The blood was next drawn into an attached syringe and injected via spring valves into tubing, which was connected to a cannula in the recipient's vein.[1] Because of his extensive experimental transfusion studies in both animals and humans, Blundell is widely regarded as the "father of blood transfusion."[1-3]

Blood clotting was a continual problem regardless of what technique was used. As far back as the 1600s, attempts were made to prevent clotting. In 1821, the French scientists Jean Louis Provost and Jean Baptiste Andre Dumas experimented with whipping blood in a churning device, which actually defibrinated the blood. They reported that using this blood for transfusion was just as effective as fibrinated (unwhipped) blood in "reviving the animals."[1,2] In 1868, Braxton-Hicks tried sodium phosphate as an anticoagulant for blood transfusion in four of his obstetric patients, none of whom survived. Over the years into the early twentieth century, other scientists/physicians experimented with different anticoagulant chemicals, including sodium bicarbonate, sulfarsenol, sodium citrate, ammonium oxalate, arsphenamine, sodium iodide, and sodium sulfate.[1,2] Sodium citrate was widely considered to be the most effective and nontoxic anticoagulant. Various scientists, Lewisohn of New York (1915), Hustin of Brussels (1914), and Weil of New York (1915), claimed credit for being the first to use it in human blood transfusion.[1,2] However, use of sodium citrate as a blood anticoagulant was well known as early as the 1890s among physiologists who needed fluid blood for their experiments.[1,5]

Successful storage of blood was first described by Rous and Turner of the Rockfeller Institute in 1916.[1,5] Their storage solution was 50% isotonic dextrose, 20% **citrate,** and 30% blood. They successfully transfused rabbits with this stored blood.[1]

Using Rous and Turner's formula for a blood storage solution, Dr. Oswald Robertson established the first recognizable blood banks in many casualty clearing stations during World War I. He was born in Britain, raised in California, and later served in the Army Medical Officer Reserve Corps during the first World War.[1,6] He was with the U.S. Army 5th Base Hospital comprised of Harvard faculty and alumni, which was the first army medical group to go to Europe. His transfusion teams drew donors, stored the blood on ice in the citrate/dextrose solution, and

---

Dr. James Blundell, an English obstetrician in the early 1800s, is considered to be the "father of transfusion medicine" for his extensive work in transfusion studies in both animals and humans. He first became interested in transfusions as a means to help women who were dying from postpartum bleeding complications.

Citrate: A calcium-chelating agent that prevents coagulation by interfering with calcium-dependent steps in the coagulation cascade. Anticoagulation is only one of the many functions of anticoagulant/preservative solutions. Refer to Chapter 9 for an additional discussion of anticoagulant/preservative solutions.

During World War I, Dr. Oswald Robertson established the first recognizable blood banks in many casualty clearing stations. His transfusion teams drew type O donors, stored the blood on ice in citrate/dextrose solutions, and were the first to type and crossmatch blood for transfusions.

successfully transfused this blood into many soldiers suffering from shock due to blood loss, which helped many survive. Based on Landsteiner's work of the different human blood types, O, A, and B,[1,2,5] Robertson's group used only type O donors and was the first to type and crossmatch blood for transfusions. For these reasons, he is credited as the "father of blood banking."[6]

In 1936, John Elliott, working with Naurice Nesset of Baxter Corporation, developed a vacuum flask, the TRANSFUSO VAC, which contained the anticoagulant sodium citrate. The bottle was used for sterile collection of whole blood and separation of plasma if the whole blood outdated. This bottle was the standard collection device, regardless of the anticoagulant used, until the invention of plastic blood bag containers. He also established a blood bank in Salisburg, North Carolina, during this time.[7] However, the credit for the first modern blood bank in the United States goes to Cook County Hospital in Chicago, Illinois, with Benard Fantus as the director and Oswald Robertson as an advisor, which opened in 1937. There, blood was collected in sodium citrate and refrigerated between 4° and 6° C, which preserved the blood for a few days.[1,2,6,7] Many U.S. cities had some type of blood bank by this time.[7]

Work continued on blood preservation and storage, and World War II provided an impetus for improvement. In the early 1940s, the anticoagulant preservative **acid–citrate–dextrose (ACD)** was developed in Great Britain by Loutit and Mollison, which extended the shelf life of refrigerated blood to 21 days due to the supply of **dextrose** for red blood cell (RBC) energy metabolism.[2] ACD was the standard anticoagulant preservative solution for many years.[8] **Citrate-phosphate-dextrose** (CPD) was developed by Gibson's group[1] in the 1950s. Because it better maintained 2,3-biphosphoglycerate (2,3-BPG) levels (a metabolite important to O_2 delivery), CPD was used for the next 20 years. By the 1960s, preservative solutions containing **adenine** were shown to greatly extend shelf life of stored, refrigerated blood as compared to ACD or CPD alone. The Food and Drug Administration (FDA) concurred and in 1978, approved the addition of adenine to CPD to create CPDA-1, which increased the shelf life of blood to 35 days. **Additive solutions (AS)** were developed and tested in the 1970s.[1] By 1983, the FDA approved additive solutions containing saline, adenine, and dextrose for RBCs, extending the shelf life of this component to 42 days.[9]

RED CELL STRUCTURE, FUNCTION, AND METABOLISM
Structure

The mature red blood cell (RBC) is a **biconcave disc,** which allows for maximum gas exchange in the tissues. It is approximately 7 to 8 μm in size with no cell organelles such as Golgi apparatus, microsomes, or a nucleus. The RBC membrane is a semipermeable, lipid bileaflet layer with proteins interspersed throughout. The lipid bilayer has equal molar parts of cholesterol and phospholipid. The membrane proteins are of two different types: integral and peripheral. Integral membrane proteins traverse the bileaflet structure and project into the plasma and/or cell cytoplasm. These proteins can function as transport proteins or receptors. Also, integral membrane proteins, such as glycophorin A or B, are part of some RBC antigen structures. Peripheral membrane proteins are found only on the cytoplasmic side of the RBC membrane. They are weakly attached to specific integral proteins and consist of proteins such as actin, ankyrin, and spectrin. They help to form the cell's cytoskeleton (Fig. 10-1). Interaction between the peripheral membrane proteins gives the RBC the flexibility and reversible deformability necessary to maintain its biconcave shape. This allows the RBC to move in the circulation and pass through the small diameters of the body's capillaries and the sinusoids of the spleen.[10,11]

Hemoglobin accounts for approximately 95% of the RBC's intracellular protein.[11] It is made of four heme rings and four polypeptide chains. Heme is a cyclic tetrapyrole ring with Fe^{2+} in the center (Fig. 10-2). In adult hemoglobin (Hgb A),

Acid-citrate-dextrose: An anticoagulant/ preservative solution containing citric acid, sodium citrate, and dextrose. Blood stored in ACD has a shelf life of 21 days. ACD is no longer used for the collection of donor blood because solutions are available that allow for extended shelf life. Owing to the acid pH, 2,3-BPG levels are not well maintained in this solution.

Dextrose: Provided as a nutrient for red cells to support the generation of ATP by glycolysis, thus enhancing red cell viability and extending shelf life.

Citrate-phosphate-dextrose (CPD): An anticoagulant/preservative solution with phosphate that is associated with higher levels of RBC 2,3-BPG when compared to RBCs stored in ACD. Blood stored in CPD has a shelf life of 21 days. Adding adenine to CPD (CPDA-1) extends the shelf life to 35 days. CPDA-1 storage results in higher levels of RBC ATP.

Adenine: Added to preservative solutions to maintain the adenine nucleotide pool and thus enhance red cell viability.

Additive solutions (AS): Solutions that contain saline, adenine, glucose, and mannitol that when added to RBCs increase the shelf life of stored blood to 42 days. The adenine and glucose increase RBC ATP levels, and the mannitol decreases RBC lysis during storage.

The mature RBC is a biconcave disc with no cell organelles and a semipermeable lipid bileaflet membrane with proteins interspersed throughout. Hemoglobin, a molecule consisting of four heme rings and four polypeptide chains, accounts for approximately 95% of the RBC's intracellular protein.

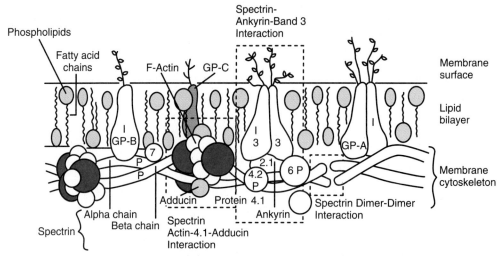

I = Integral proteins
P = Peripheral proteins

Fig. 10-1 RBC cytoskeleton. *(With permission from Harmening DM: The red blood cell: Structure and function. In Harmening DM: Clinical Hematology and Fundamentals of Hemostasis, 4th ed. Philadelphia, FA Davis, 2002.)*

the protein polypeptide, globin, consists of two α chains with 141 amino acids and two β chains with 146 amino acids.[10,12] Each polypeptide chain binds one heme group, and every hemoglobin molecule has four hemes associated with it. Therefore one hemoglobin molecule is able to bind four O_2 molecules because the O_2 binds to the Fe^{2+} in the heme's center. Hemoglobin that has oxygen bound to it is called **oxyhemoglobin,** and hemoglobin without oxygen is known as **deoxyhemoglobin** (Fig. 10-3).[12]

Function and Metabolism

Because of the large amount of intracellular hemoglobin, the major function of the RBC is gas transport. Oxyhemoglobin transports O_2 from the lungs to the tissues, and deoxyhemoglobin transports CO_2 from the tissues to the lungs for excretion. In addition, deoxyhemoglobin binds protons (H^+) to buffer the blood, preventing

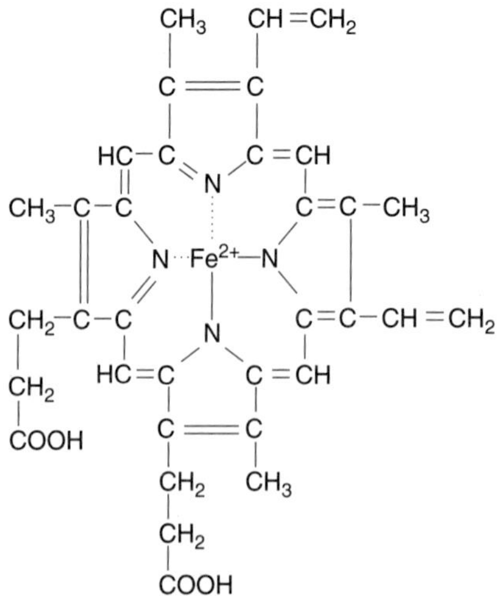

Figure 10-2 Heme molecule.

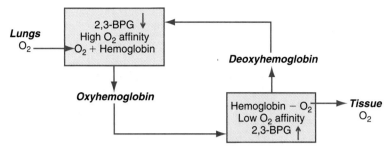

Fig. 10-3 Oxygen-dissociation cycle.

a decrease in the blood pH (Bohr effect).[12] The ability of the RBC to deliver O_2 to the tissues is dependent on many factors, such as blood pH, hemoglobin structure, 2,3-BPG levels, adenosine triphosphate (ATP) concentrations, and cooperative binding kinetics.[9]

Bohr Effect

At the tissue level, deoxyhemoglobin is able to directly bind approximately 15% of the CO_2 generated from cellular reactions through a carbamate reaction with CO_2 binding to the amino terminal nitrogen of the β chains.[12,13]

$$CO_2 + Hgb\text{-}NH_3^+ \rightarrow 2H^+ + Hgb\text{-}NH\text{-}CO_2^-$$

As CO_2 levels increase, RBC carbonic anhydrase becomes activated, generating the formation of carbonic acid (H_2CO_3) from CO_2 and H_2O, which then spontaneously dissociates into H^+ and the bicarbonate ion (HCO_3^-) (Fig. 10-4). Deoxyhemoglobin (DeoxyHgb) serves as a blood buffering system by binding the H^+ generated in this reaction to prevent the blood pH from decreasing. When the blood arrives in the lungs, the H^+ dissociates from deoxyhemoglobin as O_2 binds. The released H^+ combines with HCO_3^- to make H_2CO_3. The enzyme carbonic

Oxyhemoglobin transports O_2 to the tissues, and deoxyhemoglobin transports CO_2 to the lungs. Deoxyhemoglobin also binds protons (H^+), preventing a decrease in the blood pH. This is known as the Bohr effect.

BLOOD IN THE TISSUES

1. $2CO_2 + 2H_2O \longleftrightarrow \underset{\substack{\text{Carbonic} \\ \text{anhydrase}}}{\overset{\overset{\text{Carbonic acid}}{}}{2H_2CO_3}} \longleftrightarrow 2H^+ + \underset{}{\overset{\overset{\text{Bicarbonate}}{}}{2HCO_3^-}}$

              Spontaneous
              dissociation

2. $2H^+ + DeoxyHgb \longrightarrow \overset{\text{Buffer}}{DeoxyHgb\text{-}2H^+}$

BLOOD IN THE LUNGS

1. $4O_2 + DeoxyHgb\text{-}2H^+ \longrightarrow \overset{\text{Oxyhemoglobin}}{Hgb\text{-}4O_2 + 2H^+}$

2. $2H^+ + 2HCO_3^- \longleftrightarrow 2H_2CO_3 \longleftrightarrow \overset{\text{Exhaled}}{2CO_2 + 2H_2O}$

              Carbonic
              anhydrase

Fig. 10-4 Bohr effect. CO_2, made primarily in the citric acid cycle, and water are converted to carbonic acid, which spontaneously dissociates into hydrogen and bicarbonate ions. Deoxyhemoglobin binds the hydrogen ions and buffers the blood. As O_2 binds to deoxyhemoglobin in the lungs, the hydrogen ions are released. Carbonic acid is synthesized and it dissociates into water and CO_2, which is exhaled in the lungs. *(Modified from Rodwell VW, Kennelly PJ: Proteins: Myoglobin and hemoglobin. In Murray RK, Granner DK, Mayes PA, Rodwell VW [eds]: Harper's Illustrated Biochemistry, 26th ed. New York, McGraw-Hill, 2003.)*

anhydrase catalyzes the reverse reaction, causing the carbonic acid to dissociate into H_2O and CO_2, which is then exhaled in the lungs.[12]

2,3-Bisphosphoglycerate

The compound **2,3-bisphosphoglycerate (2,3-BPG)**, formerly known as 2,3-diphosphoglycerate (2,3-DPG), is produced in a side pathway of RBC glycolysis known as the Luebering-Rapaport shunt (Fig. 10-5). The compound 1,3-bisphosphoglycerate (1,3-BPG) is converted to 2,3-BPG by the enzyme bisphosphoglycerate mutase. 2,3-BPG can be converted into 3-phosphoglycerate (3-PG) by the enzyme 2,3-bisphosphoglycerate phosphatase and continue through the rest of anaerobic glycolysis in the RBC.[14] Certain conditions dictate whether 2,3-BPG stays in a steady-state concentration. The most important is pH, because low pH levels favor the breakdown of 2,3-BPG into 3-PG by the phosphatase enzyme and inhibit 2,3-BPG formation by the mutase reaction, and a high pH favors 2,3-BPG formation.[14] Normally, RBCs produce large amounts of 2,3-BPG through this pathway. 2,3-BPG combines with hemoglobin in the central cavity between the polypeptide chains causing a conformational change resulting in O_2 release from oxyhemoglobin to the tissues.[12,15,16]

$$OxyHgb + 2,3\text{-}BPG \rightarrow 2,3\text{-}BPG\text{-}Hgb + \uparrow O_2 \text{ delivery to tissues}$$

Storage of blood at 4° C results in a linear decrease of 2,3-BPG levels in the first 2 weeks of storage.[16] Control of RBC metabolism by pH levels is an important factor in preventing decreasing 2,3-BPG concentration during blood storage.[15] Because of the role this molecule plays in O_2 delivery to the tissue, the importance of maintaining adequate levels in stored blood is obvious.

O_2 Dissociation Curve and Cooperative Binding Kinetics

When O_2 binds to the Fe^{2+} in hemoglobin, there is a change in the conformation of the polypeptide chains because salt bonds between the four subunits are disrupted. Each time O_2 binds, the α/β polypeptide subunits rotate toward a more compact tetramer structure, pushing 2,3-BPG out of the central cavity.[12] This alteration in hemoglobin's shape makes it easier for other O_2 molecules to bind to the remaining heme molecules. Conversely, the release of one molecule of O_2 from hemoglobin facilitates the release of others.[10,12] This property is known as **cooperative binding kinetics** or **cooperativity**.

Cooperativity explains the sigmoid shape of the **hemoglobin-oxygen dissociation curve** in Fig. 10-6. The x-axis represents the partial pressure of O_2 (pO_2) measured in millimeters of mercury (mm Hg), and the y-axis represents the percent of hemoglobin that is saturated with O_2 (%Hgb-O_2). The P_{50} is the pO_2, under standard pH and temperature conditions, where the hemoglobin is 50% saturated with O_2. Normal P_{50} ranges from 26 to 30 mm Hg.[9]

When the pO_2 is 10 mm Hg, the %Hgb-O_2 is 10% (Figure 10-6, middle curve, normal oxygen dissociation curve). When the pO_2 is 20 mm Hg, the %Hgb-O_2 is approximately 40%. In other words, an increase in the pO_2 from 10 to 20 mm Hg results in an increase of hemoglobin saturated with O_2 from 10% to 40%. This illustrates the principle of cooperativity, namely, that the amount of O_2 bound to hemoglobin changes significantly with small changes in pO_2 levels due to stearic changes in the hemoglobin molecule making it easier for O_2 binding. This property facilitates maximum binding of O_2 in the lungs and maximum delivery of the gas to the peripheral tissues.[12]

Various clinical conditions in the body influence the rate of O_2 dissociation (Table 10-1). One way to evaluate normal versus abnormal O_2 release is by comparing the percent of O_2 released under various clinical conditions at a given pO_2.

2,3-bisphosphoglycerate (2,3-BPG): Produced in a side pathway of RBC glycolysis, the Luebering Rapaport shunt, it binds to hemoglobin and facilitates O_2 delivery to the tissues. 2,3-BPG was previously known as 2,3-DPG. The term 2,3-DPG still appears in much of the literature on the topic.

Cooperative binding kinetics/cooperativity: Refers to the fact that every time an O_2 molecule binds to one heme in hemoglobin, it becomes easier for other O_2 molecules to bind to the other heme subunits. This is because there is a change in the conformation or shape of hemoglobin toward a more compact tetramer, facilitating O_2 binding.

Oxygen-dissociation curve: The sigmoid relationship between the partial pressure of O_2 (pO_2) and the % O_2 saturation of hemoglobin. The P_{50} is the pO_2, under standard pH and temperature conditions, where hemoglobin is 50% saturated with O_2. The normal range for the P_{50} is 26 to 30 mm Hg.

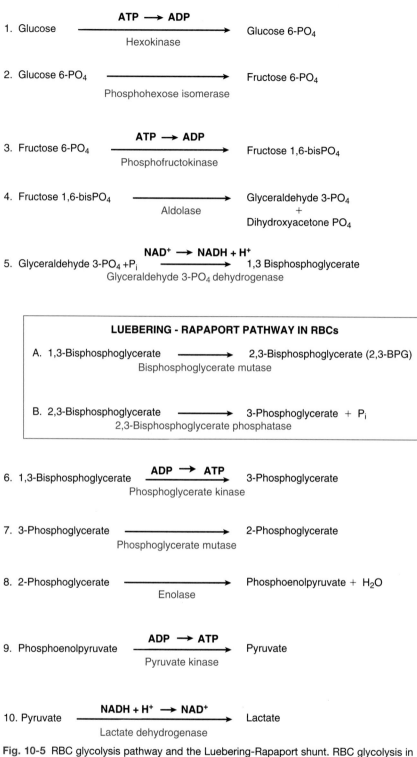

1. Glucose $\xrightarrow[\text{Hexokinase}]{\text{ATP} \longrightarrow \text{ADP}}$ Glucose 6-PO_4

2. Glucose 6-PO_4 $\xrightarrow[\text{Phosphohexose isomerase}]{}$ Fructose 6-PO_4

3. Fructose 6-PO_4 $\xrightarrow[\text{Phosphofructokinase}]{\text{ATP} \longrightarrow \text{ADP}}$ Fructose 1,6-bisPO_4

4. Fructose 1,6-bisPO_4 $\xrightarrow[\text{Aldolase}]{}$ Glyceraldehyde 3-PO_4
+
Dihydroxyacetone PO_4

5. Glyceraldehyde 3-PO_4 +P_i $\xrightarrow[\text{Glyceraldehyde 3-PO}_4 \text{ dehydrogenase}]{\text{NAD}^+ \longrightarrow \text{NADH} + \text{H}^+}$ 1,3 Bisphosphoglycerate

---

LUEBERING - RAPAPORT PATHWAY IN RBCs

A. 1,3-Bisphosphoglycerate $\xrightarrow[\text{Bisphosphoglycerate mutase}]{}$ 2,3-Bisphosphoglycerate (2,3-BPG)

B. 2,3-Bisphosphoglycerate $\xrightarrow[\text{2,3-Bisphosphoglycerate phosphatase}]{}$ 3-Phosphoglycerate + P_i

---

6. 1,3-Bisphosphoglycerate $\xrightarrow[\text{Phosphoglycerate kinase}]{\text{ADP} \longrightarrow \text{ATP}}$ 3-Phosphoglycerate

7. 3-Phosphoglycerate $\xrightarrow[\text{Phosphoglycerate mutase}]{}$ 2-Phosphoglycerate

8. 2-Phosphoglycerate $\xrightarrow[\text{Enolase}]{}$ Phosphoenolpyruvate + H_2O

9. Phosphoenolpyruvate $\xrightarrow[\text{Pyruvate kinase}]{\text{ADP} \longrightarrow \text{ATP}}$ Pyruvate

10. Pyruvate $\xrightarrow[\text{Lactate dehydrogenase}]{\text{NADH} + \text{H}^+ \longrightarrow \text{NAD}^+}$ Lactate

Fig. 10-5 RBC glycolysis pathway and the Luebering-Rapaport shunt. RBC glycolysis in mature cells is anaerobic, resulting in the production of lactate. Dihydroxyacetone PO_4, generated in step 4, is converted into another molecule of glyceraldehyde 3-PO_4 by the enzyme phosphotriose isomerase. 2,3-BPG is produced in a side pathway of RBC glycolysis, the Luebering-Rapaport shunt. *(Modified from Mayes PA: Glycolysis and the oxidation of pyruvate. In Murray RK, Granner DK, Mayes PA, Rodwell VW [eds]: Harper's Illustrated Biochemistry, 26th ed. New York, McGraw-Hill, 2003.)*

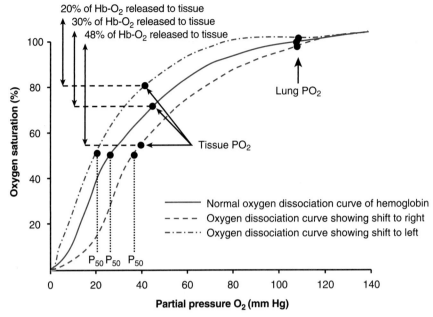

Fig. 10-6 Oxygen dissociation curves under different conditions. *(From Brecher ME: AABB Technical Manual, 14th ed. Bethesda, MD, American Association of Blood Banks, 2002.)*

For example, Fig. 10-6, middle, shows that under normal physiologic conditions where pO_2 is 30 mm Hg, normal adult hemoglobin dissociates approximately 45% of its O_2.

Clinical conditions that could result in decreased O_2 delivery to the tissues (e.g., anemia) are compensated with a shift of the curve to the right due to increased production of 2,3-BPG, which enhances hemoglobin's release of O_2 to the tissues. This is illustrated in Fig. 10-6, right. When the pO_2 is 30 mm Hg, the available hemoglobin releases close to 70% of the bound O_2. Other clinical conditions, such as transfusion of stored blood, cause the curve to shift to the left because hemoglobin has an increased affinity for O_2 regardless of what the pO_2 is. Therefore less O_2 would be released to the tissues. As shown in Fig. 10-6, left, at a pO_2 of 30 mm Hg, the hemoglobin releases close to 40% of the bound O_2. In this example, a decrease in 2,3-BPG levels in stored blood could be responsible for this change.[13,16]

RBC IN VITRO PRESERVATION

Blood transfusion is necessary to provide a means of O_2 delivery to the tissues when RBCs are low due to hemorrhage, anemia, or other pathologic conditions. While in the circulation, RBCs are provided with the nutrients required to sustain their life span of 120 days. However, stored blood continues its metabolic functions and depletes the metabolites necessary to maintain RBC viability and function.

TABLE 10-1 Clinical Conditions Causing Changes in the Oxygen-Dissociation Curve in Patients	
Shift to the Right (Favoring O_2 Release)	Shift to the Left (Favoring O_2 Binding)
Anemia	Alkalosis
Acidosis	Hemoglobinopathies
Fever	Increased levels of hemoglobin F (fetal hemoglobin)
Hypoxia	Massive transfusion of stored blood

A sterile, anticoagulant/preservative solution provides the necessary metabolic nutrients to maintain intracellular energy and decreases the possibility of bacterial contamination. Refrigeration storage temperatures slow the metabolism down and minimize bacterial proliferation. These solutions need to maintain the proper biochemical balance of glucose, pH, ATP, and 2,3-BPG in the RBC under storage conditions.[9]

Anticoagulant/Preservative Solutions

As mentioned earlier in the chapter, anticoagulant/preservative solutions for blood were investigated as early as the 1800s. Robertson's pioneering work in blood preservation and transfusion during World War I set the stage for blood banking as we know it today.[1,6] ACD, the first anticoagulant/preservative solution in modern blood banking, was in widespread use until the 1960s. Citrate, the calcium chelator in this solution, is the anticoagulant, and the dextrose serves as the RBC carbohydrate energy source for glycolysis. The shelf life of blood preserved in ACD is 21 days.[8,16]

During this time, studies using CPD as the anticoagulant/preservative demonstrated higher levels of 2,3-BPG in RBCs stored in this solution.[8] This was due to the sodium biphosphate in the solution, which buffered lactic acid production during RBC glycolysis. This resulted in a higher pH of the solution, which helped to maintain better 2,3-BPG concentrations.[16] Despite the higher levels of this metabolite, the shelf life for blood stored in this solution was limited to 21 days. However, because the role of 2,3-BPG in RBC O_2 delivery to the tissues became better understood, CPD became the storage solution of choice for the next few decades.[8] A variation of CPD, CP2D, was developed around this time. As the name suggests, this storage solution has twice the dextrose concentration of CPD. However, it too had a 21-day outdate.[16]

Shelf life for stored blood, also known as **expiration date** or outdate, is determined by ^{51}Cr survival studies, which measure how many RBCs stored in a preservative solution survive in the circulation 24 hours after transfusion. At the time these solutions were developed, the FDA established that a minimum of 70% of stored RBCs must survive in order for the CPD anticoagulant/preservative solution to be licensed for human use.[9,17] Thus an expiration date of 21 days implied that at any time during or at the end of this time period, 70% of the RBCs will still be in the patient's circulation 24 hours after transfusion. The next improvement in storage solutions came when adenine was added to CPD in the 1970s to increase ATP levels in stored blood. The FDA approved CPDA-1 in 1978 with a shelf life of 35 days.[9]

Table 10-2 compares the biochemical composition of CPD and CPDA-1. Regardless of which CPD anticoagulant/preservative is used, the ratio of the storage solution to blood is constant at 1.4:10. Blood collection bags with 63 mL of anticoagulant/preservative solutions are designed to collect 450 ± 45 mL of blood. Recently, larger blood collection bags (500 ± 50 mL of blood with 70 mL of storage solution) have been manufactured with FDA approval.[16]

Additive Solutions

Additive solutions (AS) designed to increase the shelf life of blood were introduced in the 1970s and approved by the FDA in 1983. These solutions are composed of saline, adenine, glucose (SAG), and mannitol, which was added later (SAGMAN). The adenine and glucose further increase the levels of ATP as compared to other previously described preservative solutions. The mannitol decreases RBC lysis during storage.[8,9,18] Table 10-2 lists the biochemical characteristics of the different additive solutions (AS-1, AS-3, AS-5) as compared to CPD and CPDA-1. As illustrated in Fig. 10-7, blood is initially collected in a multiple satellite bag system containing an anticoagulant/preservative solution (i.e., CPD or CPDA-1) in the

Expiration date: The last date on which stored blood can be used for transfusion. Storage periods are based on in vivo viability standards.

TABLE 10-2 Formulas for Preservative/Anticoagulant

	CPD	CPDA-1	AS-1	AS-3	AS-5
Sodium citrate ($Na_3C_6H_5O_7 \cdot 2H_2O$)	1.66 g	1.66 g	—	588 mg	—
Monobasic sodium phosphate ($NaH_2PO_4 \cdot H_2O$)	140 mg	140 mg	—	276 mg	—
Citric acid ($C_6H_8O_7 \cdot H_2O$)	188 mg	188 mg	—	42 mg	—
Dextrose ($C_6H_{12}O_6 \cdot H_2O$)	1.61 g	2.01 g	2.20 g	1.10 g	900 mg
Adenine ($S_5H_5N_5$)	—	17 mg	27 mg	30 mg	30 mg
Mannitol ($C_6H_{14}O_6$)	—	—	750 mg	—	525 mg
Sodium chloride (NaCl)	—	—	900 mg	410 mg	877 mg
Volume (mL) of solution	63	63	100	100	100

Modified with permission from Brecher ME: Preparation, storage, and distribution of components from whole blood donation.
In Brecher ME (ed): AABB Technical Manual, 14th ed, Bethesda, MD, American Association of Blood Banks, 2002.

primary bag, and 100 mL of an additive solution in one of the satellite bags.[16,19] After centrifuging to separate the plasma from the RBCs in the primary bag, the plasma is expressed into an empty satellite bag, and the additive solution is transferred from its satellite bag into the primary bag with the RBCs. Because this is a closed bag system, the integrity of the system seals is not broken, thus maintaining sterility. This process must be completed within the time frame recommended by the manufacturer.[9,16]

In 1989, the FDA ruled that RBCs stored in additive solutions had to have a minimum of 75% (previously 70%) of the RBCs survive in the circulation 24 hours after transfusion.[9,16] The shelf life of RBCs with additive solution is 42 days (American Association of Blood Banks) regardless of the type used.[9,16] This extension of the stored blood's shelf life from 21 days (ACD, CPD) to 35 days (CPDA-1) and now to 42 days with additive solutions has greatly affected the blood supply for the transfusion service, making it possible to maintain a larger inventory to meet transfusion needs.

Storage Lesion(s)

When blood sits on the shelf, RBCs are still metabolizing nutrients and producing metabolic waste products. Alterations in the RBCs' biochemistry or physical properties that occur because of storage conditions are referred to as **storage lesions.** Under normal conditions in the body's circulation, these do not occur because proper temperature, pH, nutrient concentration, and waste product removal are controlled.[9]

Because of the cold temperature (1° to 6° C) blood is stored at, RBC metabolism slows down. As RBCs sit on the refrigerator shelf, they are still breaking down

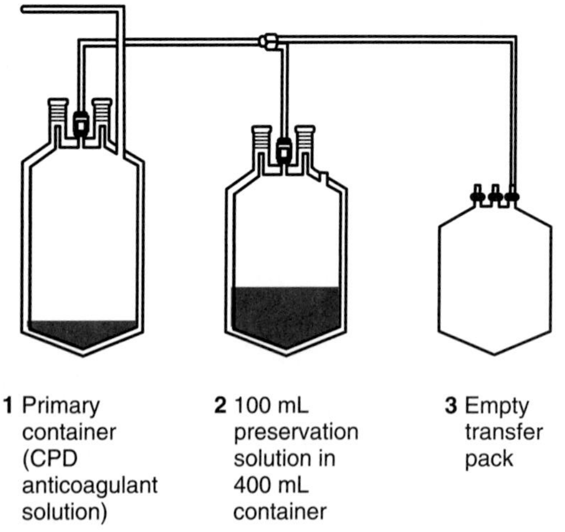

Storage lesions: Take place during blood storage and include changes in blood pH and the concentrations of 2,3-BPG, ATP, Na^+/K^+, plasma hemoglobin, NH_3, and several bioactive substances.

1 Primary container (CPD anticoagulant solution)

2 100 mL preservation solution in 400 mL container

3 Empty transfer pack

Fig. 10-7 Collection of blood in additive preservation systems.

TABLE 10-3 Biochemical Characteristics of Stored Blood

| | CPD | CPDA-1 | | AS-1 | AS-3 | AS-5 |
	Whole Blood	Whole Blood	RBCs	RBCs	RBCs	RBCs
Storage period	21	35	35	42	42	42
Percent viable cells (24 hr posttransfusion)	80	79	71	76	84	80
pH (37°C)	6.84	6.98	6.71	6.6	6.5	6.5
ATP (% of original)	86	56	45	60	59	68.5
2,3-BPG (% of original)	44	<10	<10	<5	<10	<5
Plasma K+ (mmol/L)	21	27.3	78.5	50	46	45.6
Plasma hemoglobin	191	461	658	—	386	—

Modified with permission from Brecher ME: Preparation, storage, and distribution of components from whole blood donation. In Brecher ME (ed): AABB Technical Manual, 14th ed, Bethesda, MD, American Association of Blood Banks, 2002.

glucose for energy through the glycolysis pathway. Because mature RBCs do not have mitochondria, glycolysis is anaerobic, producing two ATPs and lactic acid (lactate). Over time, lactic acid builds up in the RBCs, lowering the pH.[14,15] At day 0, regardless of which preservative solution is used, the blood pH is within normal range. However, by the expiration date, the pH for stored RBCs is below 7.0 in both the preservative solutions and additive solutions (see Table 10-3). The changes in pH decrease the activity of hexokinase and phosphofructose kinase in glycolysis, thus slowing down this metabolic pathway.[8] Alterations in pH are minimized because of the buffering capacity of both the preservative and additive solutions used today.[9]

ATP levels decline throughout the shelf life of stored blood, reaching 45% to 86% of the initial ATP concentration by the expiration date, depending on which anticoagulant/preservative solution is used (see Table 10-3). ATP is critical to maintain RBC Na+ K+ ATPase membrane pump function, RBC–plasma lipid exchange, hemoglobin function, and RBC integrity and deformability.[9] Traditionally, ATP concentrations have been used to indicate RBC viability after transfusion, but the correlation is an imprecise one.[8,9] Although low levels are associated with poor RBC viability, RBCs with high ATP concentrations do not necessarily have high viability levels because of other problems associated with storage.[8]

Na+K+ ATPase is the membrane pump that maintains RBC electrolyte balance. During refrigeration storage, it is almost stopped, but small amounts of both Na+ and K+ leak through the membrane, with Na+ entering the cell and K+ leaving it. By the expiration date, the K+ level in the solution surrounding the RBCs is elevated.[8,16]

2,3-BPG levels also decline by the expiration date of stored RBCs, regardless of the preservative or additive solution used. With any of the CPD storage solutions (CPD, CP2D, CPDA-1), 2,3-BPG levels are almost normal for the first week of shelf life, then rapidly decrease thereafter.[8,16] Because 2,3-BPG concentrations are directly related to pH levels, when the pH level drops, the 2,3-BPG does also.[8,18]

As was discussed earlier in this chapter, 2,3-BPG is of utmost importance in hemoglobin's delivery of O_2 to the tissues. Decreased levels result in a left shift of the O_2 dissociation curve, causing an increased affinity of hemoglobin for O_2.[8,18] However, when the RBCs are transfused, they continue to make 2,3-BPG while circulating in the recipient's body and synthesize normal 2,3-BPG levels within 24 hours after transfusion.[8,16,18]

By contrast, plasma hemoglobin levels increase in stored blood. This is due to the fact that there is no method to clear the blood of hemolyzed RBCs as the unit sits on the shelf. These levels can reach more than 650 mg/L depending on what preservative or additive solution is used and whether the component is whole blood or packed RBCs[16] (see Table 10-3).

Blood ammonia (NH_3) levels also increase as the stored blood sits in the refrigerator because there is no mechanism to remove this metabolite.[15,16] Ammonia is a product of protein–amino acid degradation. Normally, in the body, NH_3 is taken up by the liver, metabolized, and excreted via the urea cycle. Patients with liver problems should not be given units of blood near their expiration date for this reason, because high NH_3 concentrations can be toxic to the central nervous system.[20]

Bioactive substances such as histamine, myeloperoxidase (MPO), eosinophil cationic protein (ECP), interleukin-1β (IL-1β), IL-8, and vascular endothelial growth factor (VEGF) accumulate in a time-dependent manner as blood components sit on the shelf during storage. This is due to the cellular disintegration of platelets and the various types of white blood cells. Previous studies have demonstrated that some of these substances may enhance tumor growth and metastasis and/or are involved with immunosuppresion. This may help to explain why transfusion of various blood components is associated with reduced survival rates (increased tumor recurrence) in patients who have had surgery to remove tumors.[21,22]

RBCs also undergo physical changes during storage. Instead of the RBC's normal, biconcave shape, it can become a cell with multiple spiny projections (echinocyte)[23] or take on a spheroechinocyte shape. Membrane lipid is lost during storage and some cell hemolysis takes place. However, as mentioned earlier in the chapter, mannitol in the additive solutions very effectively decreases this problem.[8]

Rejuvenation Solutions

Even when blood reaches its expiration date, it can still be of use by adding a **rejuvenation solution** within 3 days after the outdate. This product contains pyruvate, inosine, phosphate, and adenine (PIPA). The blood needs to incubate with the solution for 1 hour to allow the RBCs to absorb the metabolites.[16,18,24] Before transfusion, the unit must be washed to remove the rejuvenation solution because inosine can be toxic since it is degraded into uric acid once it is in the circulation.[8,18] The blood can then be transfused as rejuvenated, washed RBCs within 24 hours if it has been stored at 1° to 6° C. The expiration date of the unit is 24 hours after the solution has been added because the unit seal is broken from the outside during the rejuvenation process.[16] The unit can also be glycerolyzed and frozen as RBCs,[16] but again, the rejuvenation solution must be removed before RBC freezing to prevent RBC damage during storage.[9]

The effect of this procedure is to restore the RBC ATP and 2,3-BPG levels back to acceptable levels for transfusion to have normal O_2 delivery to the tissues.[24] This is an expensive procedure and not routinely performed because it only extends the shelf life for an additional 24 hours. However, in cases of rare blood types or blood shortages, it may provide vital blood for transfusion. Units treated with these solutions must be labeled as rejuvenated and the expiration date must be changed to the new outdate.[16,18]

STORAGE OF BLOOD AND BLOOD PRODUCTS

In addition to anticoagulant preservative solutions used to preserve blood, the physical requirements for where blood is stored are also important to blood cell survival. The FDA also regulates this area, and guidelines must not only be followed, but also documented. The AABB Standards provide regulations regarding storage conditions and temperatures that also incorporate the FDA requirements as written in the Code of Federal Regulations (CFR).[9] Table 10-4 contains the appropriate storage temperatures for whole blood and blood components to ensure product viability.[25]

General Requirements for Blood Product Storage Equipment
RBC and Plasma Products

Special **refrigeration units** are required for blood storage and can only contain blood components such as Whole Blood, Red Blood Cells, Red Blood Cells Leukocyte Reduced, patient and/or donor samples, thawed plasma products, and blood bank reagents. The refrigerator must have labeled shelves or separate areas for

TABLE 10-4 Blood Component Storage Temperatures

Component	Storage Temperature	Component	Storage Temperature
Whole Blood	1° to 6° C	Cryoprecipitate Reduced Plasma	≤ −18° C
Irradiated	1° to 6° C	Thawed	1° to 6° C
RBCs	1° to 6° C	Liquid plasma	1° to 6° C
Leukocyte Reduced	1° to 6° C	Cryoprecipitated Antihemophilic	≤ −18° C
Irradiated	1° to 6° C	Factor (AHF)	
Frozen in 40% glycerol	≤ −65° C	Thawed	20° to 24° C
Frozen in 20% glycerol	≤ −120° C	Pooled plasma, solvent/detergent	≤ −18° C
Deglycerolized	1° to 6° C	treated	
Rejuvenated	1° to 6° C	Thawed	1° to 6° C
Plasma Products		**Platelets** (all platelet components	20° to 24° C
Fresh Frozen Plasma (FFP)	≤ −18° C (freezer) or	must be continuously agitated	
	≤ −65° C	during storage)	
	(liquid nitrogen)	Platelets (prepared from whole	20° to 24° C
Thawed	1° to 6° C	blood or apheresis)	
Plasma frozen within 24 hr	≤ −18° C	Irradiated	20° to 24° C
of donation		Leukocyte reduced	20° to 24° C
Thawed	1° to 6° C	Pooled/open system	20° to 24° C
		Granulocytes	20° to 24° C
		Irradiated	20° to 24° C

Modified from Fridey J (ed): Standards for Blood Banks and Transfusion Services, 22nd ed. Bethesda, MD, American Association of Blood Banks, 2003.

untested blood, tested blood separated by ABO groups and Rh types, crossmatched blood, autologous blood, and rejected or quarantined products, as well as biohazardous autologous blood. It must have fans to circulate the air throughout the unit to evenly maintain the proper temperature in all areas. The refrigerator must be clean, well lighted, and have recording thermometers/digital readout systems that continuously monitor the refrigerator's temperature with audible alarms to warn laboratory and/or other hospital personnel if the temperature required for storage goes below 1° C or above 6° C. At a minimum, temperatures should be recorded every 4 hours. Alarms should be located in areas that are continuously staffed to be sure that the necessary action is taken to ensure proper blood storage. The electrical supply for the refrigerator must be different from the one that powers the alarm system itself. In addition, a battery system or a source powered by an emergency generator is required to service the alarm system in case of a power failure.[16,25]

There must be at least two visual thermometers in the standard size blood bank refrigerators to measure the temperature. One is located in the same container with the recording sensor, which is usually on the top shelf of the unit, and the other one has to be located in the bottom shelf of the refrigerator. Both thermometers should be between 1° and 6° C at all times. In addition, the temperatures of both the recording sensor thermometer and the associated visual thermometer should be in agreement to within 2° C.[16] Larger refrigeration units may need additional thermometers to accurately monitor the temperature. All thermometers must be calibrated against a National Institute of Standards and Technology (NIST)–certified thermometer (refer to www.nist.gov/). Any necessary adjustments to the temperature interpretation must be documented.[9,16]

The temperature-recording sensor must be in a volume of liquid equal to or less than the smallest volume of blood to be stored in the refrigerator.[16] For example,

Blood bank refrigeration or freezer storage units must be clean, well lighted, and have recording systems that continuously monitor and record the units' temperature with a visual and audible alarm system to notify responsible personnel if the unit is not maintaining proper blood component storage temperatures. Alarm systems and storage units must have separate electrical power sources, as well as backup systems in case of power failure.

if the smallest blood component stored in the refrigeration unit is RBCs, with a volume of 230 mL, the recording sensor should be placed in a container (glass or plastic blood bag) with a maximum of 230 mL of liquid in it. Water is an acceptable fluid for this because water is less dense than blood and will reflect changes in temperature faster. This will alert responsible personnel to any temperature fluctuations and enable them to follow proper procedures before the blood products are affected to ensure blood safety.[9,16]

When changed, the temperature recording charts and/or digital readout hardcopies must be labeled with the start/stop dates, the proper refrigerator identification, the responsible laboratory personnel, and the institution. Finally, they must be kept in a secure place for at least 5 years or whatever the statute of limitations is in the area. All variations in temperature must be explained in writing, and any necessary corrective measures must also be documented. In addition, alarm system and power supply checks must be conducted and documented. The alarm system must be set at a temperature that will allow laboratory personnel to take corrective action before the blood is affected. The blood bank or transfusion service is required to have written policies and procedures that address what personnel must do if the alarm system is activated.[9,16]

Other areas of the hospital, such as operating rooms, trauma centers, or neonatal intensive care units, may have blood refrigeration units. These refrigerators are subject to the same regulations as described previously, and staff must also keep proper records regarding temperature monitoring, variances, and any necessary corrective actions. Usually, the blood bank or transfusion service personnel are also responsible for these refrigeration units.[16]

Units used for frozen storage of blood products such as Red Blood Cells, Fresh Frozen Plasma, or Cryoprecipitated Antihemophilic Factor (AHF) must meet the same criteria regarding organization and cleanliness, continuous temperature monitoring and recording, and alarm and power system requirements and checks as previously described for refrigeration units. This applies to liquid nitrogen storage tanks as well as freezers.[16] A minimum of two thermometers must be placed in different areas of the freezer to ensure that all frozen products are within the required temperature ranges, with one of them at the point farthest from the internal monitoring thermometer.[9] There must also be written policies and procedures, which detail the emergency procedures if there is equipment failure. Table 10-4 contains the temperature ranges that blood components must be maintained at when frozen or thawed.[26]

Platelet and Granulocyte Storage

Blood components such as Platelets and Granulocytes require room temperature storage between 20° and 24° C. This temperature must be monitored and recorded at least every 4 hours. These components can be stored on a lab bench top or in a specially designed environmental chamber (ambient room temperature incubator) that consistently maintains room temperature. These units are similar to blood refrigeration units in that they have continuous temperature monitoring and recording with an alarm system. These environmental units are subject to the same regulations as refrigeration and freezer units for blood component storage. Because refrigeration temperatures affect platelet viability and reduce the shelf life of platelets to only 24 hours, it is no longer recommended that platelets be stored at 1° to 6° C.[9,16]

Furthermore, stored Platelets need to be **continuously gently agitated** using specially designed rotators to prevent aggregation and promote gas exchange, whether they are stored on a bench top or in an environmental chamber.[16] Studies have demonstrated that platform and tumbler "face-over-face" agitators produce better platelet storage results as compared to elliptical and Ferris wheel–type agitators.[26] Expiration dates are dependent on the platelet collection system used and vary from 24 hours to 5 days.[16,26]

Blood storage records must document continuous storage unit temperature monitoring and recording, alarm and power system checks, explanation of any temperature variances, and any necessary corrective actions, as well as the blood bank's policies and procedures that address these issues. Records must be kept for at least 5 years or whatever the statute of limitations is.

Stored platelets need to be continuously gently agitated at room temperature to promote gas exchange and prevent platelet aggregation. Plastic bag composition can influence platelet storage.

Platelet storage lesions include changes in component pH, platelet shape, volume, and response to aggregating agents.

Another important aspect of platelet storage is the storage bag's plastic composition, wall thickness, and surface area.[18] Currently, plastic containers are manufactured to facilitate CO_2/O_2 exchange to maintain pH and maximum platelet metabolic activity, which increase in vitro platelet storage.[9,26] Second-generation plastics facilitate gas diffusion through the bag with CO_2 going out and O_2 coming in. These types of plastics include component bags with varying types and amounts of plasticizers, bags made of non-polyvinylchloride (e.g., polyolefin), and thinner types of polyvinylchloride storage bags.[26] Furthermore, depending on the type of plastic bag used (e.g., polyolefin with or without plasticizer, PL-732), platelets may react differently to agitation if the rotator used is elliptical vs. other types.[16]

Different types of synthetic storage media have been investigated to enhance platelet quality during storage and replace the majority of plasma in the Platelets, which could be used for further fractionation. Depending on the manufacturer, synthetic media may contain such metabolites as KCl, $MgCl_2$, or Na phosphate. Most current synthetic media contain NaCl and Na acetate, an oxidative metabolic substrate in platelets.[26,27] More work is necessary to evaluate the effects of synthetic media on platelet storage and viability before they come into widespread use.

Frozen platelet storage is available using 5% dimethylsulfoxide (DMSO) as the cryopreservative with a 40% to 50% in vivo survival rate after thawing, DMSO removal, and transfusion. Freezers must meet the criteria previously described. Because of cost and complexity of preparation, as well as reduction in platelet viability and function, this storage method is not widely used. However, it has been effectively used for autologous platelet storage for patients with platelet antibodies who are usually refractive to allogeneic platelet component transfusion.[16,26]

Platelets can develop lesions during room temperature storage over the 5-day period. They change from disc to sphere shape with a 10% decrease in mean platelet volume. This morphologic alteration is possibly due to some type of platelet activation during storage because activated platelets exhibit this type of shape change. Studies have shown that stored platelets lose membrane lipid and both α and dense granules, which could account for this alteration. Furthermore, other investigations have demonstrated that stored platelets have a decreased response to single aggregating agents (i.e., ADP, epinephrine) as compared to fresh platelets. However, they have a better, but still decreased, response to pairs of aggregating agents as compared to fresh platelets.[26,27] Recent research has suggested that stored platelets may actually be exhibiting some type of apoptosis, which can take place in nonnucleated cells.[28,29] Platelets also exhibit a decrease in pH during room temperature storage caused by lactic acid production during anaerobic glycolysis and CO_2 production during the citric acid cycle.[18,26] AABB Standards require that platelet concentrate pH be at or above 6.2 because a more acidic pH causes platelet alterations resulting in the cells not surviving after transfusion.[18,25] As mentioned earlier, the composition of the storage bag influences CO_2/O_2 gas exchange with second-generation plastics providing a more favorable environment leading to better pH levels during storage.[18,26]

Granulocytes also require room temperature storage but do not need agitation. This component is separated from whole blood during apheresis (granulocytopheresis) and needs to be transfused as soon as possible, but definitely within 24 hours after collection. Storage temperatures for this component need to be maintained and recorded as described earlier.[16] Like platelets, refrigeration temperature affects cell viability.

INSPECTING BLOOD COMPONENTS

Immediately before any blood component can be released for patient transfusion or shipped to a different institution, it must be **visually inspected** for contamination, leakage, inadequate seals, and/or abnormal appearance. RBC-containing components must be examined for areas of RBC hemolysis, visible clots, abnormal coloring (i.e.,

Blood components must be visually examined for contamination, leakage, and inadequate seals before release for transfusion or shipping. Signs of contamination include abnormal colors and turbidity. Comparison of appearance of blood in the component bag to that in attached segments is recommended because contamination may first become evident in the segments due to their smaller blood volume.

red, brown, purple) of plasma or supernatant fluid, purple RBCs, or turbidity. Any of these changes suggest contamination. Also, blood components with highly lipemic plasma (milky, mayonnaise color) are not suitable for issue. Any blood component unit that has any of these characteristics should be quarantined and not issued for patient transfusion or transport to another facility.[16]

In addition, platelet components must be examined for unusual colors and turbidity and excessive aggregates. Frozen blood components (i.e., FFP, Cryoprecipitated AHF) should be examined for bag/tubing cracks, which would result in leakage when the component is thawed. Thawed blood components must be examined for unusual colors, leaks, and turbidity. A greenish color in components containing plasma, due to exposure of bilirubin to light, generally does not require that the component be quarantined.[9,16]

It is recommended that the visual inspection of the component bag be compared to the attached segments to observe if there are any differences. In some cases of bacterial contamination, evidence was more easily observed in the bag segments because of the smaller volume of blood or plasma making the changes more obvious than in the larger bag.[9] AABB requires that all visual inspections be documented indicating the date, component type and identification number, a description of the cause for rejection and the action taken, and what laboratory personnel were involved.[16]

BLOOD PRODUCT TRANSPORT

To maintain viable blood components for transfusion, each product has specific requirements for **transport and shipping** from one facility to another, which must be monitored and documented. Shipping conditions must ensure that the products are maintained in a safe and physiologically appropriate manner at all times.[9]

Each blood bank facility must determine optimal shipping methods and conditions as well as temperature monitoring of shipped components. Working closely with the receiving institution will provide important information as to the condition and temperature of the blood components transported. Factors to be taken into consideration include such variables as time of year, weather conditions, method of transport (i.e., car, train, airplane), and distance of shipment. It is the receiving institution's responsibility to notify the shipping facility if blood products are received in a condition that makes them unsuitable for patient use. Within a facility, products must be maintained during transport within required temperature ranges.[9,16]

Shipping of Red Blood Cells

AABB Standards require that whole blood that will be used for transfusion or for red cell preparation must be maintained at 1° to 10° C during transport. All RBC components (deglycerolized, irradiated, leukocytes reduced, etc.) must also be maintained at 1° to 10° C during shipping to maintain RBC viability.[25] The best method to keep within the required temperature range is to use wet ice that is placed on the top of the blood in the transport container used for shipping. This allows the cool air to move downward around the units of blood. The ice should never come directly in contact with the cells because it can cause their hemolysis. An alternative to wet ice is approved clinical coolant packs. Transport containers are usually insulated cardboard boxes or other types of insulated containers that have been previously validated to meet requirements of temperature maintenance during shipping, meet requirements of leakage containment, and withstand various changing conditions that may occur during component transport.[9,16]

To monitor the temperature of the blood units during shipping, the blood bank technologist can use several different methods. There are products currently available that can be placed with the units in the shipping container that change color or shape if the temperature goes above 10° C. Separate high-low thermometers that will record both the high and the low temperatures during transport are also

RBC products must be transported at 1° to 10° C. Frozen blood components (e.g., frozen RBCs, FFP) are shipped with dry ice to maintain their frozen state. Components shipped with dry ice should be handled with great care because the plastic bag's physical properties may change during shipping, making it more brittle and subject to breakage. Dry ice is a miscellaneous hazardous substance and must be treated as such.

Platelets and granulocytes must be transported at 20° to 24° C. Insulated containers are available that have been validated to maintain proper transport temperatures, contain leakage, and withstand changing conditions that may occur during blood component transport.

available. An inexpensive method is to place a thermometer, secured with rubber bands, between two blood units, forming a "sandwich," to measure the blood's temperature after it has reached its destination. The sandwich is returned to the shipping container with the coolant (wet ice or coolant pack) and the temperature is recorded after at least 5 minutes have passed.[9] Regardless of what method is used to monitor the blood's temperature for transport, if it is not between 1° and 10° C, the blood must be discarded.[16] Transport of Whole Blood that will be used to provide Platelets or other room temperature components must be maintained at 20° to 24° C so that component function is not compromised.[16,25] Quality control records documenting shipping temperatures must be maintained.[16]

Frozen Red Blood Cells must be shipped in a manner that maintains the cells in a frozen state. Usually dry ice is used in properly insulated, previously validated shipping containers and placed in the top and bottom of the container, as well as around the products, to ensure proper temperatures. Padding materials (e.g., plastic air packaging, "bubbles") should be used to prevent fragile, frozen blood components from breaking. However, care must be taken to ensure that these materials do not prevent the dry ice from maintaining the required component temperatures below freezing.[9,16]

An important aspect of frozen blood transport is the plastic composition of the storage bag. A recent comparison of the different types of available bags, such as polyolefin (PO), polyethylene-co-vinylacetate (EVA), fluorinated polyethylene propylene (FEP), and polyvinyl chloride (PVC) with different plasticizers, demonstrated that the plastic's physical properties can be adversely affected by the dry ice temperatures (−70° C) resulting in bag fracture during transport.[30] The EVA bags had the best results in terms of shock resistance with the lowest rate of bag breakage as compared to the other bags.

Another issue that must be considered is that dry ice is a miscellaneous hazardous material. Any package using this as a coolant must have a diamond-shaped Class 9 symbol, be labeled as containing "dry ice" or "carbon dioxide, solid," and have its weight in kilograms (kg) and the contents of the package labeled on the outside. Additional requirements when using dry ice are in the General Laboratory Methods section of the AABB Technical Manual.[16]

Shipping of Platelets and Granulocytes

All types of Platelets (i.e., pooled, irradiated, leukocytes reduced) and Granulocyte must be transported between 20° and 24° C. Insulated containers designed to maintain these temperatures are usually used. Also, commercial coolants are available to keep these products within the required temperature range during shipping.[16,25] Wet ice is never used for transport of these components. Temperature monitoring can be conducted using the methods described in the previous section on red cell transport.

During storage, Platelets need to be continuously agitated to promote gas exchange and prevent aggregation. This is not currently possible with available transport methods. A recent study demonstrated that platelet viability and function are not affected if the Platelets are shipped, as required by AABB Standards, within 24 hours from the blood collection center to a distant facility. However, significant platelet damage results if agitation is interrupted for 2 days or more.[31]

Shipping of Plasma Products

Plasma product shipping requirements have a variety of temperature ranges depending on the product type. Fresh Frozen Plasma (FFP), Plasma Cryoprecipitate Reduced, and Cryoprecipitated AHF must be kept in the frozen state during shipping. Like frozen RBCs, these components are usually shipped with dry ice in well-insulated containers as described previously.[16,25]

Thawed FFP, liquid plasma, and all other types of thawed plasma must be transported between 1° and 10° C in the manner described for red blood cell components, and thawed cryoprecipitated AHF must be shipped between 20° and 24° C.[16,25]

CHAPTER SUMMARY

1. The notion that the removal, exchange, or transfusion of blood had some advantageous medicinal outcomes can be found in historical accounts as far back as the second and third century. Particularly important to the development of transfusion medicine was the discovery of the circulatory system by Harvey in the 1600s. James Blundell, an English physician who in the early nineteenth century became interested in transfusion for women with postpartum bleeding, is considered to be the "father of transfusion."

2. Successful blood storage was first described in the early 1900s using a formula of citrate and dextrose as the anticoagulant preservative. In World War I, the first recognizable blood banks were organized by Dr. Oswald Robertson, whose group was the first to type and crossmatch for transfusion. Dr. Robertson is considered to be the "father of blood banking." The evacuated glass bottle was developed in 1936, and by the middle of the twentieth century many U.S. cities had some type of blood bank.

3. The continued research on blood preservation and the development of sterile plastic collection sets made possible the developments in blood component preparation, storage, and transfusion that we have in today's blood banks and transfusion services.

4. The mature RBC is a 7 to 8 μm biconcave disc. The RBC membrane is a lipid bilayer with proteins both on the cytoplasmic side and extending through the membrane. The protein structures can function as transporters or receptors, serve in some instances as RBC antigens, and help maintain the RBC shape by forming part of the cytoskeleton.

5. Hemoglobin, a molecule composed of four heme rings and four polypeptide chains, accounts for approximately 95% of the RBC intracellular protein. Each hemoglobin molecule is able to bind with four O_2 molecules. Oxyhemoglobin delivers inspired O_2 from the lungs to the organs and tissues, and deoxyhemoglobin binds H^+ generated in carbonic acid dissociation, preventing the pH of the blood from decreasing.

6. The ability of hemoglobin to deliver O_2 is affected by a number of factors, including blood pH, 2,3-BPG levels, ATP concentrations, and cooperative binding kinetics (cooperativity). 2,3-BPG (formerly 2,3-DPG) facilitates the delivery of O_2 to the tissues. Low pH favors the breakdown of 2,3-BPG whereas high pH, relative to physiologic pH, favors the production of 2,3-BPG. ATP plays a role in RBC viability. Because of this, blood storage conditions should be such that levels of 2,3-BPG and ATP are maintained optimally over the course of the storage period.

7. The oxygen-dissociation curve is used to illustrate the percent O_2 saturation of hemoglobin at varying partial pressures of O_2. The sigmoid shape results from the fact that when a molecule of O_2 binds to hemoglobin there is a conformational change that facilitates the binding of another molecule. This is known as cooperativity. The P_{50} (hemoglobin 50% saturated) normally ranges from 26 to 30 mm Hg. A shift of the curve to the right facilitates the delivery of O_2; a shift to the left favors the binding of O_2.

8. Anticoagulant preservative solutions used for blood collection and storage contain three common elements: a source of nutrients for RBC metabolism, a buffer, and an anticoagulant; in addition, AS solutions may contain mannitol. The shelf life of a unit of blood is dependent on the anticoagulant preservative solution used and based on RBC viability studies. Blood collected in CPDA-1 can be stored for 35 days at 1° to 6° C. The FDA requires that at least 70% of the RBCs are viable at 24 hours after transfusion. Red cells stored in additive solutions (AS-1, AS-3, AS-5) can be stored for 42 days. For RBCs stored in AS, the FDA requires a 75% viability at 24 hours after transfusion.

9. Storage changes in Whole Blood and Red Blood Cells during the storage period include the following: decreased 2,3-BPG, decreased pH, decreased ATP, increased plasma K^+, increased plasma hemoglobin, increased NH_3, and increased levels of a number of bioactive substances. Red cells also undergo shape changes during storage, which is partially controlled by the addition of mannitol to additive solutions.

10. Rejuvenation solutions are available to extend the outdate of RBCs beyond the original expiration date. The solution must be removed by washing before transfusion. Because of the high cost of this process, it is rarely used, but is useful for extended storage of rare blood.

11. The FDA and the AABB provide regulations and standards of practice for storage of blood and components, including appropriate storage conditions and equipment. Blood bank storage devices must be clean and well organized. Temperatures must be carefully regulated throughout the unit, and records must be maintained documenting that required storage conditions have been met. Alarm systems must be maintained that alert personnel before the time that the unit is outside of the required temperature range.

12. Before release, all blood and components must be visually inspected for contamination, leakage, inadequate seals, and/or abnormal appearance. This inspection must be documented.

13. Components that are stored at 1° to 6° C must be maintained at 1° to 10° C when transported or shipped. Containers must be designed to maintain these temperatures, and some mechanism must be in place to document these conditions. Frozen components must be maintained in the frozen state. Platelets and Granulocytes must be maintained between 20° and 24° C.

REFERENCES

1. Greenwalt TJ: A short history of transfusion medicine. Transfusion 37:550-563, 1997.
2. Diamond LK: A history of blood transfusion. In Wintrobe MM (ed): Blood, Pure, and Eloquent. New York, McGraw-Hill, 1980.
3. Myhre BA: James Blundell—pioneer transfusionist. Transfusion 35:74-78, 1995.
4. Schmidt PJ: The bicentennial of transfusion in America. Transfusion 35:4, 1995.
5. Ross RE: Transfusion medicine's triumphs. Advance for Medical Laboratory Professionals, Oct 23, 2000, pp 9-11.
6. Hess JR, Schmidt PJ: The first blood banker: Oswald Hope Robertson. Transfusion 40:110-113, 2000.
7. Schmidt PJ: John Elliott and the evolution of American blood banking, 1934-1954. Transfusion 40:608-612, 2000.
8. Beutler E: Liquid preservation of RBCs. In Simon TL, Dzik WH, Snyder E, et al (eds): Rossi's Principles of Transfusion Medicine, 3rd ed. Philadelphia, Lippincott Williams & Wilkins, 2002.
9. Young JA, Rudmann SV: Blood component preservation and storage. In Rudmann SV: Textbook of Blood Banking and Transfusion Medicine. Philadelphia, WB Saunders, 1995.
10. Harmening DM: The red blood cell: Structure and function. In Harmening DM: Clinical Hematology and Fundamentals of Hemostasis, 4th ed. Philadelphia, FA Davis, 2002.
11. Murray RK: Red and white blood cells. In Murray RK, Granner DK, Mayes PA, Rodwell VW (eds): Harper's Illustrated Biochemistry, 26th ed. New York, McGraw-Hill, 2003.
12. Rodwell VW, Kennelly PJ: Proteins: Myoglobin and hemoglobin. In Murray RK, Granner DK, Mayes PA, Rodwell VW (eds): Harper's Illustrated Biochemistry, 26th ed. New York, McGraw-Hill, 2003.
13. Woodson RD: Hemglobin synthesis, structure, and oxygen transport. In Simon TL, Dzik WH, Snyder E, et al (eds): Rossi's Principles of Transfusion Medicine, 3rd ed. Philadelphia, Lippincott Williams & Wilkins, 2002.
14. Mayes PA: Glycolysis and the oxidation of pyruvate. In Murray RK, Granner DK, Mayes PA, Rodwell VW (eds): Harper's Illustrated Biochemistry, 26th ed. New York, McGraw-Hill, 2003.
15. Beutler E: Red blood cell metabolism. In Simon TL, Dzik WH, Snyder E, et al (eds): Rossi's Principles of Transfusion Medicine, 3rd ed. Philadelphia, Lippincott Williams & Wilkins, 2002.
16. Brecher ME: Preparation, storage, and distribution of components from whole blood donations. In Brecher ME: AABB Technical Manual, 50th ed. Bethesda, MD, American Association of Blood Banks, 2002.
17. Zuck TF, Bensinger TA, Peck RK, et al: The in vivo survival of red blood cells stored in modified CPD with adenine. Transfusion 17:374-382, 1977.
18. Harmening DM, Lasky L, Latchaw P: Blood preservation: Historical perspectives, review of metabolism and current trends. In Harmening DM: Modern Blood Banking and Transfusion Practices, 4th ed. Philadelphia, FA Davis, 1999.
19. Hogman CF: Additive system approach in blood transfusion: Birth of the SAV and SAGMAN systems. Vox Sang 51: 337-343, 1986.
20. Rodwell VW: Catabolism of proteins and of amino acids. In Murray RK, Granner DK, Mayes PA, Rodwell VW (eds): Harper's Illustrated Biochemistry, 26th ed. New York, McGraw-Hill, 2003.
21. Nielson HJ, Werther K, Mynster T, Brunner N: Soluble vascular endothelial growth factor in various blood transfusion components. Transfusion 39:1078-1083, 1999.
22. Buttnerova I, Baumler H, Kern F, et al: Release of WEB-derived IL-1 receptor antagonist into supernatants of RBCs: Influence of storage time and filtration. Transfusion 41:67-73, 2001.
23. Clayton LT: Taber's Cyclopedic Medical Dictionary, 18th ed. Philadelphia, FA Davis, 1997.
24. Valeri CR, Picacek LE, Cassidy PG, Ragno G: The survival, function, and hemolysis of human RBCs stored at 4° C in additive solution (AS-1, AS-3, AS-5) for 42 days and then biochemically modified, frozen, thawed, washed, and stored at 4° C in sodium chloride and glucose solution for 24 hours. Transfusion 40:1341-1345, 2000.
25. Fridey J (ed): Standards for Blood Banks and Transfusion Services, 22nd ed. Bethesda, MD, American Association of Blood Banks, 2003.
26. Murphy S: Preparation and storage of platelet concentrates. In Simon TL, Dzik WH, Snyder E, et al (eds): Rossi's Principles of Transfusion Medicine, 3rd ed. Philadelphia, Lippincott Williams & Wilkins, 2002.
27. Shapira S, Friedman Z, Shapiro H, et al: The effect of storage on the expression of platelet membrane phosphatidylserine and the subsequent impact on the coagulant function of stored platelets. Transfusion 40:1257-1263, 2000.
28. Li J, Xia Y, Bertino AM, et al: The mechanism of apoptosis in human platelets during storage. Transfusion 40:1320-1329, 2000.
29. Perotta PL, Perotta CL, Synder EL: Apoptotic activity in stored human platelets. Transfusion 43:526-535, 2003.
30. Hmel PJ, Kennedy A, Quiles JG, et al: Physical and thermal properties of blood storage bags: Implications for shipping frozen components on dry ice. Transfusion 42:836-846, 2002.
31. Hunter S, Nixon J, Murphy S: The effect of the interruption of agitation on platelet quality during storage for transfusion. Transfusion 41:809-814, 2001.

LESSONS FOR DISASTER PREPAREDNESS AFTER SEPTEMBER 11

Robert L. Jones, MD, MBA

Within an hour after the attack on the World Trade Center, the nation experienced the largest surge of blood donations in history. In the New York metropolitan area, New York Blood Center had 12,000 calls and over 5000 donations in the first 12 hours. Even more blood would have been collected had there been greater capacity to collect and process. At donor sites, lines were blocks long and auditoriums and waiting rooms crowded with willing donors, including many first-time donors. In spite of the long lines, waiting donors displayed infinite patience. After learning of the crashes into the Twin Towers, we established command centers to update and coordinate blood supply and blood donation information. Our immediate and most important priority was to ensure the blood supply to our receiving hospitals for this emergency. As such we sent 600 units of type O blood to the six hospitals that were in the immediate vicinity of the World Trade Center. This ultimately proved to be adequate for the victims of this disaster.

As the tragedy unfolded we quickly learned from the hospitals that blood needs for victims would be minimal. Most of the injuries did not require blood, and the majority of the victims were killed in the building collapse. With the long lines and with early understanding of the medical needs for trauma victims, we then prioritized donations to type O and Rh-negative donors. On day two we began telling donors and the press that donations were far exceeding the medical need and that their donations would be more beneficial if made in the following weeks to months. Managing the overwhelming surge of blood donors became our most important and demanding task. Everyone wanted to run a blood drive—despite the fact that blood was clearly not needed for medical purposes.

Collections were over four times our usual levels in the first week after the disaster, and our percentage of type O collections rose from our usual 46% to over 60% in 4 days. Type O+ ordinarily represents about 40% of our total inventory so that the peak total inventory rose to over 40,000 units, or about a 19-day supply—well above the amount that we could ever routinely distribute to our hospitals. In addition to the substantial oversupply, demand from our hospitals fell dramatically because of a marked drop in inpatient admissions. The capacity to manage products was exceeded in several operational areas when the surge in donations produced a volume that was unprecedented. Data management, nucleic acid testing

(NAT), and viral testing were overwhelmed, and significant delays occurred. Managing and storing the large volume of finished goods inventory became difficult and products were lost, especially autologous and directed donations. Ultimately these operational issues led to loss of short-dated products and longer shelf life products as well. Within 5 days after the attack, the extremes of volume led to a regional platelet shortage as viral testing capacity could not handle or prioritize the volume quickly enough. Errors in handling led to losses in red cell products as well. Although there were no documented safety issues as a result, human errors are much more likely to occur under such circumstances. In November and December 2001, the excessive blood collection volume in September led to outdating of thousands of red cell units (of a high type-O percentage) because the supply far outstripped the demand for transfusion.

A steady rate of increase in blood collections at New York Blood Center that dates back to April 1999 was suddenly interrupted by the peak in donations in September and October followed by a broad trough of reduced donations that went from November 2001 through April 2002. Declining inventories and short supply in early 2002 followed the inventory glut of late 2001. The high discard rate from expiring inventories, coupled with low distribution from low hospital demand, led to financial losses of millions of dollars at our blood center. Collections and inventory had not returned to stable levels well into the spring of 2003.

Looking back to the days just after the attack, our efforts to manage the surge of blood donations were only marginally effective. It is now clear that even when confronted with the knowledge that medical need was met and that blood had a finite shelf life, donors were compelled to give and help in some way. People who had never considered donating blood not only donated but also stayed at the donor site for hours and returned for days volunteering for any task to help in the effort. They were pensive and had a sense of helplessness along with an overwhelming need to contribute. People needed to be with one another, friends, neighbors, and strangers. Blood donation sites gave them that opportunity along with something personal to do for the cause. Blood donation assumed much more of a social value than our usual medical mission. Although the emotional aspects surrounding these events must be reckoned with, we must recognize that social value of blood donation alone can create a danger to the blood supply if not controlled to levels that are more consistent with medical need.

September 11 changed all of our lives. At the same time, it dramatically altered the landscape of blood donor recruitment and blood supply. Suddenly we were overwhelmed with a will to donate that significantly exceeded medical need. Unfortunately this short-term phenomenon has not solved the blood shortages of the United States or the New York area. Instead, significant instability of the blood supply has resulted, along with a large, unfortunate expiration of precious blood products from the September 11 donations.

An important lesson to derive from this experience is that this kind of disaster and the resultant surge in blood donations have a deleterious effect on the blood supply system, both short and long term. When any disaster of this magnitude occurs, we must manage the public's reaction in a way that recognizes these negative consequences. Dr. Paul Schmidt has written thoughtfully on this subject.[1] His conclusions from study of five such disasters, including September 11, are that the supply on the shelf before the disaster is much more medically important than that collected in response and that the mass response to a disaster is neither safe nor productive for blood collection. Ultimately disaster planning demands coordination and communication on a local and national level by a single authority. As such, the Inter-Organizational Task Force organized shortly after September 11 has made great progress to prepare for future disasters.

Hopefully the spirit of volunteerism and blood donation generated by September 11 can be crystallized and carried into the future. The tragedy of September 11 took the lives of nearly 3000 Americans. We were frightened and horrified at this sight and what it meant to us. Still, each day over 12,000 Americans face individual tragedies, illness, and injury that necessitate blood transfusions. These are the victims, our friends, family, and neighbors, on whom we can now concentrate our spirit of giving. If we can be successful in doing so, we will become a nation that no longer suffers blood shortages and the hardships they bring to patients—people in need. This could be the finest memorial of all to this tragedy and assault on our nation.

REFERENCES

1. Schmidt PJ: Blood and disaster—supply and demand. N Engl J Med 346:617-620, 2002.

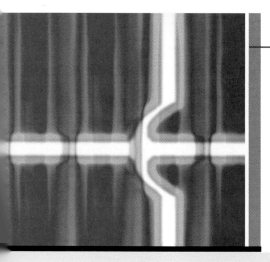

Pretransfusion Testing

The goal of transfusion medicine is to achieve an optimal patient outcome. This implies that the patient should receive the most suitable product—which in some cases is none—and that the product selected carries the lowest possible risk of adverse reaction. This can be achieved only by advancing technology, achieving technical expertise, and developing systems that minimize error.

Once a blood product has been prepared and made available for transfusion, the role of the transfusion service personnel becomes one of the ensuring that the final component selected for infusion is suitable, safe, and effective. This involves a number of important steps, including positive identification of the intended recipient; collection of appropriate blood specimens and their proper storage; development of and compliance with suitable pretransfusion testing protocols; technical accuracy and documentation of employee competence; compliance with established standards and regulations; evaluation of patterns of blood utilization and monitoring waste; review of blood transfusion practices; maintenance of thorough and

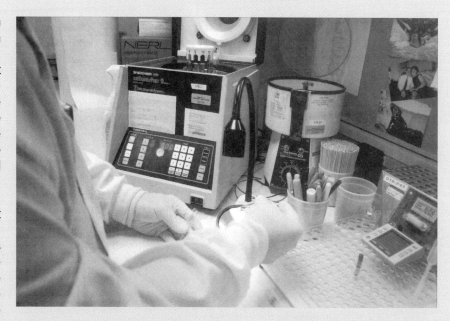

accurate procedure and policy manuals; quality control of reagents and equipment leading to quality assurance; monitoring clinical outcomes, both adverse and favorable; and record keeping and documentation.

To achieve this, blood banking personnel must develop problem-solving skills including antibody detection and identification, investigation of typing discrepancies, identification of sources of error, performance of appropriate testing, and selection of blood and components for transfusion.

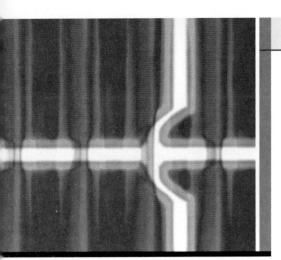

CHAPTER ELEVEN

Compatibility Testing

Mary A. Lieb and Linda Aldridge

LEARNING OBJECTIVES

After reading and studying this chapter, the student will be able to:

1. Define compatibility testing and describe seven procedures that constitute routine compatibility testing.

2. Describe the recommended standards of practice for the following:

   Information on blood/component request forms
   Information for the blood sample label
   Testing of recipient blood
   Repeat testing of donor blood
   Retention of blood samples
   Emergency release of blood
   Testing in massive transfusion
   Transfusion of neonates
   Information on blood transfusion forms and unit tag (compatibility tag)
   Inspection and issue of blood
   Reissue of blood
   Pretransfusion testing for autologous transfusion

3. Discuss the rationale for the selection of plasma versus serum for blood bank testing.

4. List four blood groups that may cause hemolysis.

5. Select the appropriate blood for emergency release in the following circumstances: Type unknown, ABO discrepancy, Rh typing problem.

6. Discuss the selection of an appropriate Rh control when using Rh testing reagents.

7. Define the terms unexpected antibody and clinically significant antibody.

8. Discuss the issues that must be considered when selecting antiglobulin reagents for compatibility testing.

9. Describe the limitations of the antibody screening procedure.

10. Briefly discuss the use of the following techniques in compatibility testing:

    Saline
    Albumin
    Low ionic strength
    Enzyme
    Low ionic polycation
    Polyethylene glycol
    Column (Gel) testing
    Solid phase red cell adherence

11. Briefly discuss the purpose of the autocontrol.

12. Define major crossmatch and minor crossmatch.

13. Describe the immediate spin versus the antiglobulin crossmatches and specify under what circumstances each would be suitable.

14. Discuss the advantages and the limitations of the electronic (computer) crossmatch.

15. Describe five criteria that should be met before implementing the electronic crossmatch.

16. Describe two possible explanations for the following serologic reaction patterns:

    Positive antibody screen; Positive major crossmatch; Negative autocontrol

    Negative antibody screen; Positive major crossmatch; Negative autocontrol

    Positive antibody screen; Positive major crossmatch; Positive autocontrol

17. Discuss the limitations of compatibility testing.

18. Describe three methods to overcome the problem of a sample that exhibited a prolonged clotting time.

19. Discuss the process of informed consent.

20. Compare and contrast the following types of blood filters:

    Standard blood filters   Leukocyte reduction filters
    Microaggregate filters

21. Briefly discuss the following aspects of blood administration:

    Compatible IV fluids   Pressure devices
    Electromechanical infusion   Blood warming devices
      pumps

22. Describe in detail the patient identification process before transfusion.

23. Apply current standards with regard to the retention of blood banking records.

24. Discuss ways in which blood usage can be conserved and utilization monitored.

OVERVIEW

The goal of pretransfusion **compatibility testing** is to provide the patient with a beneficial and safe transfusion. A compatibility test has been thought of as synonymous with the major crossmatch, but the crossmatch is just one aspect of compatibility testing. The procedures that constitute compatibility testing are briefly stated as follows:

1. Positive identification of patient and patient's blood sample.
2. Review of patient's past blood bank history and records.
3. ABO and Rh typing of patient.
4. Screening of the patient's serum or plasma for **unexpected antibodies.**
5. Confirmation of the ABO group of red cell units and the Rh type of Rh-negative red cell units.
6. Major serologic crossmatch between the donor red cells and the patient's serum/plasma or a computer crossmatch.
7. Labeling of products with the patient's identifying information.

Compatibility testing: All serologic testing and clerical checks involved in determining compatibility between a potential recipient and donor. Compatibility testing policies are based on prevailing standards of practice and ensure a high probability of a successful transfusion outcome but cannot guarantee safety.

Unexpected antibodies: Red cell antibodies that, unlike the naturally occurring anti-A or anti-B, are not routinely present in the serum and are generally a result of red cell stimulation (transfusion or pregnancy).

Requirements for donor blood collecting, processing, testing, labeling, storage, and distribution are described in Chapters 8, 9, and 10.

Properly performed compatibility procedures can usually ensure ABO-compatible blood for transfusion and detect most clinically significant unexpected antibodies that are capable of causing red blood cell (RBC) destruction. Serologic testing, however, cannot guarantee in vivo red cell survival. For example, testing cannot prevent a delayed transfusion reaction that may occur when undetected levels of antibody are present in the patient's pretransfusion specimen. However, the required review of previous records may reveal that the patient should receive specially typed "antigen-negative" units because of the presence in the past of a clinically significant antibody. Although most transfusions are tolerated without an adverse response, compatibility testing cannot prevent the patient from becoming immunized to donor antigens.

PATIENT SAMPLE COLLECTION
Patient Request Forms

Positive identification of the patient and collection of a properly labeled blood sample begin with the form requesting the blood product (Fig. 11-1). The request can be on paper or electronic but it must contain sufficient information for positive identification of the patient. American Association of Blood Banks (AABB) Standards require that the request shall contain sufficient information to uniquely identify the patient, including two independent identifiers.[1] Most facilities use the patient's first and last name and a unique identification number. Each facility should have a written policy and procedure and may routinely include other information as part of the facility's request form. The patient's location, age, and gender are frequently part of the required information on request forms used in many facilities. Request forms should also contain the amount of blood or component requested, as well as the date of request and date of anticipated transfusion. The patient's diagnosis and information concerning the patient's previous history of transfusion or pregnancy are of considerable help to the transfusion service if a problem is encountered.[2] Handwritten requests can be used, but more problems are encountered with legibility than with printed requests. Incomplete, inaccurate, or illegible forms must not be accepted by the transfusion service.

Patient Identification

Positive identification of the recipient when collecting the recipient's blood sample is critical to safe blood transfusion. Each facility must develop and implement policies and procedures for patient identification and specimen collection. Most hospitals identify patients with an identification wristband.[2] The information on the blood request form is compared with the patient's wristband identification. A blood sample must not be collected if there is a discrepancy between the two. Name plates on the door of the room, on the bed, on the wall by the bed, or on charts or records near the patient must not be used for positive identification of the recipient.

In some circumstances it may not be possible for the patient to wear an identification wristband. Circumstances making the use of wristbands difficult include patients with extensive burns, extremely premature infants, or inaccessible wristbands during surgery. Some facilities allow identifying information to be placed on a patient's ankle or forehead. Outpatients may be identified with the use of a wristband, or alternative methods may be used. Alternative methods may include use of a driver's license or other photographic identification.[2]

Bar-coded systems for increased safety are also available. The patient identifying information is contained both visually and in bar code format on both the wristband and the patient blood specimen labels. After drawing and labeling the patient sample at the bedside, a handheld bar code scanner is used to verify that the label on the patient specimen is identical to that on the patient wristband. There are also

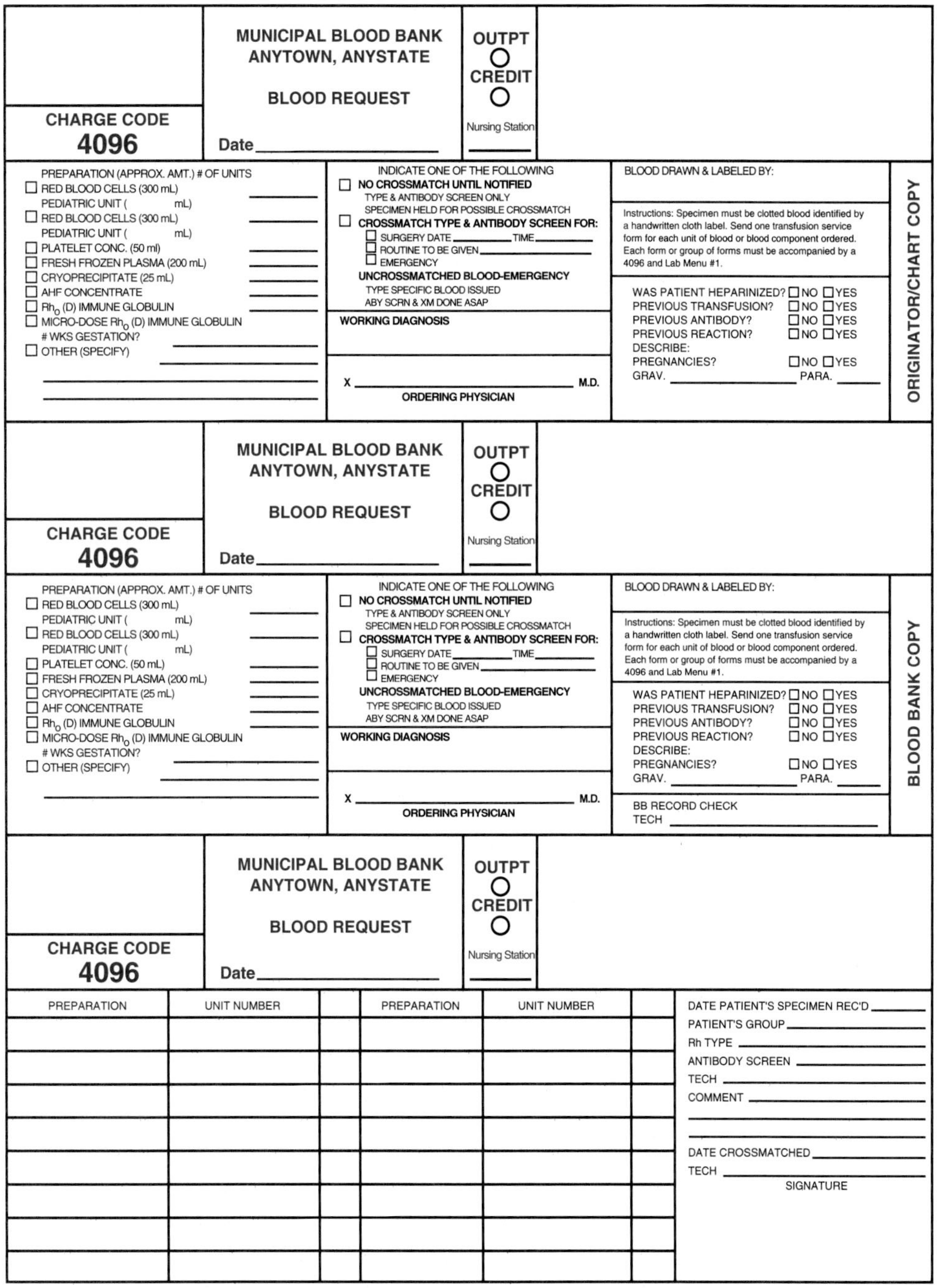

MUNICIPAL BLOOD BANK
ANYTOWN, ANYSTATE
BLOOD REQUEST
OUTPT ○ CREDIT ○ Nursing Station ____
CHARGE CODE 4096
Date ____

PREPARATION (APPROX. AMT.) # OF UNITS
☐ RED BLOOD CELLS (300 mL) ____
PEDIATRIC UNIT (mL)
☐ RED BLOOD CELLS (300 mL) ____
PEDIATRIC UNIT (mL)
☐ PLATELET CONC. (50 ml) ____
☐ FRESH FROZEN PLASMA (200 mL) ____
☐ CRYOPRECIPITATE (25 mL) ____
☐ AHF CONCENTRATE ____
☐ Rh_o (D) IMMUNE GLOBULIN ____
☐ MICRO-DOSE Rh_o (D) IMMUNE GLOBULIN
WKS GESTATION?
☐ OTHER (SPECIFY) ____

INDICATE ONE OF THE FOLLOWING
☐ **NO CROSSMATCH UNTIL NOTIFIED**
TYPE & ANTIBODY SCREEN ONLY
SPECIMEN HELD FOR POSSIBLE CROSSMATCH
☐ **CROSSMATCH TYPE & ANTIBODY SCREEN FOR:**
☐ SURGERY DATE ____ TIME ____
☐ ROUTINE TO BE GIVEN ____
☐ EMERGENCY
UNCROSSMATCHED BLOOD-EMERGENCY
TYPE SPECIFIC BLOOD ISSUED
ABY SCRN & XM DONE ASAP
WORKING DIAGNOSIS
X ____ M.D.
ORDERING PHYSICIAN

BLOOD DRAWN & LABELED BY:
Instructions: Specimen must be clotted blood identified by a handwritten cloth label. Send one transfusion service form for each unit of blood or blood component ordered. Each form or group of forms must be accompanied by a 4096 and Lab Menu #1.
WAS PATIENT HEPARINIZED? ☐NO ☐YES
PREVIOUS TRANSFUSION? ☐NO ☐YES
PREVIOUS ANTIBODY? ☐NO ☐YES
PREVIOUS REACTION? ☐NO ☐YES
DESCRIBE:
PREGNANCIES? ☐NO ☐YES
GRAV. ____ PARA. ____
ORIGINATOR/CHART COPY

MUNICIPAL BLOOD BANK
ANYTOWN, ANYSTATE
BLOOD REQUEST
OUTPT ○ CREDIT ○ Nursing Station ____
CHARGE CODE 4096
Date ____

PREPARATION (APPROX. AMT.) # OF UNITS
☐ RED BLOOD CELLS (300 mL) ____
PEDIATRIC UNIT (mL)
☐ RED BLOOD CELLS (300 mL) ____
PEDIATRIC UNIT (mL)
☐ PLATELET CONC. (50 mL) ____
☐ FRESH FROZEN PLASMA (200 mL) ____
☐ CRYOPRECIPITATE (25 mL) ____
☐ AHF CONCENTRATE ____
☐ Rh_o (D) IMMUNE GLOBULIN ____
☐ MICRO-DOSE Rh_o (D) IMMUNE GLOBULIN
WKS GESTATION?
☐ OTHER (SPECIFY) ____

INDICATE ONE OF THE FOLLOWING
☐ **NO CROSSMATCH UNTIL NOTIFIED**
TYPE & ANTIBODY SCREEN ONLY
SPECIMEN HELD FOR POSSIBLE CROSSMATCH
☐ **CROSSMATCH TYPE & ANTIBODY SCREEN FOR:**
☐ SURGERY DATE ____ TIME ____
☐ ROUTINE TO BE GIVEN ____
☐ EMERGENCY
UNCROSSMATCHED BLOOD-EMERGENCY
TYPE SPECIFIC BLOOD ISSUED
ABY SCRN & XM DONE ASAP
WORKING DIAGNOSIS
X ____ M.D.
ORDERING PHYSICIAN

BLOOD DRAWN & LABELED BY:
Instructions: Specimen must be clotted blood identified by a handwritten cloth label. Send one transfusion service form for each unit of blood or blood component ordered. Each form or group of forms must be accompanied by a 4096 and Lab Menu #1.
WAS PATIENT HEPARINIZED? ☐NO ☐YES
PREVIOUS TRANSFUSION? ☐NO ☐YES
PREVIOUS ANTIBODY? ☐NO ☐YES
PREVIOUS REACTION? ☐NO ☐YES
DESCRIBE:
PREGNANCIES? ☐NO ☐YES
GRAV. ____ PARA. ____
BB RECORD CHECK
TECH ____
BLOOD BANK COPY

MUNICIPAL BLOOD BANK
ANYTOWN, ANYSTATE
BLOOD REQUEST
OUTPT ○ CREDIT ○ Nursing Station ____
CHARGE CODE 4096
Date ____

PREPARATION	UNIT NUMBER		PREPARATION	UNIT NUMBER	

DATE PATIENT'S SPECIMEN REC'D ____
PATIENT'S GROUP ____
Rh TYPE ____
ANTIBODY SCREEN ____
TECH ____
COMMENT ____
DATE CROSSMATCHED ____
TECH ____
SIGNATURE

Fig. 11-1 Blood request form (three-part form).

systems (PatientSafe-Transfuse ID, AMTSystems) available that use a personal digital assistant (PDA) fitted with a bar code reader to interpret a bar-coded patient wristband and generate, through a portable printer, a sample label at the patient's bedside.[3,4]

In an emergency, when the patient's identity is unknown, positive identification may be accomplished by attaching a temporary wristband with an emergency identification number preprinted on the band (Fig. 11-2). Stickers with the same preprinted emergency number are placed on all samples drawn and on the blood request form. The temporary band should not be removed until proper identification has been attached to the patient and the emergency number cross-referenced with the

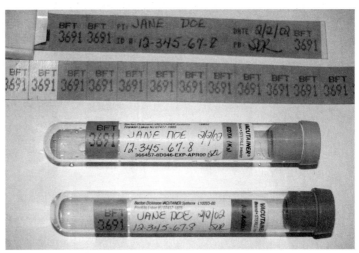

Fig. 11-2 Blood band identification system.

patient's name and identification number. Identification systems using preprinted numbers for the wristband, samples, and all forms are commercially available.

Patient Blood Samples

Compatibility testing may be performed on either serum or plasma. One or the other may be preferred depending on the method of testing. For example, plasma is the specimen of choice when using gel technology but may sometimes create technical problems in tube tests.[2] Small fibrin clots that may be difficult to distinguish from true agglutination are frequently found in plasma specimens. However, difficulty may also be encountered with a serum sample if the patient has a prolonged clotting time or has been heparinized. In these samples, clotting may be incomplete. Adding thrombin or protamine sulfate to the sample usually corrects the problem, or an anticoagulated sample can be collected.[2]

To prevent contamination of a sample with intravenous fluids, venous samples should not be drawn from above the infusion site but may be drawn from below the site or preferably from the other arm. If blood must be obtained from an infusion line, care must be taken to flush the tubing with saline and to discard the first 5 to 10 mL of blood drawn before collecting the sample to be tested.[5]

Labeling of Samples

Blood samples must be labeled with two unique patient identifiers and the date of collection.[2] Usually this will be the patient's first and last names and identification number. Handwritten labels must be legible and written with indelible ink. Preprinted labels are acceptable if the phlebotomist has compared the label with the patient's identification band item by item. The label must be applied to the stoppered test tube before leaving the patient's bedside. There must be a mechanism to identify the person who drew the blood.[1] This can be accomplished by including the phlebotomist's signature, initials, or code number on the **blood sample label** (Fig. 11-3) and/or request form. Signing the request form provides a more permanent record of this information.

When the blood sample reaches the transfusion service, a qualified person must confirm that all identifying information on the blood sample matches that on the request form. If incomplete or illegible blood request forms and/or sample labels are received or a discrepancy is found, a new blood sample must be obtained.[1,2] It is unacceptable for anyone to correct identifying information on an incorrectly labeled sample. Each laboratory should establish policies and procedures that define identifying information and describe how to document receipt of mislabeled specimens.[2]

Blood sample label: A label completed and attached to the sample before leaving the patient's bedside. This label must contain the following minimum information: two unique identifiers (usually the patient's name and identification number) and the date of collection. There must also be a mechanism to determine who drew the specimen.

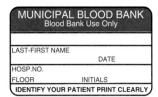

Fig. 11-3 Blood sample label.

Appearance and Age of Sample

Hemolyzed serum samples should be avoided. Mechanical hemolysis resulting from difficulty in drawing the specimen may prevent detection of hemolysis caused by the interaction of a hemolytic antibody with antigen-positive red blood cells. Antibodies capable of producing hemolysis have specificity in the ABO, P, Lewis, Kidd, or Vel blood group system. If a patient is truly hemolyzing intravascularly, either because of autoantibody, alloantibody, or another clinical condition such as hemolytic uremic syndrome, it may not be possible to obtain a sample that is not hemolyzed. If a hemolyzed sample must be used, a comparison between the size of the cell button remaining after testing the patient's serum versus a patient red cell control of saline or 6% **albumin** may demonstrate possible additional red cell destruction. Test results observed with lipemic serum can also be difficult to evaluate. Each facility should have a procedure describing the indications for using hemolyzed or lipemic specimens.

Patient blood samples used in compatibility testing should be collected no more than 3 days before the intended transfusion unless the patient has not been pregnant or transfused within the preceding 3 months. If the patient's transfusion or pregnancy history is unavailable, compatibility tests must be performed on blood samples collected within 3 days of RBC transfusions.[1] This is to ensure that the sample used for testing reflects the patient's current immunologic status because recent transfusion or pregnancy may stimulate production of unexpected antibodies. Because it is not possible to predict whether or when such antibodies will appear, a 3-day limit has been selected as an arbitrary interval expected to be both practical and safe. Each facility should establish a policy that defines the length of time specimens may be used. Many laboratories prefer to standardize their operations by setting a 3-day limit on all specimens used for pretransfusion testing. If specimens are used beyond 3 days, the transfusion service should have documentation that the patient has not been transfused or pregnant within the preceding 3 months. Testing of stored specimens must be performed with reagents approved for use with older specimens. Policies should be based on the specimen storage limitations in the reagent manufacturer's information circulars.[2]

Blood Sample Storage and Retention

The patient's stoppered blood sample, as well as a stoppered or sealed sample of each donor unit transfused, must be stored at 1° to 6° C for at least 7 days after the date of transfusion.[1,2] Because many delayed hemolytic reactions are not demonstrable clinically until 10 days after transfusion, a facility may elect to store patient blood specimens for 14 days or longer. This is done to be certain that the pretransfusion specimen and donor specimens are available if retesting becomes necessary.

COMPATIBILITY PROTOCOLS
Recipient Serologic Testing

Blood submitted for compatibility testing must be tested for ABO and RH type and unexpected antibodies to red cell antigens.[1] Past records of all patient serologic test results must be maintained and compared with testing on the current specimen

Albumin: A protein-potentiating agent that enhances the reactions of some clinically significant alloantibodies. Albumin reagents such as 22%, 30%, and polymerized bovine albumin are available commercially. Although it is of historical significance, albumin is rarely used in today's blood bank testing because newer reagents allow for similar enhancements accomplished with shorter incubation times.

and the comparison must be documented. Information must be reviewed for history of a clinically significant red cell antibody or any other problem that may affect safe transfusion of the patient.[1] Maintaining paper records and archiving patient testing information in a computerized laboratory information system are the major methods used for record retention. A backup information retrieval process must be available to recover the donor and patient's electronically captured data when the system is unavailable because of planned or unanticipated down time. Standards for record retention are established by the AABB. The reader can find the most recent requirements in the current edition of the *Standards for Blood Banks and Transfusion Services.*[1]

After completion of compatibility testing, interpretations of current testing must be compared with records of previous ABO and Rh typing performed in the last 12 months as well as previous antibody detection results. This review of historical data allows for discovery of technical or clerical errors before blood is issued for transfusion. Should a discrepancy be detected between previous results and current patient testing, the collection process must be investigated along with the patient's medical history. Transfusion fatalities can occur due to ABO incompatibility as a result of patient or sample misidentification.[6] A new sample may need to be collected from the patient to resolve the problem. Discrepancies may also occur in situations such as neonatal exchange transfusion, massive transfusion, and hematopoietic progenitor cell transplant from a donor who has a different ABO type than the patient. Transfusion of non–type-specific platelets, coagulation products, and intravenous immunoglobulin (IVIg) may result in the passive transfer of unexpected blood group alloantibodies, resulting in a discrepancy during current testing.[7]

ABO and Rh Typing

Obtaining an accurate ABO grouping for a patient is the most significant serologic test performed before transfusion. Serologic testing of the patient must include both red cell (forward) and serum tests (reverse). Slide, tube, micro plate and gel column tests can be used for routine testing of the ABO and Rh type. The ABO group must be determined by testing the recipient's red cells with anti-A and anti-B typing sera and by testing the recipient's serum or plasma for expected antibodies with A_1 and B red cells on a current sample.[1,2] If a discrepancy between the cell typing and serum/plasma confirmation is detected, the problem should be resolved by additional testing before blood is given. When time is limited and resolution of the typing discrepancy will exceed the judicious need for transfusion of the patient, type O Red Blood Cells should be transfused.

The Rh type must be determined with anti-D typing reagents. To prevent incorrect identification of an Rh-negative recipient as Rh-positive because of autoantibodies or abnormal serum proteins, a control system appropriate to the anti-D reagent in use should be followed as directed by manufacturer's instructions. For example, the manufacturer's diluent is the appropriate control system for high-protein slide and rapid tube test anti-D. Antibody-coated red cells may agglutinate spontaneously in the high-protein media of slide or rapid tube test Rh-typing reagents. The control system for low-protein chemically modified IgG anti-D or monoclonal anti-D may be a negative reaction with anti-A or anti-B, or a negative autocontrol consisting of the patient's red cells and serum. If all tests are positive (patient appears AB+) a control using 6% to 8% albumin or the manufacturer's diluent may be used as a negative control.[2] In any case in which the appropriately selected Rh control system is positive, the Rh typing is invalid and the patient should be considered an Rh-negative recipient until the problem can be resolved. Resolution of the problem may be accomplished by using washed cell suspensions or by switching to a different Rh typing reagent such as chemically modified IgG reagents, monoclonal anti-D, or saline IgM reagents. In some cases, antigen-antibody

Refer to Chapter 3 for a discussion of the ABO blood group system.

dissociation procedures that do not destroy the D antigen may be required before accurate Rh typing can be determined.

The presence of antibody-coated red cells confirmed by a positive direct antiglobulin test (DAT) is especially important to document if the patient is tested for weak D. A positive DAT would invalidate a weak D test or any other antigen typing that requires an antiglobulin procedure to demonstrate the presence of the antigen. The test for weak D is usually considered unnecessary when testing the recipient. The transfusion service may elect to extend testing for all Rh-negative patients to determine if they test positive for the weak D antigen. If so, Rh-positive blood should be selected for transfusion in patients positive for the weak D phenotype in order to conserve the Rh-negative blood inventory.

Selection of Donor Units
ABO, Rh, and Other Antigens

Selection of blood and blood components for transfusion should in most cases be the same blood type as the patient. When **type-specific blood and components** are unavailable or other circumstances do not allow their use, it may be necessary to make alternative selections. The red blood cells selected for transfusion must be compatible with the patient's plasma. This usually means that group O red cells are selected. The exception occurs when the recipient is blood group AB. The choice of an alternative blood group for a group AB recipient is extended to A, B, or O red cells. Depending on the inventory available, one of the three should be selected for a given recipient. Because group A is more often available in quantity than group B, the first choice tends to be group A. Group O should not be used if another blood group can be used. Group O is the only choice for group O recipients and the alternative choice for both group A and group B. Inventory demands and local supply will often dictate the type of compatible blood selected for a recipient at any given time.

When a component contains 2 mL or more of red cells, the donor's red cells must be ABO compatible with the recipient's plasma.[2] When possible, the ABO antibodies found in transfused plasma should be compatible with the recipient's red cells. If ABO-specific blood and components are unavailable for transfusion, alternative selections are available (Table 11-1).

Rh-positive blood components should routinely be selected for D-positive patients. Although Rh-negative blood can be given to Rh-positive patients, it should be reserved for D-negative patients. One must keep in mind that it is good inventory management to transfuse Rh-negative units nearing expiration to Rh-positive

Refer to Chapter 5 for a discussion of the Rh blood group system. Chapter 13 provides additional information on the resolution of the more commonly encountered serologic problems.

Type-specific blood and components: Refers to the selection of blood/components of the identical type as the recipient's. When transfusing whole blood, type-specific blood must be used.

TABLE 11-1 Selection of Components when ABO-Identical Donors are not Available

Component	ABO Requirements
Whole Blood	Must be identical to that of the recipient
Red Blood Cells	Must be compatible with the recipient's plasma
Granulocytes, pheresis	Must be compatible with the recipient's plasma
Fresh Frozen Plasma	Should be compatible with the recipient's red cells
Platelets, pheresis	All ABO groups acceptable; components compatible with the recipient's red cells preferred
Cryoprecipitated AHF	All ABO groups acceptable

Reprinted with permission from Brecher ME (ed): Technical Manual of the American Association of Blood Banks, 14th ed. Bethesda, MD, American Association of Blood Banks, 2002, p 389.

Refer to Chapter 16 for an in-depth discussion of the use of Rh immune globulin.

recipients rather than wasting a limited resource. Occasionally, ABO-compatible Rh-negative blood is unavailable. The risk of immunization is greater than 80% for the D antigen.[8] This is particularly important if the recipient is female and is not past childbearing age. It may be permissible to transfuse Rh-negative males and females beyond childbearing age with Rh-positive blood provided they do not have any anti-D present in their sera. When Rh-negative females of childbearing age are transfused with D-positive components it may be preferable, depending on the volume of red cell transfused, to consider administering **Rh immune globulin.** The risk versus the benefit of transfusion for the patient must always be taken into consideration when deviating from standard operating procedure. The transfusion service should have procedures to direct staff in product selection when type-specific products are unavailable. When this occurs, it usually requires the notification and/or approval with documentation from the blood bank's medical director.

Red cell antigens other than ABO and D are not routinely considered when selecting blood products for transfusion. These antigens are taken into consideration when clinically significant unexpected red cell antibodies are present or have been previously identified. In this case, antigen-negative red cell products should be selected for crossmatching and subsequent transfusion.[2] If the antibody identified reacts at a temperature below 37° C, it is considered clinically insignificant and antigen-negative blood is not required for transfusion. If the crossmatch of a cold-reacting antibody can be shown to be "crossmatch compatible" in tests performed at 37° C, the units can be safely transfused. When the antibody is found to be weakly reactive, demonstrating dosage characteristics, or was previously identified but is no longer reactive, reagent antisera must be used to screen donor units in order to select the necessary antigen-negative phenotypes before crossmatch. When the antibody in the patient's or donor's serum reacts well with known antigen-positive heterozygous red cells, it can be used for antigen-negative phenotyping when a commercial antiserum of that specificity is not available. When licensed reagents are not available, stored serum specimens from donors and/or patients may be used for screening units, especially when testing for high-incidence or uncommon antigens.[2] The blood bank medical director and the patient's physician should be consulted when compatible units cannot be found for transfusion.

Repeat Testing on Donor Units

The results of donor testing performed by the collecting facility must be clearly indicated on the label affixed to the donor unit. The transfusion service performing the crossmatch must confirm the ABO group of all units of whole blood and red blood cell components and the Rh type of units labeled Rh-negative. Testing must be performed using a sample obtained from an attached donor tubing segment.[2] Tests for weak D, tests for unexpected antibodies, and tests intended to prevent disease transmission do not have to be repeated. To detect labeling errors, confirmatory testing should be done after the original ABO and Rh label has been affixed to the units. This testing must be performed even when the units are drawn and processed by the transfusing facility because it serves as a confirmation of the testing and labeling process. Discrepancies must be reported to the collecting facility and the problem resolved before issue of the blood for transfusion.[1,2]

Antibody Screening Procedure
Overview

Clinically significant antibodies: Red cell alloantibodies that react at 37° C and are capable of causing decreased survival of transfused red cells.

Methods for detection of unexpected antibodies in the patient's serum or plasma using reagent red blood cells that are not pooled should demonstrate **clinically significant antibodies** and should include 37° C incubation and an antiglobulin test.[1] Unexpected antibodies are those present in the patient's serum in addition to the expected anti-A and/or anti-B. Red cell antibodies are produced by exposure to foreign red cell antigens by previous transfusion and/or pregnancy. These antibodies are often referred to as alloantibodies. For an antibody to be considered clinically significant, the specificity must be associated with hemolytic transfusion reactions or decreased survival of transfused incompatible red cells, or result in hemolytic disease of the newborn or some other adverse clinical event. Most of the clinically significant antibodies are optimally reactive at 37° C and/or are detected by the antiglobulin test. Occurrence of these antibodies may become evident in testing as observed agglutination or hemolysis. AABB Standards require that a control system using red blood cells sensitized with IgG must be applied to each antiglobulin test interpreted as negative in order to identify a false-negative test.[1,2] A false-negative antiglobulin test may occur as a result of failure to add the antiglobulin reagent or inactivation of the antiglobulin reagent. When a transfusion service selects an alternative methodology that has been approved by the Food and Drug Administration (FDA) that does not allow for the addition of IgG-sensitized red cells to be added to each negative antiglobulin test, controls should be used in accordance with the manufacturer's written instructions.[1] Gel column technology is an example of this type of methodology.

Antibody Detection

The patient's serum or plasma is usually tested against a set of commercially supplied single-donor group O reagent cells (Fig. 11-4) whose red cell phenotypes or antigen profiles have been carefully selected. **Single-donor screening cells** offer increased sensitivity over pooled screening cells. The following 18 antigens are required to be present on at least one of the screening cells: D, C, E, c, e, M, N, S, s, P_1, Le^a, Le^b, K, k, Fy^a, Fy^b, Jk^a, and Jk^b.[9] Because antibodies demonstrating dosage react more strongly with red cells containing a double dose (homozygous) of an antigen than with red cells containing a single dose (heterozygous) of an antigen, an effort is made to use screening cells with a double dose of the clinically significant antigens, particularly in the Rh, Duffy, and Kidd systems. This may require the use of red cells from three donors instead of two in order to be able to test donor reagent cells of the appropriate phenotypes. For example, in Figure 11-4, the two-cell set does not possess homozygous cells for Fy^b or Jk^b. There is no requirement, however, that the required antigens be a homozygous expression. In cases in which such homozygous cells are not available for testing, it is important that the technologist be aware of the effect of dosage and carefully interpret all test results, especially those of weak-reacting antibodies.

The presence of selected low-incidence antigens on reagent red cells allows for detection of antibodies directed against antigens that may be missing on donor red cells selected for crossmatch. Nevertheless, there is no requirement that low-incidence antigens such as V, C_w, or Kp^a be present on screening cells. If a low-frequency antigen is present on the donor red blood cells, it may or may not be detected depending on the method used for the crossmatch.

Methods used for pretransfusion antibody detection are selected to demonstrate clinically significant coating, hemolyzing, and agglutinating antibodies that react at 37° C. Antibodies that react at temperatures below body temperature are usually not

Single-donor screening cells: Cells from individual group O donors selected for their antigen typing configuration. Two or three unpooled cells are selected to screen for most of the commonly encountered red cell alloantibodies and are used for routine antibody detection.

VIAL	Donor	Rh-Hr								Kell						Duffy		Kidd		Lewis		P	MN				Luth-eran		Xg				
		D	C	c	E	e	f	V	C^w	K	k	Kp^a	Kp^b	Js^a	Js^b	Fy^a	Fy^b	Jk^a	Jk^b	Le^a	Le^b	P_1	M	N	S	s	Lu^a	Lu^b	Xg^a				
I	R_1R_1	+	+	0	0	+	0	0	0	+	+	0	+	0	+	+	0	+	+	0	+	0	+	+	+	+	0	+	+				
II	R_2R_2	+	0	+	+	0	0	0	0	0	+	0	+	0	+	+	+	+	0	+	0	+	+	0	+	+	+	+	0				

Fig. 11-4 Antigram of a two-cell antibody screening report.

considered to be clinically significant because the reaction does not occur during in vivo transfusion conditions.[1] For this reason, most cold-reacting antibodies such as autoanti-I, anti-IH, anti-M, anti-N, and anti-P_1 are considered to be "nuisance" antibodies.

Cold antibodies may, however, bind complement at a lower temperature. This becomes a significant consideration when a patient's body temperature is lowered during a surgical procedure such as open-heart surgery or is hypothermic as in traumas with cold exposures. Seemingly insignificant cold-reacting antibodies then become potentially clinically significant.

Selection of Antiglobulin Reagents

The selection of the antiglobulin reagent is usually based on a particular laboratory's experience with the antibody-detection technique in routine use. The ability to detect clinically significant complement-dependent antibodies that can be detected and identified only by their ability to bind complement (e.g., Kidd system) must be weighed against the problems involved with the increased detection of "nuisance" antibodies that bind complement but are not clinically significant. For this reason, some transfusion services elect to avoid complement detection in the antiglobulin phase by using monospecific anti-IgG antiglobulin rather than polyspecific antihuman globulin (AHG) containing anti-IgG and anti-C3d. If this option is selected, the possibility exists that some examples of antibodies that can be detected only by their abilities to bind complement will not be identified.[10,11] The decision to use monospecific anti-IgG to avoid complement-binding "nuisance" antibodies is usually combined with the selection of screening cells that are homozygous in antigen expression whenever possible.[10,12-14]

Depending on the type of antiglobulin reagent used, complement may be detected in the antiglobulin phase after 37° C incubation even though the cold antibody has already dissociated from the red cells. Either monospecific anti-IgG or polyspecific antiglobulin reagent containing anti-IgG and anti-C3d may be used for testing. Polyspecific AHG will detect complement bound by clinically significant antibodies, particularly in the Kidd and Duffy blood group system, but also nonspecific and/or insignificant proteins. Using polyspecific AHG routinely can result in additional testing of insignificant reactions, causing delays, increasing costs, and wasting valuable technical time, while providing little clinical importance to improve patient care.

Antibody screening of the patient's serum or plasma using the **indirect antiglobulin technique** (IAT) may be performed before or concurrently with the crossmatch. One advantage of completing the antibody screening before the selection of donor units for the crossmatch is that the antibody can be detected and identified and antigen-negative units selected for the crossmatch. If no clinically significant antibody is detected and there is no record of previous detection of such antibodies, only serologic testing to detect ABO incompatibility is required.[1]

Limitations of Antibody Screen

Antibody detection tests have proven to be very effective in the detection of potentially clinically significant antibodies. If the antibody screen is negative, the confidence level is over 99% that the crossmatch will also be compatible.[15-19] AABB Standards state that if no clinically significant unexpected antibodies are detected and there is no record of previous detection of such antibodies, only serologic testing to detect ABO incompatibility is required; that is, antiglobulin testing is not required when the crossmatch is performed. A few limitations of the antibody screen technique should be mentioned.[20] As mentioned previously, failure to detect an antibody may be due to dosage; that is, a weak antibody may be demonstrable only when a homozygous cell for the specificity is tested. Another reason for failure to detect a clinically significant antibody is that the antigen is not present on the screening cells. Low-incidence antigens such as Cw, V, Kp[a], Js[a], and Wr[a] are rarely

Antibodies that react at temperatures below 37° C are generally not clinically significant, but they interfere with the interpretation of routine serologic testing. Cold-reacting alloantibodies are discussed in Chapter 6. Cold-reacting autoantibodies are discussed in Chapters 4 and 18.

Indirect antiglobulin technique: The use of antihuman globulin reagents to detect red cell–bound antibodies. This technique is required by the AABB in routine pretransfusion testing. The antiglobulin test is described in detail in Chapter 2.

present on the screening cells. However, selection of donor units that possess the low-incidence antigen is also unlikely. Because the screening cells are group O, passive transfer of an unexpected ABO antibody in the patient's serum may not be detected until the crossmatch (in the case of non–group O) is completed.

Techniques
Saline

Several techniques are in use to detect clinically significant antibodies. The simplest and most inexpensive is the saline indirect antiglobulin technique. A ratio of two drops of the patient's serum or plasma to one drop of a 2% to 5% reagent red cell suspension constitutes the basic test. (Refer to the manufacturer's directions and your institutional procedures for testing methods.) The test may be centrifuged immediately and/or incubated at room temperature before centrifugation. However, a room temperature incubation phase is often deleted from an antibody detection test in order to avoid finding cold antibodies that are not clinically significant. Incubation of the serum-cell mixture at 37° C usually for a minimum of 30 minutes detects clinically significant antibodies that are demonstrable by direct agglutination or hemolysis. Frequently antibodies bind to red cells at 37° C but are not detected until the antiglobulin phase of testing. The sensitivity of this test is enhanced by increasing the length of incubation time at 37°C up to 1 hour. Increasing the number of drops of serum added to the test when a weak antibody is suspected can also enhance testing. Given that time is usually a critical factor in pretransfusion testing, the saline method is not routinely used by most transfusion services because of the longer incubation time.

Albumin

The addition of a potentiator before incubation at 37° C is used by many workers to shorten the required incubation time at 37° C and enhance the sensitivity of antibody-detection tests. In the 1970s and early 1980s many workers added 22% bovine albumin to the serum-cell mixture. In particular, direct agglutination by Rh antibodies appears to be enhanced after 37° C incubation of the serum-cell mixture with albumin. This test usually consists of two drops of patient serum, two drops of 22% bovine albumin, and one drop of 2% to 5% red cells. An incubation time of 30 minutes is usually the optimal time recommended for the test.

Low Ionic Strength

When low ionic strength test conditions are used, the incubation time can be shortened to 10 minutes. A low ionic strength test environment increases the rate at which an antibody binds to red cell antigens with no loss of sensitivity.[21-24] This environment may be achieved by either suspending the red cells in an isotonic low ionic strength salt (LISS) solution or by using a low ionic strength additive reagent to the traditional serum-cell mixture before incubation at 37°C. LISS solutions can be prepared in the laboratory or are available commercially for use as wash solutions or additives. To maintain a low ionic strength environment, it is extremely important to follow the procedure recommended by the manufacturer or documented by the individual laboratory. Serologic pipettes and reagent droppers must be standardized to deliver drops of equal volume. If the number of drops of serum is increased to enhance sensitivity, the number of drops of LISS must be equally increased to avoid increasing the ionic strength of the mixture. LISS-suspended screening cells should be used only on the day of preparation because some antigens, Fy[a] in particular, may deteriorate rapidly in a low ionic environment.[25]

Enzymes

Enzyme techniques are not usually used for routine pretransfusion antibody detection because enzymes destroy some red cell antigens such as M, N, S, Fy[a], and

A number of factors affect the agglutination reaction. These are described in more detail in Chapter 2. Manufacturer's directions for serologic testing are based on research that has identified the ideal conditions for testing. It is important to follow these directions and the procedures outlined in your institutional procedures manual.

Enzyme techniques: Enhancement and differential detection techniques using proteolytic enzymes. Refer to Chapter 5 for further discussion of this methodology.

Fy^b. Therefore antibodies to these specificities would not be detected. Enzyme techniques are particularly useful in the identification of antibodies in the Rh and Kidd systems and are frequently used to enhance sensitivity in antibody identification procedures.

Other Methods

Low ionic polycation tests: The combination of red cell antibody uptake in a low ionic strength, low pH medium and the use of a chemical red cell aggregating agent. If antibody has coated the cells, the aggregation does not disperse.

Low ionic polycation tests such as the manual polybrene test (MPT)[26,27] and the low ionic polycation (LIP) test[28] have proven to be very sensitive tests requiring minimal incubation times. After the uptake of antibody by the red cells under low ionic conditions at low pH, Polybrene aggregates the red cells. The aggregation can be dispersed with sodium citrate but does not disperse if antibody is able to form bridges between adjacent red cells. In the LIP procedure, the aggregation is caused by protamine sulfate, which can be dispersed by a buffered salt solution. The problem that limits the widespread acceptance of low ionic polycation tests in most transfusion services is that it takes some practice to be comfortable dispersing aggregation to a possible negative or positive end point. Although these tests are associated with enhanced detection of Rh specificities, antibodies to Kell blood group antigens do not react well at the first stage of testing and are less reactive in the antiglobulin phase. They also have significant limitations in detecting ABO incompatibilities with A$_2$ and B donor cells.[29]

Polyethylene glycol (PEG): A commercially available enhancement reagent used for the detection and identification of weak IgG antibodies.

Polyethylene glycol (PEG) has been used by several laboratories as a potentiator of red cell antigen-antibody reactions.[30-32] PEG may be prepared as an additive solution in either phosphate-buffered saline at normal ionic strength or in a low ionic strength medium. Centrifugation of PEG with the serum–red cell mixture should be avoided. Because PEG tends to aggregate red cells, the test mixture may be examined after incubation for hemolysis but cannot be examined reliably for direct agglutination at any stage of the test. Consequently, IgM antibodies, especially those of the ABO and Lewis system, may have weak reactivity or be undetectable by this technique.[2,33] PEG does enhance the sensitivity of tests for the detection of clinically significant IgG antibodies including autoantibodies at the antiglobulin phase of testing. PEG also has been helpful in enhancing reaction strength of weak-reacting IgG antibodies.

Testing can also be performed using column (gel) technology or microplate systems using solid phase red cell adherence (SPRCA). Procedures vary and must be performed as described by the manufacturer's directions.

Automated instruments are available that can perform ABO/Rh and antibody screening tests using standard gel or microplate methodologies. The patient specimen tubes are labeled with bar-coded patient identification labels, and results can be printed or interfaced with the transfusion service computer system. One advantage of using an automated testing instrument is that the chance of specimen identification error in the laboratory is reduced.

Autologous Control

Autocontrol: A control test with the patient's own serum and cells run in parallel with antibody detection and compatibility testing. Positive autocontrols require further investigation.

In pretransfusion testing, the **autocontrol** and DAT are not required tests. Some workers believe that performing an autocontrol using the patient's own cells and serum can be very helpful in determining whether or not positive antibody screen results are due to alloantibodies, autoantibodies, rouleaux, or anomalous results. Particularly when time and/or sample is limited, this information influences the approach to be used in problem solving and/or antibody identification. Others find it of little value in routine testing and perform it only with antibody identification procedure.[34]

Crossmatch

As described earlier in this chapter, compatibility testing consists of many elements. The crossmatch procedure is only one component of the compatibility process, but the terms crossmatch and serologic compatibility testing are used interchangeably. There are different approaches to crossmatching donor units for transfusion. Regardless of what approach is selected, the method must demonstrate ABO incompatibility and clinically significant antibodies to red cell antigens.

Traditional crossmatching techniques usually employ testing that uses the patient's serum or plasma with the donor's red cells. While performing the antiglobulin phase of a crossmatch, it is uncommon to detect a clinically significant unexpected antibody when the antibody screen is negative. Some workers believe that performing a serologic crossmatch provides little benefit when the blood typing is appropriately performed and there is no current serologic evidence or history of a clinically significant antibody. The benefits realized by omitting antihuman globulin testing for the crossmatch are decreased workload, improved turnaround times, and reduced reagent costs.

In the past, when whole blood was readily available, crossmatch testing incorporated testing of both the patient's cells and plasma against the reciprocal elements of the donor unit. These tests are important from a historical standpoint. The terms remain in use, and the technologist should be familiar with their meanings and significance. These tests are referred to as the **major crossmatch** and **minor crossmatch.**

The major crossmatch, using the antiglobulin technique, mixed cells suspended in saline from the originally attached donor segment with the patient's serum or plasma. This testing continues to be performed today to ensure compatibility when the patient has a history of or currently exhibits a clinically significant antibody.

The minor crossmatch involves testing the saline-suspended red cells of the patient with the plasma of the donor unit. The need for this test has been eliminated because donor units are screened for the presence of significant antibodies and are not included in general inventory if an antibody is identified. Also the majority of blood is transfused as Red Blood Cells with minimal donor plasma present in the unit. Inclusion of a minor crossmatch has little value and complicates the compatibility procedure.

Techniques

The method used for the major crossmatch may be different from that chosen for the antibody screen, but more often the same method is used. The immediate-spin crossmatch or the computer (electronic) crossmatch may be used as the primary method only if the patient has no present or previous clinically significant red cell alloantibodies.[1] If clinically significant alloantibodies are or have been present, the crossmatch technique selected must include incubation at 37° C followed by the antiglobulin test.

If possible, problems should be detected and resolved before the actual crossmatch so that appropriate units can be selected for the crossmatch. For example, if the crossmatch method chosen to demonstrate ABO compatibility is an immediate-spin room temperature reading, the same immediate-spin room temperature technique should be included as part of the antibody screen. This is done in order to anticipate what will be detected when the crossmatch is performed. The same principle holds true for the technique used to enhance antigen-antibody reactions (albumin, LISS) or the choice of an antiglobulin reagent. The results of the antibody screen should be consistent with the results obtained with the crossmatch when carried through to the AHG phase. The rationale for what method is selected is that it should provide a product that will be the safest and most beneficial to the patient. Each institution should detail these methods in its procedures manual.

Immediate-Spin Crossmatch

The immediate-spin crossmatch is the simplest and most frequently used method to demonstrate ABO compatibility. This method, also referred to as the **abbreviated**

Major crossmatch: A procedure used to determine compatibility between red cells of the donor and the serum (plasma) of the recipient.

Minor crossmatch: A procedure used to determine compatibility between the serum (plasma) of the donor and the red cells of the recipient. This test is no longer used routinely but has historical significance.

Abbreviated crossmatch: An immediate-spin, saline major crossmatch used to determine ABO compatibility in patients with no demonstrable clinically significant antibodies and a negative history of antibody formation. Under some conditions, this determination of ABO compatibility can also be accomplished by an electronic (computer) crossmatch.

crossmatch, may be performed if (1) no clinically significant unexpected antibodies are detected in the antibody screen using reagent red blood cells that are not pooled, and (2) there is no record of previous detection of clinically significant unexpected antibodies.

Studies have shown that the antibody screen is more than 99% effective in preventing the occurrence of an incompatible transfusion.[35-37] The type and antibody screen in conjunction with the immediate-spin crossmatch as a routine procedure attempts to simplify compatibility testing and encourage the use of **type and screen** ordering practices.[15-20]

The procedure requires the patient's serum to be mixed with saline-suspended red cells at room temperature. The tube is centrifuged immediately. When making the cell or red cell suspension for testing, it should be washed and resuspended to a 2% to 4% concentration in saline. Many workers prefer a weaker cell suspension in which agglutination can easily be observed.

It is important to note that the three different techniques of modified tube testing, gel column, and microplate systems using SPRCA are different methodologies and cannot be used to explain, resolve, or validate unexpected results obtained by any one method compared with the other. A number of antibodies have been shown to react by one or two methods, but not all of them. Some antibodies are reactive only in PEG/IAT, some only in solid-phase testing, and some only in gel.[33] Each of the technologies has advantages and limitations that one must know when implementing any of these methodologies into routine compatibility testing.

Antiglobulin Crossmatch

Many workers add the same potentiator (i.e., LISS, PEG, albumin) to both the antibody detection and the crossmatch. The first step of the antiglobulin crossmatch is similar to the immediate-spin crossmatch. After the immediate-spin phase of testing, the crossmatch tube is incubated at 37° C, after which the cell-serum suspension is washed. The addition of AHG is the final step before reading and interpreting the results.

Electronic Crossmatch

The electronic crossmatch, also known as the computer crossmatch, has been used in the United States and some European countries since the 1980s. Only 4% of transfusion services that use computer systems perform the electronic crossmatch.[38] Some of the benefits of using this method are job simplification, decreased turnaround times, limited handling of potentially harmful blood samples, and increased patient safety. The disadvantages of this method include confusion concerning reimbursement, process design inadequacies, inadequate validation processes, lack of knowledge of regulatory requirements, and software that lacks the desired controls to issue a safe product for transfusion. When adopting this method for crossmatching, the computer system is validated on site to ensure that ABO-compatible blood is selected before transfusion. This method is used to detect ABO incompatibility instead of an abbreviated serologic crossmatch. When the computer is not functioning, computer downtime procedures must include a serologic crossmatch. A computer crossmatch is implemented in the same circumstances as the immediate-spin crossmatch, that is, the patient shows no current evidence or history of a clinically significant antibody. Additional requirements to implement this method are as follows:[1,38]

1. The patient and the blood sample are positively identified at the time of collection.
2. Two determinations are made of the patient's ABO group, one on the current sample (serologic) and the second by one of the following methods: retesting the same sample, testing of a second current sample, or by comparison with previous records. In determining the ABO, both the forward

and reverse blood typing must be performed. If an ABO discrepancy is detected and transfusion is necessary, only group O red blood cells can be issued before resolution.

3. The computer system contains the donor unit number, the component name, ABO group and Rh type of the component, and the reconfirmed donor ABO blood group test interpretation; it also contains two unique patient identifiers (e.g., name and medical record number), ABO group, and Rh type of the recipient and antibody screen results.

4. A method is in place to verify correct entry of data before release of the unit.

5. The computer system contains logic to alert the user to discrepancies between donor ABO and RH blood type on the unit label and the interpretation of the donor unit blood group reconfirmation test, and to ABO incompatibility between the recipient and the donor unit.

In addition to the requirements listed, the literature suggests additional criteria be included to ensure safe transfusion. These criteria are not universally applied, and practice will vary from institution to institution. Some of these recommendations are included in Box 11-1.[38-42]

The limitations of the computer crossmatch depend on the accuracy of the ABO blood typing information entered into the computer. This information will be used to compare subsequent ABO/Rh typing conclusions and select component compatibility. As with all pretransfusion testing, the computer crossmatch has limitations and is not error proof. The following scenarios may occur using this method:

1. If two blood types are performed on a single sample that was initially mislabeled, or collected on the wrong patient, the error will not be detected from the second retyping.

2. Manual interpretations of ABO/Rh typing may be necessary when testing samples from patients receiving massive transfusions, neonatal exchange transfusions, donor bone marrow, or stem cell transplant with a different ABO type from the patient. Results in these cases may differ from previous records.

When deciding to select this method for crossmatching, it is important to incorporate error detection and prevention strategies, be able to meet transfusion requirements of the patients, and comply with regulatory and accrediting requirements.

Interpretation of an Incompatible Crossmatch

The major crossmatch is the final step in compatibility testing. Incompatibility between the patient's serum or plasma and the donor's red cells can usually be interpreted by reviewing the results of the antibody screening test and autocontrol. In some cases the recipient's ABO serum confirmation test results are also used in helping in the interpretation of testing results. One must remember that a negative

Box 11-1	Electronic Crossmatch Procedure: Recommended Additional Criteria

Bar code labels and armbands
Donor label information transferred by bar code
Three- to four-cell antibody screen
Two technologist perform ABO/Rh testing
Lifetime unique patient identifier
Collect second specimen for repeat ABO/Rh
Two different sources of ABO antisera
Software that prevents ABO/Rh-incompatible issue
Software that blocks or warns of a discrepancy
Printout of system warnings, overrides approved

antibody screen does not ensure that the patient's serum does not contain a clinically significant alloantibody or that the red cells being transfused will have normal red cell survival. It does indicate that the antigens present on the antibody screening cells are not reacting with the patient's serum at the time of testing using the method selected.

Historically, tube testing has been the classic methodology used in most transfusion services. Most of what we know when interpreting results has come from this methodology. With new technologies and methodologies such as micro titer plates and gel column testing becoming more popular, unexpected results of this testing will become better described and understood. It is important to note that the results of tube testing cannot always be reproduced when testing is performed using one of the alternative methodologies.[33] The following interpretations of results are based on tube testing methodology.

Positive Antibody Screen, Positive Major Crossmatch, Negative Autocontrol

The usual interpretation of this result pattern would be that the recipient has produced an alloantibody or a mixture of alloantibodies that have been detected by the screening cells, and the corresponding antigen (or antigens) is (are) also present on the donor's red cells. If all cells tested are reactive with the exception of the autocontrol, it suggests the presence of an antibody to a high-frequency antigen. Antibody identification studies should be performed on the patient's serum or plasma and units selected that are negative for the specificities involved. If antigen-negative units are incompatible, the answer may be found in the next category.

Negative Antibody Screen, Positive Major Crossmatch, Negative Autocontrol

An incompatible immediate-spin crossmatch in this situation frequently involves the ABO system, suggesting either that the patient or donor type is not correct or that a mislabeling has occurred. The ABO grouping of the patient and donor should be reviewed. It is also possible that the patient's serum may contain an ABO-system antibody such as anti-A_1 that would not be detected by group O screening cells but could be detected with known A_1 cells. A third possibility is that the patient's serum contains passively transferred anti-A or anti-B from previous alternate blood group transfusions or intravenous gamma globulin therapy. Finally, cold-reactive alloantibodies such as anti-M or anti-P may be reacting at room temperature. A careful review of the patient's transfusion history might provide information in support of this interpretation.

If the patient's serum is incompatible with only one unit in the antiglobulin phase, the donor unit may have a positive direct antiglobulin test (DAT). A DAT should be performed on the donor's red cells. If the test is positive, the unit should not be used for the transfusion. Donor red cells that are already sensitized with immunoglobulin and/or complement cannot be used for a valid indirect antiglobulin test. The result would always be positive in the antiglobulin phase of the crossmatch with all recipients tested.

A second interpretation should be pursued if the donor unit proves to be DAT negative. There may be an alloantibody in the patient's serum reacting with a low-incidence antigen present on the donor's red cells that was not present on the screening cells. Antibody identification tests should be performed that include as many low-incidence antigen specificities as possible.

Another possible solution is the presence of an antibody that is reacting only with homozygous donor red cells showing dosage. In this particular circumstance, the screening cells do not react because they are heterozygous for the antibody specificity demonstrating dosage. Again, antibody identification using enhancement techniques should resolve the problem.

Positive Antibody Screen, Positive Major Crossmatch, Positive Autocontrol

Three possible interpretations must be investigated when all three tests are positive. The first is the presence of autoantibody. Most autoantibodies react with all cells tested because of the high incidence of the antigen specificities involved. This is true of either a cold autoantibody, such as autoanti-I, or a warm autoantibody, such as those with broad Rh system specificity. Techniques for removal of the autoantibody must be performed in order to determine whether or not an alloantibody masked by the reactions of the autoantibody is also present in the patient's serum. See Chapter 18 for a discussion of the techniques to be used.

If the patient has been recently transfused, the second possible interpretation is that an alloantibody is reacting with transfused donor cells, resulting in a positive autocontrol. In these cases the autocontrol and the DAT will show mixed-field agglutination. Antibody identification studies, including antigen phenotyping of a pretransfusion specimen, should be performed to resolve the incompatibility.

The third line of investigation includes abnormalities in the patient's serum and/or anomalous reagent-related serologic reactions.[43] A reversal in the normal ratio of albumin and gamma globulin in the patient's serum may cause red cells to stick together in "coin-like" stacks that can be recognized microscopically as rouleaux formation. All tests, including the autocontrol, appear to be agglutinated at the room temperature and 37° C phases of testing. Rouleaux formation does not affect the antiglobulin test because the cells are washed free of serum before the addition of the antiglobulin reagent. This phenomenon is associated with diseases such as myeloma and macroglobulinemia. A saline replacement technique can be used if it is necessary to differentiate strong rouleaux from antibody-mediated agglutination.

Reagent-related problems can occur when the patient has produced an antibody to substances present in reagent red cell preservative solutions or in reagent additives.[43] An antibody to a red cell preservative would not react in the autocontrol or crossmatch. Washing the reagent red cells before use or switching to another manufacturer's cells usually identifies the causative agent. However, an antibody to a reagent additive is reactive in the autocontrol and crossmatch, as well as in the antibody screen. A positive autocontrol antiglobulin test should be confirmed with a DAT on the patient's red cells. If the DAT is negative, the difference in result may be related to the additive used in the autocontrol test. If an antibody to a substance in the reagent is suspected, one should switch to another additive or use saline antibody detection techniques. Two examples of substances that have caused this phenomenon are thimerosal, which is used as a preservative for some LISS reagents, and sodium caprylate, which is a stabilizing substance added to albumin reagents.

Refer to Chapters 12 and 13 for a discussion of antibody identification and serologic problem solving.

Compatibility in Unique Circumstances
Massive Transfusion/Emergencies

When the amount of blood transfused to a patient within 24 hours is equal to or greater than the patient's total blood volume, compatibility testing may be shortened or eliminated. Because the patient's circulation contains predominantly donor blood, the primary concern is to ensure that ABO-incompatible blood is not transfused. Therefore before urgent issue, performing an immediate-spin test for ABO compatibility or confirming the donor's ABO group by testing with reagent blood grouping sera is done. The physician responsible for the transfusion service must provide written policy guidelines that include the criteria for abbreviated compatibility testing.[1,2]

If the patient is known to have a clinically significant unexpected antibody, blood selected for transfusion should be antigen negative. Although the antibody in the patient's serum may not be demonstrable, the antibody production increases after secondary exposure to the corresponding antigen and subsequently destroys donor cells from antigen-positive units present in the patient's circulation.

It is very important that a recipient be given antigen-negative blood for **all antigens** that correspond to antibodies that may have been evident in the patient's serum at any time in his or her medical history. This is true even in cases in which the antibody is currently not demonstrable in laboratory testing.

Samples with Prolonged Clotting

Samples from patients who have prolonged clotting times, as a result of anticoagulation due to disease processes or medication, may cause difficulty for the transfusion service. Patients who are on heparin therapy may not clot at all, and serum separated from an incompletely clotted sample can continue to generate fibrin, especially during 37° C incubation. To accelerate clotting of these samples, a number of different approaches can be used depending on the reason for the anticoagulation. One drop of thrombin solution per 1 mL of blood or dry thrombin that adheres to the tip of an applicator stick may be added to a sample of whole blood.[2] Care must be taken when interpreting results using serum treated with thrombin because some preparations may contain anti-A and/or anti-B. A second approach allows separation of the serum using the addition of small glass beads incubating at 37° C for several minutes followed by centrifugation and recovery of the serum. If heparin is causing the anticoagulation in the specimen, one drop of protamine sulfate solution to 4 mL of whole blood incubating at 37° C for 5 to 10 minutes will allow for clotting to occur. Protamine used excessively can promote rouleaux formation and could also inhibit clotting.[2]

Autologous Compatibility Testing

Removal and storage of blood or components from a donor/patient for his or her own use, normally for a surgical procedure, is referred to as a predeposit autologous collection. A patient scheduled to receive autologous units should be treated in a similar manner to patients who receive homologous transfusion. Repeat testing of autologous donor blood by the transfusion service should include confirmation of the ABO group and the Rh type of autologous units labeled Rh negative using a sample obtained from an attached segment. Required testing on the patient's pretransfusion sample must include the ABO and Rh typing procedures, but testing for unexpected antibodies and the major crossmatch are optional.[1] It is usually good practice to perform the test for unexpected antibodies in order to be prepared, particularly in a surgical situation, for a request for homologous blood. Many transfusion services perform at least an abbreviated crossmatch to document ABO compatibility, especially if the autologous unit was drawn at another facility.[1] When issuing autologous blood, the oldest unit(s) should be issued first; allogeneic units should be administered last. All transfusion records remain the same as for a homologous transfusion.

Neonatal Compatibility Testing

Neonate: An infant less than 4 months of age.

An initial pretransfusion specimen from the **neonate** first must be tested to determine the ABO group (forward grouping with anti-A and anti-B reagents only) and the Rh type. The serum or plasma of either the neonate or the mother may be tested for unexpected antibodies. If the initial screen is negative, it is unnecessary to crossmatch donor red cells for the initial or subsequent transfusions during any one hospital admission for infants less than 4 months old. If the cells selected for transfusion are not group O, the neonate's serum or plasma must be tested for the presence of passive transfer of maternal anti-A or anti-B by methods that include the antiglobulin phase using either known reagent A_1 or B cells or donor cells. If anti-A or anti-B is detected, ABO-compatible red blood cells must be transfused.[1] These units do not need to be crossmatched.

There are a number of unique transfusion issues associated with neonatal and pediatric transfusion. Refer to Chapter 17 for a thorough discussion of this topic.

Serologic compatibility testing should be performed every 3 days when unexpected antibodies are demonstrated in the patient's serum or plasma and/or units containing incompatible plasma are transfused, for example, group O red cells to a group A patient. If the initial screen demonstrates clinically significant unexpected red cell antibodies, appropriately selected antigen-negative units must be prepared for transfusion until antibody is no longer demonstrable in the neonate's serum.[1] When selecting blood for intrauterine or exchange transfusion it should as fresh as possible and no older than 7 days old. Blood selected for replacement therapy should take into consideration limiting donor exposures for the neonate and using aliquots of the same donor unit until expiration date or exhausted.

Limitations of Compatibility Testing

In some cases, the transfusion of apparently compatible blood results in a transfusion reaction or accelerated clearance of the transfused red cells. There are several reasons why this might occur. A check of the patient's previous blood bank record may reveal that a clinically significant antibody, for example, anti-Jk[a], was detectable at some time in the past. Unfortunately, the antibody can disappear only to be detected again when the antibody develops rapidly in an anamnestic response to the specific antigen present on donor cells. Studies show that approximately one third of potentially hemolytic alloantibodies are not detected after 5 years.[35] Specialized techniques may or may not be able to demonstrate the antibody in the pretransfusion specimen, but there is usually no difficulty in demonstrating the antibody after the delayed transfusion reaction. For this reason, previous records of alloantibody production dictate that antigen-negative blood should be transfused even though the antibody cannot be detected in the pretransfusion sample.

In the investigation of unexpected hemolysis, the laboratory should try to use a different enhancement medium, incubation time, or enzyme technique or simply increase the serum to red cell ratio. Because no single serologic technique detects all antibodies, reagents for other techniques should be available for use. A routine method is chosen by a laboratory because it is practical to use one technique that detects almost all clinically significant antibodies without detecting an appreciable number of antibodies that are not clinically significant. However, what is routine for one laboratory may be a special technique for another.

In a few cases, the antibody cannot be serologically identified.[44] If possible, the red cells of these patients should be phenotyped for antigens in the Rh, Ss, Kell, Duffy, and Kidd systems. Blood should be selected for transfusion that is negative for the antigens that the patient's red cells lack. A particular specificity may be suspected if an antigen known to be present on a donor's red cells but absent from the patient's red cells cannot be detected in the posttransfusion specimen. In vivo compatibility studies with radio-labeled red cells are used to document accelerated red cell clearance with antigen-positive red cells and normal survival with antigen-negative red cells. In vivo studies may also be used when it is not known whether or not the antibody specificity present would cause red cell destruction. When a patient is in dire need of transfusion and all units are incompatible, it may be necessary to transfuse incompatible blood. Consultation between the blood bank medical director and the patient's attending physician should occur when this is being considered. Transfusing incompatible blood in this scenario should be done slowly with the patient being carefully monitored.

Chapter 15 provides a more complete discussion of the clinical signs, laboratory investigation, and management of adverse reactions to transfusion.

Blood Shortages

For various reasons, there are times of the year when blood shortages occur. Inclement weather, coupled with holidays and/or the flu season, often results in a reduced number of people donating blood. At times there may be a sufficient shortage of blood such that there is not enough blood available to fill all routine orders. This is particularly true of group O red blood cells. Each facility should have a policy defining the minimum number of stock blood products available to meet its specific needs and a procedure it will follow if the inventory falls below this required minimum. The reason this is important is that you never want to totally deplete your supply so that there is none left for a critical patient who may require an immediate life-saving transfusion. This policy must be tailored to the specific needs of the facility. It will be different for trauma facilities, which may need a higher number of group O red cells available at all times, or specialty hospitals such as cancer treatment facilities, which may face special challenges due to platelet shortages. Triage procedures should be implemented whenever inventory falls below the facility's predetermined minimum quantity. The specifics of the triage procedure will vary depending on the needs of each facility. Some facilities may need to cancel elective surgeries. Other facilities may implement a procedure where each requested transfusion is discussed with the patient's physician to determine if the transfusion can be delayed. These requests are then filled when inventory levels are sufficient. The goal is to keep enough blood products available at all times so that a product will always be on hand for the patient who critically requires it.

BLOOD RELEASE FOR TRANSFUSION

Each facility should have written policies about pickup and delivery of blood products. Documented training programs should be in place for staff assigned to these functions. Blood is not routinely dispensed from the controlled environment of the blood bank until all testing is completed, the patient is properly prepared, and the transfusionist is ready to begin the procedure. There must be a mechanism to identify the intended recipient and the requested component at the time of issue.[2]

Blood Transfusion Form

> **Blood transfusion form:** A form completed for each unit of crossmatched blood that contains the following minimum information: two unique identifiers (usually the patient's name and identification number), ABO and Rh type of the recipient and the donor, donor unit number, pool number (if applicable), interpretation of compatibility testing, and identification of the person performing the tests.

The **blood transfusion form** is completed for each unit of blood, component, or component pool (Fig. 11-5). This form becomes a part of the patient's permanent medical record after completion of the transfusion. The form must include the following information:[1,2]

1. Recipient's name, identification number, ABO group, and Rh type
2. Donor unit or component pool identification number, ABO group, and Rh type
3. Interpretation of compatibility testing—possible options:
   a. Compatible
   b. Status of compatibility testing indicated conspicuously if incomplete at time of issue
   c. Incompatible (medical consultation required)
   d. No crossmatch required if the component contains less than 2 mL of red cells

In some institutions the transfusion form is attached to the unit and therefore serves as the required unit tag.[2] This form typically will have fields to identify the transfusionist and co-identifier and other information, such as pretransfusion and posttransfusion vital signs, amount of blood given, whether a reaction occurred, and other relevant information as determined by the institution.

A label or tag must be securely attached to the blood container before the unit is released for transfusion. This must include the following information:[1,2]

1. The patient's two independent identifiers, usually the first and last names and ID number
2. Donor unit number or pool number
3. Interpretation of compatibility tests, if performed

Final Inspection of Blood

A visual inspection of the blood or component for color, appearance, and expiration date must be completed and a record made of this inspection before issue.[1,2] An abnormal color or appearance may be an indication of contamination. The unit should not be used for transfusion unless specifically authorized by the medical director. Checking the expiration date avoids inadvertent issue of an outdated component. A record must be kept of the unit inspection at the time of issue. This is often documented electronically in a computer system, or a manual form may be used.

MUNICIPAL BLOOD BANK
ANYTOWN, ANYSTATE 10000

TRANSFUSION SERVICE FORM

Instructions: Send one form for **each** unit ordered. Each form or group of forms must be accompanied by a blood request form (4096).

Before starting transfusion, I certify that I have identified the recipient from inspection of the wristband and that the name and hospital number are the same as on this form. I further certify that the blood or blood preparation label has the same donor number, ABO group, and Rh type as stated on this form.

_____

SIGNATURES

DATE:	BLOOD WARMED ☐NO ☐YES

TIME BEGUN:	TIME COMPL:	REACTION: ☐NO ☐YES
AMOUNT GIVEN: ☐1/4 ☐1/2 ☐3/4 ☐ALL		IF A REACTION OCCURS, STOP THE TRANSFUSION, NOTIFY BLOOD BANK AND PHYSICIAN, AND SUBMIT TRANSFUSION REACTION FORM.

HOSPITAL NO.

PATIENT

SERVICE	AGE

HOSP. LOCATION

BLOOD GROUP AND Rh TYPE	RECIPIENT	DONOR	DONOR NUMBER

PREPARATION (Blood Bank completes)
RBC _____
WB _____
PLT _____
FFP _____
CRYO _____
OTHER _____

CROSSMATCH
☐**COMPATIBLE**
☐INCOMPATIBLE
☐NOT INDICATED

DONE BY: _____
DATE: _____

☐ Unit issued before crossmatch completed per physicians order

TIME AND DATE ISSUED	INSPECTED AND ISSUED BY

INSERT IN PATIENT'S CHART

MUNICIPAL BLOOD BANK
ANYTOWN, ANYSTATE 10000

TRANSFUSION SERVICE FORM

Instructions: Send one form for **each** unit ordered. Each form or group of forms must be accompanied by a blood request form (4096).

Before starting transfusion, I certify that I have identified the recipient from inspection of the wristband and that the name and hospital number are the same as on this form. I further certify that the blood or blood preparation label has the same donor number, ABO group, and Rh type as stated on this form.

_____

SIGNATURES

DATE:	BLOOD WARMED ☐NO ☐YES

TIME BEGUN:	TIME COMPL:	REACTION: ☐NO ☐YES
AMOUNT GIVEN: ☐1/4 ☐1/2 ☐3/4 ☐ALL		IF A REACTION OCCURS, STOP THE TRANSFUSION, NOTIFY BLOOD BANK AND PHYSICIAN, AND SUBMIT TRANSFUSION REACTION FORM.

HOSPITAL NO.

PATIENT

SERVICE	AGE

HOSP. LOCATION

BLOOD GROUP AND Rh TYPE	RECIPIENT	DONOR	DONOR NUMBER

PREPARATION (Blood Bank completes)
RBC _____
WB _____
PLT _____
FFP _____
CRYO _____
OTHER _____

CROSSMATCH
☐**COMPATIBLE**
☐INCOMPATIBLE
☐NOT INDICATED

DONE BY: _____
DATE: _____

☐ Unit issued before crossmatch completed per physicians order

TIME AND DATE ISSUED	INSPECTED AND ISSUED BY

RETURN THIS SLIP TO BLOOD BANK

MUNICIPAL BLOOD BANK
ANYTOWN, ANYSTATE 10000

TRANSFUSION SERVICE FORM

Instructions: Send one form for **each** unit ordered. Each form or group of forms must be accompanied by a blood request form (4096).

Before starting transfusion, I certify that I have identified the recipient from inspection of the wristband and that the name and hospital number are the same as on this form. I further certify that the blood or blood preparation label has the same donor number, ABO group, and Rh type as stated on this form.

_____

SIGNATURES

DATE:	BLOOD WARMED ☐NO ☐YES

TIME BEGUN:	TIME COMPL:	REACTION: ☐NO ☐YES
AMOUNT GIVEN: ☐1/4 ☐1/2 ☐3/4 ☐ALL		IF A REACTION OCCURS, STOP THE TRANSFUSION, NOTIFY BLOOD BANK AND PHYSICIAN, AND SUBMIT TRANSFUSION REACTION FORM.

HOSPITAL NO.

PATIENT

SERVICE	AGE

HOSP. LOCATION

BLOOD GROUP AND Rh TYPE	RECIPIENT	DONOR	DONOR NUMBER

PREPARATION (Blood Bank completes)
RBC _____
WB _____
PLT _____
FFP _____
CRYO _____
OTHER _____

CROSSMATCH
☐**COMPATIBLE**
☐INCOMPATIBLE
☐NOT INDICATED

DONE BY: _____
DATE: _____

☐ Unit issued before crossmatch completed per physicians order

TIME AND DATE ISSUED	INSPECTED AND ISSUED BY

LAB COPY

Fig. 11-5 Transfusion service form (three-part form).

Issuing

At the time of issue, there must be a final check of transfusion service records and each unit of blood or component.[1] The records that identify the intended recipient and requested component are reviewed and compared to the unit being issued. The following information must be checked:

1. The patient's two independent identifiers, usually the first and last names and ID number, ABO group, and Rh type.
2. The donor unit or pool identification number and the donor ABO group and Rh type.

3. The interpretation of crossmatch tests, if performed.
4. Special transfusion requirements. If, for example, an order has been received for irradiated or leukocyte-reduced blood products, it must be verified that the unit has been processed and labeled appropriately.

Each facility must have a written policy for these steps. Any discrepancies must be resolved before the unit is issued.[1] Transfusion service personnel and the person to whom the unit is released are responsible for confirmation of the identification of the recipient and the blood or component to be issued as stated on the request form, the transfusion form, **compatibility label,** and the donor unit or component label.

In addition to the information listed previously, the following must be documented. This documentation is often recorded electronically in a computer system, or a paper form may be used.

1. Name of the person issuing the blood or component
2. Date and time the blood was issued
3. Name of the person to whom the blood or component was issued

Reissuing of Blood

Ideally, blood should be requested from the blood bank only at the time when it is intended to be administered. If the transfusion cannot be initiated promptly, the blood should be returned to the blood bank for storage. Blood should not be stored in unmonitored refrigerators. Red cell units that have warmed to greater than 10° C should not be reissued because of the possible risk of bacterial growth. Many blood banks set a time limit past which issued blood will not be accepted back into inventory, usually after 30 minutes of exposure to room temperature.

Blood may remain at room temperature for up to 4 hours during transfusion with no harmful effects. However, if the transfusion is expected to take longer than 4 hours, the unit should be divided into smaller aliquots that can be given within the 4-hour time frame.[2] If blood is returned to the blood bank, a record must be kept of the date and time returned.

Blood may be returned to the transfusion service or collecting facility for reissue if the following conditions are met:[1]

1. The container closure has not been disturbed.
2. Blood components have been maintained at the appropriate temperature.
3. At least one sealed segment of integral donor tubing has remained attached to the container. Removed segments can be reattached only after confirming that the tubing identification numbers on both the removed segment and the container are identical.
4. The records indicate that the blood has been inspected and that it is acceptable for reissue.

Emergency Release of Blood

When blood is urgently needed, the patient's physician must weigh the risk of transfusing uncrossmatched or partially crossmatched blood against the risk of delaying transfusion until compatibility testing is complete.[2] The transfusion service should establish a standard operating procedure for emergency provision of blood when a delay in transfusion could be detrimental to the patient.[1] When blood is released before pretransfusion testing is complete, the records must contain a signed statement of the requesting physician indicating that the clinical situation was sufficiently urgent to require release of blood.[1,2] This statement does not need to be signed before the blood is issued; it can be completed after the emergency is dealt with.[2]

When emergency release of blood is requested, the blood bank personnel should do the following:

1. Issue uncrossmatched blood. ABO and Rh compatible should be given if there is time to test a current patient specimen. Previous records of a

---

Compatibility label: A firmly attached unit label that contains the following minimum information: two unique identifiers (usually the recipient's name and identification number), donor number, interpretation of compatibility testing, and identification of person who performed the tests.

patient's blood type cannot be used. If there is not sufficient time to perform ABO and Rh testing on the patient's current blood sample, group O Red Blood Cells must be given. It is preferable to give Rh-negative Red Blood Cells, especially if the patient is a female of childbearing age.[2] ABO and Rh typing should be completed as soon as possible and the patient switched to group-specific blood so that group O units, which are often in short supply, are not transfused unnecessarily.

2. Indicate in a conspicuous fashion on the attached tag or label that compatibility testing has not been completed.

3. Begin compatibility testing immediately and complete promptly. If incompatibility is detected at any stage of testing, the patient's physician and the transfusion service physician should be immediately notified.[2]

It is important that patient identification procedures are strictly followed in emergency situations. Increased attention to patient identification is warranted particularly in situations of multiple trauma in which there is an increased risk of patient mixups.[2] Records must include all of the following:

1. Positive identification of the patient
2. The unit number, ABO group, and Rh type of the blood issued
3. Identity of personnel who issued the blood

BLOOD ADMINISTRATION

Good transfusion practice requires that comprehensive policies and procedures for blood administration be designed to prevent and reduce errors. The development of these policies should involve the medical director of the transfusion service, the directors of the clinical services, both nursing and medical personnel, and all personnel involved in blood administration. Policies and procedures must be accessible, monitored for compliance, and periodically reviewed for appropriateness.[2]

Patient Education and Informed Consent

The patient's physician has a responsibility to explain the benefits and risks of transfusion therapy, as well as alternative treatment, in a manner that the patient can understand.[2] The patient should understand the procedure, the blood or component to be given, the length of transfusion, and the expected outcome, as well as possible adverse effects of transfusion. The patient should be given the opportunity to ask questions. This type of dialog allows the patient to make an informed decision regarding the transfusion of blood products. The patient has the right to accept or refuse transfusion.[1] This informed choice should be documented. Some states have specific requirements for blood transfusion consent. Institutions should be careful to ensure that their individual processes and procedures comply with applicable laws.[2]

Equipment and Supplies
Administration Sets and Filters

Blood and components must be administered through a filter designed to retain clots and other debris.[1,2] Standard in-line blood filters typically have a pore size of 170 microns, which traps large blood clots. The administration set may be a Y type that is commonly used to start transfusions with 0.9% normal saline or to dilute a red blood cell transfusion to reduce viscosity and enhance flow. The red blood cells should not be diluted if the patient cannot tolerate the extra volume. Multiple units may be given with a Y-type administration set, but it is not recommended that the set be used for longer than 4 hours because of the risk of bacterial growth at room temperature. A straight-line administration set is appropriate when only blood or a blood component is to be infused. Other specialty sets that are available include a component recipient set that has a shorter line and a smaller filter. The set is used for infusion of Platelets, Fresh Frozen Plasma, and Cryoprecipitate AHF. An even

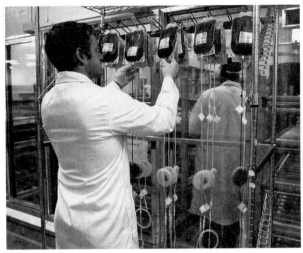

Fig. 11-6 Red cell leukocyte-reduction filters.

smaller component infusion set can be used for direct-syringe intravenous push of small amounts of a blood component.

Blood and blood components are usually infused to an adult through a 19-gauge or larger needle. A 23-gauge or larger thin-walled scalp vein needle may be used for pediatric transfusions and for adults whose large veins are inaccessible. Care should be taken to avoid red cell hemolysis when external pressure to speed infusion is applied to a red cell component infused through a high-gauge (small-bore) needle.[45]

Filters that have a pore size of 20 to 40 microns are designed to remove microaggregates composed of degenerating platelets, white cells, and fibrin strands.[46] Microaggregates form in blood after 5 or more days of storage and range in size from 20 to 200 microns. Most microaggregates are too small to be trapped by a standard 170-micron filter. Microaggregate blood filters have been used extensively during cardiopulmonary bypass. The concern is that microaggregates from transfused blood may accumulate in pulmonary capillaries, causing adult respiratory distress syndrome or other pulmonary dysfunction. The smaller pore size of these filters results in a slower infusion rate than may be desirable in situations requiring rapid massive transfusions. **Microaggregate filters** should not be used in the administration of a granulocyte component.[1,46] Microaggregate filters are not needed if leukocyte reduced blood products are transfused.

Special "third-generation" leukocyte reduction filters are available that can reduce the number of leukocytes in red cell or platelet components to less than 5×10^6, a level that reduces the risk of HLA (human leukocyte antigen) alloimmunization and the transmission of cytomegalovirus, as well as the incidence of febrile nonhemolytic transfusion reactions[47] (Figs. 11-6 and 11-7). The filters are currently manufactured from a number of natural and synthetic media. These filters contain multiple layers of synthetic nonwoven fibers that selectively retain leukocytes but allow red cells or platelets to pass, depending on the filter type. Selectivity is based on cell size, surface tension characteristics, the differences in surface charge, density of the blood cells, and possibly cell-to-cell interactions and cell activation/adhesion properties.[48] Red cell and platelet leukocyte-reduction filters are not interchangeable. They have strict priming and flow rate requirements, and they must be used only with their intended component and only according to the manufacturer's directions.[49]

Depending on the filter used, leukocyte reduced blood and blood components are prepared by blood bank personnel or filtered at the bedside at the time of

Microaggregate filters: Screen- or depth-type filters that remove aggregates smaller than 170 microns. Microaggregate screen filters have pore sizes ranging from 20 to 40 microns and effectively remove 70% to 90% of the leukocytes.

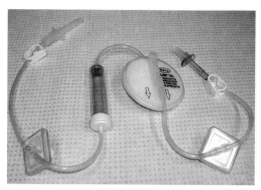

Fig. 11-7 Platelet leukocyte-reduction filter.

blood administration. Using these filters at the bedside is more complex than the use of standard infusion sets. The filters are ineffective if improperly primed or used.[50] There are also filter sets available that come integrally attached to the whole blood collection set, so that Red Blood Cells Leukocytes Reduced and/or Platelets are produced at the time of component preparation. A quality control program that measures the effectiveness of leukocyte reduction is important but impractical at the beside; therefore adherence to proper protocol is all the more important if using a bedside leukocyte reduction filter.[2] Each facility should have a policy regarding the use of leukocyte reduced blood components.[1]

Leukocyte reduced plateletpheresis products are now also commonly manufactured by apheresis instruments that separate the white cells from the platelet product during collection. Methods used by the blood bank or transfusion service to prepare leukocyte reduced products must be validated and quality control tested.[1] Routine methods of automated blood cell counting are not sensitive enough to enumerate the small numbers of leukocytes in leukocyte-reduced components. High-volume manual counting chambers or flow cytometry procedures must be used, but these techniques can only be used if the products are leukocyte reduced before issuing.[51,52]

Intravenous Solutions

AABB *Standards for Blood Banks and Transfusion Services* and the *Circular of Information for the Use of Human Blood and Blood Components* specifically state that medications must not be added to blood or components.[1,53] A solution of 0.9% sodium chloride for intravenous use may be added to reduce viscosity and enhance flow rate or to rinse the blood or blood component out of the bag. This is not ordinarily needed for red cells prepared with an additive solution because these units have a hematocrit of approximately 60%.[2] Drugs or medications, including those intended for intravenous use, must not be added to blood or components. Crystalloid solutions other than 0.9% **normal saline** and medications may cause agglutination, hemolysis, or other unanticipated changes in the blood or component or in the drug or medication. Lactated Ringer's solution or other calcium-containing solutions contain enough calcium to overcome the chelating agents in the anticoagulant or additive solutions and cause clotting of the blood or component in the bag or in the infusion set tubing. Hypotonic sodium chloride solutions and 5% dextrose in water cause hemolysis of red cells. Solutions intended for intravenous use other than 0.9% sodium chloride, such as 5% albumin or 2% dextrose in saline, may be in contact with blood or components in the administration set or added to blood or components if one or both of the following conditions are met:[1,2]

1. They have been approved for this use by the FDA.
2. There is documentation available to show that addition is safe and does not adversely affect the blood or component.

Normal saline: A volume expander (0.9% saline) that is compatible with red blood cells.

Electromechanical infusion devices: Devices that control the flow of intravenous fluids.

Electromechanical Infusion Devices

Electromechanical infusion devices permit infusion at controlled rates and may also alert the transfusionist when an infusion problem has occurred (Fig. 11-8). These are particularly useful for very slow rates of infusion used for pediatric, neonatal, and selected adult patients.[2] Some pumps use a mechanical screw drive to advance the plunger of a syringe filled with blood; others use roller pumps or other forms of pressure applied to the infusion tubing. Standard blood administration sets can be used with some, whereas others require special plastic disposables or tubing supplied by the manufacturer. Blood filters can be added to the required setups.[2] Because red cells may undergo hemolysis when infused under pressure, an infusion pump designed for use with crystalloid or colloid solution may not be suitable for blood products. Platelets and granulocytes appear to sustain no adverse effects when infused with a pumping device.[54,55] The infusion device should be used only if the manufacturer can provide documentation on safety of use for blood and blood component infusion. Proper training of personnel and appropriate policies for maintenance and quality control should reduce the chances of damage to transfused components.[2]

Pressure Devices

In cases of massive hemorrhage, it is often necessary to infuse large quantities of red cells in a short amount of time. These situations require flow rates faster than gravity can provide. A simple method to speed the infusion rate is the use of a blood administration set with an in-line pump that can be squeezed by hand.[2] Another option is the use of a compression device. These operate similar to a blood pressure cuff but entirely encase the bag.[2] Care should be taken when using these devices; the pressure should be monitored because pressures greater than 300 mm Hg may cause the seams of the blood bag to rupture or leak.[2] Standard **sphygmomanometers** apply uneven pressure and should not be used.[45] Studies have shown that there is some red cell hemolysis when external pressure is used. However, the amount is not considered to be clinically significant.[56]

Sphygmomanometers: Blood pressure measurement devices with inflatable pressurized cuffs.

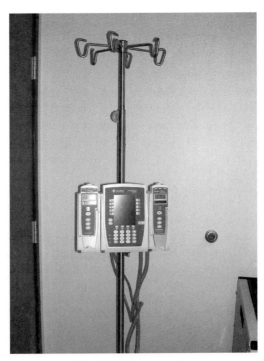

Fig. 11-8 Infusion device.

Blood Warmers

Patients who are rapidly transfused with large amounts of blood are at increased risk of hypothermia, cardiac arrhythmias, and/or cardiac arrest.[57] Transfusion of large volumes of cold blood can lower the temperature of the sinoatrial node to below 30° C, at which point an arrhythmia can occur.[2] Also, cardiac output decreases and ventricular irritability increases, possibly leading to ventricular fibrillation and cardiac arrest.[58] Hemostatic abnormalities from impaired platelet function and slowed enzymatic reactions in the coagulation cascade, vasoconstriction, dehydration, lack of oxygen to tissues, increased red cell release of potassium, and citrate toxicity are also possible side effects of hypothermia. The metabolism of drugs may also be impaired, prolonging the duration of some pharmacologic effects.[58]

Blood warmers are used to prevent these side effects. Since there is no evidence that patients receiving a few units of blood over several hours are at any increased risk of developing hypothermia, routine warming of blood is not recommended.[59] Blood must be warmed under controlled conditions using a device FDA approved or validated for this purpose (Fig. 11-9). There are many devices available on the market today. Some are combined with rapid infusion pumps, but most fall into one of four general technologies:[58]

- Countercurrent heat exchange
- Dry heat
- Thermostatically controlled water bath
- In-line microwave

Regardless of the technology used, blood warmers must have precise temperature control to prevent hemolysis caused by excessive heat. Warming devices must be equipped with a warning system to detect malfunctions and prevent hemolysis

Blood warmers: Devices that warm blood to 37° C in line during infusion.

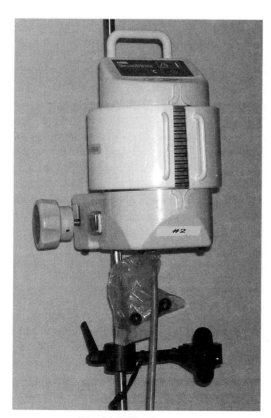

Fig. 11-9 Blood warmer.

or other damage.[1] As with all equipment used in blood bank and transfusion processes, there must be procedures for equipment operation, validation, routine preventive maintenance, and quality control. Training and competency of staff must be documented.[58] A unit of blood that has been warmed but not used cannot be reissued and must be discarded.

Patient Identification Procedure

Accurate identification of the transfusion component and the intended recipient is probably the single most important step in ensuring transfusion safety.[2] Most fatal hemolytic transfusion reactions occur because of misidentification of the patient or donor.[6,60] The transfusionist who administers the blood represents the last point at which identification errors can be detected before the blood is transfused. All identifying information must be checked immediately before beginning the transfusion. If a discrepancy is found, the transfusion cannot be started until it is resolved. It is common practice in many institutions that there is a two-person check to confirm the identity of the patient with the information on the blood unit tag and the blood unit tag with the information on the unit label. Some facilities also require the transfusionist to check for informed consent before starting the transfusion.[2]

The following information must be checked:

1. Physician's order. The blood component should be checked against the physician's order to verify that the correct component and amount are being given.
2. Patient identification. The name and ID number on the patient's wristband must be identical to the name and ID number on the unit tag. If the patient's identity is not known, the emergency identification number that was attached to the patient before collection of samples must be used for positive identification and becomes part of the permanent record of transfusion. Some facilities also ask patients to state their name if they are able. This should not be done by stating the patient's name in a question that can be answered "yes" or "no."
3. Unit identification. The unit number on the product label, attached tag, and/or transfusion form must be identical. The identifying information attached to the unit must remain on the unit until the transfusion has been completed.
4. ABO and Rh. The ABO and Rh type on the primary label of the product must match the ABO and Rh recorded on the transfusion form.
5. Expiration date. It should be verified that the expiration date on the product label is acceptable and the product has not expired.
6. Compatibility. If compatibility testing has been performed, the interpretation must be recorded on the transfusion form and/or unit tag. It should be verified that the unit is compatible.

Engineering Controls

Any procedure performed by human beings is always at risk of human error. In terms of error prevention, it is always safer if a system can be developed that will stop the process if it is being performed incorrectly. One example of an engineering control for blood administration is a mechanical barrier system (Bloodloc). In this system a sticker with a random three-letter code is affixed to the patient's wristband, and the code is written on the patient's pretransfusion blood sample tube by the phlebotomist. This code is not written on the patient's chart or any place other than the patient's wristband. This code is used to lock a plastic lock over the outlet ports of the red cell unit or through a hole in the top of an over-wrap bag by the transfusion service staff who perform compatibility testing. The only place for the transfusionist to obtain the code to open the lock is from the arm of the patient who gave the pretransfusion blood specimen.[6,61]

Another available safety control system is PatientSafe-Transfuse ID (AMTSystems). This system uses a PDA fitted with a bar code reader to interpret a bar-coded patient wristband and compare to the intended patient on a bar-coded unit tag. If they do not match, the transfusionist would be warned not to continue. These types of safety control systems are not required but certainly reduce the risk of error.

Infusion Rate

The desirable infusion rate varies with the patient's condition and should be specified by the physician. Because symptoms of a severe transfusion reaction usually occur during the first 50 mL or less of blood infused, the infusion should be started slowly at approximately 2 mL/min for the first 15 minutes. Infusion rates are calculated by counting the drops per minute in the drip chamber and dividing by the drop/ml rating of the infusion system.[2] The patient should be closely observed for the first 15 minutes. Vital signs are usually repeated at 15 minutes and compared with the previous baseline vital signs; if no problem is observed in the first 15 minutes, the infusion rate may be increased to the rate specified by the physician. A unit of Red Blood Cells is usually given to an adult over 2 to 3 hours but should not exceed 4 hours. A typical pediatric infusion rate is 2 to 5 mL/kg/hr.[45] The date and time that the transfusion was started should be recorded.

Patient Monitoring

The patient must be observed frequently throughout the transfusion and for an appropriate time after completion of the transfusion for signs and symptoms of an adverse reaction. A facility policy may be to record vital signs every 30 minutes or as the patient's condition requires. If outpatient transfusion services are provided, they must be done under medical supervision in accordance with the standards that apply to inpatient transfusion. Specific written instructions for possible adverse reactions should be provided for the outpatient. This should include signs and symptoms of a reaction and who to notify if any of these symptoms appear. If a transfusion reaction occurs, the transfusion must be immediately stopped and the infusion site kept open with 0.9% normal saline. The reaction should be reported to both the transfusion service and the attending physician immediately. The blood or component container, administration set, and attached containers of intravenous solutions, if any, are sent to the transfusion service. Transfusion reactions are discussed in detail in Chapter 15.

Termination of Transfusion

On completion or termination of the transfusion, a record is kept of the start and end times, posttransfusion vital signs, volume transfused, and whether or not an adverse reaction occurred.[1] The identity of the person who stopped the transfusion and observed the patient should be documented. The transfusion service form or a copy should be placed in the chart as a permanent record of the transfusion. In many facilities, a copy of the completed transfusion service form is returned to the transfusion service. The empty blood bag with attached forms need only be returned if an adverse reaction has occurred.[2]

RECORD KEEPING

According to AABB Standards,[1] a record system must make it possible to trace any unit of blood or blood component from source to final disposition. The "source" means the donor. The "final disposition" means recipient ID or discard information. Records may be stored written, in a computer or on computer disks, on microfilm or microfiche, or in some other storage medium. There must also be a means to identify persons performing each significant step in collecting, processing, and compatibility testing, and distributing blood or blood components. Records concerning donors and donor blood are retained indefinitely because of the potential transmission of disease to a recipient. Patients' records must be retained for a minimum of 5 years. Because final disposition of each unit of blood or component must be kept indefinitely, patient transfusion records are frequently maintained indefinitely.

Before blood is issued for transfusion, interpretations of current tests must be compared with patient records to detect error or potentially dangerous situations.[1] The following records must be immediately available for the record check:

1. ABO grouping and Rh typing done during the past 12 months
2. Difficulty in blood typing, clinically significant unexpected antibodies, and severe adverse reactions to transfusion during the past 5 years (minimum)

All blood bank and transfusion service records must be readable and, if hand written, must be done with indelible ink. If an error is made, a single line is made through the error, and the initials of the person making the correction and the date must be written alongside the corrected items. Erasing, overwriting, and using "white-out" liquids are not acceptable. There must also be a means to document computer record corrections of previously transmitted information.

BLOOD UTILIZATION

Type and Screen

A transfusion service may follow any of several policies that lead to more efficient use of blood inventory levels and consequently a reduction in blood bank operating costs.[62] The most important is a type and screen policy whereby compatibility testing is completed up to the point of the major crossmatch. Units are not crossmatched until an actual need for transfusion occurs. This works extremely well for surgical procedures that rarely require transfusion. However, the transfusion service must be in a position to respond immediately to the request for blood. Blood of the appropriate type must be in inventory and available for issue. An immediate-spin or electronic (computer) crossmatch to demonstrate ABO compatibility can usually be completed before issue or before transfusion of the blood. If an abbreviated crossmatch is the policy of the transfusion service, the compatibility test is complete. Otherwise, a full major crossmatch can be completed with greater than 99% confidence that no significant antibody will be found in the antiglobulin phase of testing.[14,15-20,36,37,42] It is important that the physician have total confidence that blood will be immediately available on request. Any problem that may interfere with an immediate response should be communicated to the physician. For example, the patient may have an unexpected antibody present that would require selecting antigen-negative blood of the appropriate blood type and the completion of a full crossmatch. The physician should be notified of the problem and given an estimate of the additional time that may be required before blood could be issued. Usually, the appropriate decision is to crossmatch the units before surgery rather than leave the order as a "type and screen."

Maximum Surgical Blood Order

Another policy that has proven to be successful in many facilities is the practice of establishing a **maximum surgical blood order schedule (MSBOS)** (Table 11-2).[63,64] Data concerning blood usage for each procedure performed in the hospital should be reviewed over several months. In particular, a crossmatch-to-transfusion (C:T) ratio of greater than 2:1 would indicate excessive requests for crossmatches for that procedure. Based on the utilization review, the blood bank

There are a number of requirements for the retention of blood bank records. These are discussed more completely in Chapter 22. The technologist should be aware of all regulations that relate to the maintenance of records, and these should be detailed in the institutional procedures manual.

Maximum surgical blood order schedule (MSBOS): Criteria developed from institutional usage statistics providing a figure for the number of units to be crossmatched for any given surgical procedure.

TABLE 11-2 Example of a Maximum Surgical Blood Order Schedule

Procedure	Units	Procedure	Units
General Surgery		**Orthopedics**	
Breast biopsy	T/S	Arthroscopy	T/S
Colon resection	2	Spinal fusion	3
Exploratory Laparotomy	2	Total hip replacement	3
Gastrectomy	2	**Obstetrics/Gynecology**	
Pancreatectomy	4	Cesarean section	T/S
Splenectomy	2	D&C	T/S
Cardiac-Thoracic		Hysterectomy, radical	2
Aneurism resection	6	**Urology**	
CABG	2	TUR, bladder	T/S
Lobectomy	T/S	Nephrectomy	3
Lung biopsy	T/S	Renal transplant	2
Vascular			
Aortic bypass with graft	4		
Endarterectomy	T/S		

Modified with permission from Brecher ME (ed): Technical Manual of the American Association of Blood Banks, 14th ed. Bethesda, MD, American Association of Blood Banks, 2002, p 84.
CABG, coronary artery bypass graft; *D&C,* dilation and curettage; *T/S,* type and screen; *TUR,* transurethral resection.

medical director, staff surgeons, and anesthesiologists establish realistic ordering levels for each procedure. Some facilities have modified the MSBOS concepts into a "standard" blood order system (SBO) representing the average number of units transfused for each surgical procedure. The MSBOS often defines the number of units needed to meet the transfusion needs of 80% to 90% of patients undergoing a specific surgical procedure.[2] Once the transfusion guidelines are established for each of the surgical procedures, the transfusion service crossmatches the designated number of units. Use of "type and screen" is recommended for procedures that have an average transfusion level of 0.5 unit or less. Maximum surgical blood orders may be modified by the physician if the patient's condition indicates that increased blood use is expected.[2] The implementation of an MSBOS or SBO can reduce unnecessary crossmatching and help in inventory management, saving reagents, supplies, resources, and technical time and resulting in improved efficiencies for the transfusion service.

Blood Utilization Review

Blood utilization review programs that monitor the transfusion practices and appropriate use of all blood and blood components are required by accrediting agencies such as the Joint Commission on Accreditation of Healthcare Organizations (JCAHO) and the AABB.[1,63,65-67] Generally, blood utilization review is performed by the **transfusion committee,** which consists of representatives from all the major departments that transfuse blood products, as well as the medical director of the transfusion service. Areas of review may include ordering, distribution, handling, dispensing, administration, and monitoring the effectiveness of the transfusion. The committee establishes written criteria for evaluating justification for transfusion of all blood and blood components. All transfusions are reviewed until documentation of blood use has demonstrated consistent

Transfusion committee: The process by which physicians review transfusion practice within the institution using a set of predetermined criteria. The goal of peer review is improvement in the quality of blood transfusion practice.

compliance with the written "audit" criteria. Then periodic review of an adequate sample of cases is acceptable. Frequently, the audit criteria may be used by medical records or quality assurance personnel to select patient charts for review by the transfusion committee. All committee activities should be documented by written minutes of meetings and reports forwarded to other hospital committee services, departments, and hospital staff.

Most often, transfusion episodes are reviewed several days to months after the occurrence. This is referred to as a retrospective review. It is most helpful in identifying trends and overall practice patterns. The retrospective audit is the easiest to perform but is the least useful in changing physician ordering practice.[63] In addition to retrospective review of transfusion practices, the transfusion service may be able to evaluate product utilization by a prospective or concurrent review of ordering practices. For example, if justification for transfusion of blood or blood components is not within the previously approved acceptable range, the medical director consults with the ordering physician before the product is issued for transfusion. This is a prospective audit. Appropriate transfusion therapy expertise is immediately provided, and the patient receives the correct component or avoids an unnecessary transfusion. Concurrent audit is performed within the previous 12 to 24 hours of transfusion, and the patient's laboratory and clinical data are reviewed. This is useful especially when reviewing blood products that have been transfused on an emergency basis and a prospective audit is unable to be completed. The transfusion events being evaluated are current for the physicians who have ordered the products. When selecting what process will be performed for transfusion review, each transfusion committee or its equivalent is responsible for the development of its procedures and audit criteria. Medical staff participation and approval is essential for a successful process. Finally, the process and procedures for transfusion utilization review should be reviewed and revised on a regular basis.

CHAPTER SUMMARY

1. A procedure must be in place to identify persons performing each significant step in collecting, processing, compatibility testing, and administration of blood or blood components.

2. The determination of ABO and Rh of donor blood and detection of clinically significant donor antibodies done by the collecting facility are integral parts of compatibility testing. Repeat testing of donor blood by the transfusion service confirms the ABO group of all units of whole blood and red blood cell components and the Rh type of units labeled Rh negative, using a sample obtained from an attached segment.

3. Positive identification of the recipient and collection of a properly labeled blood sample must be confirmed by a qualified person in the transfusion service before a sample can be used for compatibility testing. The sample must be tested for ABO group and Rh type and for clinically significant unexpected antibodies.

4. A review of previous transfusion service records for ABO and Rh typing, difficulty in blood typing, clinically significant unexpected antibodies, and severe adverse reactions to transfusion is done to detect possible error or potentially dangerous situations. Interpretations of current test results must be compared with prior serologic results before blood is issued for transfusion.

5. A major crossmatch using donor cells from the originally attached whole blood or component segment and the recipient's serum or plasma must be done before administration of whole blood and red blood cell components, except for urgent blood requirements. The crossmatch should use methods that demonstrate ABO incompatibility and clinically significant unexpected antibodies and should include an antiglobulin test.

6. Transfusion must be done under medical direction. Development and approval of written policies and procedures relating to the distribution, handling, use, and administration of blood and blood components are the responsibility of the medical staff.

7. Positive identification of the recipient and blood container must be verified by the transfusionist in writing immediately before transfusion in the presence of the recipient. The patient must be observed during the transfusion and for an appropriate time thereafter for adverse reactions.

8. The record system should make it possible to trace any unit of blood or blood component from source (the donor or the collecting facility) to final disposition (transfused, shipped, discarded), to recheck the records applying to a specific component, and to investigate adverse reactions manifested by the recipient.

9. Blood must be transfused through a filter no larger than 170 microns to eliminate potential clots or storage debris. Infusion devices that are FDA approved can be used to control the flow rate and temperature of products for safe transfusion.

10. Type and screen protocols, along with the development of maximum surgical blood ordering protocols, allow for better inventory management; savings in reagents, supplies, and technical time; and improved efficiencies for the transfusion service.

11. Blood utilization practices are important for performance improvement and in evaluating the utilization of the blood bank services, physician ordering practices, and the efficacy of the transfusions.

REFERENCES

1. Fridey JL (ed): Standards for Blood Banks and Transfusion Services, 22nd ed. Bethesda, MD, American Association of Blood Banks, 2003.

2. Brecher ME (ed): Technical Manual of the American Association of Blood Banks, 14th ed. Bethesda, MD, American Association of Blood Banks, 2002.

3. Dzik WH: Emily Cooley Lecture 2002: Transfusion safety in the hospital. Transfusion 43:1190-1199, 2003.

4. Jensen NJ, Crosson JT: An automated system for bedside verification of the match between patient identification and blood unit identification. Transfusion 36:216-221, 1996.

5. Procedures for the Collection of Diagnostic Blood Specimens by Venipuncture; Approved Standard, 4th ed. NCCLS document H3-A2. National Committee for Clinical Laboratory Standards, 1998.

6. Sazama K: Reports of 355 transfusion-associated deaths: 1976-1985. Transfusion 30:583-590, 1990.

7. Garratty G: Problems associated with passively transfused blood group antibodies. Am J Clin Pathol 109:169-177, 1998.

8. Mollison PL, Englefreit CP, Contreras M: Blood Transfusion in Clinical Medicine, 9th ed. Oxford, Blackwell Scientific, 1993.

9. US Department of Health and Human Services, Food and Drug Administration: The Code of Federal Regulations, 21 CFR 660.3-660.36, current edition. Washington, DC, US Government Printing Office.

10. Howard JE, Winn LC, Gottlieb CE, et al: Clinical significance of the anti-complement component of antiglobulin antisera. Transfusion 22:269-272, 1982.

11. Shulman IA, Petz LD: Red cell compatibility testing: Clinical significance and laboratory methods. In Petz LD, Swisher SN, Klienman S (eds): Clinical Practice of Transfusion Medicine, 3rd ed. New York, Churchill Livingstone, 1996.

12. Judd WJ, Butch SH: Cost-containment in the blood bank: Eliminating unnecessary serological testing. J Med Technol 1:484-495, 1984.

13. Petz LD, Garratty G: Antiglobulin sera—past, present and future. Transfusion 18:257-268, 1978.

14. Shulman IA: Controversies in red blood cell compatibility testing. In Nance SJ (ed): Immune Destruction of Red Blood Cells. Arlington, VA, American Association of Blood Banks, 1989.

15. Oberman HA, Barnes BA, Friedman BA: The risk of abbreviating the major crossmatch in urgent or massive transfusion. Transfusion 18:137-141, 1978.

16. Heisto H: Pretransfusion blood group serology: Limited value of the antiglobulin phase of the crossmatch when a careful screening test for unexpected antibodies is performed. Transfusion 19:761-763, 1979.

17. Roualt C: Appropriate pretransfusion testing. In Treacy M (ed): Pretransfusion Testing for the 80's. Washington, DC, American Association of Blood Banks, 1980.

18. Walker RH: On the safety of the abbreviated crossmatch. Pathologist 35:543-547, 1981.

19. Garratty G: The role of compatibility tests. Transfusion 22:169-172, 1982.

20. Judd WJ, Butch SH: Streamlining serological testing: Scientific considerations. In Smith D, Judd WJ (ed): Blood Banking in a Changing Environment. Arlington, VA, American Association of Blood Banks, 1984.

21. Low B, Messeter L: Antiglobulin test in low-ionic strength salt solution for rapid antibody screening and crossmatching. Vox Sang 26:53-61, 1974.

22. Moore HC, Mollison PL: Use of low ionic strength medium in manual tests for antibody detection. Transfusion 16:291-296, 1976.

23. Wicker B, Wallas CH: A comparison of a low ionic strength saline medium with routine methods for antibody detection. Transfusion 16:469-472, 1976.

24. Fitzsimmons JM, Morel PA: The effects of red blood cell suspending media on hemagglutination and the antiglobulin test. Transfusion 19:81-85, 1979.

25. Allan JC, Bruce M, Mitchell R: The preservation of red cell antigens at low ionic strength. Transfusion 30:423-426, 1990.

26. Lalezari P, Jiang AF: The manual polybrene test: A simple and rapid procedure for detection of red cell antibodies. Transfusion 20:206-211, 1980.

27. Mintz PD, Anderson G: Comparison of a manual hexadimethrine bromide-antiglobulin test with saline- and albumin-antiglobulin test for pretransfusion testing. Transfusion 27:134-137, 1987.

28. Rosenfield RE, Shaikh SH, Innella F, et al: Augmentation of hemagglutination by low ionic conditions. Transfusion 19:499-510, 1979.

29. Shulman IA, Petz LD: Red cell compatibility testing: Clinical significance and laboratory methods. In Petz LD, Swisher SN, Klienman S (eds): Clinical Practice of Transfusion Medicine, 3rd ed. New York, Churchill Livingstone, 1996.

30. Nance S, Garratty G: Polyethylene glycol: A new potentiator of red blood cell antigen-reactions. Am J Clin Pathol 87: 633-635, 1987.

31. Wentz B, Apuzzo J, Shah DP: Evaluation of the polyethylene glycol-potentiated indirect antiglobulin test. Transfusion 30:318-321, 1990.

32. Slater JL, Griswold DJ, Wojtniak LS, Reisling MJ: Evaluation of the polyethylene glycol-indirect antiglobulin test for routine compatibility. Transfusion 29:686-688, 1989.

33. Issitt PD: From kill to overkill: 100 years of (perhaps too much) progress. Immunohematology 16(1):18-25, 2000.

34. Judd WJ, Barnes BA, Steiner EA, et al: The evaluation of a positive direct antiglobulin test (autocontrol) in pretransfusion testing revisited. Transfusion 26:220-224, 1986.

35. Ramsey G, Smietana SJ: Long term follow-up testing of red cell alloantibodies. Transfusion 34:122-124, 1994.

36. Oberman HA: The present and future crossmatch. Transfusion 32:794-795, 1992.

37. Beck ML, Tilzer LL: Red cell compatibility testing: A perspective for the future. Transfus Med Rev 10:118-130, 1996.

38. Scientific Section Coordinating Committee: Guidelines for Implementing an Electronic Crossmatch. Bethesda, MD, American Association of Blood Banks, 2003.

39. Butch SH, Judd WJ, Steiner EA, et al: Electronic verification of donor-recipient compatibility: The computer crossmatch. Transfusion 34:187, 1994.

40. Butch SH, Judd WJ: Requirements for the computer crossmatch (letter). Transfusion 34:187, 1994.

41. Safwenberg J, Hogman CF, Cassemar B: Computerized delivery control: A useful and safe complement to the type and screen compatibility testing. Vox Sang 72:162-168, 1997.

42. Butch SH, Oberman HA: The computer or electronic crossmatch. Transfus Med Rev 11:256-264, 1997.

43. Pierce SR: Anomalous blood bank results. In Dawson RD (ed): Trouble-shooting the Crossmatch. Washington, DC, American Association of Blood Banks, 1976.

44. Issitt PD, Gutgsell NS: Clinically significant antibodies not detected by routine methods. In Nance SJ (ed): Immune Destruction of Red Blood Cells. Arlington, VA, American Association of Blood Banks, 1989.

45. US Department of Health and Human Services: Transfusion Therapy Guidelines for Nurses. Publication No. (NIH) 90-2668, National Blood Resource Education Program, September, 1990.

46. Snyder EL, Bookbinder M: Role of microaggregate blood filtration in clinical medicine. Transfusion 23:460-470, 1983.

47. Stack G, Judge JV, Snyder EL: Febrile and non-immune transfusion reactions. In Rossi EC, Simon TL, Moss GS, Gould SA (eds): Principles of Transfusion Medicine, 2nd ed. Baltimore, Williams & Wilkins, 1995.

48. Buril A, Beugeling T, Feijen J, van Aken WG: The mechanisms of leukocyte removal by filtration. Transfus Med Rev 9: 145-166, 1995.

49. Dzik WH: Leukoreduced blood components: Laboratory and clinical aspects. In Rossi EC, Simon TL, Moss GS, Gould SA (eds): Principles of Transfusion Medicine, 2nd ed. Baltimore, Williams & Wilkins, 1995.

50. Sprogre-Jakobsen U, Saetre AM, Georgsen J: Preparation of white cell-reduced red cells by filtration: Comparison of a bedside filter and two blood bank filter systems. Transfusion 35:421-426, 1995.

51. Lutz P, Dzik WH: Large-volume hemacytometer chamber for accurate counting of white cells (WBCs) in WBC-reduced platelets: Validation and application for quality control of WBC-reduced platelets prepared by apheresis and filtration. Transfusion 33:409-412, 1993.

52. Vachyla M, Simpson SJ, Martinson JA, et al: A flow cytometric method for counting very low levels of white cells in blood and blood components. Transfusion 33: 262-267, 1993.

53. American Association of Blood Banks, America's Blood Centers, American Red Cross: Circular of Information for the Use of Human Blood and Blood Components. Bethesda, MD, American Association of Blood Banks, 2002.

54. Snyder EL, Ferri PM, Smith EO, Ezekowitz MD: Use of electromechanical infusion pump for transfusion of platelet concentrates. Transfusion 24:524-527, 1984.

55. Snyder EL, Malech HL, Ferri PM, et al: In vitro function of granulocyte concentrates following passage through an electromechanical infusion pump. Transfusion 26:141-144, 1986.

56. Frelich R, Ellis MH: The effect of external pressure, catheter gauge, and storage time on hemolysis in RBC transfusion. Transfusion 41:799-802, 2001.

57. Boyan CP, Howland WS: Cardiac arrest and temperature of bank blood. JAMA 183:58-60, 1963.

58. Hrovat TM, Passwater M, Palmer RN: Guidelines for the Use of Blood Warming Devices. Bethesda, MD, American Association of Blood Banks, 2002.

59. Calhoun L: Blood product preparation and administration. In Petz LD, Swisher SN, Kleinman S (eds): Clinical Practice of Transfusion Medicine, 3rd ed. New York, Churchill Livingstone, 1996.

60. Linden JV, Wagner K, Voytovich AE, Sheehan J: Transfusion errors in New York State: An analysis of 10 years' experience. Transfusion 40:1207-1213, 2000.

61. Wenz B, Burns ER: Improvement in transfusion safety using a new blood patient identification system as part of safe transfusion. Transfusion 32:401-403, 1991.

62. AuBuchon JP: Blood transfusion options: Improving outcomes and reducing costs. Arch Pathol Lab Med 121: 40-47, 1997.

63. Scientific Section Coordinating Committee: Guidelines for Blood Utilization Review. Bethesda, MD, American Association of Blood Banks, 2001.

64. Boral LJ, Henry JB: The type and screen: A safe alternative and supplement in selected surgical procedures. Transfusion 17:163-168, 1977.

65. Medical staff monitoring functions: Blood usage review. In Accreditation Manual for Hospitals. Chicago, Joint Commission on Accreditation of Healthcare Organizations, 1993.

66. US Department of Health and Human Services, Food and Drug Administration: The Code of Federal Regulations, Title 21 CFR 482.27(d)(6), current edition. Washington, DC, US Government Printing Office.

67. Commission on Laboratory Accreditation: Inspection Checklist. Chicago, College of American Pathologists, 1992.

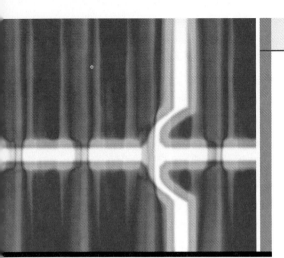

CHAPTER TWELVE

Antibody Identification

Karen Rodberg

LEARNING OBJECTIVES

After reading and studying this chapter, the student will be able to:

1. Discuss alloimmunization and situations that may stimulate it.
2. Discuss serologic situations in which antibody identification is indicated.
3. When given a diagram, accurately grade agglutination reactions.
4. Discuss the difference between the direct and indirect antiglobulin test.
5. Given a case study, correctly apply the use of enhancement media and alternative techniques in antibody problem solving.
6. Discuss the purpose of IgG-coated RBCs (check cells) in indirect antiglobulin testing.
7. Discuss the age limitations of the sample used for antibody identification and the differences that may be seen when using serum vs. plasma.
8. Explain the process of antibody exclusion when interpreting a red cell panel.
9. When given a case study, properly select additional rule-out and confirmatory cells for testing in a selected cell panel.
10. Discuss the role of antigen typing of the patient's red blood cells.
11. Describe the use of enzyme-treated RBCs and two situations in which they would be useful.
12. Describe the use of DTT-treated RBCs and give an example of a case in which they would be useful.
13. Describe two situations in which the direct antiglobulin test might be positive.
14. Discuss the role of autologous and allogeneic adsorption in antibody identification.
15. Discuss the role of elution in antibody identification.
16. Explain the term *potentially clinically significant antibody*.
17. Explain why the patient's ethnicity is important if an antibody to a high-incidence antigen is suspected.
18. Explaih why the identification of antibodies to low-incidence antigens is often of academic interest only.
19. Discuss examples of passively acquired antibodies.
20. Select the appropriate red cell component(s) for patients with alloantibodies.

THE SEROLOGIC DETECTIVE

Introduction

Antibody identification is the next logical step in pretransfusion testing following the discovery of a positive antibody screen. Other circumstances encountered in pretransfusion testing, such as an ABO serum/cell discrepancy or an incompatible crossmatch, may also indicate that antibody identification should be performed. The ability to identify atypical antibodies in the patient's serum is necessary in order to select appropriate blood products for transfusion, ideally products that are serologically compatible, to minimize the risk of adverse reaction to the transfusion.

The serologic techniques used for antibody identification include those used in routine pretransfusion testing, that is, standard agglutination and indirect antiglobulin techniques. More complicated investigations, however, may require chemical treatment of the patient's red cells or serum, **neutralization, titration, adsorption,** and/or **elution**, depending on the nature of the serologic picture. The identification of atypical antibodies may be further aided by additional information, such as the patient's transfusion history, diagnosis, clinical status, previous antibody history, and ethnicity. The technologist must analyze the serologic clues in light of the patient's medical history and clinical status in order to solve the puzzle, much as a detective would do. Skills that aid in being a good serologic sleuth, then, are knowledge of and technical expertise in various serologic techniques, knowledge of expected reactivity of common antibodies, background knowledge in clinical diagnosis, logical thought processes, and perhaps a touch of intuition.

The Basics

All serologic tests are based on testing knowns against unknowns. In most instances, the patient's sample, either cells or serum depending on the test being done, is the unknown. Well-characterized, licensed reagents, either antisera or reagent red cells, are the knowns. For example, in ABO testing the anti-A and anti-B reagents are the knowns. They are used to test the patient's red blood cells (RBCs) to identify whether A or B antigens (the unknowns) are present. If anti-A reagent reacts with (agglutinates) the RBCs being tested, the logical conclusion is that A antigen is present; conversely, if anti-A does not react with the red cells, A antigen is absent. In ABO serum grouping the A and B reagent red cells are the knowns. If the patient's serum agglutinates the group A reagent red cells, anti-A is present in the patient's serum; if the patient's serum is nonreactive with group A red cells, anti-A is absent.

Likewise, in antibody detection (screening) and antibody identification the patient's sample, in this case the serum or plasma, is the unknown and the reagent

Neutralization: Inactivation of an antibody resulting from binding with a soluble antigen. Blood group substances in saliva, for example, bind with their corresponding antibody, thus reducing the ability of the antibody to bind with particulate antigen (red cells).

Titration: A technique involving the serial dilution of an antiserum to determine the range of antibody activity (titer). In a mixture of antibodies, specificities can sometimes be distinguished by titration methods.

Adsorption: The attachment of antibody to the red cell surface via binding with specific antigen. For example, A cells adsorb anti-A from solution. Adsorption is a blood bank technique in which red cells and plasma are mixed, and antibody is adsorbed onto the red cell surface.

Elution: The process by which adsorbed antibody (on the red cell surface) is removed and returned to solution. Elutions can be performed by a number of physical and chemical procedures.

RBCs (antibody detection cells or antibody identification panel cells) are the knowns. The primary sources of antibody identification cells are typically commercially prepared panels of group O red cells, which have been well characterized by the manufacturer. The phenotype of each donor's RBCs is supplied by the manufacturer on a printed antigram (worksheet) that accompanies the panel. As with the antibody detection cells, the red cell panel suspensions are supplied in an isotonic diluent containing a preservative so that the shelf life of the panel on receipt is approximately 3 weeks. Typically, antibody identification panels contain 10 to 16 vials of red cell suspensions, each containing RBCs from a single group O donor, as compared to the set of two or three vials supplied for antibody screening.

The process of testing the red cell panel is technically similar to setting up the antibody screen; there are just more tubes in the "batch." The initial panel is usually tested using the laboratory's routine method, for example, albumin, low ionic strength saline (LISS), gel, or polyethylene glycol (PEG) indirect antiglobulin test (IAT). Several additional methods used in problem solving will be introduced later in this chapter. The ability to perform tests using these additional methods is dependent on the availability of such reagents in each laboratory and the experience and expertise of the technologist.

The interpretation of the results of the antibody identification panel is made by systematically analyzing the agglutination reactivity noted (positive or negative) as compared to the antigens present on each panel donor's RBCs as indicated on the antigram. The serologist is then able to determine with some element of confidence which atypical antibodies are present in the patient's serum. Based on the antibody identification the technologist can then select appropriate red cells for transfusion that lack the antigen(s) to which the patient has made antibody(ies).

Alloantibodies

Alloantibodies are antibodies that react with antigens absent from the patient's own red cells. Some alloantibodies may be naturally occurring (similar to naturally occurring anti-A and/or anti-B), but most are produced in response to stimulus of "foreign" (non-self) red cells that have been introduced into the patient's circulation as a result of a transfusion or pregnancy. For example, if the patient's RBCs are E− and the patient is transfused with RBCs that are E+, the patient's immune system may recognize the E antigen as foreign and produce alloanti-E. If the patient's serum containing anti-E is mixed with E+ RBCs (either in the test tube or in the patient's circulation), the anti-E will react with (sensitize or directly agglutinate) the E+ RBCs. If this were to happen in vivo (i.e., in the body) the patient would probably experience a hemolytic transfusion reaction and the transfused cells would be removed from circulation. In vitro pretransfusion tests (i.e., tests performed in the laboratory), such as antibody screening and antibody identification, are designed to try to prevent this kind of adverse outcome from transfusion.

Alloimmunization has been reported to occur in 0% to 34% of multitransfused individuals, although the average rate of response is between 11% and 12.5%.[1] This means that some patients, the nonresponders, do not appear to form alloantibodies whereas others, the responders, make one or more alloantibodies. The highest rates of alloimmunization are found in patients with sickle cell disease (8% to 35%) or those with autoimmune hemolytic anemia (15% to 41%). These high rates of response are caused in part by the frequency of exposure to foreign antigens through multiple transfusions of red blood cell components for these chronic anemias.

Direct vs. Indirect Agglutination

Refer to Chapter 2 for a discussion of the factors that affect agglutination.

RBCs may be agglutinated directly by an antibody if the antibody, which binds to a specific antigen on one red cell, can also bind to that antigen on multiple adjacent RBCs and bridge the gap between them, bringing the red cells together. If this happens with many adjacent RBCs, visible agglutinates form. This type of reactivity is most often seen with IgM antibodies because the IgM molecules are large enough to span the gap between two RBCs. Although it is characteristic of IgM antibodies to agglutinate RBCs directly, it cannot be assumed that all antibodies that directly agglutinate cells are IgM. Additional testing is needed to determine the class of the antibody.

RBCs may also be sensitized with antibody, meaning that antibody has bound to a specific antigen on one red cell, but cannot span the gap between two red cells to bring them together in an agglutinate. This type of reactivity is typical of IgG antibodies, which are smaller molecules than IgM. For the sensitization to be visible, another antibody must be added to bridge the gap between the IgG molecules bound to RBCs. Antihuman globulin (AHG) does this. The method, known as the indirect antiglobulin test (IAT), was reported by Coombs and colleagues in 1945.[2] Its discovery was responsible for subsequent discoveries of most of the blood group antigens and antibodies central to blood banking today. The performance and control of the IAT in pretransfusion testing is vital to minimizing the risk of transfusion.

Reading and Grading Agglutination

Consistency in determining the strength of agglutination is necessary both from test to test and technologist to technologist; therefore a standardized grading or scoring scheme is used that assigns semiquantitative results to the reactions observed. The agglutination observed constitutes the visible endpoint of the antigen-antibody reaction. In conventional test tube methods, this endpoint must be read immediately after centrifugation and recorded concurrently on the appropriate worksheet. **Optical aids,** such as an agglutination viewer or a microscope, which magnify the image, may be useful in visualizing the endpoint (Fig. 12-1).

Optical aids: Devices that enhance the reading of test tube agglutination reactions.

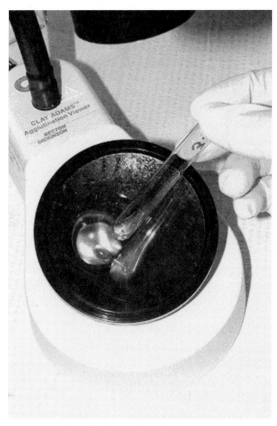

Fig. 12-1 Agglutination viewer.

TABLE 12-1 Reading and Grading of Serologic Reactions

Grade	Score	Description of Appearance
4+	12	One solid clump, no free cells, clear supernatant
3+	10	Several large clumps, clear supernatant
2+	8	Many medium-sized clumps, clear supernatant
1+	5	Numerous small clumps, cloudy red supernatant
±	3	Numerous very small clumps easily dispersed, cloudy red supernatant
(+)	1	Appears negative macroscopically, but agglutination visible microscopically
0	0	Negative, no agglutination seen macroscopically or microscopically
H		Complete hemolysis, no intact RBCs remaining
PH		Partial hemolysis, some RBCs still intact, but hemolysis visible in supernatant
mf		Mixed field—mixtures of agglutinated and unagglutinated cells

Sometimes the notations "S" for strong or "W" for weak are used to denote slight variations between reaction grades. For example, a reaction between 1+ and 2+ might be noted as 1+^{s} or 2+^{w}.

Conventionally, agglutination reactions are graded from negative (0) if no agglutination took place to strongly positive (4+) if all RBCs are agglutinated in one tight clump. Mixed-field (mf) reactivity is the notation used when one population of RBCs is agglutinated but another is not. Mixed-field reactivity is often seen when phenotyping the RBCs from a recently transfused patient where some RBCs are antigen positive and others are antigen negative. Hemolysis of the test RBCs, if observed, is also a positive reaction. Because complement is necessary for hemolysis, it cannot occur if the sample being tested is plasma, because calcium, necessary for the complement cascade, is chelated by the anticoagulant, or serum that is several days old, because complement is labile and decreases during storage of the sample. Table 12-1 summarizes the grading scheme recommended by Race and Sanger[3] and popularized by Marsh[4] that has become the industry standard (Fig. 12-2).

Each laboratory can decide to routinely use serum or plasma, understanding the differences between them. The American Association of Blood Banks (AABB) *Standards for Blood Banks and Transfusion Services* requires that a blood sample for pretransfusion testing be less than 3 days old if the patient is pregnant or has been recently transfused.[5] This requirement helps ensure that clinically significant antibodies stimulated by recent sensitizing events will have the best chance of being detected. Most hospital laboratories find it easier to follow that policy for all samples for pretransfusion testing in order to be on the conservative side, because a reliable patient history is not always available.

TESTING A PANEL OF RED BLOOD CELLS

Each laboratory should have its own set of written policies and procedures to follow for routine testing. The following example of an antibody identification method is given for the purpose of explanation of the sample panels used in this chapter. It includes one set of test tubes carried through three phases of testing: room temperature (RT); incubation at 37° C in LISS, which enhances antibody uptake; and IAT. It also includes an autologous control tube (consisting of the patient's own RBCs) tested in parallel with the commercial panel cells. Although

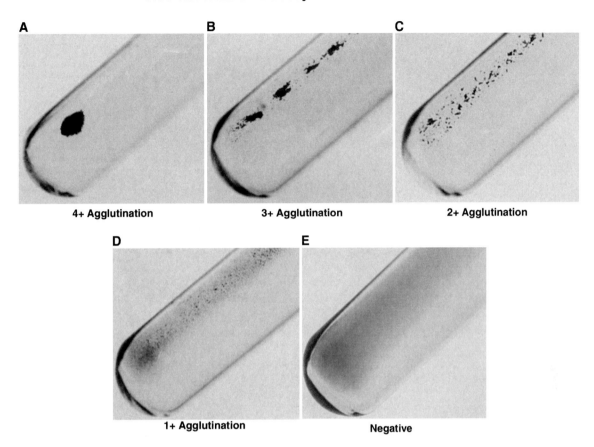

Fig. 12-2 Grading agglutination. *(Courtesy Organon Teknika, Inc.)*

incubation at room temperature is not recommended for routine antibody detection or identification, it may be helpful in problem solving if the initial panel results are difficult to interpret. It is included in the following example as an option. Similarly, an autologous control (auto control) is not routine to pretransfusion testing, but is of major importance in problem solving, so it is highly recommended when performing antibody identification studies.

An Example of an Antibody Identification Test Tube Method

1. Label one 10×75 mm test tube for each example of panel RBCs to be tested and one additional tube for the auto control.
2. Add 2 drops of the patient's serum or plasma to each tube. Inspect the tubes to ensure that serum/plasma is present in each.
3. To each tube, add 1 drop of 2% to 5% RBC suspension from the appropriate vial of panel cells. Add 1 drop of 2% to 5% patient RBCs to the auto control tube. Mix tubes thoroughly by gentle agitation.
4. Perform immediate spin (IS) (or incubate for 5 to 15 minutes at RT [optional]).
5. Centrifuge all tubes for the time specified by calibration of the serologic centrifuge in use (approximately 15 seconds).
6. Inspect the supernatant for hemolysis; then resuspend the cell button using gentle agitation. Use an optical aid (e.g., agglutination viewer) if available. Grade the reaction from 0 to 4+ and record concurrently in the appropriate space on the worksheet. (i.e., when reading tube 1 for RT phase, record the reaction on Row 1 of the antigram under the RT column).
7. Add 2 drops LISS reagent to each tube. Mix by agitation and incubate for 10 to 15 minutes (per manufacturer's instructions) at 37° C in a water bath or heat block.

8. Centrifuge, read, and record reactions for each tube in the appropriate space on the antigram as in steps 5 and 6.

9. Proceed with IAT by washing each tube three or four times with physiologic saline. (This may be done manually or by use of an automated serologic cell washer.)

10. Add 1 or 2 drops of AHG, according to manufacturer's instructions, to the dry button of RBCs in each tube. Mix.

11. Centrifuge, read, and record reactions for each tube in the appropriate space on the antigram as in steps 5 and 6.

12. To each test tube with a negative IAT, add 1 drop of IgG-coated "check" cells. Mix.

13. Centrifuge, read, and record.

Note: The check cells give a mixed-field positive reaction that may be recorded as a check mark next to the appropriate negative IAT reading ($0^{\sqrt{}}$) as an alternative to grading the reaction. Results of the IAT are only considered valid if the check cells reacted as expected, indicating that the saline washing was sufficient to remove serum proteins not bound to the test RBCs (which, if present, could neutralize the AHG) and that AHG was functional and was added to the test.

Initial Impressions

Before the actual interpretation of the panel begins, the technologist should review the results obtained in order develop an initial hypothesis about the antibody specificity. Questions that should be addressed include the following: Does the antibody directly agglutinate some panel red cells or are the positive reactions seen in IAT only? Are both positive and negative reactions seen with the panel RBCs or are all RBCs reactive, suggesting an antibody to an antigen of high incidence in the population? Are all reactions of similar strength, suggesting a single antibody, or is there a variety of reaction grades, suggesting multiple antibodies? Is the auto control reactive or nonreactive, suggesting autoantibody or alloantibody? The serologist can form a first impression about the nature of the antibody from these first clues, but identification of the antibody specificity(ies) is done by a process of exclusion.

The Principle of Exclusion

Interpretation of the antibody identification panel is made by analyzing in a logical step-by-step manner the panel cells that were nonreactive with the patient's serum and those that were reactive. This process, in blood banking jargon, is called "ruling out" antibodies. The serologic reactions documented during testing of the patient's serum, the unknown, will be compared to the phenotype of each panel donor, the known. This is best illustrated by using an example of a completed antibody identification panel (Case 12-1).

Case 12-1 shows a simplified version of a commercial red cell panel that characterizes (provides the phenotype of) the donor RBCs for the common antigens that the U.S. Food and Drug Administration (FDA) requires to be present on antibody detection and antibody identification RBCs.[6] These common antigens are D, C, E, c, e, P_1, M, N, S, s, Le^a, Le^b, K, k, Fy^a, Fy^b, Jk^a, and Jk^b. Actually, the reagent RBCs have many additional antigens on them, for example, antigens of high incidence in the population such as Js^b, U, Jr^a, Lu^b, and At^a, which are present on the RBCs of nearly 100% of donors. Commercial panels often list some of these high-incidence antigens in additional columns on the antigram or in a footnote on the page. RBCs of individual donors may also contain antigens of low incidence, for example, C^w, Kp^a, Js^a, Lu^a, or Co^b. If additional phenotype information about the reagent cell donor is known, it will be listed in a separate column on the worksheet or provided by the manufacturer in another format.

In Case 12-1, note that there were no positive reactions with any of the panel RBCs in the IS or LISS 37° C phases. All positive reactions occurred only in the

Case 12-1

	Cell ID	D	C	E	c	e	P₁	M	N	S	s	Le^a	Le^b	(K)	k	Fy^a	Fy^b	Jk^a	Jk^b	IS	LISS 37° C	Anti -IgG
1	R₁R₁–1	+	+	0	0	+	0	+	0	+	0	0	+	0	+	+	0	+	+	0	0	0✓
2	R₁R₁–2	+	+	0	0	+	+	+	+	0	+	0	+	0	+	+	0	+	+	0	0	0✓
3	R₂R₂	+	0	+	+	0	+	0	+	0	+	0	+	0	+	0	+	+	0	0	0	0✓
4	R₂r	+	0	+	+	+	+	+	+	+	+	0	0	+	0	+	+	0	+	0	0	3+
5	rr–1	0	0	0	+	+	+	+	0	+	+	+	0	0	+	+	+	0	+	0	0	0✓
6	rr–2	0	0	0	+	+	+	+	0	+	+	0	0	+	+	+	0	+	+	0	0	2+
7	r'r	0	+	0	+	+	0	0	+	+	0	0	+	0	+	+	+	+	0	0	0	0✓
8	r"r	0	0	+	+	+	+	+	+	0	+	0	+	0	+	0	+	+	0	0	0	0✓
9	R₁r	+	+	0	+	+	+	0	+	0	+	+	0	0	+	+	0	0	+	0	0	0✓
10	R₁R₂	+	+	+	+	+	0	+	0	+	+	0	+	0	+	0	+	+	0	0	0	0✓
11	R₀r	+	0	0	+	+	+	+	+	0	+	0	0	0	+	0	0	+	+	0	0	0✓
12	Auto Control													0✓						0	0	0✓

Anti-K can be identified. All K+ RBCs are reactive and all K– RBCs are nonreactive. All other common alloantibodies can be excluded. The patient's RBCs type K–.

IAT (column headed Anti-IgG), suggesting that the antibody is IgG in nature. The next step is to exclude from consideration antibodies to all antigens present on the RBCs of panel cells that were nonreactive with the patient's serum. The first example of nonreactive RBCs is with panel cell 1.

Using a ruler, isolate the first row of pluses and zeros on the grid that correspond to the phenotype of panel cell 1 and the results of the patient's serum with these RBCs. Cross out (rule out) each antigen in the header column where there is a plus sign (+) on the antigram. Using the first row, the following antigens can be crossed out: D, C, e, M, S, Le^b, k, and Fy^a. Although these RBCs are also Jk(a+) and Jk(b+), it is preferable to exclude these antibodies using RBCs that are from RBCs homozygous for Jk^a and Jk^b. The zygosity of the reagent red cell donor is important because the amount of antigen present on the red cells may be dependent on whether the individual has a "double dose" of that antigen or a "single dose" and some antibodies may react more strongly with RBCs from homozygous donors than with RBCs from heterozygous donors. This phenomenon is called "dosage" and is seen most often with antibodies in the Rh, MNS, Duffy, and Kidd blood group systems. Exclusion should be done on RBCs from donors presumed homozygous for these antigens whenever possible.

Next move the ruler down the panel to the row of the grid for panel cell 2. Following the same logic, the following additional antigens can be crossed out: P₁ and s. (Do not rule out N, Jk^a, and Jk^b until RBCs from homozygous donors are available.) Now focus on the row of the next nonreactive panel cells, row 3. The following antigens can be crossed out: E, c, N, Fy^b, and Jk^a. The patient's serum reacted strongly by IAT with the RBCs of panel cell 4, so skip over row 4 and focus on row 5. Le^a and Jk^b can be ruled out, leaving only one antigen, K, remaining in the column headings not excluded thus far. Following the same rule-out process for the remaining nonreactive cells, 7 through 11, no additional exclusions can be done on this particular panel.

Next evaluate the panel RBCs that were reactive with the patient's serum (panel cells 4 and 6) for the presence of the antigen(s) not excluded. In this case, both panel cells are K+, which is consistent with the only antigen not excluded by the rule-out process. Because the patient's serum reacted with all K+ RBCs on the

Refer to Chapter 1 for a discussion of zygosity and applications in blood banking.

TABLE 12-2 Serologic Characteristics of Common Antibodies

Blood Group System	Antibody	Reactive at RT?	Reactive by IAT?	Reactive with Enzyme-Treated RBCs?	Associated with HDN?	Associated with HTR?
Rh	–D	Some	Yes	Yes	Yes	Yes
	–C	Some	Yes	Yes	Yes	Yes
	–E	Some	Yes	Yes	Yes	Yes
	–c	Some	Yes	Yes	Yes	Yes
	–e	Some	Yes	Yes	Yes	Yes
P	–P₁	Most	Rare	Yes	No	Rare
MNS	–M	Most	Rare	No	No	Rare
	–N	Most	Rare	No	No	No
	–S	Few	Yes	No	Rare	Yes
	–s	No	Yes	Variable	Rare	Rare
Lewis	–Leᵃ	Yes	Some	Yes	No	Rare
	–Leᵇ	Yes	Some	Yes	No	No
Kell	–K	Rare	Yes	Yes	Yes	Yes
	–k	No	Yes	Yes	Rare	Yes
Duffy	–Fyᵃ	Rare	Yes	No	Yes	Yes
	–Fyᵇ	No	Yes	No	Rare	Yes
Kidd	–Jkᵃ	No	Yes	Yes	Yes	Yes
	–Jkᵇ	No	Yes	Yes	Rare	Yes

panel and was nonreactive with all donors who were K–, the antibody identified in Case 12-1 appears to be anti-K. This is referred to as a "perfect fit." Next consider the degree of fit between the hypothesized antibody, in this case K, and the typical reactivity patterns of this antibody. Anti-K typically reacts by IAT, so the identification of anti-K is highly probable. Refer to Table 12-2 for the typical reactivity phase for common antibodies.

If the patient has formed anti-K it is expected that the patient's RBCs are K–. To further strengthen the hypothesized solution (anti-K), the patient's RBCs should be phenotyped for the K antigen using a commercial anti-K reagent. To further increase the probability that the solution is correct, many blood banks recommend that a third example of K+ donor RBCs be tested, if available. In this case, or any example of a single alloantibody, looking back at the cells reactive by the antibody screen and comparing them to the antigram provided with the antibody detection cells would provide a third example of antigen-positive cells.

The practice of testing three antigen-positive cells to confirm the antibody specificity is often called the "three-plus-three" rule; antibody identification is made based on a minimum of three antigen-positive RBCs that react with the unknown antibody and a minimum of three antigen-negative RBCs that do not react. It is based on the statistical probability recommended by Fisher ($p < 0.05$).[7] A more practical approach using two positives and two negatives is also acceptable.[8] In any case, whether a laboratory chooses a policy to use two or three antigen-positive RBCs, the minimum of nonreactive RBCs that need to be tested will vary depending on the number of panel cells necessary to exclude all other common alloantibodies. In many cases this will be more than two or three.

Case 12-2 is an example of anti-D, the most common alloantibody found in Rh-negative individuals. All other common antibodies can be excluded by using the nonreactive donor RBCs, panel cells 5, 6, 7, and 8. Note that anti-C and anti-E must be excluded on RBCs from heterozygous panel cells (i.e., whose donors who are either C+c+ or E+e+). This is because the rarity of Rh-negative donors who are homozygous for C or E (D–C+c– and D–E+e– phenotypes, respectively) is such that manufacturers of commercial panels cannot supply them. In Case 12-2, there

Case 12-2

Cell ID	D	C	E	c	e	P₁	M	N	S	s	Leᵃ	Leᵇ	K	k	Fyᵃ	Fyᵇ	Jkᵃ	Jkᵇ	IS	LISS 37°C	Anti-IgG
1 R₁R₁–1	+	+	0	0	+	0	+	0	+	0	0	+	0	+	+	0	+	+	0	0	3+
2 R₁R₁–2	+	+	0	0	+	+	+	+	0	+	0	+	0	+	+	0	+	+	0	0	3+
3 R₂R₂	+	0	+	+	0	+	0	+	0	+	0	+	0	+	0	+	+	0	0	0	3+ˢ
4 R₂r	+	0	+	+	+	+	+	+	+	+	0	0	+	0	+	+	0	+	0	0	3+
5 rr–1	0	0	0	+	+	+	+	0	+	+	+	0	0	+	+	+	0	+	0	0	0√
6 rr–2	0	0	0	+	+	+	+	0	+	+	0	0	+	+	+	0	+	0	0	0	0√
7 r'r	0	+	0	+	+	0	0	+	+	0	0	+	0	+	+	+	+	0	0	0	0√
8 r"r	0	0	+	+	+	+	+	+	0	+	0	+	0	+	0	+	+	0	0	0	0√
9 R₁r	+	+	0	+	+	+	0	+	0	+	+	0	0	+	+	0	0	+	0	0	3+
10 R₁R₂	+	+	+	+	+	0	+	0	+	+	0	+	0	+	0	+	+	0	0	0	3+
11 Rₒr	+	0	0	+	+	+	+	+	0	+	0	0	0	0	+	0	0	+	+	0	2+
12 Auto Control	0																		0	0	0√

Anti-D can be identified. All D+ RBCs are reactive and all D− RBCs are nonreactive. All other common alloantibodies can be excluded. The patient's RBCs type D−.

are more than three examples each of antigen-positive and antigen-negative cells already on the panel, so additional cells do not need to be tested to confirm the identification of anti-D. The patient's D phenotype may already be known if the laboratory has performed ABO and Rh typing of this patient for pretransfusion testing. A small number of individuals who are Rh positive (D+) but whose RBCs have only partial D antigen are capable of forming alloanti-D because they can form antibody to the D epitopes that are lacking from their own RBCs. Partial D individuals who have formed alloanti-D must be transfused with Rh-negative red blood cells.

Case 12-3 shows reactivity at RT only. Using panel cell 1, anti-D, anti-C, anti-e, anti-M, anti-S, anti-Leᵇ, anti-k, and anti-Fyᵃ can be excluded. The next nonreactive panel cell is 7. Anti-N and anti-Jkᵃ can be ruled out. Panel cell 9 allows for exclusion of anti-Fyᵇ. This leaves anti-E, anti-c, anti-P₁, anti-s, anti-Leᵃ, anti-K, and anti-Jkᵇ not ruled out. The pattern of panel cells reactive with the patient's serum matches the pattern of phenotype results for P₁ (all P₁+ RBCs were reactive and all P₁− RBCs were nonreactive), but there is a degree of variability of reactivity (some P₁+ RBCs reacted 1+ and some 2+). Anti-E, anti-c, anti-s, and anti-Jkᵇ cannot be excluded using double-dose panel cells, but anti-E, anti-c, anti-s, and anti-Jkᵇ, as well as anti-K, would be expected to react by IAT, so are unlikely to be present. Anti-Leᵃ cannot be excluded and would be most likely to be reactive at RT like anti-P₁.

Phenotyping the patient's RBCs for various antigens may be helpful, but all the necessary antisera may not be available in a hospital laboratory. For the sake of example, assume that the antisera are available and the patient is c+ s+ Jk(b+). If that information is known, the corresponding antibodies (anti-c, anti-s, and anti-Jkᵇ) can be excluded; however, because the patient types E− Le(a−) K−, as well as P₁−, an additional panel of selected RBCs must be tested to confirm anti-P₁ and to exclude anti-E, anti-Leᵃ, and anti-K.

Case 12-3, Selected Cell Panel, is an example of an additional panel that could be constructed to complete the exclusion process. By selecting specific panel RBCs from additional panels, anti-E, anti-c, anti-s, anti-Leᵃ, anti-K, and anti-Jkᵇ could be excluded and anti-P₁ confirmed. The variability in reactivity noted earlier is probably due to varying P₁ antigen strength on individual panel donors'

Refer to Chapter 5 for a discussion of the inheritance and serology of the Rh system.

Refer to Chapter 6 for a discussion of the unique serologic characteristics of many of the more commonly encountered blood group antigens.

Case 12-3

	Cell ID	D	C	E	c	e	P_1	M	N	S	s	Le^a	Le^b	K	k	Fy^a	Fy^b	Jk^a	Jk^b	15' RT	LISS 37°C	Anti-IgG
1	R_1R_1–1	+	+	0	0	+	0	+	0	+	0	0	+	0	+	+	0	+	+	0	0	0√
2	R_1R_1–2	+	+	0	0	+	+	+	+	0	+	0	+	0	+	+	0	+	+	1+	0	0√
3	R_2R_2	+	0	+	+	0	+	0	+	0	+	0	+	0	+	0	+	+	0	1+	0	0√
4	R_2r	+	0	+	+	+	+	+	+	+	+	0	0	+	0	+	+	0	+	2+	0	0√
5	rr–1	0	0	0	+	+	+	+	0	+	+	+	0	0	+	+	+	+	0	1+	0	0√
6	rr–2	0	0	0	+	+	+	+	0	+	+	0	0	+	+	+	0	+	+	2+	0	0√
7	r'r	0	+	0	+	+	0	0	+	+	0	0	+	0	+	+	+	+	0	0	0	0√
8	r''r	0	0	+	+	+	+	+	+	0	+	0	+	0	+	0	+	+	0	1+	0	0√
9	R_1r	+	+	0	+	+	+	0	+	0	+	+	0	0	+	+	0	0	+	1+	0	0√
10	R_1R_2	+	+	+	+	+	0	+	0	+	+	0	+	0	+	0	+	+	0	0	0	0√
11	R_or	+	0	0	+	+	+	+	+	0	+	0	0	0	+	0	0	+	+	2+	0	0√
12	Auto Control	3+	4+	0	4+	4+	0				3+	0		0√					3+	0	0	0√

Anti-P_1 is tentatively identified. All P_1+RBCs are reactive and all P_1– RBCs are nonreactive. The patient is P_1–. Not all other common alloantibodies can be excluded by the rule-out process. Anti-E, anti-c, anti-s, anti-K, and anti-Jk^b would be expected to react by IAT, so are not likely to be present. Anti-c, anti-s, and anti-Jk^b can be excluded based on the patient's RBC phenotype. Anti-Le^a cannot be excluded and would also be most likely to react at RT. Le(a+) P_1– RBCs would need to be tested to confirm or exclude anti-Le^a.

Selected Cell Panel

	Cell ID	D	C	E	c	e	P_1	M	N	S	s	Le^a	Le^b	K	k	Fy^a	Fy^b	Jk^a	Jk^b	15' RT	LISS 37°C	Anti-IgG
1	R_or	+	0	0	+	+	0	+	0	+	0	+	0	0	+	+	0	+	+	0	0	0√
2	R_1R_1–3	+	+	0	0	+	0	+	+	0	+	0	+	+	+	+	0	0	+	0	0	0√
3	R_2R_2–2	+	0	+	+	0	0	0	+	0	+	0	+	0	+	0	+	+	0	0	0	0√
4	R_2r	+	0	+	+	+	+	+	+	+	+	+	0	0	+	+	0	0	+	1+	0	0√
5	rr–1	0	0	0	+	+	0	+	0	+	+	0	+	0	+	+	+	0	+	0	0	0√
6	rr–2	0	0	0	+	+	+	+	0	+	+	0	0	0	+	+	+	+	+	2+	0	0√

Anti-P_1 is confirmed and anti-E, anti-c, anti-Le^a, anti-K, and anti-Jk^b can be excluded.

RBCs. This type of variability in antigen strength, which is unrelated to zygosity, is known to occur with P_1 and other antigens, including A, I, Le^a, Le^b, and Sd^a.

Enhancement Media and Alternative Methods

In addition to the LISS IAT method used in the previous section to illustrate antibody identification, there are various other acceptable methods used routinely in pretransfusion testing. Other common **enhancement** reagents, such as 22% or 30% bovine albumin and PEG, are examples of alternative antibody enhancement media. Although the principle use of enhancement media is to reduce incubation time or to increase reaction strength, there are advantages and disadvantages of each medium. For example, albumin is often used to enhance direct agglutination of Rh antibodies but may also enhance detection of "nuisance" antibodies, such as cold-reacting antibodies, that are not usually considered clinically significant. PEG can enhance reactivity of weak Kidd or Duffy system antibodies but may also enhance detection of warm autoantibodies, causing additional testing to resolve the

Enhancement: Strengthening antigen-antibody reactions through a variety of chemical and nonchemical techniques. In some cases, the most convenient and least expensive of these techniques involve no special reagents or equipment, such as increasing the serum-cell ratio.

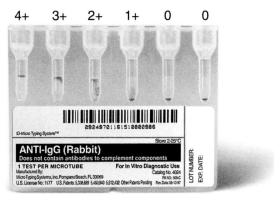

4+   3+   2+   1+   0   0

ID-Micro Typing System™

Store 2-25°C

ANTI-IgG (Rabbit)
Does not contain antibodies to complement components

1 TEST PER MICROTUBE   For In Vitro Diagnostic Use
Manufactured By: Catalog No. 4024
Micro Typing Systems, Inc, Pompano Beach, FL 33069   PK NO: 009-C
U.S. License No: 1177   U.S. Patents: 5,338,689 5,460,940 5,512,432 Other Patents Pending   Rev. Date: 06-13-97

LOT NUMBER:
EXP. DATE:

Fig. 12-3 Grading agglutination: ID-MTS gel card. *(Courtesy Ortho Clinical Diagnostics, Raritan, NJ.)*

serology. No single testing protocol is perfect and none will detect every example of a clinically significant antibody. Problem solving often involves the use of more than one method of testing in order to increase or decrease sensitivity.

As mentioned briefly in Chapter 11, technologic advances have resulted in the introduction of alternative methodologies such as solid-phase and column agglutination techniques to the blood bank. Solid-phase technology uses microplates in which a monolayer of RBCs or RBC stroma containing the target antigen is fixed to the well of the microplate. The patient's unknown antibody is incubated in the well to allow for the antigen-antibody reaction to take place. For indirect antiglobulin testing, the microplate is then washed to remove unbound antibody. Antiglobulin reagent bound to indicator cells (RBCs coated with IgG) is added to each well and the microplate is centrifuged. Adherence of the indicator cells to the surface of the well is a positive reaction whose strength can be graded.

Column agglutination technology, also known as the gel test, uses microtubes prepared by the manufacturer. The most commonly used application of the gel test is the anti-IgG card for indirect antiglobulin testing. Serum/plasma and RBCs are added to the reaction chamber of the microtube and incubated at 37° C to allow for sensitization of the red cells. The gel card is then centrifuged, which brings the RBCs in contact with the antiglobulin reagent contained in the gel in the lower half of the microtube. If the RBCs are sensitized with IgG antibody, the cells will agglutinate and subsequently be trapped in the gel. Depending on the size of the agglutinate, the RBCs are trapped on top of the gel layer or at varying points throughout the gel. This agglutination can be graded. Unsensitized RBCs pass through the gel and are pelleted at the bottom of the microtube (Fig. 12-3).

These techniques have advantages and disadvantages as well. Both have the advantage of a stable endpoint, which allows a more objective measure of grading the agglutination. Both have the option to be automated or semiautomated. Column agglutination has the disadvantage of requiring acquisition of some dedicated equipment, and both systems require some specialized training for their use.

Chemical Treatment of Test RBCs

In addition to different enhancement media, treatment of test cells with various chemicals may be a good alternative to testing selected cell panels. Two of the most widely used groups of chemicals in blood banking are **proteolytic enzymes** (e.g., ficin, papain, bromelin, trypsin) and **sulfhydryl reagents** (e.g., dithiothreitol [DTT], 2-mercaptoethanol [2-ME]). Enzymes cleave certain proteins from the surface of the RBCs, destroying some antigens while enhancing others. Sulfhydryl reagents cleave disulfide bonds that are necessary in maintaining some antigens' physical conformation. For example, ficin treatment of RBCs will destroy the

Enzymes: The use of proteolytic enzymes in in vitro test systems to facilitate antibody identification. Blood group antigen antibody reactions are differentially affected by enzyme treatment.

Sulfhydryl reagents: Substances that cleave the disulfide bonds of IgM molecules, abolishing the ability of the molecule to agglutinate or bind complement. Thiol and sulfhydryl reagents (DTT and 2-ME) are useful in differentiating IgM antibodies from IgG antibodies.

TABLE 12-3 Effect of Enzymes and DTT on Blood Group Antigens

Reaction with 0.1% Ficin- or Papain-treated RBCs	Reaction with 0.2M DTT-treated RBCs	Possible Specificity of Antibody
Negative	Positive	M, N, S, s,* Ge2, Ge4, Xg^a, Fy^a, Fy^b, Ch/Rg
Negative	Negative	Indian, JMH
Positive	Weak	Cromer, Knops (weak or negative in ficin), Lutheran, Dombrock
Variable	Negative	Yt^a
Positive	Negative	Kell, LW, Scianna
Positive	Positive	A, B, H, P$_1$, P, Rh, I, i, Lewis, Kidd, Fy3, Diego, Colton, Ge3, At^a, Cs^a, Er^a, Jr^a, Lan, Ok^a, Vel, Sd^a
Positive	Enhanced	Kx

Modified from Reid ME, Lomas-Francis C: Blood Group Antigen Facts Book, San Diego, Academic Press, 2004.
*s variable with ficin/papain.

common antigens M, N, S, s, Fy^a, and Fy^b but will enhance Rh and Lewis antigens. DTT treatment of RBCs will destroy all Kell blood group system antigens. Table 12-3 summarizes the action of these chemicals on additional antigens or whole blood group systems.

Case 12-4 shows an example of anti-Fy^a, which is reactive by LISS IAT but which is not reactive if the same panel RBCs are ficin treated because ficin destroys the Fy^a antigen. The ficin-treated panel shows an underlying anti-K. Testing selected cell panels should have also revealed the anti-K, but if additional panels are not available, the second antibody could have been missed. This illustrates the concept of a "masked" antibody, that is, an antibody hidden by the reactivity of another. This further emphasizes the importance of doing a complete rule-out process. This patient should receive red cells that are both Fy(a−) and K−.

Case 12-5 shows an example of anti-k and anti-E. Note that an antigen of high incidence in the population, such as k, is present on all, or nearly all, the RBCs on a panel. In Case 12-5, the patient's serum reacts with the RBCs of all panel cells by LISS IAT, but the reactivity with cell 4 is weaker than with the other panel cells. This pattern of reactivity suggests multiple alloantibodies.

When the panel RBCs are ficin treated and tested with the patient's serum, all panel donors are still reactive, so it does not appear that the target antigens of these antibodies are ficin sensitive. Next, the panel cells are DTT treated and tested with the patient's serum. Anti-E is evident in the DTT-treated panel. The patient is E−, which is consistent with anti-E in the serum. The antigens in the Kell, LW, and Scianna blood group systems are destroyed by DTT but not by ficin. No commercial antisera exist to test RBCs for LW or Scianna antigens, but most blood banks have access to anti-K and many also stock anti-k. The patient in Case 5 types K + k− so is capable of making anti-k. Panel cell 4 is also K + k− and was the weakest reacting panel cell by LISS IAT, but was apparently reactive due to anti-E. All other common alloantibodies can be excluded by the results of testing with the DTT-treated panel cells.

The anti-E and anti-k should be confirmed by testing a minimum of two examples of antigen-negative (E−k−) RBCs. Confirmation of anti-k may need to be performed by an immunohematology reference laboratory that has access to rare reagent red cells. If the patient requires transfusion, red cell products that are E−k− must be provided. Compatible red cell components may need to be obtained by a regional blood center with access to the American Rare Donor Program (the combined registry of rare donors for the American Association of Blood Banks and the American Red Cross).

Case 12-4

	Cell ID	D	C	E	c	e	P₁	M	N	S	s	Leᵃ	Leᵇ	K	k	Fyᵃ	Fyᵇ	Jkᵃ	Jkᵇ	LISS 37C	LISS -IgG	Ficin 37°C	Ficin -IgG
1	R₁R₁−4	+	+	0	0	+	0	+	0	+	0	0	+	0	+	+	0	+	+	0	3+	0	0√
2	R₁R₁−5	+	+	0	0	+	+	+	+	0	+	0	+	0	+	+	0	+	+	0	3+	0	0√
3	R₂R₂	+	0	+	+	0	+	0	+	0	+	0	+	0	+	0	+	+	0	0	0√	0	0√
4	R₂r	+	0	+	+	+	+	+	+	+	+	+	0	+	0	+	+	0	+	0	3+	0	2+
5	rr−3	0	0	0	+	+	+	+	0	+	+	0	0	0	+	+	+	0	+	0	2+	0	0√
6	rr−4	0	0	0	+	+	+	+	0	+	+	0	+	+	+	+	0	+	+	0	3+	0	2+
7	Rₒr	+	0	0	+	+	+	+	+	0	+	+	0	0	+	0	0	+	+	0	0√	0	0√
8	R₁R₂	+	+	+	+	+	0	+	0	+	0	0	+	0	+	0	+	0	+	0	0√	0	0√
9	Auto Control											0√	0√							0	0√	0	0√

Anti-D, anti-E, anti-c, anti-e, anti-P₁, anti-M, anti-N, anti-S, anti-s, anti-Leᵃ, anti-Leᵇ, anti-k, anti-Fyᵇ, anti-Jkᵃ, and anti-Jkᵇ can be excluded by LISS IAT using panel cells 3, 7, and 8.
Anti-C can be excluded using panel cells 1 or 2 by ficin IAT.
Anti-K is detectable by ficin IAT. Anti-Fya is detectable by LISS IAT. The patient's RBCs are K−Fy(a−).

Case 12-5

	Cell ID	D	C	E	c	e	P₁	M	N	S	s	Leᵃ	Leᵇ	K	k	Fyᵃ	Fyᵇ	Jkᵃ	Jkᵇ	LISS 37°C	LISS -IgG	Ficin -IgG	DTT -IgG
1	R₁R₁−1	+	+	0	0	+	0	+	0	+	0	0	+	0	+	+	0	+	+	0	3+	3+	0√
2	R₁R₁−2	+	+	0	0	+	+	+	+	0	+	0	+	0	+	+	0	+	+	0	3+	3+	0√
3	R₂R₂	+	0	+	+	0	+	0	+	0	+	0	+	0	+	0	+	+	0	0	3+	3+	2+
4	R₂r	+	0	+	+	+	+	+	+	+	+	0	0	+	0	+	+	0	+	0	1+	3+	1+
5	rr−1	0	0	0	+	+	+	+	0	+	+	+	0	0	+	+	+	0	+	0	3+	3+	0√
6	rr−2	0	0	0	+	+	+	+	0	+	+	0	0	+	+	+	0	+	+	0	3+	3+	0√
7	r'r	0	+	0	+	+	0	0	+	+	0	0	+	0	+	0	+	+	0	0	3+	3+	0√
8	r"r	0	0	+	+	+	+	+	+	0	+	0	+	0	+	+	+	+	0	0	3+	3+	1+
9	R₁r	+	+	0	+	+	+	0	+	0	+	+	0	0	+	+	0	0	+	0	3+	3+	0√
10	R₁R₂	+	+	+	+	+	0	+	0	+	+	0	+	0	+	0	+	+	0	0	3+	3+	1+
11	Rₒr	+	0	0	+	+	+	+	+	0	+	0	0	0	+	0	0	+	+	0	3+	3+	0√
12	Auto Control			0								4+	0√							0	0	0√	0√

The initial panel tested by LISS IAT shows all donor RBCs reactive, but a negative Auto Control. Ficin-treated RBCs are also all reactive.
DTT-treated panel RBCs reveal anti-E underlying an antibody to an antigen of high incidence. The patient's RBCs phenotype is E−k−.
The identification of anti-E and anti-k should be confirmed by testing E−k− RBCs.

Not all alloantibodies identified by the process of analyzing a panel are clinically significant. Alloantibodies that do not react at 37° C generally do not require the use of antigen-negative blood for transfusion. Common alloantibodies that tend to fall into this category of clinically insignificant antibodies are anti-Leᵇ, anti-P₁, anti-M, anti-N, and anti-A₁. The expected clinical significance of these and other antibodies is listed in Table 12-4. It should be emphasized, however, that any example of an alloantibody that is reactive at 37° C (i.e., body temperature) is potentially clinically significant.

TABLE 12-4 **Clinical Significance of Some Alloantibodies to Blood Group Antigens**

Usually Clinically Significant	Sometimes Clinically Significant	Clinically Insignificant if Nonreactive at 37° C	Generally Clinically Insignificant
A and B	At^a	A_1	HLA/Bg
Di^a and Di^b	Co^a and Co^b	H	Ch/Rg
Fy^a, Fy^b, Fy3	Cr^a	I	Cs^a
H in O_h (Bombay)	Do^a, Do^b, Hy, Gy	Le^a	JMH
K, k, Kp^a, Kp^b, Js^a, Js^b	Ge^2, Ge^3	Lu^a and Lu^b	Kn^a/McC^a
Jk^a and Jk^b	Jr^a	M and N	Le^b
P and PP_1P^k	Lan	P_1	Xg^a
D, C, E, c, e, C^w	LW	Sd^a	
S, s, U	Sc1 and Sc2		
Vel	Yt^a		

Modified from Reid ME, Lomas-Francis C: Blood Group Antigen Facts Book, 2nd. San Diego, Academic Press, 2004.

Refer to Chapter 2 for a discussion of antiglobulin testing.

INVESTIGATING THE POSITIVE DIRECT ANTIGLOBULIN TEST

Direct Antiglobulin Test

Thus far, all the pretransfusion testing discussed has focused on the indirect antiglobulin test (IAT), in which the test red cells are incubated with serum to determine if IgG has coated the red cells in vitro. In contrast, the direct antiglobulin test (DAT) involves adding antihuman globulin reagent directly to a patient's washed red cells to determine if IgG or complement coating has occurred in vivo. Although direct antiglobulin testing is not necessary for routine pretransfusion testing, it is of particular value in antibody identification, especially when evaluated according to the patient's recent transfusion history. Although the DAT results are often similar to the autologous control tested with an antibody identification panel, the DAT performed on an anticoagulated whole blood sample (e.g., EDTA tube) reflects the status of red blood cells circulating in the patient. (RBCs from a clotted blood sample stored in the cold may have in vitro–bound complement, resulting in misleading information if reported to the physician.)

When the DAT is positive it indicates that the red cells in the patient's circulation are coated with IgG and/or complement. Hospital patients are known to have a higher rate of a positive DAT than the normal blood donor population (1% to 15% vs. 0.1%). The finding of a positive DAT in a random patient may be anomalous, but if there is clinical evidence that the patient's red cells are not surviving normally (such as an elevated reticulocyte count, elevated bilirubin, decreased hematocrit with no evidence of bleeding, etc.) the presence of a positive DAT is significant.[9] If the patient has recently been transfused, the patient may have specific alloantibody coating circulating transfused red cells and the antihuman globulin reagent used in the DAT is detecting the IgG-coated transfused cells. If the patient has not recently been transfused, the patient may have autoantibody coating his or her RBCs.

Delayed Hemolytic Transfusion Reactions

In all the examples of panels studied thus far, the autologous control has been negative. If the auto control is positive, a DAT should be performed, because it correlates better with the patient's clinical status. A positive DAT should be investigated if there is evidence of a hemolytic process in the patient. The patient may not have overt symptoms of a hemolytic transfusion reaction, but if a patient was recently transfused and is not currently bleeding but the hematocrit is dropping, there may be increased red cell destruction of circulating transfused red cells by the reticuloendothelial (RE) system if the transfused RBCs are sensitized with alloantibody and/or coated with complement. In many cases, the positive DAT in this situation will have a mixed-field appearance, because some of the patient's RBCs are DAT+ (antibody-coated transfused RBCs) and some are DAT− (autologous RBCs).

When a transfusion reaction is suspected, the serologic evaluation should include the preparation and testing of an eluate of the patient's RBCs. An eluate should recover antibody that is coating the patient's red cells. To prepare an eluate, RBCs are thoroughly washed with saline, and then treated with heat, chemicals, or acids to dissociate RBC-bound IgG. Eluate preparation methods may be found in the current edition of the AABB *Technical Manual*.[10] Alternatively, eluates may be prepared using commercially available kits. Antibody identification, using an eluate prepared from the patient's RBCs, may be done by testing it with the reagent red cell panel. It is most useful if this is done in parallel with the patient's serum for comparison. Rarely, an antibody is identified in the eluate that is not yet present in the serum, presumably because it is not of high enough titer (quantity) to both sensitize the transfused red cells and be present in detectable quantities in the serum. As a control on the adequacy of the washing of the red cells before the elution of RBC-bound antibody, a "last wash" control (consisting of the supernatant from the last time the RBCs are washed) is tested with the RBC panel and should be nonreactive.

Case 12-6 is an example an eluate tested in parallel with a recently transfused patient's serum following the detection of a positive DAT.

In Case 12-6, anti-E is detected in the patient's serum at the 37° C agglutination phase and is enhanced by LISS IAT. There is additional weak reactivity by LISS IAT. Using the exclusion process, all common alloantibodies except anti-E and anti-Jk^a can be ruled out. The patient's RBCs are typed and found to be E−, but the Jk^a phenotyping (using monoclonal anti-Jk^a reagent) shows mixed-field reactivity, similar to the auto control. The eluate contains anti-Jk^a but not anti-E. This serologic picture is consistent with a patient recently transfused with E− Jk(a+) RBCs. Either E− RBCs were chosen because the blood bank detected and identified anti-E in the pretransfusion sample or the patient had a historical record of it, or because up to 70% of donors are E− so E− RBCs happened to be transfused. Some Jk(a+) RBCs appear to still be in the patient's circulation, but are probably in the process of being cleared.

Case 12-6

	Cell ID	D	C	E	c	e	P₁	M	N	S	s	Leᵃ	Leᵇ	K	k	Fyᵃ	Fyᵇ	Jkᵃ	Jkᵇ	Serum LISS 37° C	Serum LISS anti-IgG	Eluate Eluate Anti-IgG	Eluate L. Wash Anti-IgG
1	R₁R₁−1	+	+	0	0	+	0	+	0	+	0	0	+	0	+	+	0	0	+	0	0$^{\sqrt{}}$	0$^{\sqrt{}}$	0$^{\sqrt{}}$
2	R₁R₁−2	+	+	0	0	+	+	+	+	0	+	0	+	0	+	+	0	+	+	0	±	2+	0$^{\sqrt{}}$
3	R₂R₂	+	0	+	+	0	+	0	+	0	+	0	+	0	+	0	+	+	0	2+	4+	2+	0$^{\sqrt{}}$
4	R₂r	+	0	+	+	+	+	+	+	+	+	0	0	+	+	+	+	0	+	1+	3+	0$^{\sqrt{}}$	0$^{\sqrt{}}$
5	rr−1	0	0	0	+	+	+	+	0	+	+	+	0	0	+	0	+	0	+	0	0$^{\sqrt{}}$	0$^{\sqrt{}}$	0$^{\sqrt{}}$
6	rr−2	0	0	0	+	+	+	+	0	+	+	0	0	+	+	+	0	+	+	0	±	2+	0$^{\sqrt{}}$
7	r'r	0	+	0	+	+	0	0	+	+	0	0	+	0	+	+	+	+	0	0	1+	2+	0$^{\sqrt{}}$
8	r"r	0	0	+	+	+	+	+	+	0	+	0	+	0	+	0	+	+	0	1+	3+	2+	0$^{\sqrt{}}$
9	R₁r	+	+	0	+	+	+	0	+	0	+	+	0	+	+	+	0	0	+	0	0$^{\sqrt{}}$	0$^{\sqrt{}}$	0$^{\sqrt{}}$
10	R₁R₂	+	+	+	+	+	0	+	0	+	+	0	+	0	+	0	+	+	0	1+	3+	2+	0$^{\sqrt{}}$
11	R₀r	+	0	0	+	+	+	+	+	0	+	0	0	0	+	0	0	+	+	0	±	2+	0$^{\sqrt{}}$
12	Auto control			0												mf		0	1+mf	mf	0	1+mf	

Refer to Chapter 17 for a discussion of autoimmune hemolysis.

ZZAP: A reagent that combines enzymes and a thiol reagent and inactivates the Kell antigens (except for K_x) on the red cell surface.

Warm Autoantibodies

Thus far, the antibodies described in this chapter have been alloantibodies, that is, antibodies to antigens that the patient lacks. Sometimes individuals form autoantibodies, which by definition are antibodies to antigens on their own red blood cells. Some of these are clinically significant and cause the patient to experience autoimmune hemolytic anemia (AIHA) whereas others are benign. Over 90% of patients with AIHA have a positive DAT. The patient's RBCs may be coated with IgG antibody and/or complement (C3). (Rarely RBCs may be coated with IgM or IgA, but these globulins may not be detectable with routine antiglobulin reagents.) In 50% to 90% of the patients with AIHA there is also autoantibody present in the serum; higher percentages of detection are dependent on the enhancement medium used (e.g., PEG). Sometimes the specificity of the autoantibody is obvious when a panel of red cells is tested, but most often the antibody has a broad specificity and reacts with all RBCs tested, including the patient's own.

Selecting blood for patients with warm autoantibodies requires that any alloantibodies that might be masked by the presence of the autoantibody be excluded. This is most often accomplished by the process of adsorption, where the autoantibody is removed from the serum by in vitro adsorption onto antigen-positive RBCs. The patient's serum is incubated with an aliquot of adsorbing cells, usually using a ratio of one volume of serum to one volume of RBCs. Often the adsorbing cells are chemically treated (e.g., with ficin or ZZAP,[11] a combination of enzyme and DTT) to enhance antibody uptake. After an appropriate incubation period (usually 30 minutes at 37° C), the mixture is centrifuged and the adsorbed serum is harvested and retested, either with antibody detection cells or a red cell panel. Sometimes multiple adsorptions must be subsequently performed on the aliquot of serum in order to remove all autoantibody.

If the patient has not been recently transfused (i.e., within the last 3 months), autologous adsorption using the patient's own RBCs is the method of choice; however, if the patient has been recently transfused, there is danger of adsorbing alloantibody onto the circulating transfused RBCs in the process, so allogeneic adsorptions must be done. Allogeneic adsorptions, sometimes called differential adsorptions, use aliquots of donor red cells chosen by their phenotypes for Rh, MNS, Kell, Duffy, and Kidd antigens, to differentiate alloantibodies underlying the warm autoantibody. As an alternative, if the blood bank knows the patient's phenotype for the common Rh, MNS, Kell, Duffy, and Kidd antigens and is able to obtain RBCs that are phenotypically identical to the patient's own, adsorptions may be performed on aliquots of those RBCs. Differential adsorptions are beyond the scope of most hospital blood banks, and may require an immunohematology reference laboratory. Autologous adsorption methods are considered routine and are performed in most hospital transfusion services.

Case 12-7 is an example of a warm autoantibody that reacts equally with all RBCs tested. When the patient's serum is adsorbed with ficin-treated autologous RBCs and retested, an alloantibody is detectable. Using the exclusion process and focusing on the adsorbed serum columns, anti-S can be identified in the adsorbed serum. It is assumed that the anti-S detected is an alloantibody, but in order to prove that, the patient's RBCs should be phenotyped for S. This poses a problem because the patient's autologous RBCs are DAT positive (i.e., already coated with IgG) and anti-S reagent requires indirect antiglobulin testing. In Case 12-6 this sort of problem, phenotyping of DAT+ RBCs, could be circumvented using monoclonal anti-Jk[a], which does not require the IAT, but no monoclonal examples of anti-S are currently available.

Problems Encountered with DAT-Positive Red Blood Cells

If DAT+ RBCs are used for phenotyping using antisera that require the use of the indirect antiglobulin test, false-positive reactions will result. Sometimes false-

Case 12-7

	Cell ID	D	C	E	c	e	P₁	M	N	S	s	Le^a	Le^b	K	k	Fy^a	Fy^b	Jk^a	Jk^b	Serum LISS 37°C	Serum Anti-IgG	Autoadsorbed Serum LISS 37°C	Autoadsorbed Serum Anti-IgG
1	R₁R₁-1	+	+	0	0	+	0	+	0	+	0	0	+	0	+	+	0	+	+	0	3+	0	2+
2	R₁R₁-2	+	+	0	0	+	+	+	+	0	+	0	+	0	+	+	0	+	+	0	3+	0	0^v
3	R₂R₂	+	0	+	+	0	+	0	+	0	+	0	+	0	+	0	+	+	0	0	3+	0	0^v
4	R₂r	+	0	+	+	+	+	+	+	+	+	+	0	+	+	+	+	0	+	0	3+	0	1+
5	rr-1	0	0	0	+	+	+	+	0	+	+	0	0	0	+	+	+	0	+	0	3+	0	1+
6	rr-2	0	0	0	+	+	+	+	0	+	+	0	0	0	+	+	0	+	+	0	3+	0	1+
7	r'r	0	+	0	+	+	0	0	+	+	0	0	+	0	+	+	+	+	0	0	3+	0	2+
8	r"r	0	0	+	+	+	+	+	0	0	+	0	+	+	+	0	+	+	0	0	3+	0	0^v
9	R₁r	+	+	0	+	+	+	0	+	0	+	+	0	0	+	0	+	0	+	0	3+	0	0^v
10	R₁R₂	+	+	+	+	+	0	+	0	+	+	0	+	0	+	0	+	+	0	0	3+	0	1+
11	R₀r	+	0	0	+	+	+	+	+	0	+	0	0	0	+	0	0	+	+	0	3+	0	0^v
12	Auto control						*0^v													0	3+		

* CDP-treated RBCs used for S typing.

positive reactions may even occur with reagents that directly agglutinate RBCs, such as monoclonal reagents[12] or high-protein Rh antisera, if the antibody-coated cells spontaneously agglutinate (i.e., agglutinate without the addition of antiglobulin serum) when centrifuged.

Chemicals that dissociate IgG from RBCs and leave the treated red cells intact are useful in blood banking to render DAT+ red cells DAT−. The treated RBCs can then be used to perform antiglobulin-dependent phenotyping. One of these chemicals is **chloroquine diphosphate** (CDP).[13] Choloroquine solutions may be prepared by the laboratory but are also commercially available. Chloroquine treatment of RBCs may weaken Rh antigens, so positive and negative control cells should be treated in parallel. RBCs should never be CDP treated for more than 2 hours. Chloroquine is also known to denature residual human leukocyte antigens (HLAs) that may be present on some RBCs; therefore this chemical can also be useful in the investigation of Bg (HLA-related) antibodies. Methods for preparing CDP and CDP treatment of RBCs may be found in the current edition of the AABB *Technical Manual*[10] or other textbooks.

Glycine acid EDTA treatment of RBCs also dissociates RBC-bound IgG and has the advantage of taking a few minutes instead of an hour. It is also commercially available in a kit. The disadvantage of using glycine acid EDTA–treated RBCs for phenotyping is that all antigens in some blood group systems (i.e., Kell, Cartwright, Er, and Bg) are destroyed. The most notable example is the Kell blood group system, because nearly all transfusion services stock anti-K reagent. Typing EGA-treated RBCs for the K antigen would give invalid results. Fortunately, monoclonal anti-K is commercially available and may be used to test DAT+ RBCs so long as no spontaneous agglutination is observed in a direct agglutination control tube (e.g., 10% albumin). Although this effect of glycine acid may be a disadvantage for RBC phenotyping for K and other affected antigens, this "destructive" property of glycine acid EDTA can be used as an investigative tool in selectively denaturing antigens for selected cell panels.

ANTIBODIES TO ANTIGENS OF HIGH OR LOW INCIDENCE

Blood group antigens vary tremendously in their frequency of representation on human RBCs. Most antigens are of moderate frequency within the population, but

Chloroquine diphosphate and glycine acid EDTA: Reagents that dissociate IgG from the red cell membrane while retaining membrane integrity. This technique is useful for removing bound antibody so that cells can be antigen typed using antisera that require the indirect antiglobulin phase of testing.

some antigens are of low incidence (less than 1%) and some are of high incidence (greater than 99%.) There are sometimes ethnic differences that are associated with the incidence of antigens within a specific blood group. Although the incidence of Jk^a antigen in a general population is approximately 75%, that is, three out of four individuals would be expected to type as Jk(a+), if the population being studied is predominantly black, the incidence of Jk(a+) individuals would be much higher, approximately 92%.

In some blood groups these ethnic differences are not noticeable; in others they are extreme. For example, the Fy(a–b–) phenotype is virtually nonexistent in Caucasians and Asians but is common (approximately 68%) in blacks. The unusual phenotypes At(a–), U–, and Js(b–) are rare in all populations, but are most frequently associated with blacks; the rare phenotypes Kp(b–), k–, PP$_1$P^k–, and Vel– are most frequently seen in Caucasians; the rare phenotypes Jr(a–), Jk(a–b–), and Ok(a–) are seen predominantly or exclusively in Asians; the rare phenotype Di(b–) is most frequently seen in Hispanics and Asians. The ethnic background of a patient may be an important clue if an antibody to an antigen of high incidence is suspected. (Caution: Although the sound or spelling of the patient's name may be a clue to his or her ethnicity, it is not as reliable as a short visit to the patient's bedside.)

Refer to Case 12-8 for an example of an antibody to an antigen of high incidence, anti-U. In this panel, an extra column called "Special" has been added. Note that in Case 12-8, panel cell 1 is Kp(a+), panel cell 2 is C^w+, panel cell 4 is Co(b+), and panel cell 11 is Js(a+); these are examples of antigens of low incidence. Panel cell 9 is noted to be Bg(a+). Bg antigens are residual HLA (white blood cell) antigens that have varying expression on some people's RBCs, but will be noted on a panel in the special information column if a particular panel donor's RBCs would be likely to react with sera containing Bg antibodies. Technically, Bg antigens are not of low incidence, but because Bg expression is so variable, the pattern of reactivity with anti-Bg^a, for example, might be similar to the pattern of reactivity seen for an antibody to a low-incidence antigen.

Panel cell 11, in addition to being Js(a+), is also U–. U is an antigen of high incidence in the MNS system; so all panel cells would be assumed to be U+ unless otherwise noted. The example of anti-U in Case 12-8 reacts equally with all panel RBCs tested except the RBCs of panel cell 11. (If any of the previous panels in Cases 12-1 through 12-7 had been tested, all panel cells would have reacted because all would have been U+.) Since the auto control is negative, the antibody is assumed to be an alloantibody. If the patient is African American, the likelihood that the anti-

Case 12-8

	Cell ID	D	C	E	c	e	P$_1$	M	N	S	s	Le^a	Le^b	K	k	Fy^a	Fy^b	Jk^a	Jk^b	Special	IS	LISS 37°C	Anti-IgG
1	R$_1$R$_1$–1	+	+	0	0	+	0	+	0	+	0	0	+	0	+	+	0	+	+	Kp(a+)	0	0	2+
2	R$_1$R$_1$–2	+	+	0	0	+	+	+	+	0	+	0	+	0	+	+	0	+	+	C^w+	0	0	2+
3	R$_2$R$_2$	+	0	+	+	0	+	0	+	0	+	0	+	0	+	0	+	+	0		0	0	2+
4	R$_2$r	+	0	+	+	+	+	+	+	+	+	0	0	+	0	+	+	0	+	Co(b+)	0	0	2+
5	rr–1	0	0	0	+	+	+	+	0	+	+	+	0	0	+	+	+	0	+		0	0	2+
6	rr–2	0	0	0	+	+	+	+	0	+	+	0	0	+	+	+	0	+	+		0	0	2+
7	r'r	0	+	0	+	+	0	0	+	+	0	0	+	0	+	+	+	+	0		0	0	2+
8	r"r	0	0	+	+	+	+	+	+	0	+	0	+	0	+	0	+	+	0		0	0	2+
9	R$_1$r	+	+	0	+	+	+	0	+	0	+	+	0	0	+	+	0	0	+	Bg(a+)	0	0	2+
10	R$_1$R$_2$	+	+	+	+	+	0	+	0	+	+	0	+	0	+	0	+	+	0		0	0	2+
11	R$_o$r	+	0	0	+	+	+	+	+	0	0	0	0	0	+	0	0	+	+	Js(a+) U–	0	0	0$^√$
12	Auto control	4+	0	0	4+	4+				0$^√$	0$^√$			0$^√$		0$^√$	3+	3+	0$^√$		0	0	0$^√$

body is anti-U is increased. Exclusion of other alloantibodies using the only nonreactive cell on the panel, cell 11, rules out anti-D, anti-c, anti-e, anti-P₁, and anti-k. The patient is Fy(b+) and Jk(a+), so anti-Fy^b and anti-Jk^a can also be excluded. Additional selected cells must be tested to exclude the presence of anti-C, anti-E, anti-K, anti-Fy^a, and anti-Jk^b, because these antibodies would be clinically significant, if present. Many transfusion services would not require that antibodies generally considered clinically insignificant (e.g., anti-M, anti-N, anti-Le^a, or anti-Le^b) to be serologically excluded in a case like this. Because almost all U– RBCs are also S–s–, exclusion of anti-S and anti-s would be nearly impossible.

The ability to test appropriate selected cells, that is, to put together a panel of U– RBCs that are also C+, E+, K+, Fy(a+), and Jk(b+) and to type the patient's RBCs with anti-U, is beyond the scope of most hospital transfusion serivces. A sample that contains an antibody to an antigen of high incidence will often have to be sent to an immunohematology reference laboratory for antibody identification or confirmation and for provision of the rare blood components if a transfusion is ordered.

Case 12-9 is an example of an antibody to an antigen of low incidence, anti-C^w. Note that all panel cells, with the exception of panel cell 2, are nonreactive. Exclusion of common alloantibodies is not a problem with this panel because all antigens in the column headers can be ruled out; but in order to match the pattern of reactivity with an antigen, the information in the "Special" column must be noted. Since the only additional information available about panel cell 2 is that the RBCs are C^w+, the antibody most likely to be causing the reactivity is anti-C^w. The identification is not confirmed until one or two more examples of C^w+ RBCs are found to be similarly reactive. Since the C^w antigen is of low incidence in the donor population, finding compatible blood is no problem.

Although the mechanism is not understood, blood bankers have noted that sera containing an antibody to one antigen of low incidence often contain additional antibodies to other low-incidence antigens, so confirmation of these antibodies is not always simple. If an antibody to a low-incidence antigen is confirmed, there may not be a commercial antiserum available to screen for antigen-negative components for transfusion. Consolation for this type of frustration, however, must be that the antibody specificities in these cases are often of academic interest only, because compatible blood is readily available. Whether or not antibodies to antigens of low incidence can be identified, the transfusion recommendation is the same: transfusion of crossmatch-compatible blood is acceptable.

Refer to Chapter 6 for additional information about the MNSs blood group system.

Case 12-9

	Cell ID	D	C	E	c	e	P₁	M	N	S	s	Le^a	Le^b	K	k	Fy^a	Fy^b	Jk^a	Jk^b	Special	IS	LISS 37° C	Anti -IgG
1	R₁R₁–1	+	+	0	0	+	0	+	0	+	0	0	+	0	+	+	0	+	+	Kp(a+)	0	0	0^v
2	R₁R₁–2	+	+	0	0	+	+	+	+	0	+	0	+	0	+	+	0	+	+	C^w+	0	0	3+
3	R₂R₂	+	0	+	+	0	+	0	+	0	+	0	+	0	+	0	+	+	0		0	0	0^v
4	R₂r	+	0	+	+	+	+	+	+	+	+	0	0	+	0	+	+	0	+	Co(b+)	0	0	0^v
5	rr–1	0	0	0	+	+	+	+	0	+	+	+	0	0	+	+	+	0	+		0	0	0^v
6	rr–2	0	0	0	+	+	+	+	0	+	+	0	0	+	+	+	0	+	+		0	0	0^v
7	r'r	0	+	0	+	+	0	0	+	+	0	0	+	0	+	+	+	+	0		0	0	0^v
8	r''r	0	0	+	+	+	+	+	+	0	+	0	+	0	+	0	+	+	0		0	0	0^v
9	R₁r	+	+	0	+	+	+	0	+	0	+	+	0	0	+	+	0	0	+	Bg(a+)	0	0	0^v
10	R₁R₂	+	+	+	+	+	0	+	0	+	+	0	+	0	+	0	+	+	0		0	0	0^v
11	R₀r	+	0	0	+	+	+	+	+	0	0	0	0	0	+	0	0	+	+	Js(a+)U–	0	0	0^v
12	Auto control																				0	0	0^v

Also, many antibodies to antigens of low incidence routinely go undetected because antibody detection RBCs (screening cells) are not mandated to contain these antigens. Unless the blood bank detects an incompatible crossmatch due to the random selection of an antigen-positive unit of blood, the antibody will be overlooked. Since transfusion services commonly employ the practice of using an immediate-spin crossmatch for patients with a negative antibody screen, and since the antibody screen in patients with antibodies to low-incidence antigens would usually be negative, there is a small probability that such antibodies would be missed in routine testing. Because the incidence is extremely low, the risk is likewise extremely low.

PASSIVELY ACQUIRED ANTIBODIES

Occasionally the serum of a patient contains an antibody that was acquired from a source other than the patient's own immune system. Newborns may have maternal IgG antibodies that crossed the placenta from the mother's plasma into the circulation of the fetus. Patients receiving transfusions of non–ABO-identical platelets may have "unexpected" anti-A or anti-B. Obstetric patients who have received antenatal Rh immune globulin may have anti-D still detectable in their serum at delivery. Patients receiving intravenous IgG (IVIG) or intravenous anti-D (e.g., WinRho) for treatment of autoimmune cytopenias may have anti-D or a host of other antibodies that have been passively acquired from these medications, which are prepared from a large pool of donor plasmas.[14] Knowing the patient's medical history and recent transfusion history is vital to provide clues to identify antibodies that may either be coating the patient's RBCs (if they are antigen positive) or free in the serum (if the patient's RBCs are antigen negative) or a combination of both.

The most frequently seen passive antibodies are in newborns. Since IgG antibodies cross the placenta, any IgG antibody present in the mother is also likely to be present in the newborn. This includes the usual suspects: anti-A, anti-B, or anti-A,B; anti-D (alloantibody or Rh immune globulin); or alloantibody produced by the mother (e.g., anti-K, anti-E, anti-c, etc.). If hemolytic disease of the newborn (HDN) is suspected, the blood bank will be asked to perform a DAT on the baby's RBCs, either by testing the cord blood or by obtaining a heelstick sample. If the baby's RBCs are DAT+, the blood bank may be asked to prepare an eluate from the baby's RBCs to identify the coating antibody. If this is required, group A and B RBCs should be included in the cells selected to test the eluate, because ABO antibodies are likely to be present. If both mother and baby are of the same ABO group, the suspected HDN is not due to ABO antibodies and the eluate may contain maternal alloantibody. Since the RBC sample from the baby is likely to be quite small, identifying the alloantibody in the mother's serum should be the first order of business. This information can expedite confirmation of the antibody in the eluate, if indeed even necessary.

Case 12-10 is an example of the pattern of reactivity seen in a patient receiving intravenous anti-D, which is used to treat idiopathic thrombocytopenia purpura (ITP). The exclusion process in Case 12-10 is exactly the same as in Case 12-2; anti-D is identified in both panels. The difference between the panels is that the autologous control is positive in Case 12-10 and the patient is antigen positive (D+). These results might indicate autoanti-D, but if the blood bank has the medication history and knows that the patient is receiving WinRho, it is almost certain that the anti-D was passively acquired. An eluate of the patient's RBCs would almost certainly contain anti-D. There is some controversy as to whether patients receiving intravenous anti-D, should they require transfusion, should receive Rh-negative blood, which would be serologically compatible, or Rh-positive blood, because the patient is D+ and transfusion of D+ RBCs will not stimulate more antibody production or cause a transfusion reaction. The medical director for each laboratory should make the decision about transfusion protocols for these patients.

Refer to Chapter 16 for a discussion of hemolytic disease of the newborn (HDN).

Case 12-10

	Cell ID	D	C	E	c	e	P₁	M	N	S	s	Leᵃ	Leᵇ	K	k	Fyᵃ	Fyᵇ	Jkᵃ	Jkᵇ	IS	LISS 37° C	Anti -IgG
1	R₁R₁-1	+	+	0	0	+	0	+	0	+	0	0	+	0	+	+	0	+	+	0	0	3+
2	R₁R₁-2	+	+	0	0	+	+	+	+	0	+	0	+	0	+	+	0	+	+	0	0	3+
3	R₂R₂	+	0	+	+	0	+	0	+	0	+	0	+	0	+	0	+	+	0	0	0	3+ˢ
4	R₂r	+	0	+	+	+	+	+	+	+	+	0	0	+	0	+	+	0	+	0	0	3+
5	rr-1	0	0	0	+	+	+	+	0	+	+	+	0	0	+	+	+	0	+	0	0	0√
6	rr-2	0	0	0	+	+	+	+	0	+	+	0	0	+	+	+	0	+	+	0	0	0√
7	r'r	0	+	0	+	+	0	0	+	+	0	0	+	0	+	+	+	+	0	0	0	0√
8	r"r	0	0	+	+	+	+	+	+	0	+	0	+	0	+	0	+	+	0	0	0	0√
9	R₁r	+	+	0	+	+	+	0	+	0	+	+	0	0	+	+	0	0	+	0	0	3+
10	R₁R₂	+	+	+	+	+	0	+	0	+	+	0	+	0	+	0	+	+	0	0	0	3+
11	R₀r	+	0	0	+	+	+	+	+	0	+	0	0	0	+	0	0	+	+	0	0	3+
12	Auto control	4+																		0	0	4+

SELECTION OF APPROPRIATE RED BLOOD CELLS FOR TRANSFUSION

When patients have alloantibodies that are potentially clinically significant (i.e., those that react at 37° C or by the indirect antiglobulin test) the red cells selected for transfusion should lack the corresponding antigen(s) and be crossmatch compatible.[5] Once antibodies are identified, they should be made a part of the patient's permanent blood bank records. The information that composes the patient's serologic history must be checked each time pretransfusion testing is done so that clinically significant historical antibodies will be honored, even if not currently demonstrable.

Depending on the antigen profile needed (e.g., E−, c−, K−) and the incidence of those antigens in the donor population, the hospital may be able to find appropriate units in its inventory by screening the units with the appropriate antisera. Various blood bank texts contain tables of antigen frequencies, but a rough guide, if such a text is not immediately available, is the panel worksheet itself. If one or two donor cells are antigen positive, such as "K," it might be expected that only about 10% of the random donor population is antigen positive and a compatible unit would be relatively easy to find. On the other hand, if one or none of the panel cells is antigen negative, such as "e," the likelihood that any random donor unit would be compatible is poor.

In Case 12-1, the patient's serum contains alloanti-K, so units for transfusion must be K−. Approximately 91% of blood donors are K−, so if the laboratory has anti-K reagent, screening the red cell components in its inventory and finding K− units should be easy to do. The patient in Case 12-2 has anti-D. Any ABO-compatible Rh-negative unit of red cells should be compatible with this patient, and because Rh-negative units are routinely confirmed for their ABO and Rh type on receipt into the blood bank, screening for units that lack the D antigen has already been done.

In Case 12-3, anti-P₁ was identified; but because anti-P₁ is not clinically significant unless it is reactive at 37° C, random units (i.e., P₁+) may be transfused. For any patient with antibodies that are primarily cold reacting (e.g., anti-P₁, anti-M, anti-N, anti-Leᵇ, anti-A₁, etc.), the blood bank technologist may wish to be sure that the room temperature incubation is not performed and that anti-IgG (rather than polyspecific antiglobulin) is used for the IAT phase of the crossmatch in order to have the best chance of finding random units that are serologically compatible.

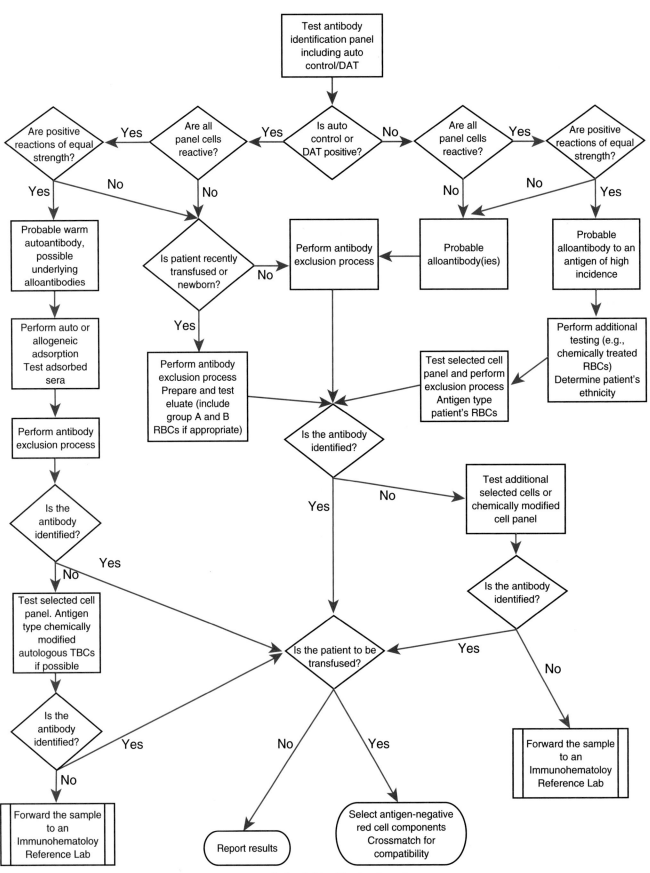

Fig. 12-4 Antibody identification flow chart.

The patient in Case 12-4 has two alloantibodies, anti-Fy^a and anti-K. Units for this patient must typed and found to be both Fy(a–) and K–. Approximately 35% of random donors will be Fy(a–) and 91% will be K–. As discussed in Chapter 2, calculating the percentage of random donors that will lack both antigens is done by multiplying the percentages: $0.35 \times 0.91 = 0.32$, so 32% of ABO-compatible donors should be Fy(a–) and K– and serologically compatible for the patient in Case 12-4.

The patient in Case 12-5 also has two alloantibodies, anti-E and anti-k. Approximately 70% of random donors are E–, but only 0.2% will be k–. Calculating the percentage of antigen-negative donors in a random population $(0.7 \times 0.002 = 0.0014)$ reveals that only about 1 in 1000 donors would be suitable for this patient. Unless the blood bank has a huge inventory, a lot of antiserum, and a lot of time, screening blood for this patient will be a wasted effort. Rare donor files, such as the American Rare Donor Program, will probably need to be accessed. If the blood need is for an elective surgical procedure, the patient may be able to donate autologous units. Also, since inheritance of blood types is genetic, siblings are a good source of additional rare units. Within the family, the odds of finding E– k– donors are reduced from 1 in 1000 in the general population to 1 in 4.

Fig. 12-4 is a flow chart that summarizes the major decision points encountered in antibody identification.

PRACTICAL CONSIDERATIONS

While this chapter contains the basic principles for antibody identification, the scientific literature is filled with example of antibodies that "didn't read the book" ... And while the principles of exclusion and examples of antibody reaction characteristics can be done as "paper problems," there is no substitute for actual laboratory experience to become proficient in antibody identification. Practical application in a laboratory setting will reinforce the didactic material. Antibodies do not always present themselves at times convenient for the technologist to work on them, but the ability to efficiently choose and perform the appropriate tests and analyze the clues to solve the serologic puzzle is its own reward. Finding a compatible crossmatch after hours of slaving over racks of test tubes and multiple panel worksheets is a wonderful feeling, both for the technologist and the transfusion recipient.

REFERENCES

1. Petz LD, Garratty G: Immune Hemolytic Anemias. Philadelphia, Churchill Livingstone, 2004.
2. Coombs RRA, Mourant AE, Race RR: Detection of weak and "incomplete" Rh agglutinins: A new test. Lancet 2:15-16, 1945.
3. Race RR, Sanger R: Blood Groups in Man. Oxford, Blackwell, 1950.
4. Marsh WL: Scoring of hemagglutination reactions. Transfusion 12:352-353, 1972.
5. Fridey J (ed): Standards for Blood Banks and Transfusion Services, 20th ed. Bethesda, MD, American Association of Blood Banks, 2003.
6. Code of Federal Regulations, 21 CFR 660.33.
7. Fisher RA: Statistical Methods and Scientific Inference, 2nd ed. Edinburgh, Oliver & Boyd, 1959.
8. Kanter MH, Poole G, Garratty G: Misinterpretation and misapplication of p values in antibody identification. Transfusion 37:816-822, 1997.
9. Petz LD, Garratty G: Immune Hemolytic Anemias. Philadelphia, Churchill Livingstone, 2004.
10. Brecher ME (ed): Technical Manual, 14th ed. Bethesda, MD, American Association of Blood Banks, 2002.
11. Branch DR, Petz LD: A new reagent ZZAP having multiple applications in immunohematology. Am J Clin Pathol 78: 161-167, 1982.
12. Rodberg K, Tsuneta R, Garratty G: Discrepant Rh phenotyping results when testing IgG-sensitized RBCs with monoclonal Rh reagents. Transfusion 35(Suppl):67S, 1995.
13. Edwards JM, Moulds JJ, Judd WJ: Chloroquine diphosphate dissociation of antigen-antibody complexes. Transfusion 22: 59-61, 1982.
14. Garratty G: Problems associated with passively transfused blood group alloantibodies. Am J Clin Pathol 109:769-777, 1998.

FURTHER READING

Issitt PD, Anstee DJ: Applied Blood Group Serology, 4th ed. Durham, Montgomery Scientific Publications, 1998.

Reid ME, Lomas-Francis C: Blood Group Antigen Facts Book, 2nd ed. San Diego, Academic Press, 2004.

Expert Opinion

DO WE HAVE TO WORRY ABOUT NOT DETECTING ANTIBODIES TO LOW-INCIDENCE ANTIGENS?
George Garratty, PhD, FRCPath.

Some antibodies to low-incidence antigens are relatively common. For instance, anti-Wr[a] has been detected in 3% to 12% of patients and 1% to 3% of donors.[1,2] Antibodies to low-incidence antigens have been reported to sometimes cause hemolytic transfusion reactions (HTRs) and hemolytic disease of the fetus and newborn (HDFN).[3] Antibody detection RBCs do not possess low-incidence antigens; the Food and Drug Administration (FDA) only mandates that such RBCs possess C, c, D, E, e, M, N, S, s, P[1], Le[a], Le[b], K, k, Fy[a], Fy[b], Jk[a], and Jk[b]. Thus antibodies to low-incidence antigens are usually detected by the crossmatch (including an antiglobulin test [AGT]) or because a baby is born with HDFN and the mother has no antibodies detectable by routine procedures. In the late 1970s and early 1980s, the question posed by the title of this section became commonly debated following the suggestion that the crossmatch could be abbreviated by not performing the AGT if the antibody screen was negative.[4,5] Many data have been accumulated to show that this is a safe approach, and it is approved by all regulatory authorities in the United States.[4,5] It is interesting that in this new century the debate has begun again. I believe that this is because the electronic/computer crossmatch has been gaining popularity and the same questions arise as no serologic crossmatch is being performed. Unfortunately, I believe that the new generation has not related to the extensive (sometimes old) data in the literature suggesting that detection of antibodies to low-incidence antigens is not necessary, based on cost-benefit-risk calculations.[1,2]

For instance, seven studies from the 1970s and 1980s[6-12] showed that the risk of missing an antibody of potential significance, by using an abbreviated crossmatch, was 1 in 5494 recipients' sera, or 1 in 10,615 crossmatches.[1,2] About half of the antibodies detected by the crossmatch but not the antibody screen were antibodies to low-incidence antigens.

Although antibodies to low-incidence antigens may not be detected by the abbreviated crossmatch, the real risk to a patient is whether the patient will receive a unit that possesses a particular low-incidence antigen and whether the antibody to that low-incidence antigen is clinically significant. The incompatibility frequency (antigen frequency times antibody frequency) has been calculated to range from .000160 (or 1 of 6250 units incompatible) for Lu[a] to .000020 (or 1 of 50,000 units incompatible for Wr[a]).[13] Table EO3-1 shows the incompatibility frequencies for some low-frequency antigens.

In 1990, Shulman[14] gathered data from 20 hospitals in different parts of the United States. These hospitals had issued blood for transfusion based on 1.3 million negative antibody screens and negative immediate-spin crossmatches. Only five patients experienced an acute overt HTR (a risk of 1 overt HTR per 260,000 crossmatches). The antibodies associated with the HTRs, and undetected by the antibody screen, were one example each of an anti-Jk[a], anti-C, anti-c, anti-Wr[a], and anti-Kp[a]. Thus the risk of an overt HTR associated with antibodies to low-incidence antigens (anti-Wr[a] and anti-Kp[a]) was 1 per 650,000 crossmatches. In a 19-year period, the Mayo Clinic found that only 4 of 197 HTRs were associated with antibodies to low-incidence antigens (3 anti-C[w], and 1 anti-Wr[a]).[15,16] One HTR was caused by anti-Lu[a]; although Lu[a] is not officially a low-incidence antigen, Lu[a] is often not present on antibody detection RBCs.

In Europe, the experience has been similar. Rouger[17] reported that, in a 30-year period involving 600,000 antibody screens, he has only encountered two HTRs due to antibodies to low-incidence antigens. If we consider only anti-Wr[a], which is the most common antibody to low-incidence antigens in Europe and the United States, HTRs are rare. De La Rubia and colleagues[18] encountered only one mild HTR in a 5-year period when 100,000 antibody screens were performed. Arriaga and colleagues[19] reported that in a 10-year period, when 300,000 units of RBCs were transfused, only three HTRs due to anti-Wr[a] were encountered. Wallis and colleagues[20] reported that over a 34-month period, they detected 10 antibodies, of potential clinical significance, that were detected by the crossmatch but not the antibody screen; 7 of these were anti-Wr[a] and anti-Kp[a]. Anti-Wr[a] was detected, with no other unexpected antibodies, in 8% of 1112 patients and 1% of 5098 blood donors. Only 2 of 5253 (1 in 2600) donors were found to be Wr(a+). Wallis and colleagues[20] concluded that it was not practical to include Wr(a+) RBCs in a set of antibody detection RBCs. They suggested either performing an AGT crossmatch, Wr[a] type all donors, and only perform AGT crossmatches on Wr(a+) donors, or assume the risk. Schonewille and colleagues[21] reviewed the records of 1795 patients, during a period when a complete crossmatch was used, and a period when an abbreviated crossmatch was used. These patients' sera contained 2257 antibodies; 89 (5%) patients had 94 antibodies to low-incidence antigens (4% of all antibodies). Anti-Wr[a] was the most common antibody to low-incidence antigens. In a prospective study, 12.3% of the patients were shown to have anti-Wr[a]. Thirty-nine patients had antibodies to low-incidence antigens, together with other antibodies; 20

TABLE EO3-1 Antibodies to Some Low-Incidence Antigens Often Not Present on Antibody Detection RBCs That Have Been Reported to Cause Hemolytic Transfusion Reactions

Specificity	Antigen Frequency*	Antibody Frequency[†]	Incompatibility Frequency (# Units Incompatible)*
Lu[a]	0.080	0.0020	0.000160 (1 of 6250)
f (ce)[‡]	0.650	0.0002	0.000130 (1 of 7692)
C[w]	0.020	0.0100	0.000100 (1 of 10,000)
Kp[a]	0.020	0.0017	0.000034 (1 of 29,000)
Js[a]	0.010	0.0017	0.000017 (1 of 50,000)
Wr[a]	0.001	0.0200	0.000020 (1 of 50,000)

*Based on predominantly Caucasian populations. Marked differences of some antigens exist in Asian or black populations (see reference 3).
[†]Only rough estimate (see reference 13).
[‡]Not present if only R_1R_1 and R_2R_2 RBCs are used as antibody detection RBCs: will be present if rr RBCs are used.

(51%) of these patients had autoantibodies. Fifty-one antibodies to low-incidence antigens were found as solitary antibodies in 50 patients; 14 were detected by crossmatching when a complete crossmatch was used; 37 were detected by antibody screening tests. Six hundred and sixty-four patients who had alloantibodies detected received 7792 transfusions. Only one anti-Wr[a] was detected by crossmatching; anti-C[w] was detected posttransfusion in an eluate from DAT+ RBCs, but the patient had no signs of an HTR. Although 5% of patients were found to have antibodies to low-incidence antigens, no HTRs were reported as being due to antibodies to low-incidence antigens. The authors concluded that the risk to recipients was no different in the period when the abbreviated crossmatch was used compared to the period when a complete crossmatch was performed.

Thus the risk of an obvious HTR due to antibodies to low-incidence antigens in patients who receive blood crossmatched using an abbreviated method (i.e., no AGT in the crossmatch phase), and using antibody detection RBCs, not especially selected to have low-incidence antigens, is somewhere in the region of 1 in 500,000. Such a risk hardly justifies the expense and trouble of supplying antibody detection RBCs containing C[w], Wr[a], and Kp[a]. The choice to use an abbreviated crossmatch (including an electronic crossmatch) is based on cost benefit/risk calculations, and people not comfortable with the risk/benefit ratio cited here should use a complete crossmatch that includes an AGT.

REFERENCES

1. Garratty G: Screening for RBC antibodies—what should we expect from antibody detection RBCs. Immunohematology 18:71-77, 2002.
2. Garratty G: How concerned should we be about missing antibodies to low incidence antigens? Transfusion 43:844-847, 2004.
3. Issitt PD, Anstee DJ: Applied Blood Group Serology, 4th ed. Durham, NC, Montgomery Scientific, 1998.
4. Garratty G: The role of compatibility tests. Transfusion 22: 169-172, 1982.
5. Beck ML, Tilzer LL: Red cell compatibility testing: A perspective for the future. Transfus Med Rev 10:118-130, 1996.
6. Boral LI, Henry JB: The type and screen: A safe alternative and supplement in selected surgical procedures. Transfusion 17: 163-168, 1977.
7. Boral LI, Hill SS, Apollon CJ, et al: The type and antibody screen, revisited. Am J Clin Pathol 71:578-581, 1979.
8. Oberman HA, Barnes BA, Friedman BA: The risk of abbreviating the major crossmatch in urgent or massive transfusion. Transfusion 18:137-141, 1978.
9. Oberman HA: Abbreviation or elimination of the crossmatch. Clin Lab Med 2:181-192, 1982.
10. Lown JAG, Barr AL, Jackson JM: A reappraisal of pre-transfusion testing procedures in a hospital blood bank. Pathology 17:489-492, 1985.
11. Mintz D, Haines AL, Sullivan MF: Incompatible crossmatch following nonreactive antibody detection test. Transfusion 22:107-110, 1982.
12. Shulman IA, Nelson JM, Saxena S, et al: Experience with the routine use of an abbreviated crossmatch. Am J Clin Pathol 82:178-181, 1984.
13. Walker RH: On the safety of the abbreviated crossmatch. In Polesky HF, Walker RH (eds): Safety in Transfusion Practices. Skokie, IL, College of American Pathologists, 1982.
14. Shulman IA: The risk of an overt hemolytic transfusion reaction following the use of an immediate spin crossmatch. Arch Pathol Lab Med 114:412-414, 1990.
15. Vamvakas EC, Pineda AA, Reisner R, et al: The differentiation of delayed hemolytic and delayed serologic transfusion reactions: Incidence and predictors of hemolysis. Transfusion 35:26-32, 1995.
16. Pineda AA, Vamvakas EC, Gorden LD, et al: Trends in the incidence of delayed hemolytic and delayed serologic transfusion reactions. Transfusion 39:1097-1103, 1999.
17. Rouger PH: International forum. Do you think that the cross match with donor red cells can be omitted when the serum of a patient has been tested for the presence of red cell alloantibodies with a cell panel? Vox Sang 43:151-168, 1982.
18. De la Rubia J, Sempere A, Arriaga F, et al: Safety of the antibody screening test as the sole method of pretransfusion testing. Vox Sang 63:141, 1992.
19. Arriaga F, Alvarez C, Llopis F, et al: Incidence and clinical significance of Wright antigen and antibody. In Book of Abstracts of the ISBT VII Paris, European Congress, 2001.
20. Wallis JP, Hedley GP, Charlton D, et al: The incidence of anti-Wr[a] and Wr[a] antigen in blood donors and hospital patients. Transfus Med 6:361-364, 1996.
21. Schonewille H, van Zijl AM, Wijermans PW: The importance of antibodies against low incidence red blood cell antigens in complete and abbreviated crossmatching. Transfusion 43: 939-944, 2003.

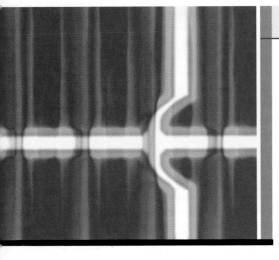

CHAPTER THIRTEEN

Resolving ABO Typing Discrepancies and Other Typing Problems

Kerry Burright-Hittner and Sally V. Rudmann

CHAPTER OUTLINE

LEARNING OBJECTIVES

After reading and studying this chapter, the student will be able to:

1. Discuss various sources of technical error as potential causes of an ABO discrepancy.
2. Discuss testing useful in the resolution of weak subgroups of A and B.
3. Describe the clinical ramifications of inability to detect weak antigens, such as subgroups of A and B.
4. Discuss the clinical conditions responsible for the presence of mixed populations of red cells.
5. Discuss possible causes of ABO discrepancies due to weakly reactive or missing antigens.
6. Discuss possible causes of ABO discrepancies due to weakly reactive or missing antibodies.
7. Discuss possible causes of ABO discrepancies due to unexpected antigens.
8. Discuss possible causes of ABO discrepancies due to unexpected antibodies.
9. Given the history and serology of a patient with an ABO discrepancy, discuss the possible causes for the reactivity observed and determine what further testing is necessary to resolve the problem.
10. Formulate a testing strategy to follow when performing serologic investigation of an ABO discrepancy.
11. Discuss factors that might interfere with accurate Rh and other antigen typings and testing strategies necessary to determine the correct antigen typing results.
12. Choose the appropriate units of blood to be transfused to a patient before typing problems can be resolved.

In this chapter, the student will begin to use the theory and skills learned from the previous chapters and apply it to a variety of problem-solving situations. Knowledge gained from study is invaluable, but experience is the best teacher. The flow charts included in this chapter are designed to assist in processing and categorizing information, resulting in discrepancy resolution and safe and effective transfusion.

TECHNICAL ERRORS

Collection and Patient Variables

Technical errors are caused by a variety of scenarios, discussed in detail in the paragraphs that follow. Refer to Table 13-1 for a list of common technical errors.

Sample Collection Error

The accuracy of serologic testing is dependent on careful patient identification and appropriate sample collection; thus it is dependent on the individual collecting the sample. If the phlebotomist collects the sample from the wrong patient or mislabels the tubes with incorrect patient identifiers, the careful control of serologic testing means nothing. A technologist should accept only accurately and legibly labeled samples. The American Association of Blood Banks (AABB) publishes standards for sample suitability.[1] Transfusion services are responsible for developing procedures that provide explicit guidance for sample suitability and

TABLE 13-1 Examples of Technical Errors	
Clerical errors	Sample/patient misidentification
	Mislabeling of test tubes
	Error in recording results
	Transcription error
	Computer entry error
Reagent/equipment variables	Use of outdated reagents
	Inappropriate storage temperatures
	Contaminated reagents
	Use of an uncalibrated centrifuge
Procedural errors	Improper cell suspensions
	Reagents not added
	Failure to recognize or record hemolysis
	Fibrin clots in serum
	Misinterpretation of results
	Failure to follow manufacturer's directions

for implementing a system of process control to ensure the accuracy of patient identification, specimen collection, and blood transfusion.

Patient Exhibits a Clotting Deficiency

Sometimes patient serum does not clot efficiently. This may be due to a decreased platelet count, anticoagulant therapy, or factor deficiencies. Plasma may be used for routine testing to prevent this problem. If serum is used, it should be allowed to clot completely before centrifugation. If the serum sample is not completely clotted, fibrin clots may continue to form in the serum, appearing as clear, gel-like clumps in the bottom of the tube. These may or may not contain red cells, and can mimic the appearance of agglutination. The addition of protamine sulfate to neutralize the effects of heparin therapy and/or thrombin to the serum will facilitate complete clotting.[2] With the advent of the use of plastic blood collection tubes, serum samples cannot be obtained without the use of clot activators added to the tubes by the manufacturers. It is important to review the manufacturer's package insert to determine the suitability of the sample for blood bank testing.

Contaminated Samples

Contamination of samples may be attributed to bacterial growth within the tube or the presence of some other unexpected contaminant. Collection of blood samples above an intravenous (IV) catheter may introduce the presence of a contaminant. It is important to stopper all tubes when not in use, especially during storage, to prevent contamination. Bacterial contamination of red cells may manifest as polyagglutination. This phenomenon is discussed later in this chapter.

Testing Variables
Glass Fragments in the Tube

If tube testing is routinely performed, borosilicate glass tubes are likely to be used for testing. Excessive breakage experienced during transportation and storage may distribute glass fragments in the unbroken tubes. If glass fragments are observed in testing tubes, they should not be used.

Contaminated Reagents

Contamination of reagents may be due to bacterial growth or cross contamination with another reagent. Reagents for serologic testing should be stored in accordance with the manufacturer's package insert. Do not use reagents with an abnormal appearance, such as reagents that appear cloudy or discolored. To avoid cross contamination between reagents, do not touch the sides of the testing tubes when adding reagents. Saline bottles used for preparing cell suspensions should be clearly labeled, changed frequently, and washed regularly to avoid the possibility of bacterial growth. The AABB requires the institution of a quality control (QC) program to ensure that all reagents function as expected.[1] Although the periodicity of QC is not stipulated, it is generally performed on each reagent at least once each day of use.

Equipment Performance

Testing should always be performed using qualified, validated equipment.[1] This traditionally includes serologic centrifuges, cell washers, incubators, agglutination viewers, timers, and thermometers. It may also include other equipment, such as that used for gel or solid phase testing. If the serologic centrifuge is not operating appropriately, false-negative or false-positive results may be observed. Optimum times of centrifugation (functional calibration) for each individual centrifuge should be available to the technologist for use in the performance of testing. Procedures for functional calibrations can be found in the AABB *Technical Manual*.[2] Periodic speed and timer verifications should be performed to ensure optimum equipment performance. Thermometers and timers should be calibrated to ensure conformance to acceptable industry standards. For a comprehensive discussion of quality control, quality assurance, and required documentation, refer to Chapters 21 and 22.

Human Error
Manufacturer's Directions Not Followed

The AABB Standards require that all materials shall be used in accordance with the manufacturer's directions.[1] Testing performed contrary to the package insert may invalidate test results obtained. Critical elements in any procedure include such variables as the serum/cell ratios, media, temperature, incubation time, sample type, and length/revolutions per minute of centrifugation. The reagent manufacturer's technical support staff can provide useful information regarding the reagents the company manufactures. In rare situations where testing is performed outside the limits of the package insert, laboratory validation must be performed and documented to ensure accurate results.

Failure to Recognize Hemolysis as a Positive Reaction

Both agglutination and hemolysis are visible endpoints of red cell antigen/antibody reactions.[2] Hemolysis is the endpoint of complement binding resulting in red cell destruction and release of hemoglobin. This is generally seen with strong complement binding antibodies, such as anti-A, anti-B, anti-H, and anti-Le[a]. This hemolysis may be partial (some red cells left intact) or complete (no intact red cells). The technologist should observe the color of the supernatant serum after removing the tube from the centrifuge. Hemolysis observed at the time of test interpretation should always be noted. Documentation should include the degree of hemolysis.[2] Care must be taken to ensure that hemolysis is a result of antigen/antibody reactions rather than some other testing variable such as bacterial contamination.[3]

Clerical Error

A high percentage of fatal transfusion reactions are the result of clerical as opposed to technical errors.[2] The beginning serologist should develop a careful routine; a standard method of performing testing, in a set order, with a routine workflow will help to prevent errors. If a discrepancy is observed, the technologist will be wise to repeat the testing. This is often the most effective and easiest way to resolve a discrepancy. In the case of error, the blood bank or transfusion service must have a process for collecting and analyzing data and for initiating corrective and preventive action.[1] The goal of all transfusion facilities should be the reduction of error.

ABO DISCREPANCIES
Overview

ABO grouping is the most important pretransfusion test performed. Transfusion of ABO-incompatible blood can result in significant morbidity and mortality. As described in Chapter 3, individuals generally form naturally occurring antibodies to the ABO antigens they lack. The ability to test both the red blood cells (RBCs) for ABO antigens (forward grouping) and the serum for antibodies (reverse grouping) provides a useful check on the accuracy of ABO testing results. The interpretations of the cell and serum grouping should match (Landsteiner's rule).[4] If they do not match, technical/human error must be ruled out. If no error is detected, the technologist should proceed with antibody detection testing. It is important to note that ABO typing results cannot be interpreted until the forward and reverse typing match.[4] If the transfusion must precede the resolution of the discrepancy, group O RBCs should be selected for transfusion.[1]

This chapter introduces the student to some of the basic techniques used in the resolution of ABO discrepancies and other typing problems. For a more in-depth

Box 13-1	ABO Typing Discrepancies and Some Associated Causes

WEAK-REACTING OR MISSING ANTIGENS
ABO subgroups
Acquired weak expression of ABO antigens
HPC transplants and other mixed cell populations
Excess blood group substances

WEAK-REACTING OR MISSING ANTIBODIES
Neonatal specimens
Elderly/immunosuppressed patients
Prozone

UNEXPECTED ANTIGEN REACTIONS
Rouleaux
Polyagglutination (including acquired B phenotype)
Antibody-coated cells (e.g., cold autoantibody)
Wharton's jelly
Mixed cell populations (chimerism)
Contaminating antibody in reagent

UNEXPECTED ANTIBODY REACTIONS
Rouleaux
ABO subgroups (e.g., A_2 with anti-A_1)
Cold-reactive or room temperature–reactive autoantibodies
Cold-reactive or room temperature–reactive alloantibodies

treatment of these problems, refer to Issitt and Anstee,[5] Judd,[4] and the AABB *Technical Manual*.[2] A summary of ABO typing discrepancies and some common causes can be found in Box 13-1.

Initial Steps

Some basic initial steps are suggested for every ABO discrepancy.

Strength of Reactions

Monoclonal A and B antiserum produced in the United States has been manufactured according to good manufacturing practices (GMPs) of the Food and Drug Administration (FDA).[6] It is very potent, and positive reactions are generally very strong (4+). As a rule of thumb, the technologist should look at the strength of reactivity when considering steps to take in the resolution of a discrepancy. The strongest reactivity generally is correct, and using this rule of thumb the technologist can hypothesize the most likely solution to the problem. Focus on the reason for weak or missing reactivity, keeping in mind that there are always exceptions to every rule.

Previous Records

Additional information from the patient's medical/serologic history is important during the resolution of a discrepancy. Obtain the patient's age, diagnosis, transfusion history, history of pregnancy (if applicable), medications, and the results of previous serologic testing (e.g., ABO typing, antibody detection and identification, and direct antiglobulin test). These may provide clues to assist with problem solving.

Wash Patient Cells

A number of serologic problems are associated with the use of unwashed patient cells.[7] Wash the red cells at least once with normal saline and resuspend to a concentration compatible with the manufacturer's package insert directions. This will reverse some problems, such those associated with excess blood group–specific substance.

Weak-Reacting or Missing Antigens

The following is an example of a missing antigen:

Case A: Missing Antigen Reaction			
Anti-A	Anti-B	A₁ Cells	B Cells
0	0	0	4+

In this example, the reverse grouping suggests that the patient is group A. The strength of the reaction with anti-B would support this hypothesis. If this hypothesis is correct, the A antigen reactivity in the forward typing is missing. Some situations that may result in the missing antigen pattern are discussed here.

ABO Subgroups

Problem

A number of inherited subgroups of A and B have been identified serologically, and more recently many of these have been defined by molecular techniques.[2,4,5] These subgroups are generally associated with discrepant ABO serologic findings. The major concern with ABO subgroups is the risk that a donor unit could be mislabeled due to the failure to detect a weak-reacting A or B antigen. Refer to Chapter 3 for a more extensive discussion of ABO subgroups.

Resolution

ABO subgroups can be classified based on the strength of agglutination with ABO antisera; serum grouping results; the presence or absence of anti-A₁; secretion of A, B, and H substances; the presence of A or B transferase in the serum; and the number of antigen sites on the RBCs. Techniques such as the use of anti-A,B and adsorption/elution procedures may be useful in the resolution of these problems. These are briefly described in the following section on acquired weak expressions of A and B antigens. Refer to Chapter 3, Tables 3-5 and 3-6, for the common serologic results of selected subgroups of A and B.

With the exception of A₂, the resolution of A and B subgroups is outside the scope of the routine transfusion service and generally requires consultation with an immunohematology reference laboratory. The reader is encouraged to refer to the AABB *Technical Manual*[2] and Judd[4] for a discussion of procedures used in the investigation of ABO discrepancies and other serologic problem solving.

Acquired Weak Expressions of ABO Antigens

Problem

ABO antigen expression may be weakened in certain chronic disease states.[2,4]

Resolution

A review of the patient history (clinical and serologic) will provide useful information to help determine possible reasons for such discrepancies. If, for example, previous records indicated that the patient in the preceding case had been previously typed as group A, it can be concluded that the current findings are either in error or a result of some acquired disorder as opposed to an inherited weak subgroup of A.

In all missing ABO reactions, a recommended early step in resolution would be to repeat testing with extended incubation at room temperature or below. Because

TABLE 13-2 Enhancement of ABO Reactions Using Extended Room Temperature Incubation and Incubation at 4° C

	CELL GROUPING			SERUM GROUPING			
	Anti-A	Anti-B	Anti-A,B	A_1 Cells	B Cells	O Cells*	Auto Control*
Immediate spin	0	0	0	0	4+	0	0
Room temperature (15 min)	0	0	1+	0	4+	0	0
4° C (15 min)	1+	0	2+	0	4+	0	0

*O cells and autologous controls are run as negative controls.

ABO antigens react most strongly in the cold, 4° C incubation may demonstrate otherwise weak-reacting antigens (Table 13-2). An auto control and an antibody screen (group O cells) should be performed with all such testing to ensure that any reactions noted at 4° C are not due to cold-reacting autoantibodies or alloantibodies. Enzyme treatment of the patient's cells will also enhance ABO antigen-antibody reactivity. Extended room temperature incubation may be sufficient to detect weakly expressed ABO antigens.[2]

Extended incubations, decreased temperatures, and enzyme-treated cells have been used for many years for the resolution of ABO discrepancies. The procedures require variations from the manufacturer's directions and can produce erroneous results if not carefully controlled. For a brief discussion of the limitations of such techniques, refer to Kowalski.[7]

Testing with another manufacturer's antiserum may also be useful in the resolution of these types of ABO missing antigen reactions. Each antiserum is manufactured using a unique blend of clones selected by the manufacturer to conform to their specifications. No single reagent will detect all A or B antigens. Consult the package insert to determine the clone used.

If not routinely used, testing with anti-A,B may detect a weak expression of the A or B antigen not detected by routine anti-A and/or anti-B. Anti-A,B is an antibody produced by group O individuals. Unlike a mixture of anti-A plus anti-B, anti-A,B is inseparable with adsorption techniques. Monoclonal anti-A,B may be manufactured as a combination of the clones used in the manufacture of anti-A and anti-B, or it may be enhanced by the addition of other clones.

Adsorption-elution techniques may be used as an indirect method for determining the presence of the A or B antigen when routine ABO testing results suggest a missing antigen.[7] Because of a number of variables, human sources of antisera are preferred for adsorption/elution techniques. Use of monoclonal antisera with this technique is not supported by the manufacturer's package insert, so testing must be validated and strictly controlled. The basic principle for this procedure is as follows: A sample of the patient's red cells is washed and all residual saline removed. An equal amount of reagent antiserum is added to the test and incubated at refrigerator temperature (1° to 6° C). During this time, antibody binds to the antigen (if present). The antibody-coated cells are washed several times and an eluate prepared and tested for the desired antigen. If the patient cells in the preceding example were weakly positive for the A antigen, those cells would adsorb anti-A onto their surface.[5]

Approximately 78% of the population are secretors. If the patient is a secretor, the saliva can be tested for A- and B-soluble antigens. The antigens are demonstrated by their ability to inhibit ABH antisera. A detailed procedure for saliva testing can be found in the AABB *Technical Manual*.[2]

Hematopoietic Progenitor Cell Transplants
Problem

A hematopoietic progenitor cell (HPC) transplant may introduce a temporary ABO discrepancy.[2] For some period after transplant, two different populations of cells (for example, group O transplanted to group A or B) exist in the individual,

TABLE 13-3 Mixed Field (mf) Agglutination

CELL GROUPING			SERUM GROUPING			
Anti-A	Anti-B	Anti-A,B	A₁ Cells	B Cells	O Cells	Auto
2+ mf*	0	2+ mf*	0	4+	0	0

*Mixed field reactions with anti-A and anti-A,B in what appears to be a group A patient could be due to a mixed cell population or to a subgroup of A.

those of the original marrow and those of the transplanted marrow. **Mixed field agglutination** may be observed to varying degrees, depending on the length of time required for the transplanted marrow to begin cellular production.

Resolution

Reviewing a patient's history can reveal information useful to the resolution of ABO discrepancies. If, for example, a patient's serologic findings were normal during a previous admission, it can be concluded that the discrepancy is acquired rather than inherited. This would eliminate the possibility of an inherited ABO subgroup. The history is particularly useful in determining acquired discrepancies such as mixed cell populations resulting from allogeneic bone marrow transplant.

Careful examination of agglutination may be useful to identify the presence of mixed-field agglutination. The presence of mixed-field agglutination, suggesting the presence of mixed cell populations, should be documented (Table 13-3).

Excess Soluble Blood Group Substances
Problem

Infrequently, an excess of ABH soluble blood group substance produced by the patient may neutralize antisera in the forward grouping. This has been observed in patients with gastrointestinal carcinoma or obstruction.[4] These substances neutralize commercial antisera.

Resolution

A simple step to the resolution of missing antigen ABO discrepancies is to wash patient cells with saline. In the case of excess ABH soluble substances, this will remove antigen and resolve the discrepancy.

Resolution of Case A

Case A is an example of a group A patient with excess soluble blood group substance in the patient's serum that resulted in the neutralization of the anti-A. The patient's clinical history of gastrointestinal carcinoma was consistent with this hypothesis. Previous serologic records indicated that the patient had typed as group A 3 years previously. The technologist washed the patient's RBCs in saline and repeated the initial testing. This resulted in removal of the soluble A substance and resolution of the discrepancy.

Missing or Weak-Reacting Antibodies

An example of a missing antibody is presented next. In this example, the strong reaction with anti-B in the forward typing would suggest that the patient is group B with a missing antibody (anti-A).

Mixed field agglutination: The appearance of agglutinated cells in a background of nonagglutinated cells, often indicating the presence of mixed cell populations.

Case B: Missing Antibody Reaction

Anti-A	Anti-B	A₁ Cells	B Cells
0	4+	0	0

Neonatal Specimens
Problem

Missing reactivity in reverse grouping is found when testing neonatal specimens. Infants do not demonstrate anti-A or anti-B at birth (with the exception of passively acquired maternal antibody). Antibody production is generally minimal during the first 4 months of life. Titers of anti-A and anti-B increase and peak at about age 10, after which they decrease with age. Reverse grouping performed on a cord sample will demonstrate weak or no reactivity. If reactivity is observed, it is likely of maternal origin.[2,4]

Resolution

To avoid serologic discrepancies in specimens from neonates (first 4 months of life), ABO reverse typing is not performed.[1,2]

Elderly or Immunosuppressed Patients
Problem

Elderly patients may also demonstrate decreased reactivity in the reverse grouping, due to a decrease in antibody production. Immunosuppresion due to chemotherapy or associated with disease may also diminish ABO antibody production.[2]

Resolution

Incubation of the patient's reverse (serum) grouping at room temperature (20° to 24° C), 18° C, or 4° C may enhance the missing reactivity. An auto control and antibody screening cells should be tested at the same time to rule out the possibility of mistaking a cold autoantibody or alloantibody for the missing anti-A or anti-B.

Patient demographic information and history (clinical and serologic) are useful in the resolution of these reactions in cases that are related to patient age, treatment, or disease state.

Prozone
Problem

Prozone is a phenomenon associated with antibody excess.[2,4] Sera with high-titer antibodies (anti-A and/or anti-B) may not cause the agglutination of A or B cells due to the fact that all antigen sites have bound antibody, leaving no sites available for cross-linking with another red cell. Antibody is bound to the cells, but visible agglutination will not take place. A similar inhibition of agglutination can be due to the binding of complement components to the bound antibody, resulting in a steric hindrance and no lattice formation.[4]

Resolution

If prozone is suspected, techniques can be used to reduce the complement in the specimen (such as collection of an EDTA [ethylenediaminetetraacetic acid] specimen) and/or reduce the antibody titer (such as dilution of the serum in saline).[4]

Resolution of Case B

Case B is an example of a discrepancy due to prozone. The patient had a high-titer anti-A that interfered with lattice formation and therefore inhibited RBC agglutination. The test was repeated using serial dilutions of patient serum and the anti-A was demonstrated at a 1:8 dilution. The patient was group B.

Unexpected Antigen Reactions

An example of an unexpected antigen reaction is presented next. In this case, based on the strength of the reactions, the reverse grouping would suggest that the patient is group O and the weak reactions with anti-A and anti-B manifest as unexpected antibody reactions.

Case C: Unexpected Antigen Reactions			
Anti-A	Anti-B	A₁ Cells	B Cells
1+^{w}	1+^{w}	4+	4+

Rouleaux

Problem

Rouleaux can be responsible for both unexpected antigen and unexpected anti-body reactions.[4] When viewed microscopically, rouleaux is described as "coin-like stacking" of the red cells (Fig. 13-1). **Rouleaux** formation is often observed in the serum of patients diagnosed with multiple myeloma or other dysproteinemias. Intravenous therapy with high molecular weight fluids, such as fibrinogen, dextran, or hydroxyethyl starch, has also been associated with this phenomenon. Macroscopically, strong rouleaux may appear as agglutination. Characteristically, rouleaux is strongest at immediate spin, is weaker at 37° C, and is not usually observed at the antihuman globulin phase of testing.

Resolution

Rouleaux is brought about by abnormal proteins in the serum, and therefore the resolution is accomplished by removing the offending protein. In the forward grouping reactions, unexpected reactions can be generally resolved by washing the patient's cells and repeating the testing. In reverse grouping or other tests that use patient serum, the saline replacement technique will generally resolve this discrepancy. When performing this technique, the serum and cells are added together and centrifuged. Antigen-antibody reactivity, if present, is allowed to take place during this step. The serum is removed from the tube and saline added to "replace" the serum. The tube is mixed, recentrifuged, and reexamined for agglutination. Rouleaux will be dispersed, but true agglutination will not be affected.[8]

Polyagglutination

Problem

Red cells that are agglutinated by ABO-compatible adult human sera and are not agglutinated by cord sera are defined as polyagglutinable. In these patients, the autocontrol is usually negative. **Polyagglutinable cells** result from the exposure of normally sequestered red cell membrane structures (antigens) by the action of bacterial enzymes or as a result of a somatic mutation of hematopoietic tissue, or an inherited condition. These exposed antigens react with naturally occurring

Polyagglutinable cells: Cells that are agglutinated by most normal sera and not by cord sera.

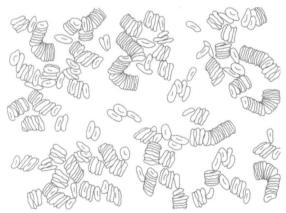

Fig. 13-1 Rouleaux formation: microscopic appearance. (*Adapted from Harmening D: Modern Blood Banking and Transfusion Practices, 2nd ed. Philadelphia, FA Davis, 1989.*)

antibodies in the serum of all adult humans. These antibodies are lacking in cord serum, explaining the serologic presentation described previously.[9,10]

A number of polyagglutinable states have been identified, which differ from each other with regard to etiology, serologic characteristics, and clinical significance. Multiple types of polyagglutination may occur in the same individual, making precise identification difficult. Reactivity observed may range from strong to weak. The variability is due to antibody strength and amount of red cell antigen exposed. Reactions may appear mixed field in nature.[10]

Monoclonal reagents do not contain these antibodies, but human source reagents may react weakly at room temperature with polyagglutinable cells, because the antibodies are IgM, saline-reactive agglutinins. These cells, therefore, may be responsible for discrepant serologic results when tested with human sera.

The most common form of polyagglutination is associated with bacterial or viral infections and is transient, disappearing when the infection is eliminated. The action of bacterial enzymes results in the exposure of a number of hidden (crypt) antigens on the red cell surface, including T, Tk, Th, and VA. Of these, activation of the T **cryptantigen** (T activation) was the first of the acquired polyagglutinable states to be characterized. T activation can take place in vivo and in vitro, resulting from the cleavage of sialic acid by bacterial neuraminidase. Other bacterial enzymes reveal different hidden antigens (Tk, Th, and VA).

Cryptantigen: An antigen hidden from detection on normal red cells.

Resolution

Presumptive evidence for polyagglutination includes the following: reactivity of cells with normal, ABO-compatible human sera; nonreactivity with cord sera and aged antisera; reactivity with most human source reagent antisera; and nonreactivity with monoclonal antisera. Unlike normal red cells, some polyagglutinable cells, such as T-activated cells, that have reduced levels of sialic acid, will not aggregate in the presence of positively charged polymer reagents such as hexadimethrine bromide (Polybrene).[2,4,5,9,10] Polyagglutination is confirmed and further characterized by running cells against a panel of lectins.[11]

Because most routine ABO testing is now performed with monoclonal reagents, polyagglutinable cells do not generally interfere with ABO forward typing as they did when antisera were of human origin.

Polyagglutinable states include the following:[9,10]

1. **T polyagglutination** is associated with bacterial contamination/infection. *Arachis hypogea*, the peanut lectin, detects this type of polyagglutination.

2. **Tk polyagglutination** is associated with *Bacteroides fragilis, Serratia marcescens, Escherichia coli*, and *Aspergillus niger* infections. Unlike other types of polyagglutination, these cells demonstrate normal sialic acid levels. *Arachis hypogea* and *Glycine max (soja)* lectins demonstrate positive reactivity when tested against Tk polyagglutinable cells.

3. **Tn polyagglutination** may be associated with hematologic disorders, such as leukemia, thrombocytopenia, or hemolytic anemia. Tn polyagglutination is usually permanent. Mixed-field agglutination of the auto control has been observed. This type of polyagglutination reacts with *Salvia horminum, Salvia schlera*, and *Glycine max (soja)* lectins. Non–group A individuals experiencing Tn polyagglutination will react with *Dolichos biflorus* (anti-A₁ lectin).

Dolichos biflorus: A lectin with anti-A₁ specificity.

4. **Inherited polyagglutination:** There are inherited forms of polyagglutination, characterized by abnormal RBC membranes, such as Cad and HEMPAS (hereditary erythroblastic multinuclearity with a positive acidified serum lysis test). Cad cells are agglutinated by *Salvia horminum* and *Glycine max (soja)* lectins; HEMPAS cells are agglutinated by anti-HEMPAS, present in 30% of adult serum.

For additional discussion of polyagglutination, refer to Judd[9] and Horn.[10]

Cold Autoantibody
Problem

In the case of potent, high-titer cold autoantibodies, a patient's cells may agglutinate spontaneously even without the addition of antiserum or enhancement. Careful observation of the EDTA blood sample of these patients will be sufficient to demonstrate the presence of agglutinated cells. This is particularly true at room temperature and below. The patient's auto control will be positive and the DAT positive with anticomplement reagents.

Resolution

Warming the tube at 37° C and washing cell suspensions several times with 37° C saline is helpful in dispersing this agglutination.[4,8] Special specimen collection protocols can reduce the titer of cold antibody in specimens. To achieve this, two specimens are drawn: an EDTA tube that is incubated immediately at 37° C and a clotted specimen that is maintained at 4° C until the serum is separated from the cells. Cells from the 37° C EDTA tube should be washed with 37° C saline to minimize the binding of cold antibody to the cells. When stored at 4° C, the cold antibody in the clotted specimen will adsorb to the RBCs. If the serum is removed from the cells at 4° C, the antibody will be retained on the cells and the serum will have reduced titers of antibody. The EDTA cells can be used for forward grouping and the serum for reverse grouping and other pretransfusion testing.

Sometimes, cells must be treated with a reducing agent, such as dithiothreitol (DTT) or 2-mercapto ethanol (2-ME), to disperse spontaneous agglutination and allow for typing of the red cells.[5] Procedures for the use of these reagents can be found in the AABB *Technical Manual*.[2]

Wharton's Jelly
Problem

In cord blood samples, Wharton's jelly may cause red cells to agglutinate, giving the appearance of unexpected antigen reactions.[7] Wharton's jelly is primitive connective tissue of the umbilical cord. It is rich in hyaluronic acid, and may contaminate cord blood samples collected by cutting the cord and allowing the sample to drain into a tube. Wharton's jelly contamination will spontaneously aggregate the red cells and be observed as positive reactivity with all reagent antisera (Table 13-4).

Resolution

Washing cord blood samples several times (usually four to six washes) with saline before testing is a good practice, but may not always reverse this clumping. To prevent Wharton's jelly interference, collect cord blood samples from the umbilical vein using a needle and syringe. If Wharton's jelly contamination is suspected in a cord sample, a new sample from the infant's heel or umbilical catheter may be required.

TABLE 13-4 Group A Cord Blood Contaminated with Wharton's Jelly

	CELL GROUPING			SERUM GROUPING			
	Anti-A	Anti-B	Anti-A,B	A₁ Cells	B Cells	O Cells†	Auto†
Cord blood	3+	2+	2+	ND*	ND*	2+	2+
Venous blood	3+	0	0	ND*	ND*	0	0

*ND, Not done (ABO reverse grouping is not performed on neonatal samples).
†O cells and autologous control (auto) are negative controls.

Chimerism
Problem

Multiple cell populations or chimeras may cause mixed-field reactivity. Chimerism may be acquired or inherited. Acquired chimerism is temporary and may result from transfusion, such as when group O units are transfused to a group A or B individual, excessive fetal-maternal hemorrhage, intrauterine transfusion, or exchange transfusion. A genetic chimera can result from the in utero exchange of erythropoietic tissue in fetal twins. A mosaicism chimera, also know as dispermy, can result when two sperm fertilize one ovum with two nuclei. The resulting fetus may have two blood groups, both recognized as self. Such an individual will demonstrate immune tolerance: A genetically group O individual with implanted A cells does not produce anti-A. There are two distinct red and white blood cell lines.

Resolution

As mentioned previously, detection of mixed-field agglutination is an important skill for the serologist. When performing tube testing, roll/shake and observe the entire cell button until it has been resuspended before making an agglutination determination. Mixed-field agglutination will appear as some cells exhibiting negative reactivity and a population of cells exhibiting a positive reaction. Depending on the percentage of antigen-positive cells in the sample, this reactivity may be obvious, or very subtle.

Acquired B
Problem

Acquired B is a type of polyagglutination.[2,4,9,10] Acquired B is seen only in a subpopulation of group A_1 patients.[9] Some manufacturers' reagents detect this reactivity better than others, probably due to the pH of the reagent. Patients demonstrating acquired B have a history of colon cancer or septicemia. It has been suggested that bacteria in the group A individual's gut escapes into the bloodstream and deacetylates the patient's A terminal sugar (*N*-acetyl-galactosamine). The resulting sugar cross-reacts with B antisera and has been noted with increased frequency in tests with certain monoclonal reagents containing the ES-4 clone.[2] Patients demonstrating acquired B possess anti-B, but this anti-B does not react with the acquired B antigen; therefore the auto control is negative. The forward grouping resembles group AB, and the reverse resembles group A. These patients should be transfused with group A or O blood.[10]

A(B) and B(A) Phenotypes
Problem

Some monoclonal anti-A and anti-B detect trace amounts of A and B antigen on red blood cells.[7] Two such aberrations of monoclonal testing are the A(B) and B(A) phenotypes. The first case is an A individual with trace amounts of B antigen that is not detected by polyclonal reagents but is detected by some monoclonal reagents. In the A(B) phenomenon the reverse is true. Most examples react very weakly and are easily dispersed.

Resolution

Again, attention to the strength of reactivity is important in the identification of these phenotypes; in apparent AB patients weak reactions with anti-A or B should be suspect. So, too, serologic histories are useful in identifying inconsistencies in typing over time using different reagents. Because the aberration is reagent specific, it can often be resolved by repeating testing with another manufacturer's monoclonal serum or using antisera of human origin.[7]

Contaminating Antibody in Reagent
Problem

Contaminating specificities in reagent antisera may cause discrepancies. This is most frequently observed when human source antisera are used. An antibody to a low-frequency antigen might be present in the serum of the donor, providing reagent-grade plasma for manufacture.[3] This antibody could cause a false-positive typing of a patient or donor, demonstrating the corresponding low-frequency antigen on the red cells. For example, a human source anti-M reagent could also contain anti-V^w, a low-frequency antigen in the MNSs system. If the reagent were used for M antigen typing of an M antigen–negative patient positive for V^w, the M typing would be interpreted as positive because of the contaminating specificity, rather than the presence of the M antigen on the red cells.

Resolution

Repeating testing with another lot of antiserum or a different manufacturer's antiserum will generally resolve this problem. Manufacturers should be contacted regarding any such reagent contamination.

Resolution of Case C

The patient's history indicated that the patient suffered from multiple myeloma. On microscopic examination, it was clear that the apparent agglutination in the forward grouping tubes was rouleaux formation. The patient's cells were washed three times with saline and the forward grouping was repeated. After washing, the rouleaux no longer interfered with the testing and the problem was resolved.

Unexpected Antibody Reactions

An example of an unexpected antibody reaction is presented next. In this case, based on the strong reactions with anti-A and with B cells, the hypothesized ABO type is A. The discrepant result is the weaker 2+ reaction with A_1 cells.

Case D: Unexpected Antibody Reaction			
Anti-A	Anti-B	A_1 Cells	B Cells
4+	0	2+	4+

A_2 Patient with Anti-A_1
Problem

The patient may inherit a weak subgroup of A and form anti-A_1. The most common of these is the A_2 patient (or A_2B patient) with a naturally occurring IgM Anti-A_1. The antibody reacts with A_1 cells, but not A_2 cells.[2]

Resolution

Resolving this problem involves two steps, one to confirm that the cells are not A_1 and the second to confirm that the antibody is anti-A_1. This can be accomplished by typing of the patient's red cells with A_1 lectin *(Dolichos biflorus)* and by repeating the reverse grouping using A_2 rather than A_1 reverse grouping cells. Both of these will be negative if the hypothesis is correct (Table 13-5).

Room Temperature–Reactive Alloantibody
Problem

The patient may demonstrate an IgM alloantibody. These antibodies usually react best at room temperature or below, making it possible for them to react at room

TABLE 13-5 Resolution of Subgroup of A with Anti-A₁

	CELL GROUPING				SERUM GROUPING			
Anti-A	Anti-B	Anti-A,B	Anti-A₁ Lectin	A₁ Cells	A₂ Cells	B Cells	O Cells*	Auto*
4+	0	4+	0	2+	0	4+	0	0

*O cells serve as negative controls (control for the possibility of a cold autoantibody and/or an alloantibody in the serum of the patient).

temperature with reverse grouping cells that are positive for the corresponding antigen. Some examples of these antibodies are anti-P₁, anti-M, and anti-Le^b.[7]

Resolution

Perform an antibody screen and identification to determine the antibody. Type the reverse grouping cells for the corresponding antigen to confirm the cause of the discrepancy. Then select antigen-negative reverse grouping cells and repeat the reverse grouping to resolve the discrepancy (Table 13-6).

Rouleaux
Problem

As described previously, abnormal or excessive serum proteins can result in rouleaux formation.

Resolution

The saline replacement method will generally reverse rouleaux formation. Refer to the previous discussion of rouleaux in the section on unexpected antigen reactions.

Passive Infusion of Antibody
Problem

Antibody may be introduced passively as a result of intravenous administration of antibody or the transfusion of ABO-incompatible plasma-containing components.[2,8] An example of this is intravenous immunoglobulin (IVIg) administration. Prepared from large pools of donor plasma, this product may contain significant titers of ABO antibody. In rare instances, it may cause a positive direct antiglobulin test and red cell hemolysis. Group O platelet components transfused to group A patients could result in sufficient titers of anti-A to react with A₁ reverse grouping cells.

Resolution

A complete patient history should be sufficient to identify the source of passive ABO antibody. Previous serologic records, if available, may help further clarify the reason for the discrepancy. So long as the passive antibody is present, the ABO type of transfused cells should be compatible with both naturally occurring and passively administered antibody. If transfusion is necessary before resolution, group O cells should be selected.

Bombay Phenotype
Problem

The Bombay phenotype results when a patient does not inherit a gene that codes for the production of the H antigen, which is necessary for normal ABO gene

TABLE 13-6 Room Temperature–Reactive Alloantibody: Anti-M

	CELL GROUPING			SERUM GROUPING		
Anti-A	Anti-B	Anti-A,B	A₁ Cells	B Cells	O Cells	Auto
0	4+	4+	4+	2+	2+	0

Course of action: Panel identification = anti-M.
Reverse grouping was repeated using M-negative B cells and was nonreactive.

TABLE 13-7 Bombay Phenotype O$_h$

CELL GROUPING				SERUM GROUPING				
Anti-A	Anti-B	Anti-A,B	Anti-H*	A$_1$ Cells	B Cells	O Cells	O Cells (Cord)	Auto
0	0	0	0	4+	4+	4+	4+	0

*Bombay individuals lack the *H* gene and therefore are unable to produce A and B antigens. Because of this, Bombay serum contains naturally occurring anti-A, anti-B, anti-A,B, and anti-H.

expression. As a result, the classic Bombay individual has no H or ABO antigens. This rare individual demonstrates anti-H, anti-A, anti-B, and anti-A,B and thus forward types as group O and reverse types as group O. All reactions will be very strong (3 to 4+). The potent IgM anti-H of Bombay individuals reacts with all O cells such as those routinely used for antigen screening and antibody identification. Refer to Chapter 3 for additional discussion of the Bombay phenotypes.

Resolution

Suspected Bombay cells should be typed with anti-H. The further resolution of this problem is outside of the scope of the routine transfusion service and should be referred to an immunohematology reference laboratory. Bombay individuals must be transfused with blood from other Bombay individuals or receive autologous blood. Rare-donor databases will be necessary to locate compatible blood for transfusion (Table 13-7).

Reactions to Drugs, Dyes, and Other Additives
Problem

Patient serum may react with components of the enhancement or solutions in which reagent red cells are suspended. Most of these are IgM antibodies, appearing to agglutinate all cells tested. The auto control is negative unless suspended in the same medium, and may mimic an antibody to a high-frequency antigen. Several substances have been reported to cause non–blood group specific agglutination. Reactivity with antibiotics used to retard bacterial growth in reagent red cell panels, EDTA anticoagulant, saline, sodium caprylate (used as a stabilizer in albumin preparations), and thrombin have been reported as the cause of agglutination observed during antibody investigation. These are generally observed only during in vitro testing, but may require considerable time and resources to investigate. It is not always necessary to identify the causative agent. During the production of the cells, each manufacturer uses different drugs to retard bacterial growth, so one panel may demonstrate reactivity, but a different panel will not.

Resolution

Performing testing using cells with no enhancement (such as donor cells) or substituting a second source of reagent antisera may assist in resolution of the problem.[5]

Resolution of Case D

Case D is an example of an A$_2$ individual with anti-A$_1$. The patient cells were tested with anti-A$_1$ lectin, and the reverse typing was repeated with A$_2$ reagent red cells. The results of both were negative, resolving the discrepancy.

Rh DISCREPANCIES

Rh antisera have evolved through time. Understanding the various types of antisera developed over time is helpful in understanding pitfalls and cautions of current test performance.

Reagents
Human Anti-D[12]

Human source anti-D had a high protein content, greater than 22% albumin. Because of the high protein content, this reagent caused false-positive agglutination in some instances (for example, patients with positive direct antiglobulin tests). It required the use of a high-protein inert control to detect the possibility of false-positive typings. When a patient demonstrated a positive control, which was commonly seen in cases of warm autoantibody, the Rh typing was considered invalid.

Chemically Modified Anti-D

Production of this reagent included the addition of chemicals, which modified the Y shape of the IgG molecule to a T shape, and enhanced the potency of the reagent by decreasing the distance between antigen-antibody binding sites. It had the benefit of low protein content, and no inert control was required to validate positive reactions.

Saline Anti-D[13]

This antiserum was derived from human source IgM antibody. It was reactive at immediate spin and contained low protein content. No inert control was required. Production of the reagent was dependent on a source of IgM antibody, not often found in Rh antibodies.

Monoclonal Anti-D[14]

This was the first nonhuman source of Rh IgM antibody. It contained a low protein content and no control was required. A very potent reagent, it detected more D-positive typings at immediate spin. Fewer "Du" phenotypes were reported, and many weak D individuals were considered D positive with this reagent. It was not successful at detecting some D mosaics—specifically category VI D-positive individuals.

Monoclonal-Polyclonal Blend[14]

This blend of reagents contained IgM monoclonal antibody to detect D-positive cells at immediate spin and IgG human (polyclonal) antibody to detect D-positive cells at the antiglobulin phase of testing (such as category VI D). Because of the low protein content, no inert control is required. However, human source antibodies can be difficult to maintain, because human source antibodies may drop to titers unsuitable for reagent manufacture, or donors may become unavailable due to health or personal reasons.

Monoclonal-Monoclonal Blend[14]

IgM monoclonal antibody detects D-positive cells at immediate spin, and IgG monoclonal antibody detects D-positive cells at the antiglobulin phase of testing (category VI). No control is required and the source is easier to maintain, because it is not dependent on a human component for production.

Causes/Indications of Discrepant or Incorrect D Typings

1. **Cold agglutinin.** A cold autoantibody may cause spontaneous agglutination of cells. Refer to the ABO discrepancies section of this chapter for a discussion of ways to resolve this problem.
2. **Positive direct antiglobulin test (DAT).** A positive DAT indicates the presence of antibody coating the red blood cells. This can invalidate test results of weak D testing performed at the antiglobulin phase of testing. If an Rh control was run, it will generally be positive, indicating that the positive result with anti-D is invalid.

3. **Rare Rh phenotypes.** R_o^{Har}, also known as Rh32, is a low-frequency anti-gen in the Rh system. This individual may type as D positive or D negative, depending on the composition of the D antisera. Weak positive reactivity is observed with this phenotype. Refer to Chapter 5 for a discussion of other rare Rh phenotypes.

4. **Historical mismatch.** This may be seen when a previously D-negative indi-vidual is now found to be D positive based on testing with newer, more potent reagents. Care must be taken to rule out misidentification of the sample before accepting the new typing.

FLOW CHARTS

Refer to flow charts 13-1 through 13-6 for a systematic approach to the resolu-tion of ABO typing discrepancies.

CHART 13-1

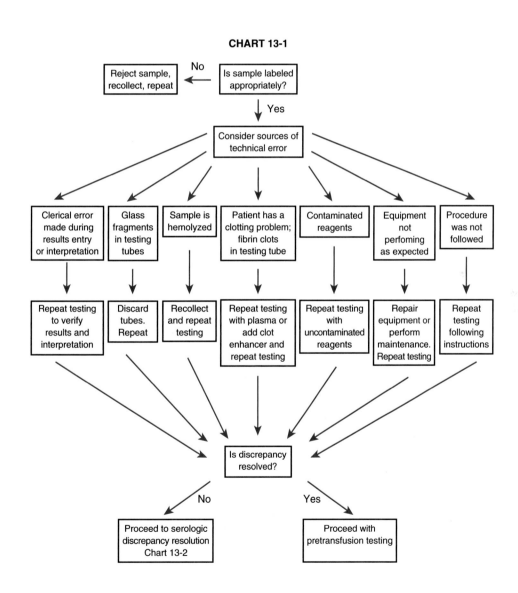

CHART 13-2

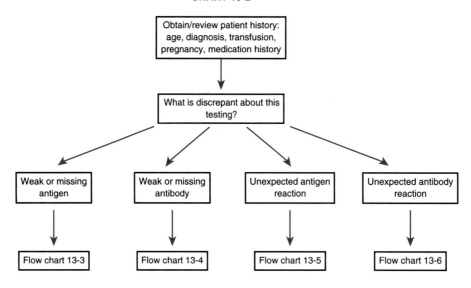

Obtain/review patient history:
age, diagnosis, transfusion,
pregnancy, medication history

↓

What is discrepant about this
testing?

Weak or missing antigen	Weak or missing antibody	Unexpected antigen reaction	Unexpected antibody reaction
↓	↓	↓	↓
Flow chart 13-3	Flow chart 13-4	Flow chart 13-5	Flow chart 13-6

CHART 13-3

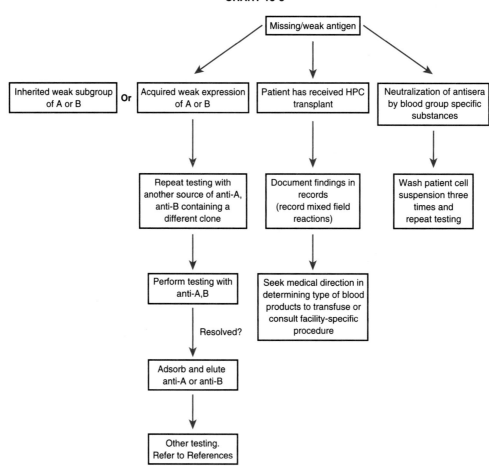

Missing/weak antigen

Inherited weak subgroup of A or B   **Or**   Acquired weak expression of A or B

Patient has received HPC transplant

Neutralization of antisera by blood group specific substances

Repeat testing with another source of anti-A, anti-B containing a different clone

Document findings in records (record mixed field reactions)

Wash patient cell suspension three times and repeat testing

Perform testing with anti-A,B

Resolved?

Seek medical direction in determining type of blood products to transfuse or consult facility-specific procedure

Adsorb and elute anti-A or anti-B

Other testing. Refer to References

CHART 13-4

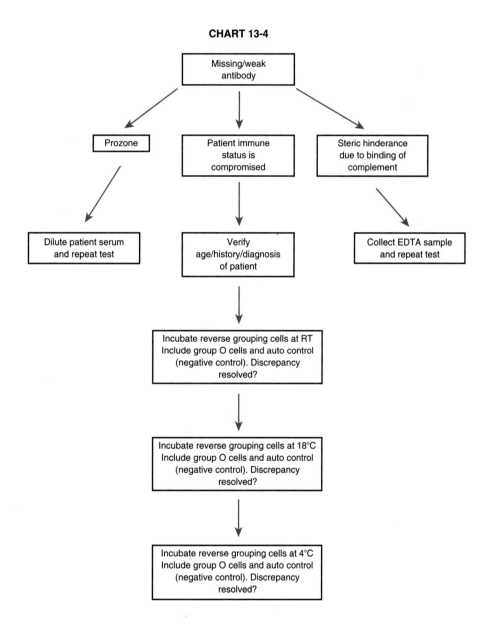

CHART 13-5

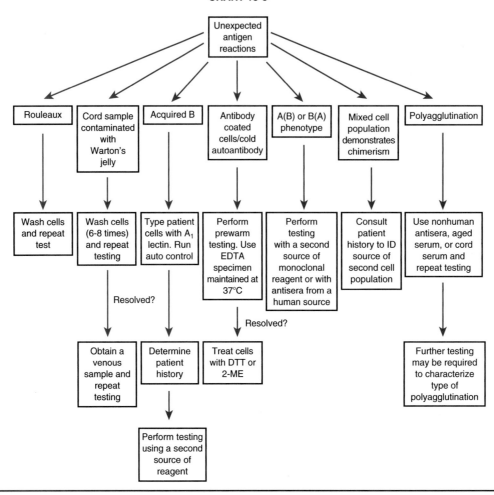

Unexpected antigen reactions

- **Rouleaux** → Wash cells and repeat test
- **Cord sample contaminated with Warton's jelly** → Wash cells (6-8 times) and repeat testing → Resolved? → Obtain a venous sample and repeat testing
- **Acquired B** → Type patient cells with A₁ lectin. Run auto control → Determine patient history → Perform testing using a second source of reagent
- **Antibody coated cells/cold autoantibody** → Perform prewarm testing. Use EDTA specimen maintained at 37°C → Resolved? → Treat cells with DTT or 2-ME
- **A(B) or B(A) phenotype** → Perform testing with a second source of monoclonal reagent or with antisera from a human source
- **Mixed cell population demonstrates chimerism** → Consult patient history to ID source of second cell population
- **Polyagglutination** → Use nonhuman antisera, aged serum, or cord serum and repeat testing → Further testing may be required to characterize type of polyagglutination

CHART 13-6

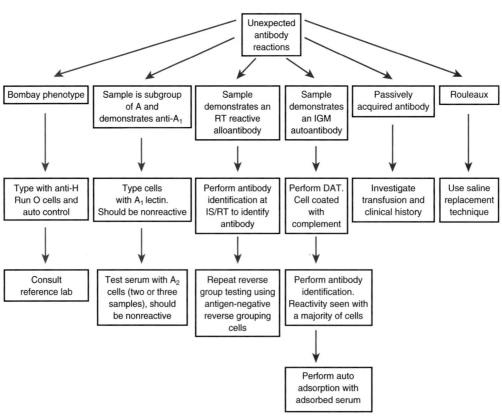

Unexpected antibody reactions

- **Bombay phenotype** → Type with anti-H Run O cells and auto control → Consult reference lab
- **Sample is subgroup of A and demonstrates anti-A₁** → Type cells with A₁ lectin. Should be nonreactive → Test serum with A₂ cells (two or three samples), should be nonreactive
- **Sample demonstrates an RT reactive alloantibody** → Perform antibody identification at IS/RT to identify antibody → Repeat reverse group testing using antigen-negative reverse grouping cells
- **Sample demonstrates an IGM autoantibody** → Perform DAT. Cell coated with complement → Perform antibody identification. Reactivity seen with a majority of cells → Perform auto adsorption with adsorbed serum
- **Passively acquired antibody** → Investigate transfusion and clinical history
- **Rouleaux** → Use saline replacement technique

CASE STUDIES
Case Study 1
Presentation

Patient KB's sample was received from the outpatient clinic. Her physician has ordered a transfusion of two units of blood. Her ABO/Rh typing results are as follows:

Anti-A	Anti-B	Anti-D	A$_1$ Cells	B Cells
0	0	4+	+3	0

Initial Hypothesis

The forward grouping appears to be group O. The reverse group appears to be group B. The D typing is positive. An unexpected antibody reaction is noted with A$_1$ cells. An ABO discrepancy exists.

Resolution

The requisition and all tubes are reverified for positive identification. No errors are found. This patient has historic information on file. She was crossmatched 5 years ago and was typed as B positive.

A new sample is requested to investigate the potential of a mislabeled sample. All testing is repeated. The results are the same.

The patient's physician is contacted for a patient history. This 45-year-old patient had been pregnant three times. She had been transfused more than 20 times in the past 5 years with red cells and platelets. She was the recipient of a bone marrow transplant due to aplastic anemia. The donor was a group O, D-positive sibling.

As a result of her HPC transplant, this patient was producing group O, D-positive red cells in the bone marrow. She has continued to produce anti-A, but her anti-B production has not begun. The patient should be transfused with group O red cells.

Case Study 2
Presentation

Patient JEH is scheduled for surgery, and a type and screen is ordered in preparation for potential transfusion during surgery. The ABO and D typing are as follows:

Anti-A	Anti-B	Anti-D	A$_1$ Cells	B Cells
4+	0	4+	0	0

Initial Hypothesis

The forward grouping appears to be group A. The reverse grouping appears to be group AB. The D typing is positive. The category of ABO discrepancy noted is a missing antibody.

Resolution

The patient's samples are reverified. No discrepancies are noted. It is noted on the patient's demographic data that she is 95 years old. The patient's medical history reveals that she has been pregnant six times. She was transfused with three units of red cells 20 years ago during bowel surgery resulting in a colostomy. Surgery is scheduled for colostomy revision.

Because of the patient's age, it is suspected that the discrepancy is caused by a missing/weak antibody. JEH has decreased production of anti-B due to her age. To prove this theory, room temperature incubation for 15 minutes is performed testing the patient's serum against A1 and B cells, an auto control, and antibody screening cells. The tubes are centrifuged and examined. No reactivity is detected. The cells are incubated at 18° C for 15 minutes, centrifuged, and examined. Weak reactivity is observed with only the B cells. To enhance the agglutination, the cells are incubated at 4° C for 10 minutes, centrifuged, and examined. Incubation at 4° C strengthened B cell reactivity to 2+. This indicates that anti-B is present. The negative auto control indicates that no autoantibody is present at room temperature, 18° C, or 4° C. The negative screening cells indicate that no cold-reactive alloantibody is present in the sample. The patient's ABO type is group A.

Case Study 3
Presentation

SPH was admitted from the emergency department. His hemoglobin is 5.3 g/dL. A transfusion is ordered for infusion as soon as possible. Following are the results of ABO/Rh testing performed:

Anti-A	Anti-B	Anti-D	Anti-A$_1$	Anti-B
4+	4+	4+	0	0

Because the manufacturer's insert requires the performance of a direct antiglobulin test (DAT) whenever the AB typing is determined, a DAT is performed with the following result:

Polyspecific Antihuman Globulin	Anti-IgG	Anti-C3d	Anti-C3d (5 min incubation)	Saline Control
4+	4+	0	1+	0

Resolution

This patient exhibits a positive DAT. This result calls into question the positive cell typing results with anti-A, anti-B, and anti-D. Because the patient's condition warrants immediate transfusion, group O, Rh-negative Red Blood Cells are released for transfusion while the serologic investigation proceeds. The patient's cells are treated with EDTA glycine acid, to attempt to remove antibody coating his cells. After treatment, the DAT is nonreactive. ABO/Rh typing is repeated on the treated cells with the following result:

Anti-A	Anti-B	Anti-D	A$_1$ Cells	B Cells
4+	4+	0	0	0

This demonstrates that the D typing initially observed was falsely positive. This patient is AB negative.

Case Study 4
Presentation

Patient LSH's sample arrives in the blood bank with a request for a type and screen in preparation for surgery. Following are the results of ABO/Rh typing and antibody screening performed:

Anti-A	Anti-B	Anti-D	A₁ Cells	B Cells
4+	0	3+	2+	2+

Cell	Immediate Spin	LISS/37° C	LISS/AHG
Cell I	2+	0	0
Cell II	2+	0	0
Cell III	2+	0	0
Auto control	2+	0	0

An ABO discrepancy and a positive antibody screen are observed. From the strength of reactivity observed, it appears that this discrepancy fits the category "additional antibody."

Resolution

Because the auto control is positive, a direct antiglobulin test is performed. The DAT is nonreactive, indicating that the patient's red cells are not coated with antibody in vivo.

Surgery is contacted to determine additional history for this patient. This patient is undergoing surgery for the implantation of a catheter. His admitting diagnosis is multiple myeloma. The antibody screen is repeated at immediate spin and examined under the microscope. Coin-like stacking of the red cells is observed, rather than the traditional appearance of random clumping of red cells seen in agglutination. The reactivity observed in the tubes is rouleaux. A saline replacement is performed at immediate spin and the type and screen repeated. Here are the results:

Anti-A	Anti-B	Anti-D	A₁ Cells	B Cells
4+	0	3+	0	2+

Cell	Immediate Spin
Cell I	0
Cell II	0
Cell III	0
Auto	0

The patient is A positive and demonstrates a nonreactive antibody screen.

Case Study 5
Presentation

WKH is scheduled for a 2-unit red cell infusion during his next dialysis. The whole blood sample is received from the dialysis unit and prepared for testing. After centrifugation, it is noted that the serum is milky and contains a large fibrin clot. This clot is manipulated, and the tube is recentrifuged.

During the performance of antibody screening, strange agglutination is noted. The agglutinates are translucent. There are many free red cells present in the tube.

Resolution

This is an example of an incompletely clotted sample. Fibrin clots have formed during the testing. It is difficult to determine the results of the tube testing. An EDTA anticoagulated sample is obtained and plasma is used for all testing. No fibrin clots are noted when testing with plasma.

Case Study 6

Patient SPH requires a type and screen for surgery. Following are the results of ABO and D typing performed:

Anti-A	Anti-B	Anti-D	A_1 Cells	B Cells
4+	w+	0	0	4+

Based on the strength of the reaction, the patient's forward group appears to be group A; however, there is weak reactivity with anti-B. The reverse group appears to be group A. The D typing is negative. This discrepancy appears to be an additional antigen.

Resolution

The patient's samples are verified. No discrepancies are noted. The nursing floor is notified to obtain history. The patient has been prescribed some pain medication. He has not been transfused in the past. Surgery is scheduled to investigate a potential bowel obstruction. The antibody screen, including an auto control, is nonreactive.

A_1 lectin typing is performed on the patient's red cells. This patient types as A_1 positive. An additional source of monoclonal anti-B is used to type the patient's red cells. It is nonreactive with this source. The auto control is negative. This appears to be an example of acquired B antigen, possibly caused by the bacteria from the obstruction entering the patient's bloodstream and deacetylating the patient's group A terminal antigen sugar. This patient is group A_1. Group A red cells should be selected for the patient's transfusion.

REFERENCES

1. Fridey J (ed): AABB Standards for Blood Banks and Transfusion Services, 22nd ed. Bethesda, MD, American Association of Blood Banks, 2003.
2. Brecher ME (ed): Technical Manual, 14th ed. Bethesda, MD, American Association of Blood Banks, 2002.
3. Anti-A, Anti-B and Anti-A,B Murine Monoclonal Blend. Reagent package insert, 6402F. Houston, TX, Gamma Biologicals, January 2004.
4. Judd WJ: Methods in Immunohematology, 2nd ed. Durham, NC, Montgomery Scientific, 1994.
5. Issitt PD, Anstee DJ: Applied Blood Group Serology, 4th ed. Durham, NC, Montgomery Scientific, 1998
6. FDA, CBER, 21 CFR Sections 200–299. Washington, DC, US Government Printing Office, April 2000.
7. Kowalski MA: ABO and Rh typing discrepancies. In. Johnson ST, Rudmann SV, Wilson SM (eds): Serologic Problem-Solving Strategies: A Systematic Approach. Bethesda, MD, American Association of Blood Banks, 1996.
8. Silva MA: ABO and Rh typing discrepancies. In Pierce SR, Wilson JK (eds): Approaches to Serological Problems in the Hospital Transfusion Service. Arlington, VA, American Association of Blood Banks, 1985.
9. Judd WJ: Review: Polyagglutination. Immunohematology 8(3):58-69, 1992.
10. Horn KD: The classification, recognition and significance of polyagglutination in transfusion medicine. Blood Rev 13: 36-44, 1999.
11. Lectin System. Package insert, 7027B. Houston, TX, Gamma Biologicals, March 1997.
12. Anti-D (Human). Package insert, 6004H. Houston, TX, Gamma Biologicals, March 2000.
13. Anti-D (Saline). Package insert, 356-2. Immunocor, March 1990.
14. Anti-D (Monoclonal Blend). Package insert, 6404D. Houston, TX, Gamma Biologicals, July 2000.

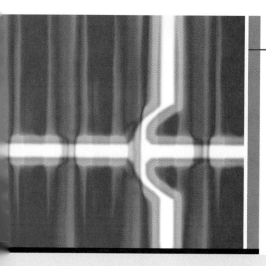

Transfusion Therapy

The goal of transfusion therapy is to provide the safest and most suitable blood product to meet the desired clinical outcome. This requires knowledge of the component composition, indications for use, dosage calculations, and contraindications and risks. All of these factors are assessed while considerations of cost, donor resources, and environmental impact are kept in mind.

Blood components can be divided into those that contain red cells (whole blood, red blood cells, leukocyte-poor red cells, and deglycerolized red cells) and those that do not contain red cells (platelets, granulocytes, and plasma components). In addition, a number of commercially prepared blood derivatives are available, such as volume expanders and coagulation factor concentrates.

The risks associated with the infusion of allogeneic blood—particularly the transmission of viral disease—have resulted in expanded research in the areas of autologous salvage and reinfusion and in providing the safest possible blood product for the recipient and the most efficient use of the nation's blood resources.

All component transfusion is associated with the risk of adverse reactions, including

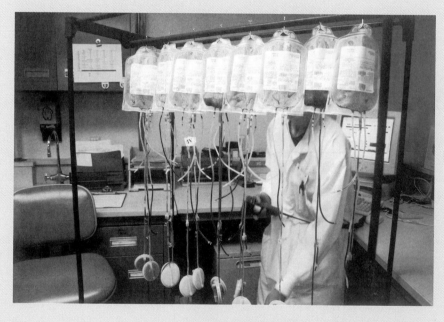

hemolytic, febrile, and allergic reactions; noncardiogenic pulmonary edema; bacterial contamination; circulatory overload; disease transmission; graft-versus-host disease; and others. The discovery of additional infectious risks that are theoretically transmissible by blood and blood components further challenges our ability to balance safety with an adequate blood supply. For each patient, the possible unfavorable consequences of transfusion must be weighed against the benefits of the therapy. Adverse hemolytic reactions should be carefully investigated and documented.

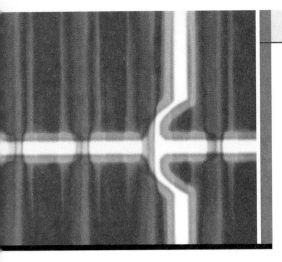

CHAPTER FOURTEEN

Component Therapy

Deborah T. Firestone and Christine Pitocco

CHAPTER OUTLINE

OVERVIEW

COMPONENTS CONTAINING RED CELLS

Whole Blood
Red Blood Cells
Alternatives to Red Blood Cells
Red Blood Cells Leukocytes Reduced
Red Blood Cells Deglycerolized
Red Blood Cells Washed
Pretransfusion Testing of Red Cell
　Components
Maximum Surgical Blood Order
　Schedule

TRANSFUSION OF OTHER BLOOD
COMPONENTS

Platelets
Granulocytes

PLASMA COMPONENTS

Fresh Frozen Plasma
Plasma Products with Reduced Levels
　of Labile Coagulation Factors
Cryoprecipitated AHF
Blood and Blood Product Precautions
Plasma Substitutes
Intravenous Immunoglobulins

TREATMENT OF COAGULATION
DEFICIENCIES

Congenital Disorders of Coagulation
Acquired Disorders of Coagulation

AUTOLOGOUS TRANSFUSION

Acute Normovolemic Hemodilution
Intraoperative Salvage
Postoperative Blood Salvage

LEARNING OBJECTIVES

After reading and studying this chapter, the student should be able to:

1. Describe the goals of blood transfusion therapy.
2. List the four major indications for the transfusion of blood or blood components/products.
3. Describe the composition, indications and contraindications, and required pretransfusion testing for each of the following red cell components:
   Whole Blood
   Red Blood Cells
   Red Blood Cells Leukocyte Reduced
4. Given a patient scenario, select the appropriate red cell component and defend that selection.
5. Describe the AABB standards for pretransfusion testing of red cell components for routine transfusion.
6. Describe the rationale for the use of a maximum surgical blood order schedule.
7. Describe the composition, indications, contraindications, and pretransfusion testing for the following non–red cell components:
   Platelets　　　　　Fresh Frozen Plasma
   Platelets Pheresis　Plasma products
   Granulocytes　　　Cryoprecipitated AHF
8. Discuss nonimmune and immune mechanisms that may result in patient refractoriness to the administration of platelets.
9. Briefly describe the current guidelines for the irradiation of blood components for the prevention of transfusion-associated graft-versus-host disease.
10. Given a patient scenario, select the appropriate non–red cell component and defend that selection.
11. Describe the composition, indications, and contraindications for the following plasma substitutes:
    Albumin
    Plasma protein fraction
12. Discuss the transfusion therapy commonly associated with the support of patients with the following congenital hemostatic disorders:
    von Willebrand's disease
    Hemophilia A
    Hemophilia B
13. Given patient body weight, initial Factor VIII level, and desired Factor VIII outcome, calculate the number of units of Factor VIII concentrates to administer.
14. Describe the treatment of hemophiliacs with inhibitors to Factor VIII.

15. Briefly describe the transfusion therapy of patients with the following acquired disorders of coagulation:
    Liver disease
    Disseminated intravascular coagulation
    Coumarin overadministration
16. Briefly describe the current standards of practice for acute normovolemic hemodilution, intraoperative salvage, and postoperative salvage/reinfusion of blood-containing fluids.

OVERVIEW

The goal of transfusion therapy is to provide the most appropriate blood product for the patient. Critical initial questions that need to be asked before a blood transfusion are as follows: Will the patient's condition be improved by a blood transfusion? Do any alternative therapies to a blood transfusion exist? Do the potential benefits of a blood transfusion outweigh the potential risks?

The major indications for the transfusion of blood or blood products are to restore or maintain (1) blood volume, (2) oxygen-carrying capacity, (3) hemostasis, and/or (4) leukocyte function. A patient's clinical condition, not a laboratory result, is the most important factor to consider when determining the transfusion needs of the patient. Once it has been determined that a transfusion is necessary, it then becomes crucial to ascertain which blood product or products will best serve the needs of the patient.

A variety of components can be produced from one unit of donated Whole Blood, each with its own indications and contraindications for transfusion (Table 14-1). Thus, with component therapy, many patients can benefit from one volunteer blood donor.

COMPONENTS CONTAINING RED CELLS
Whole Blood

Whole Blood contains 450 ± 45 mL of blood collected into a suitable anticoagulant/preservative solution such as CPDA-1, CPD1, or CP2D. **Whole Blood, Modified,** is prepared by returning plasma to the red blood cells after cryoprecipitate and/or platelets have been removed. The hemostatic properties of both these products are essentially the same; however, the added advantage of Whole Blood, Modified, is that cryoprecipitate and/or platelets can be collected and still leave a unit of Whole Blood available for transfusion.

Indications

Administration of Whole Blood restores or maintains blood volume, increases oxygen-carrying capacity, and provides stable coagulation factors. There are only

Whole Blood: Blood collected (450 ± 45 mL) into anticoagulant/preservative solutions for the purpose of transfusion and/or component preparation. Whole blood is indicated for hypovolemic patients with clinical symptoms associated with poor oxygen-carrying capacity.

Whole Blood, Modified: Whole blood from which cryoprecipitate and/or platelets have been removed.

TABLE 14-1 Indications and Contraindications of Blood and Blood Products

Blood and Blood Components	Indications for Use	Contraindications for Use
Whole Blood (WB)	Restore/maintain blood volume and red cell mass in acute, massive blood loss	Volume replacement Correct anemia in normovolemic patients
Red Blood Cells (RBCs)	Increase red cell mass of symptomatic, normovolemic patients	
Red Blood Cells Leukocytes Reduced	Increase red cell mass Prevent febrile reactions due to leukocyte antibodies in patients with severe and/or recurrent nonhemolytic febrile transfusion reactions Decrease the likelihood of alloimmunization to leukocyte or HLA antigens Decrease transmission of viral infections	
Red Blood Cells Deglycerolized	Increase red cell mass Storage of rare and autologous blood for more than 42 days Minimize allergic/febrile reactions	Cost precludes routine use in transfusion therapy
Fresh Frozen Plasma (FFP)	Reversal of Coumadin drugs Replace antithrombin III Thrombotic thrombocytopenic purpura Replace isolated factor deficiencies Correct multiple coagulation factor deficiencies secondary to DIC, liver disease, and massive transfusion	Volume expander Nutritional source of protein Source of immunoglobulins
Cryoprecipitated AHF	von Willebrand's disease, hemophilia A, factor XIII deficiency, and congenital/acquired fibrinogen deficiency Source of fibrin glue	
Factor VIII concentrate	Prevent/control bleeding in hemophilia A patients with moderate to severe deficiency of factor VIII Hemophilia A patients with low levels of factor VIII inhibitors	Treat von Willebrand's disease
Factor IX complex	Hemophilia B Patients with factor VIII or IX inhibitors Congenital factor VII or X deficiency	Patients with liver disease
Coagulation Factor IX complex	Hemophilia B	
Anti-inhibitor coagulation complex (AICC)	Hemophilia A patients with high titer of factor VIII antibodies	
Desmopressin acetate (DDAVP)	Mild/moderate forms of hemophilia A Certain types of von Willebrand's disease	
Platelets Random donor	Prophylaxis Dilutional thrombocytopenia	Autoimmune idiopathic thrombocytopenic purpura

TABLE 14-1 Indications and Contraindications of Blood and Blood Products—cont'd

Blood and Blood Components	Indications for Use	Contraindications for Use
Platelets—cont'd	Active bleeding due to thrombocytopenia or thrombocytopathy	Drug-induced thrombocytopenia Untreated DIC Thrombocytopenia due to septicemia/hypersplenism in nonbleeding patient Thrombotic thrombocytopenic purpura
Platelets single donor (Pheresis)	Thrombocytopenia in alloimmunized patients	
Granulocyte concentrates (GC)	Documented granulocyte dysfunction Infections unresponsive to antibiotics	Patients with poor chance of bone marrow recovery Infections responsive to antibiotic therapy
Plasma substitutes: albumin, plasma protein	Volume expansion, colloid replacement	Correct nutritional deficiency

limited clinical settings in which the patient needs all of these attributes; therefore, the use of Whole Blood has decreased precipitously in favor of individual component therapy. Currently, Whole Blood is rarely used for allogeneic transfusion and is minimally available in most regions; however, it may be indicated in cases of acute massive blood loss and in exchange transfusions.

In the case of exchange transfusion, fresh Whole Blood is usually selected. The definition of "fresh" varies from institution to institution, but generally refers to blood no more than 5 days old. Fresh blood is selected to limit potassium levels (to limit the risk of potassium toxicity), and to provide adequate levels of 2-3-diphosphoglycerate (2,3-DPG) to facilitate oxygen delivery to the tissues.

Contraindications and Complications

Whole Blood is not indicated solely to replace volume. **Crystalloid** and **colloid** solutions provide blood volume expansion without the associated disease transmission risks associated with Whole Blood or other blood components. An acute blood loss of approximately 20% of the total blood volume can usually be compensated for by the infusion of crystalloid solutions (e.g., normal saline and Ringer's lactate). When blood loss exceeds one third of the patient's blood volume, crystalloid therapy is no longer sufficient to sustain blood volume and may be replaced by colloid solutions (e.g., dextran, hydroxyethyl starch [HES]). Colloids, owing to their oncotic properties, stay within the vasculature for a longer time and serve to expand blood volume more effectively than similar volumes of crystalloid solutions.

Whole Blood is also not indicated to correct anemia in normovolemic patients. Although transfusion of Whole Blood to a chronically anemic patient will correct the anemia, the additional volume of plasma is unnecessary and may cause volume-related complications in certain populations of patients, such as infants and patients with chronic renal failure or congestive heart failure.

In cases of acute, massive blood loss, where a patient has received many units of stored Whole Blood, the patient may experience **dilutional coagulopathy.** After storage, units of Whole Blood do not contain functional platelets or sufficient levels of labile coagulation factors (V and VIII). As a result, hemostatic function may be impaired. Laboratory tests to determine hemostatic function (e.g., platelet count, prothrombin

Refer to Chapter 17 for a more in-depth discussion of transfusion in the perinatal period.

Crystalloid solution: A solution that can be diffused through animal membranes. Crystalloids such as normal saline can be used to restore blood volume up to approximately 20% blood loss.

Colloid solution: A solution with particles too large to pass through animal membranes. Colloids therefore remain in the vasculature and exert an oncotic effect, drawing water into the vascular space. Colloids are indicated for volume expansion.

Dilutional coagulopathy: Dysfunction of hemostasis due to the dilution of coagulation factors and platelets during the massive administration of blood, components, and derivatives. Refer to Chapter 17 for a discussion of massive transfusion.

time [PT], activated partial thromboplastin time [aPTT], and fibrinogen levels) along with clinical signs in the patient should be monitored to determine whether additional blood components are necessary to correct the hemostatic abnormality.

Red Blood Cells

Red Blood Cells: The blood component prepared by the removal of 200 to 250 mL of plasma from a unit of whole blood. Red cells are indicated for the treatment of anemia in normovolemic patients.

Red Blood Cells are prepared by removing 200 to 250 mL of plasma from a unit of Whole Blood, leaving a product with an approximate volume of 250 mL.[1] Red Blood Cells do not contain functional platelets or granulocytes. The hematocrit of a unit of Red Blood Cells varies according to the suspending medium. The hematocrit of Red Blood Cells in additive solutions (AS) is between 55% and 65%, and between 70% and 80% for Red Blood Cells stored in a CPDA-1 anticoagulant/preservative solution.[3]

Red Blood Cells with AS added are prepared by partially replacing the removed plasma with 100 to 110 mL of a solution that contains dextrose, adenine, sodium chloride, and either sodium phosphate or mannitol. Red Blood Cells with AS have a lower viscosity than red cells without the additive and an extended shelf life (42 days).

Red Blood Cells and Whole Blood have the same oxygen-carrying capacity because the number of red blood cells is the same in both products. However, infusion of a unit of Whole Blood (approximately 450 mL) produces a greater expansion in blood volume, whereas a unit of red blood cells (approximately 250 mL) produces an increase in the hemoglobin concentration with less risk of volume overload. One unit of Red Blood Cells increases the hemoglobin level by approximately 1 g/dL (10 g/L) and the hematocrit by 3% in an adult who is not actively bleeding and has no other predisposing factors (e.g., alloantibodies) that would shorten the survival of the transfused red blood cells.[2]

Indications

Red Blood Cell transfusions are indicated to increase the oxygen-carrying capacity of anemic patients who require an increase in their red cell mass without concomitant increase in their blood volume. This population includes patients who have congestive heart failure, who are elderly or debilitated, or who have chronic anemia due to renal failure or malignancy.

No universal hemoglobin threshold exists at which patients should be transfused. At one point, it was widely accepted that a hemoglobin value less than 10 g/dL (100 g/L) or a hematocrit less than 30% indicated a need for transfusion in the perioperative period. The decision to transfuse a patient in the perioperative period should take into consideration the presence of coexisting conditions (e.g., impaired pulmonary or myocardial function), duration of the anemia, intravascular volume, hemostatic function, and anticipated blood loss. Otherwise healthy patients with hemoglobin values of 10 g/dL (100 g/L) rarely require transfusions in the perioperative period, whereas those with acute anemia resulting in hemoglobin values less than 7 g/dL (70 g/L) frequently require perioperative transfusion.[4] A comparison of mortality rates in patients undergoing elective surgery found no difference in mortality rates between patients with preoperative hemoglobin levels above 10 g/dL and those between 6 and 10 g/dL (3.2% and 5%, respectively).[5]

Blood transfusions should be used to correct symptoms that are a direct result of anemia only when it has been determined that other treatment regimens (e.g., nutritional replacement therapy) are either not indicated or ineffective. It must first be determined if the patient has adequately compensated for the low hemoglobin level. The body has the ability to compensate for chronic anemia that has developed over a long period of time by increasing cardiac output and shifting the oxygen-hemoglobin dissociation curve to the right to increase the delivery of oxygen to the tissues. These compensatory mechanisms lessen the physiologic effects of a low hemoglobin level and explain why some patients with chronic anemia (e.g., chronic renal failure) have low hemoglobin levels yet are asymptomatic. It is more important in such cases to treat the underlying cause of the anemia than to use a blood transfusion to restore hemoglobin levels.

Alternatives to Red Blood Cells

Erythropoietin is produced primarily by the kidney and stimulates the proliferation, maturation, and differentiation of erythroid precursors. The production of this hormone is decreased in patients with kidney disease.[6] Erythropoietin has been produced using recombinant DNA technology and is known as recombinant human erythropoietin. Recombinant erythropoietin therapy has been shown to reduce the need for allogeneic transfusions by stimulating red blood cell (RBC) production (see Expert Opinion).

Erythropoietin: A hormone produced predominantly by the kidneys in response to hypoxia.

Expert Opinion

RECOMBINANT ERYTHROPOIETIN IN SURGERY
Lawrence T. Goodnough, MD

Interest in recombinant human erythropoietin (EPO) therapy as a surgical blood conservation intervention has been stimulated by recent emphasis on issues of blood safety, blood inventory, and alternatives to allogeneic blood transfusion. Published guidelines have recommended that if elective surgical patients require transfusion, autologous blood is the preferred therapy.[1] The effectiveness of preoperative autologous blood donation has been demonstrated for open heart surgery, orthopedic surgery, and urologic patients. Despite autologous blood donation, however, 15% to 20% of elective orthopedic patients receive allogeneic blood transfusions.[2] Studies of endogenous erythropoietin levels in autologous blood donors suggested that treatment of autologous blood donors with EPO would diminish or prevent the development of anemia in these patients and increase the volume of autologous blood that could be collected before surgery.[3,4] This was demonstrated in a randomized, placebo-controlled study in which patients receiving EPO twice weekly (600 μ/kg intravenously) donated 41% greater red blood cell (RBC) volume than placebo-treated patients.[5] Further analysis of preoperative RBC production (taking into account both in vivo and ex vivo [stored] RBC volumes) indicated that patients who underwent aggressive autologous blood phlebotomy (procurement of six units beginning 25 to 35 days before surgery) had a significant (27%) expansion of RBC volume preoperatively, along with accelerated erythropoiesis at the time of surgery.[6] As illustrated in Fig. EO4-1, the RBC volume expansion (47%) in the patients treated with EPO was significantly greater, generating the equivalent of nearly five blood units preoperatively, compared with three blood units for the control group.[7] The major difference in RBC

expansion between the placebo and erythropoietin groups occurred early in the collection period; by the time of surgery, the endogenous erythropoietin effect in the placebo patients diminished the differences between groups. However, not all patients can tolerate an aggressive blood donation schedule. Because the increased erythropoiesis can be attributed to the drug rather than to the aggressive phlebotomy program in EPO-treated patients, a more modest autologous blood procurement program of three to four units, coupled with administration of EPO to maintain hematocrit, may be a preferable approach.

Many issues remain in need of definition for the use of EPO therapy in the surgical setting. First, mobilization of iron stores and/or iron deficiency may limit the response to EPO through iron-restricted erythropoiesis. This has been analyzed for nonanemic autologous blood donors undergoing elective orthopedic surgery, in which premenopausal females treated with EPO were demonstrated to need oral iron supplementation.[8] Additionally, for autologous blood donors who are anemic at the time the first unit of blood is donated, approximately one third of such patients are iron depleted and require iron supplementation.[9] One study suggests that even with oral iron supplementation, autologous blood donors treated with EPO may have functional iron deficiency.[10] Alternative forms of oral or intravenous iron supplementation may be needed to optimize the erythropoietic response to EPO therapy.[11]

Finally, questions of optimal dose, route, and interval of administration for EPO therapy in the surgical setting have yet to be established. Each of these issues is important in determining the cost-effectiveness of EPO therapy. The response to EPO administered

Continued

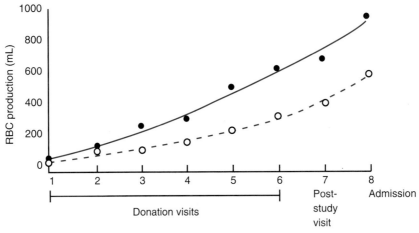

Fig. EO4-1 Red blood cell (RBC) production during autologous blood donation, in 23 placebo-treated (open circles) and 21 erythropoietin-treated (closed circles) patients. Data points represent calculated RBC production from donation visits 1 through 6, post-study visit, and hospital admission. *(From Goodnough LT: Preoperative blood phlebotomy with and without erythropoietin therapy. Transfusion 32:441-445, 1992.)*

intravenously occurs within 3.5 days,[5] with the equivalent of one blood unit produced within 7 days.[6] The EPO dosage (600 μ/kg given twice) for a 70 kg patient to achieve this effect is 84,000 units; at current costs of $0.01/unit, EPO therapy to produce the equivalent of one blood unit can be estimated to cost $840. Alternative routes of iron administration may significantly improve the cost-benefit ratio of EPO therapy.[12] Subcutaneous administration may be superior to an intravenous route, in that lower doses of EPO may be sufficient for the desired effect on erythropoiesis.[13] Recent estimates of the high effectiveness of preoperative autologous blood donation[14,15] emphasize that blood conservation interventions, including pharmacologic agents, need to be considered in light of their costs as well as their benefits.

The use of EPO in patients with surgical anemia should similarly be restricted to clinical settings in which need for avoidance of allogeneic blood transfusion has been demonstrated. Therapy should be linked to ongoing blood losses to avoid potential complications related to polycythemia and hyperviscosity. The use of this agent to correct preoperative anemia should be coupled with autologous blood procurement not only for these safety concerns but to enhance effectiveness in reducing perisurgical allogeneic blood transfusions. For example, most blood transfusion support in coronary artery bypass surgery and orthopedic surgery is given on the day of operation and could be avoided if autologous blood were available preoperatively.[16,17] Emerging issues related to blood availability will make alternatives to allogeneic blood such as erythropoietin therapy increasingly attractive.[18]

SUMMARY

Recombinant human erythropoietin (EPO) has been approved for use in patients undergoing autologous blood donation in Japan, the European Union, and Canada since 1993, 1994, and 1996, respectively, and is now approved for perisurgical adjuvant therapy in Canada, Australia, the United States, and the European Union (Table EO4-1).[1] Emerging strategies to improve the dose-response relationship between erythropoietin therapy and red cell production include low-dose EPO and intravenous iron therapy, to be addressed in this discussion.

TABLE EO4-1 Approval Status of Recombinant Human Erythropoietin Therapy in Surgical Anemia

	United States	Canada	European Union*	Australia	Japan
Autologous blood donation	—	1996	1994	1996	1993
Surgery	1996[†]	1996	1998[‡]	1996	Under review

*Approval dates for France, Germany, Italy, and the United Kingdom are the same as for other countries of the European Union.
[†]Noncardiac, nonvascular surgery.
[‡]Orthopedic surgery.

REFERENCES

1. American College of Physicians: Practice strategies for elective red blood cell transfusion. Ann Intern Med 116:403-406, 1992.
2. Goodnough LT, Vizmeg K, Verbrugge D: The impact of autologous blood ordering and blood procurement practices of allogeneic blood exposure in elective orthopedic patients. Am J Clin Pathol 101(3):354-357, 1994.
3. Kickler TS, Spivak JL: Effect of repeated whole blood donations on serum immunoreactive erythropoietin levels in autologous donors. JAMA 260:65-67, 1988.
4. Goodnough LT, Brittenham G: Limitations of the erythropoietic response to serial phlebotomy: Implications for autologous blood donor programs. J Lab Clin Med 115:28-35, 1990.
5. Goodnough LT, Rudnick S, Price TH, et al: Increased collection of autologous blood preoperatively with recombinant human erythropoietin therapy. N Engl J Med 312:1163-1167, 1989.
6. Goodnough LT, Price TH, Rudnick S: Preoperative red blood cell production in patients undergoing aggressive autologous blood phlebotomy with and without erythropoietin therapy. Transfusion 32:441-445, 1992.
7. Goodnough LT: Erythropoietin therapy as a surgical blood conservation intervention. Lab Med 23:457-461, 1992.
8. Goodnough LT, Price TH, Rudnick S: Iron-restricted erythropoiesis as a limitation to autologous blood donation in the erythropoietin-stimulated bone marrow. J Lab Clin Med 188:289-295, 1991.
9. Goodnough LT, Vizmeg K, Riddell J, Soegiarso W: Prevalence of anemia in autologous blood donors prior to elective orthopaedic surgery: Implications for blood conservation programs. Vox Sang 63:96-101, 1992.
10. Brugnara C, Chambers LA, Malynn E, et al: Red blood cell regeneration induced by subcutaneous recombinant erythropoietin: Iron-deficient erythropoiesis in iron-replete subjects. Blood 81:956-964, 1993.
11. Goodnough LT, Skikne B, Brugnara C: Erythropoietin, iron, and erythropoiesis. Blood 96:823-833, 2000.
12. Goodnough LT, Soegiarso RW, Birkmeyer JD, Welch HG: The economic impact in inappropriate blood transfusions in coronary artery bypass graft surgery. Am J Med 94:1-5, 1993.
13. Hughes RT, Cotes PM, Oliver DO, et al: Correction of the anemia of chronic renal failure with erythropoietin: Pharmacokinetic studies in patients on haemodialysis and CAPD. Contrib Nephrol 76:122-130, 1989.
14. Birkmeyer JD, AuBuchon JP, Littenberg B, et al: The cost-effectiveness of preoperative autologous blood donation in coronary bypass grafting. Ann Thorac Surg 57(1):161-168, 1994.
15. Birkmeyer JD, Goodnough LT, Aubuchon JP, et al: The cost-effectiveness of preoperative autologous blood donation for total hip and knee replacement. Transfusion 33(7):544-551, 1993.
16. Goodnough LT, Soegiarso RW, Geha AS: Blood lost and blood transfused in coronary artery bypass graft operations as implications for blood transfusion and blood conservation strategies. Surg Gynecol Obstet 177(4):345-351, 1993.
17. Goodnough LT, Vizmeg K, Marcus RE: Blood lost and blood transfused in patients undergoing elective orthopedic operation. Surg Gynecol Obstet 176:235-238, 1993.
18. Goodnough LT, Shander A, Brecher ME: Transfusion medicine: Looking to the future. Lancet 361:161-169, 2003.

Red Blood Cells Leukocytes Reduced

Red Blood Cells Leukocytes Reduced are prepared by a method that reduces the leukocyte number in the final components while retaining at least 85% of the original red cells. Leukocyte reduction can be accomplished at any of a number of times, including during collection, after collection but before storage, in the laboratory before issue, or during infusion. The American Association of Blood Banks (AABB) *Standards for Blood Banks and Transfusion Services* states that leukocyte components shall be prepared by a method known to reduce the leukocyte number to less than 5×10^6.[7]

Red Blood Cells Leukocytes Reduced: A red cell component from which white cells have been removed by one of a number of leukocyte-reduction processes. This component is useful for patients who have exhibited severe febrile reactions.

Indications

Red Blood Cells Leukocytes Reduced are indicated for those patients who have experienced recurrent and/or severe nonhemolytic febrile transfusion reactions. Red Blood Cells Leukocytes Reduced also decrease the risk of alloimmunization to human leukocyte antigen (HLA) class I antigens, and reduce the transmission of cytomegalovirus (CMV) infection.[2]

Multiply transfused patients and multiparous women may develop antibodies to leukocyte and/or platelet antigens by virtue of their repeated exposure to cells (e.g., leukocytes, platelets) expressing foreign antigens. Patients with leukocyte antibodies may experience a febrile nonhemolytic transfusion reaction (FNHTR) on receiving blood or blood products (e.g., Platelets) containing incompatible leukocytes. The severity and frequency of these reactions are proportional to the volume of leukocytes transfused. Leukocyte antibodies are directed against the Human Leukocyte Antigens and are responsible for the majority of FNHTRs. Considerable evidence indicates that peripheral blood leukocytes are a site of latent infection for CMV. It has been demonstrated through clinical studies that leukocyte-reduced blood components prepared by third-generation filters are as effective in preventing transmission of CMV infection as are blood components that are tested to be CMV negative.[2] Leukocyte-reduced components are termed "CMV safe."

Red Blood Cells Deglycerolized

Red Blood Cells Deglycerolized: A component prepared by thawing and washing red cells that have been stored in a cryoprotective agent for up to 10 years. This freezing process is especially useful for rare blood storage.

Red Blood Cells Deglycerolized (RBCs Deglycerolized) are red blood cells that have been frozen at optimal temperatures in a cryoprotective agent, which is then removed by a washing process before transfusion. The method used to prepare RBCs Deglycerolized ensures adequate removal of the cryoprotective agents and minimal free hemoglobin in the supernatant solution. At least 80% of the original red blood cells should be recovered following the deglycerolization process, and viability of at least 70% of the transfused cells must be established 24 hours after transfusion. AABB Standards allow frozen red cells that will be used for routine transfusion to be stored for 10 years at temperatures $\leq -65^\circ$ C.[7]

Indications

The use of this component is most commonly reserved for the storage of rare and autologous blood for a longer period of time than can be achieved with anticoagulant/preservative (35 days) or additive (42 days) solutions. Virtually all of the plasma and most of the leukocytes and platelets have been removed from a unit of RBCs Deglycerolized.

Contraindications

The requirements for the preparation, storage, and deglycerolization of RBCs Deglycerolized make the cost of this component two to three times that of liquid-stored Red Blood Cells. RBCs Deglycerolized are not, therefore, a cost-effective component for routine use in transfusion therapy. For example, transfusing RBCs Deglycerolized prevents reactions in patients with leukocyte and/or platelet antibodies, but other less costly blood components (e.g., RBCs Leukocytes Reduced) may be just as effective.[2]

Disease Transmission

It was once believed that freezing and deglycerolizing red blood cells would eliminate the transmission of viral diseases. Unfortunately this has not proven true, because RBCs Deglycerolized have been found to transmit both hepatitis B and C. RBCs Deglycerolized contain reduced numbers of leukocytes and have been used in place of blood that is negative for CMV to decrease the rate of CMV seroconversion in susceptible individuals; however, cost remains an issue and other components may be equally effective.

Red Blood Cells Washed

Red Blood Cells Washed: Red cells that are washed with sterile saline, resulting in the removal of plasma proteins, platelets, leukocytes and cellular debris.

Red cells may be washed with sterile saline to remove plasma proteins. The saline washing process results in the reduction of the number of leukocytes and the removal of platelets and other cellular debris.[1]

Indications

RBCs Washed may be used for neonatal and intrauterine transfusions. They are also indicated for patients who have experienced severe allergic transfusion reactions to components contained in plasma.[1]

Pretransfusion Testing of Red Cell Components

The transfusion service performing the crossmatch must confirm the ABO group of all Whole Blood or Red Blood Cell donor units and the Rh type of such units labeled Rh negative. Weak D confirmation testing on Rh-negative units is not required. The sample used for confirmatory testing of ABO and Rh type must be obtained from a segment attached to the donor unit.[2]

The recipient's blood sample must be tested for ABO and Rh type; weak D testing is not required. Methods for screening the recipient's serum or plasma for unexpected antibodies must be able to detect clinically significant antibodies and include a 37° C incubation preceding an antiglobulin phase. Reagent red blood cells may not be pooled, and negative reactions at the antiglobulin phase must be confirmed with IgG-sensitized control cells (unless the manufacturer states otherwise).[2]

If no clinically significant antibodies are detected and there is no record of such antibodies having been previously detected, an abbreviated serologic crossmatch, capable of detecting recipient/donor major ABO incompatibility, may be performed. An electronic crossmatch may be used to substitute for this serologic crossmatch so long as there are two separate determinations of ABO type and the computer system used has been suitably validated for this purpose.

If clinically significant antibodies are identified or the patient has a record of such antibodies, a crossmatch must be performed that is capable of detecting ABO compatibility and clincally significant antibodies. Minimally such a crossmatch must include a 37° C incubation followed by an indirect antiglobulin test.[2]

Whole Blood units issued for transfusion must be ABO-group identical, whereas red cell components may be ABO-group compatible (Fig. 14-1). Rh-negative recipients should receive Rh-negative Whole Blood or red cell components except in reasonable extenuating situations when this cannot be accomplished. Rh-positive recipients may receive either Rh-negative or Rh-positive Whole Blood or red cell components.[2] Transfusion of Rh-negative blood to an Rh-positive individual is usually reserved for situations where Rh positive blood is not available or when the unit of Rh-negative blood is due to expire and would otherwise be discarded.

Maximum Surgical Blood Order Schedule

The implementation of a maximum surgical blood order schedule (MSBOS) allows for the designation of the appropriate number of units to be crossmatched for commonly performed surgical procedures. It is important to differentiate between procedures that most commonly require blood transfusions and those that do not. An MSBOS can be established by analyzing blood use for all commonly performed elective surgical procedures and comparing the number of units crossmatched with the number of units transfused (C/T ratio). Utilization may vary among institutions, surgical practice, and patient populations. Guidelines are published for comparison and to ensure acceptable quality and standard of care. The goal of an MSBOS is to limit the number of units crossmatched to the usual number of units that are transfused for a particular surgical procedure. Surgical procedures with a C/T ratio greater than 2.0 to 2.5 are generally considered to have an excessive number of units crossmatched. A type and antibody screen (without a crossmatch) are performed for invasive procedures that rarely require transfusion.[2]

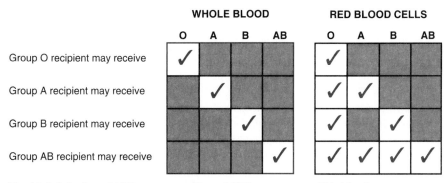

Fig. 14-1 Selection of ABO group–specific and ABO group–compatible blood.

Ultimately, an MSBOS decreases patient care costs by reserving crossmatches for surgical procedures that are most likely to require blood.

TRANSFUSION OF OTHER BLOOD COMPONENTS
Platelets

Platelets can be prepared by cytapheresis or by separating platelet-rich plasma from a unit of whole blood within 8 hours of collection and recentrifuging to remove the majority of the supernatant plasma. Platelets are suspended in a sufficient amount of plasma to ensure a pH of 6.2 or higher at the end of the allowable storage period. The mean life span of donated platelets is approximately 4 to 5 days. **Platelets** prepared from a single unit of whole blood (random-donor platelet) usually contain a minimum of 5.5×10^{10} platelets suspended in 40 to 70 mL of plasma. One unit of **Platelets Pheresis** (single-donor platelets) contains a minimum of 3×10^{11} platelets and is equivalent to six to eight units of random-donor platelets.[2] In a hematologically stable adult with 1.8 m^2 body surface area, each unit of platelets is expected to increase the platelet count by approximately 5 to 10 $\times$ 10^8/L (5 to 10 $\times 10^3$/mm^3) and one unit of Platelets Pheresis increases the platelet count by approximately 30 to 60 $\times 10^9$/L (30 to 60 $\times 10^3$/mm^3).

As with Red Blood Cells, Platelets and Platelets Pheresis can be leukocyte reduced at the time of collection, prestorage, at the time of issue, or during infusion. The storage conditions remain the same for leukocyte-reduced platelet components.

Indications

Many factors must be considered before initiating platelet therapy. The clinical condition of the patient, the number and functional ability of the patient's own platelets, and the cause of the thrombocytopenia must all be evaluated. Before platelet therapy is initiated, it is important to determine if platelets are necessary to prevent or correct the bleeding episode.

Most commonly platelets are transfused prophylactically to prevent spontaneous life-threatening hemorrhage in individuals with transient **thrombocytopenia** due to treatment regimens for malignancy, or marrow aplasia. The literature contains much controversy about what the platelet count should be before Platelets are administered prophylactically. Patients with uncomplicated thrombocytopenia generally do not require platelet transfusions until the count falls below 10×10^9/L (10×10^3/mm^3).[8] Serious complications (e.g., major gastrointestinal bleeding, central nervous system hemorrhage) do not arise until the platelet count is below $5 \times$ 10^9/L (5×10^3/mm^3).[8,9] Lowering the "trigger value" for prophylactic platelet transfusions decreases the overall requirement for platelet transfusions and presumably diminishes the risk of alloimmunization. The use of Platelets Pheresis (single donor) rather than Platelets (random donor) offers potential advantages to this population by limiting exposure to infectious agents and reducing the likelihood of alloimmunization. Studies have indicated, however, that Platelets Pheresis is no more effective than Platelets in raising the platelet count in patients who have not yet become alloimmunized.[9]

During massive transfusion, dilutional thrombocytopenia can result from the multiple units of blood (e.g., Whole Blood or Red Blood Cells) transfused to replace that lost through hemorrhage. The degree of dilutional thrombocytopenia is usually predictable with regard to the number of volume replacements the patient has sustained. Generally, 35% to 40% of the patient's own platelets remain following replacement of one blood volume. Although dilutional thrombocytopenia may lead to microvascular bleeding, this does not occur in the majority of patients who receive replacement of one to two volumes of blood. Following massive transfusion, Platelets should be given only when there is evidence of thrombocytopenia and clinically abnormal bleeding.[10] It is important to remember that each unit of Platelets contains approximately 50 mL of relatively fresh plasma, and,

Platelets: A blood component prepared by centrifugation from a unit of donor blood before refrigeration. Platelets are indicated for patients who are at risk of hemorrhage or who are bleeding secondary to low platelet number or dysfunctional platelets.

Platelets Pheresis: A component separated by pheresis techniques allowing for large platelet yields from a single donor, making this product valuable for the patient who requires HLA-matched platelets.

Thrombocytopenia: Decreased platelet numbers.

according to the general guidelines for plasma therapy, this would provide 50 mL of stable coagulation factors.[2]

Patients with chronic thrombocytopenia caused by impaired platelet production (e.g., aplastic anemia) generally do not require prophylactic platelet transfusion.[9] However, when thrombocytopenia and/or **thrombocytopathy** is present in a patient experiencing uncontrollable blood loss (e.g., major surgery, gastrointestinal bleed), Platelets are indicated to help control bleeding and avoid life-threatening hemorrhages.

Contraindications

Platelet transfusions are not indicated in patients with autoimmune idiopathic thrombocytopenia purpura, drug-induced thrombocytopenia, untreated disseminated intravascular coagulation (DIC), and thrombocytopenia due to **septicemia** or **hypersplenism** unless uncontrolled active bleeding is present. In these situations, platelets are rapidly cleared from the circulation and are of relatively little benefit. Platelets are contraindicated in patients with **thrombotic thrombocytopenic purpura** (TTP) because of the risk of potentially serious thrombotic episodes.[9] Platelet transfusion should also be avoided in the case of active heparin-induced thrombocytopenia except in life-threatening conditions.[2]

ABO and Rh Type in Platelet Transfusion

The donor plasma of Platelets and Platelets Pheresis units should be ABO compatible with the recipient's red blood cells, especially when the product is being transfused to neonates.[2] ABO agglutinins in donor plasma may cause a positive direct antiglobulin test (DAT) or, rarely, hemolysis if the volume of ABO-incompatible plasma transfused is large in relation to the recipient's red cell mass. It may be advisable to reduce the volume of ABO-incompatible plasma in pooled Platelets or Platelets Pheresis, particularly if the transfusion is for a child or neonate. Shortly before transfusion, the majority of plasma may be removed from stored Platelets, leaving only an appropriate amount for resuspension. These modified Platelets must remain at room temperature without agitation, then be resuspended and transfused within 4 hours of the time the bag was entered.[2] ABO antigens are present on the surface of platelets, and transfusion of ABO-incompatible platelets (e.g., A platelets to an O recipient) may have a slightly diminished 24-hour recovery. It is preferable to transfuse ABO-compatible platelets. However, the ABO type of the Platelets becomes inconsequential if the clinical condition of the patient dictates that Platelets be given in a timely manner. In this case, it is unacceptable to delay the transfusion to wait for ABO-compatible Platelets.

It is not necessary to routinely crossmatch Platelets and Platelet Pheresis products. Each unit of random-donor Platelets that has been properly prepared contains 0.5 mL or less of red blood cells. Even if the recipient had alloantibodies, the small volume of red cells transfused would not be sufficient to result in significant hemolysis. A major crossmatch is required for Platelets if they contain 2 mL or more of red blood cells.[7]

The D antigen is not present on the platelet surface. However, Rh-positive platelets containing 0.5 mL or less of red blood cells carry a small risk of immunizing Rh-negative individuals. It is therefore not desirable to transfuse Rh-positive platelets to Rh-negative females of childbearing age. If this is unavoidable, Rh immune globulin (RhIG) may be administered. Each 300 g vial of RhIG provides protection against the administration of 15 mL of red blood cells.

Alloimmunization

Appropriate posttransfusion monitoring is essential to determine the efficacy of the platelet transfusion. This is done by measuring the pretransfusion and posttransfusion platelet count and noting the clinical effect of the platelet transfusion

Thrombocytopathy: Functionally abnormal platelets.

Septicemia: A serious condition marked by the presence of pathologic microorganisms in the blood.

Hypersplenism: Enlargement of the spleen.

Thrombotic thrombocytopenic purpura: A disorder characterized by decreased platelet numbers, hemolytic anemia, and thrombosis.

(prevention or cessation of bleeding). If the posttransfusion platelet count deviates from the expected value on two or more occasions, the patient may no longer be responsive to the platelet transfusions. An inadequate platelet response can be documented by comparing a corrected count increment (CCI) (Fig. 14-2) and the expected minimum response from the platelet transfusion.[10] "In the clinically stable patient, the CCI is typically greater than 7500 at 10 minutes to one hour after transfusion and remains above 4600 at 24 hours."[3]

Repeated failure to see the expected posttransfusion increment in the platelet count is generally due to antiplatelet antibodies, anti-HLA antibodies, or some aspect of the clinical condition of the patient that would result in decreased survival of the platelets (e.g., fever, infection, DIC, sepsis). The 10- to 60-minute CCI is considered to be diminished primarily by alloimmunization and splenomegaly, whereas a decrease in the 18- to 24-hour CCI is most commonly due to nonimmune causes such as fever, infection, or DIC.[1,10] Studies have indicated, however, that some nonimmune causes may result in such a rapid destruction or sequestration of platelets that the decrease would be reflected in the 10- to 60-minute CCI.[10]

When a patient becomes refractory because of alloimmunization, subsequent platelet transfusions from random donors fail to produce the expected therapeutic results. The majority of these patients are immunized to HLA antigens. Leukocytes present in routinely prepared platelet components, as well as the platelets themselves, express HLA antigens that can provoke HLA antibody formation. A lymphocytotoxicity test (LCT) can be used to document the presence of (HLA) antibodies. This assay is widely available, and the percentage of reactive cells (cells injured by an antigen-antibody-complement reaction that are detected by dye exclusion) correlates well with transfusion outcome.[10] To improve the effectiveness of platelet transfusions in this alloimmunized population, HLA-matched platelets may be transfused. Family members are the most likely source of HLA-identical or HLA-compatible donors because of the considerable homology of HLA antigens that usually exists.

Reports have appeared in the literature of fatal transfusion-associated graft-versus-host disease (TA-GVHD) in recipients of cellular blood transfusions from closely related donors. This may be due to the fact that the HLA homology that produces a better increase in the posttransfusion platelet count may also result in the recipient's immune system being unable to recognize these lymphocytes as foreign, especially when donor HLA antigens are identical at multiple loci.[10] The AABB has responded by recommending that blood and cellular products be irradiated with a minimum of 2500 cGy (25 Gy) to reduce the risk of TA-GVHD in bone marrow transplant recipients, as well as in recipients of donor units known to be from a blood relative.[2] Irradiation has had no adverse effects on the recovery, survival, and hemostatic efficiency of platelets following transfusion.[11,12]

When it is not possible to find an HLA-compatible donor from family members, transfusions of HLA-matched Platelets Pheresis from unrelated donors can be arranged. Files of HLA-matched donors are kept by many organizations, including the AABB and American Red Cross.

$$CCI = \frac{(\text{Post-tx plt ct}) - (\text{Pre-tx plt ct}) \times BSA}{\text{Platelets transfused } (\times 10^{11})}$$

where Post tx plt ct = post-transfusion platelet count
Pre-tx plt ct = pretransfusion platelet count
BSA = body surface area in square meters

Minimum acceptable CCI values[2]:
$>7.5 \times 10^9$/L from a sample drawn 10 to 60 minutes post-transfusion
$>4.5 \times 10^9$/L from a sample drawn 18 to 24 hours post-transfusion

Fig. 14-2 Corrected count increment (CCI).

Failure of HLA-matched Platelets Pheresis units to produce the expected post-transfusion platelet count increment in alloimmunized patients suggests that the refractory state of the patient may be due to alloimmunization to platelet-specific antigens. A platelet crossmatch can be used to detect antibodies to specific platelet antigens and thereby improve the responsiveness to platelet transfusions.[10]

Granulocytes

Granulocytes are prepared by cytapheresis and contain greater than 1.0×10^{10} granulocytes suspended in 200 to 300 mL of plasma.[1] There are variable amounts of lymphocytes, platelets, and red blood cells in this product.

Indications

The number of Granulocyte transfusions has decreased in recent years because of the availability of a broad spectrum of antibiotics to treat infections and reports of adverse reactions (e.g., pulmonary and febrile transfusion reactions) to the product.

Granulocyte therapy should be initiated only in patients with documented infections after it has been established that the infection is unresponsive to antibiotic therapy and that a reasonable quality of life is expected after the patient recovers from the infection. Because Granulocytes are only a temporary form of therapy, it should be determined that the bone marrow is likely to recover.

Patients with documented granulocyte dysfunction (e.g., neutropenia, chronic granulomatous disease) may be candidates for Granulocyte therapy. The absolute granulocyte count should be less than 0.5×10^9/L (0.5×10^3/mm³), because counts higher than this are not believed to place the patient at an increased risk of infection. The length of time for which Granulocytes are administered is controversial, but generally they are given for at least 4 to 6 days unless the bone marrow recovers or the patient has an adverse reaction to the product.

Contraindications

Granulocytes are not indicated for the treatment of infections when the organism is responsive to antibiotic therapy and the patient can be satisfactorily treated. In addition, patients with a poor prognosis (e.g., terminal malignancies) are not candidates for Granulocyte therapy because the temporary beneficial effects of Granulocytes do not alter the patient's clinical condition.

Pretransfusion Testing

The red blood cells in the Granulocyte product must be ABO compatible and preferably Rh compatible with the recipient's plasma. Granulocytes must be crossmatched if they contain 2 mL or more of red blood cells or the recipient's plasma contains clinically significant alloantibodies.[7] Because Granulocytes from an Rh-positive donor contain sufficient red blood cells to immunize an Rh-negative individual, consideration should be given to administering RhIG if this situation arises. Granulocytes contain a large volume of plasma and therefore should contain no clinically significant antibodies. Plasma volume should be minimized to reduce the risk of fluid overload when the transfusion recipient is a pediatric patient. Pretransfusion testing should be performed in a timely manner, and the granulocytes should be transfused as soon as possible and always within 24 hours of collection.[1] Because Granulocytes contain large numbers of lymphocytes, they need to be irradiated to prevent GVHD before transfusion to bone marrow recipients or otherwise immunocompromised recipients and if the intended recipient is a blood relative of the donor from whom the Granulocytes were prepared.[1] Leukocyte-reduction filters are contraindicated when administering granulocytes.

The efficacy of Granulocyte transfusions is best judged by observing the clinical condition of the patient. Cell counts are not a good indicator because following transfusion, granulocytes rapidly leave the vascular compartment.

Granulocytes: A component prepared by cytapheresis and indicated for patients with overwhelming sepsis and insufficient numbers of circulating neutrophils for normal phagocytic activity.

PLASMA COMPONENTS
Fresh Frozen Plasma

Fresh Frozen Plasma (FFP) is prepared by removing plasma from blood drawn from an individual donor and placing it at −18° C or lower within 8 hours of collection. FFP contains water, carbohydrates, fats, minerals, and proteins (which include all the labile and stable clotting factors) in a volume of 200 to 225 mL.[1]

Indications

Transfusion of FFP is justified for the (1) replacement of coagulation factors when specific concentrates are not available (e.g., Factors V and XI), (2) management of multiple factor deficiency (e.g., liver disease), and (3) treatment of antithrombin deficiency and TTP.

Deficiencies of any single coagulation factor other than Factors VIII and IX are rare. For example, bleeding due to acquired Factor V deficiency is not common, and hereditary Factor V deficiency is rare. In addition, only 10% to 15% of Factor V levels are needed to maintain hemostasis. (Table 14-2 identifies the hemostatic levels of coagulation factors.) If the level of Factor V drops below 10% to 15%, FFP can be used to replace the deficient coagulation factor and restore hemostasis.

Antithrombin, also known as heparin cofactor, is a serine protease inhibitor that circulates in plasma and has a normal range of 84% to 116%. It is a circulating protein that is an important inhibitor of coagulation and acts by inhibiting thrombin and other factors (IX, X, XI, and XII) and by potentiating the in vivo effect of heparin.[2] Antithrombin deficiencies may be hereditary or acquired (e.g., chronic liver disease, consumptive coagulopathy, burns) and are associated with spontaneous thrombosis.[13] Antithrombin is approved for use in hereditary deficiencies and also for prophylactic use in perioperative and postoperative settings.[2]

Contraindications

FFP is not appropriate as a volume expander, and its use for this purpose should be strongly discouraged. More appropriate volume expanders include crystalloid and colloid solutions, which, in contrast to FFP, are more cost-effective and are free of the risk of disease transmission. FFP should not be given as a nutritional source of protein and is no longer indicated as a source of immunoglobulins because of the availability of intravenous serum immune globulin. It should also not be given if there is a more effective treatment for the coagulopathy such as vitamin K or factor concentrates.

TABLE 14-2 Coagulation Factors		
Factor	Common Name	Minimum Hemostatic Level
I	Fibrinogen	50–100 mg%
II	Prothrombin	30%–40%
V	Proaccelerin	10%
VII	Proconvertin	10%
VIII	Antihemophilic factor	30%
IX	Christmas factor	30%–50%
X	Stuart-Prower factor	10%
XI	Plasma thromboplastin antecedent (PTA)	20%–30%
XIII	Fibrin stabilizing factor	1%

Data from Harmening DM: Clinical Hematology and Fundamentals of Hemostasis, 4th ed. Philadelphia, FA Davis, 2002.

Dose and Administration

FFP should be ABO compatible with the recipient's red blood cells and can be given without regard to Rh type because it is a cell-free product. Crossmatching is not required.[1]

The amount of FFP transfused depends on the clinical situation and any extenuating circumstances (e.g., underlying disease process). One milliliter of FFP contains one unit of coagulation factor activity.[2] The efficacy of transfusion should be assessed with routine coagulation tests (PT, aPTT) or specific factor assays. Hemostatic effectiveness is generally achieved with the PT and aPTT when factor levels are 30% or higher. Results of coagulation tests and the clinical status of the patient indicate whether additional therapy is needed.

Plasma Products with Reduced Levels of Labile Coagulation Factors

Plasma that does not meet the preparation requirements for FFP (separation within 8 hours of collection and storage at −18° C) has diminished levels of labile coagulation factors. Included in this category are **Plasma, Liquid Plasma, Thawed Plasma, and Plasma Frozen Within 24 Hours After Phelebotomy.** Plasma and Liquid Plasma are separated no later than 5 days after the expiration of the Whole Blood. Plasma is stored at −18° C and Liquid Plasma at 1° to 6° C. These components can be used to replace coagulation factors in patients with deficiencies other than Factors V and VIII.

Plasma Cryoprecipitate Reduced is a by-product of the production of Cryoprecipitated AHF. This product is deficient in Factor VIII, von Willebrand Factor (vWF), fibrinogen, cryoglobulin, and fibronectin. Other coagulation factors remain at the same concentration as FFP. This component can serve as a source of coagulation proteins except for Factor VIII, von Willebrand Factor, and fibrinogen.

Cryoprecipitated AHF

Cryoprecipitated AHF is the cold-insoluble portion of plasma that remains after FFP has been thawed at 1° to 6° C. Each bag of Cryoprecipitated AHF contains Factor VIII:C (procoagulant activity), fibrinogen, Factor XIII, and Factor VIII:vWF (von Willebrand factor) in approximately 10 to 15 mL of plasma (see Summary 14-1).[2]

Indications

Cryoprecipitated AHF is the only product that contains a concentrated amount of fibrinogen, which may be indicated for the treatment of congenital or acquired fibrinogen deficiencies (e.g., DIC). Cryoprecipitated AHF may also be used for the treatment of severe **von Willebrand's disease** and Factor XIII deficiency, as well as for Factor VII deficiencies if factor concentrates are not available. Cryoprecipitated AHF has received widespread acceptance as a source of **fibrin glue.** Fibrin glue has been used in procedures such as cardiopulmonary bypass, colostomy closure, and other surgical procedures. In 1998, the Food and Drug Administration approved the first commercial product (Tisseel) that can be used as a fibrin sealant.[14]

Plasma, Liquid Plasma, Thawed Plasma, and Plasma Frozen Within 45 Hours After Phlebotomy: Plasma components that lack labile coagulation factors but contain stable coagulation factors.

Plasma Cryoprecipitate Reduced: A plasma product deficient in Factor VIII, von Willebrand Factor (vWF), fibrinogen, cryoglobulin, and fibronectin.

Cryoprecipitated AHF: A component derived from donor plasma that is rich in Factor VIII:C, fibrinogen, Factor XIII, and Factor VIII:vWF. This component is indicated for patients with von Willebrand's disease, Factor XIII deficiency, obstetric accidents, and hemophilia A.

von Willebrand's disease: An inherited disorder characterized by decreased levels of Factors VIII:C, VIII:vWF, and VIII:Ag.

Fibrin glue: Cryoprecipitate used as a topical hemostatic agent.

Summary 14-1

Contents of Cryoprecipitated AHF*

80 to 120 units of Factor VIII:C (procoagulant activity)
≥150 mg fibrinogen
20% to 30% of the Factor XIII in the original unit
40% to 70% of the Factor VIII:vWF (von Willebrand factor) in the original unit

---

*Note: All values are approximations.

Administration

Cryoprecipitated AHF contains small amounts of plasma, and although the volume of each individual unit is small, most patients receive many units. The plasma should therefore be ABO compatible with the recipient's blood type when possible. Hemolysis of recipient red blood cells has been observed following transfusion of large amounts of ABO-incompatible Cryoprecipitated AHF. Infusions of smaller amounts of ABO-incompatible Cryoprecipitated AHF have been reported to cause a positive DAT in the recipient. Cryoprecipitated AHF may be transfused without regard to Rh type, and crossmatching is not required.

Blood and Blood Product Precautions

The risk of transfusion reaction (hemolytic, allergic, febrile, GVHD, fluid overload, viral transmission) and alloimmunization should be considered with each unit of blood or blood component transfused.

Plasma Substitutes

Plasma substitutes and synthetic volume expanders do not carry the risk of viral disease transmission and should be used when volume replacement is the desired patient outcome. Because of the associated risk of viral transmission with fresh-frozen plasma, it is not suitable for this purpose.

Albumin is available in 5% and 25% solutions and contains 96% albumin and 4% globulins and other proteins. Plasma protein fraction (PPF), available as a 5% solution, contains 83% albumin and 17% globulins. The 5% solution is osmotically and oncotically equivalent to plasma, whereas the 25% solution is five times that of plasma. The preparation of both of these products includes an extended heating period that eliminates the risk of transmission of viral diseases.[1]

Indications

Enteric administration, parenteral administration, or hyperalimentation: The administration of nourishment through a variety of routes (enteric: small intestine; parenteral: subcutaneous/intramuscular) or in greater than optimum (hyper) amounts.

Albumin and PPF solutions are indicated for volume expansion and colloid replacement for patients in hypovolemic shock, burn patients, and patients undergoing retroperitoneal surgery in which large volumes of protein-rich fluid may pool in the bowel. The indications for using PPF parallel those for 5% albumin. Albumin solutions are not indicated to correct nutritional deficiencies when **enteric administration, parenteral administration, or hyperalimentation** would be more appropriate.[1,2] These products provide volume expansion and colloid replacement without the risk of transfusion-transmitted viruses.

Contraindications

Oncotic pressure: Osmotic pressure that is exerted by colloids in solution.

The rapid infusion of PPF may lead to hypotensive episodes. It is therefore not indicated in clinical situations involving the rapid restoration of volume (e.g., hypovolemic shock).[2] Infusion of 25% albumin rapidly increases the **oncotic pressure** by drawing large volumes of water from the tissues to the vascular space. This carries the risk of cardiac overload and/or intestinal dehydration.[1,2]

Administration

Albumin and PPF do not contain ABO antigens or antibodies, so compatibility testing is not required.

Intravenous Immunoglobulins

Intravenous immunoglobulin: A plasma product produced by Cohn fractionation and treated to inactivate viruses. The IV preparation contains monomeric IgG molecules almost exclusively.

Intravenous immunoglobulins (IVIGs) are manufactured from pooled plasma and contain all subclasses and allotypes of IgG, immune aggregates, and anticomplement activity. IVIG has been shown to be beneficial in the treatment of many diseases, such as idiopathic thrombocytopenia purpura (ITP), thrombotic thrombocytopenia purpura, warm autoimmune hemolytic anemia, hypogammaglobulinemia, agammaglobulinemia, and acquired antibody deficiency. WinRho SDF, a form of **intravenous immunoglobulin,** has been used in the treatment of acute and chronic cases of ITP for both children and adults.[15]

TREATMENT OF COAGULATION DEFICIENCIES

Congenital Disorders of Coagulation

von Willebrand's Disease

Von Willebrand's disease is the most common of the inherited coagulopathies.[16] It is inherited in an autosomal dominant pattern, both sexes are affected, and the clinical severity is variable. Patients with von Willebrand's disease have decreased levels of all components of the Factor VIII molecule (VIII:C, VIII:vWF, and VIII:Ag), which results in a prolonged aPTT and template bleeding time.[8] Platelet aggregation in response to ristocetin is impaired because von Willebrand factor mediates platelet adhesion to the subendothelial tissue.[1,2]

Mild cases may be treated with **desmopressin (DDAVP)**, which causes the release of endogenous stores of Factor VIII and vWF. A number of commercial virus–inactivated concentrates are available that contain satisfactory levels of vWF. Cryoprecipitate can be used to replace both the von Willebrand factor necessary for normal platelet function and Factor VIII:C levels, and may also be used if factor concentrates are not available. The amount of cryoprecipitate transfused to treat a bleeding episode or prepare for surgery varies with the patient. Generally, it is advisable to achieve Factor VIII levels greater than 50% in preparation for major surgery and to maintain levels at 30% during convalescence. Efficacy of treatment can be monitored by Factor VIII assays and evaluating the clinical condition of the patient.[2]

Hemophilia A–Factor VIII Deficiency

Hemophilia A is a sex-linked disorder (the gene is present on the X chromosome) that is transmitted by females and manifested in males (Fig. 14-3). Factor VIII:C levels are decreased, whereas Factor VIII:Ag levels are normal. The clinical severity of hemophilia A is variable. Mild hemophiliacs have Factor VIII levels between 6% and 30%, moderate hemophiliacs between 1% and 5%, and severe hemophiliacs less than 1%. Laboratory findings include a prolonged aPTT, normal PT and template bleeding time, and deficient Factor VIII levels as determined by specific factor assays. (See Table 14-3 for a comparison of von Willebrand's disease and hemophilia A.)

Desmopressin (DDAVP): An analogue of vasopressin that is used for the management of patients with mild hemophilia A and von Willebrand's disease.

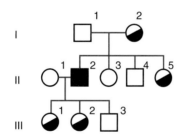

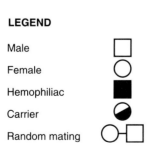

LEGEND

Male	□
Female	○
Hemophiliac	■
Carrier	◑
Random mating	○–□

Fig. 14-3 Inheritance pattern for hemophilia A, an X-linked recessive trait. Affected male (II-2) transmits the gene to his daughters (III-1 and III-2), who then become carriers. Each son of a carrier has a 50% chance of being affected, and each daughter of a carrier has a 50% risk of being a carrier. There is no male-to-male transmission.

TABLE 14-3 Comparison of Von Willebrand's Disease and Hemophilia A

	Von Willebrand's Disease	Hemophilia A
Mode of inheritance	Autosomal dominant	X-linked recessive
Gender predilection	Both sexes affected	Primarily males
Deficiency		
Factor VIII:C	Yes	Yes
Factor VIII:vWF	Yes	No
Factor VIII:Ag	Yes	No
Laboratory abnormalities		
aPTT	Abnormal	Abnormal
Template bleeding time	Abnormal	Normal
Ristocetin aggregation	Abnormal	Normal

Factor VIII concentrate: A lyophilized commercial product prepared from the fractionation of plasma that contains Factor VIII:C. The product is treated to reduce the risk of viral transmission and is indicated for the management of hemophilia A.

Factor VIII Concentrate (Antihemophilic Factor or Factor FVIII:C)

Factor VIII concentrate is a sterile, lyophilized source of Factor VIII:C that provides a product of known dosage in a small volume. The quantity of Factor VIII coagulant activity in International units (IU) is stated on the vial, and reconstitution is performed aseptically with the diluent provided. (Note: One IU is the Factor VIII activity present in 1 mL of normal, pooled human plasma less than 1 hour old.)[1]

A variety of methods are employed to inactivate viruses in Factor VIII concentrates. These include heat treatments, solvents/detergents, and purification with monoclonal antibodies. These methods reduce the levels of Factor VIII recovered and substantially decrease, but do not completely prevent, the risk of viral transmission.[1] Recombinant DNA technology, which has been proven to be both safe and effective, is currently being used to manufacture Factor VIII concentrate.

Factor VIII concentrates are indicated prophylactically or therapeutically to prevent or control bleeding episodes in hemophilia A patients with a moderate to severe congenital deficiency of Factor VIII and in those hemophilia A patients with low levels of **inhibitors** to Factor VIII.

Inhibitor (circulating anticoagulant): An endogenous substance in the blood that directly inhibits the activity of plasma coagulation factors. Most Factor VIII inhibitors are IgG immunoglobulins.

Calculating Factor VIII Dosage

The amount of Factor VIII transfused depends on the nature of the bleeding episode and the severity of the initial Factor VIII deficiency. The dose of Factor VIII to be administered can be calculated as follows:

$$\text{Weight (kg)} \times 70 \text{ mL/kg} = \text{blood volume (mL)}$$

$$\text{Blood volume (mL)} \times (1.0 - \text{Hematocrit}) = \text{Plasma volume (mL)}$$

$$\text{Plasma volume (mL)} \times (\text{Desired Factor VIII level [IU/mL]} - \text{Initial Factor VIII level [IU/mL]}) = \text{Units of Factor VIII required}$$

Factor VIII levels are reported as a percentage of normal. Note: Divide the number of units of Factor VIII by 80 (average of 80 IU of Factor VIII per bag of cryoprecipitate) when calculating the number of bags of cryoprecipitate to be administered.[2]

Example

A 45 kg boy with moderate hemophilia A is scheduled for a dental extraction. He has a hematocrit of 39%, his initial Factor VIII level is 1%, and his physician has requested that his Factor VIII level be 40% immediately preceding surgery.

$$45 \text{ kg} \times 70 \text{ mL/kg} = \text{Blood volume of 3150 mL}$$

$$3150 \text{ mL} \times (1.0 - 0.39) = \text{Plasma volume of 1921.50 mL}$$

$$1921.50 \text{ mL} \times (0.4 - 0.01) = 750.0 \text{ IU}$$

In the previous example, a dose of 750.0 IU of Factor VIII is expected to produce a Factor VIII level of 40% immediately following transfusion. Factor VIII has a half-life of 8 to 12 hours, and administration of Factor VIII would have to be repeated every 8 to 12 hours to maintain the desired level of Factor VIII activity. If no additional Factor VIII were administered, after 12 hours the patient would have a Factor VIII level of 20%, after 24 hours 10%, and so on.

The aPTT can be used to monitor Factor VIII levels. The aPTT is within normal range if Factor VIII levels are above 30% and prolonged if levels are below 30%. It is advised that Factor VIII levels be maintained above 30% following dental extraction or major surgery for hemophilia A patients.

Factor VIII concentrates contain anti-A, anti-B, and anti-A,B, and positive DATs have been reported following intensive use of this product.[1]

Inhibitors to Factor VIII

Approximately 10% to 35% of patients with hemophilia A develop an inhibitor to Factor VIII, and the majority of inhibitors develop in severe hemophiliacs. The amount of Factor VIII exposure needed to induce the development of an inhibitor is variable. In persons with hemophilia A, an inhibitor to the Factor VIII molecule should be suspected if administration of Factor VIII concentrates no longer produces the expected therapeutic results. Persons who develop inhibitors can be divided into two groups: low and high responders. Low responders have a low concentration of antibody and can be treated with standard or slightly higher than normal doses of Factor VIII concentrates. The majority of responders are classified as high responders. These individuals have high concentrations of Factor VIII antibodies; although their bleeding episodes are particularly difficult to treat, Factor IX products have been found to be effective. There are products available, such as Porcine Factor VIII (made from porcine plasma), HYATE:C, and recombinant VIIa (NovoSeven), that are generally only used in patients with high titers of inhibitors.[14]

Desmopressin

Desmopressin (DDAVP) is a synthetic analogue of vasopressin that induces the release of endogenous Factor VIII and von Willebrand factor. DDAVP has been shown to be effective in the treatment of mild forms of hemophilia A, classic (type I) von Willebrand's disease, and platelet function disorders, such as cirrhosis and uremia. Desmopressin has also been used prophylactically in patients undergoing surgical procedures in which large blood loss may occur.[17] Levels of Factor VIII and von Willebrand factor increase within 30 minutes after administration of DDAVP. The rise in Factor VIII/von Willebrand factor is usually transient, and infusions are repeated every 8 to 12 hours. A diminishing response may be seen following repeat doses of DDAVP owing to temporary depletion of the storage sites. Side effects of DDAVP are mild when the recommended dosage is administered and include facial flushing and, rarely, fluid retention, allergic reactions, hypertension, hyponatremia, and seizures.

Hemophilia B (Factor IX Deficiency)

Hemophilia B, a sex-linked disorder, is caused by an abnormal gene on the X chromosome that results in the defective synthesis of Factor IX. This disorder causes a prolonged aPTT with a normal PT and bleeding time. It can be distinguished from hemophilia A with specific factor assays.

Factor IX is stable in plasma, but no single blood component is available to treat this disorder. FFP, Plasma, and Plasma Cryoprecipitate Reduced all contain Factor IX, but large amounts of plasma need to be infused to supply sufficient quantity of Factor IX, and this places the patient at risk of circulatory overload.

Hemophilia B: An inherited (sex-linked) disorder associated with a deficiency of Factor IX.

Factor IX concentrate: A commercial product similar to Factor IX complex except that it is more highly purified and the final concentration of Factor IX is 30%. Both products are indicated for the management of Factor IX deficiency.

Factor IX complex (prothrombin complex): A commercial lyophilized product containing Factors II, VII, IX, and X. Factor IX makes up about 5% of this product.

Ischemic: Characterized by a local deficiency in the blood supply to a tissue or organ.

Warfarin sodium: The generic name for 3-(alpha-acetonylbenzyl)-4-hydroxycoumarin, an anticoagulant drug that acts by inhibiting the synthesis of the vitamin K–dependent Factors (II, VII, IX, and X). Product names include Coumadin, Panwarfin, and Sofarin.

Factor IX Concentrate

Factor IX concentrate is available in activated, recombinant, affinity purified, and immunoaffinity purified form. **Factor IX complex** contains Factor IX and quantities of Factors II, VII, X, and other proteins.[1] Activation of coagulation factors may occur when administering these concentrates.[1]

Indications

Factor IX concentrate products are indicated for the treatment of patients with hemophilia B. They are also used to treat congenital Factor VIII or X deficiency, as well as for patients with Factor VIII or IX inhibitors.[1] The exact mechanism of action of these products is unknown but is speculated to involve activated Factor X, which bypasses the portion of the coagulation cascade that requires Factor VIII, so clotting occurs in spite of the deficiency.[1,18]

Administration

One activity unit is the amount of Factor IX present in 1 mL of pooled normal human plasma, and the dose administered depends on the patient's symptoms. The half-life is approximately 24 hours, and the amount of Factor IX concentrate infused is calculated by determining the number of Factor IX units needed to achieve desired levels. The same formula used for calculating dosages of Factor VIII can be used for Factor IX, but the observed posttransfusion increments are often half of what would be expected (even in patients without inhibitors), presumably because a large portion of Factor IX is being distributed to the extravascular space.[1,2]

Acquired Disorders of Coagulation
Liver Disease

Several factors may contribute to the bleeding episodes in patients with severe hepatic disease. These include deficiencies of multiple coagulation factors (especially Factors I, II, V, VII, IX, and X) due to reduced synthesis by the liver, chronic consumptive coagulopathy (DIC), and platelet function abnormalities. These multiple defects are frequently subclinical, yet when the patient is hemostatically challenged (e.g., surgery, trauma), bleeding may result. FFP infusion is theoretically appropriate, and its use has been advocated even though data to support its efficacy are limited. See Chapter 17 for a more extensive discussion of transfusion in liver disease.

Disseminated Intravascular Coagulation

Disseminated intravascular coagulation (DIC) is another condition associated with multiple coagulation factor deficiencies. In DIC, the normal coagulation response may be accentuated and the normal inhibitory mechanisms overwhelmed. Coagulation factors are activated and consumed in DIC as are platelets, resulting in the formation of small thrombi that are deposited throughout the body.[19]

Common clinical conditions leading to DIC include obstetric complications, metastatic cancer, and septicemia. DIC can be manifested clinically by diffuse hemorrhage (resulting from platelet and coagulation factor consumption) and/or **ischemic** tissue damage (from the occlusion of the vasculature by thrombi).[19]

Therapy should be aimed at identifying and treating the cause of the initiating disorder and maintaining blood volume and hemostatic function. Packed Red Blood Cells, Platelets, plasma, and/or cryoprecipitate infusion may be used to maintain the blood volume and correct the bleeding caused by coagulation factor and platelet deficiency. It is advisable to consult a hematologist first if heparin therapy is being considered to inhibit thrombin generation.

Reversal of Coumarin Drugs

Warfarin sodium (Coumadin) interferes with the hepatic synthesis of the vitamin K–dependent coagulation Factors II, VII, IX, and X. Patients given this anticoagulant are deficient in these factors, which is manifested in vitro by an abnormal aPTT. The effect of this drug can be reversed by the administration of vitamin K, with a subsequent correction in the deficiencies of the vitamin K–dependent factors. Vitamin K injections neutralize the effects of Coumadin within several hours to a day. When patients on Coumadin are in an emergency situation (e.g., actively bleeding), FFP can be administered to rapidly achieve hemostasis.[2]

AUTOLOGOUS TRANSFUSION

Autologous transfusion conserves the blood bank's limited homologous blood supply and provides products with therapeutic benefits that are safe in that the risks of transfusion-transmitted infection and alloimmunization are eliminated. Certain categories of autologous donation that apply to operative and postoperative situations are discussed in the following sections.

Acute Normovolemic Hemodilution

For some operations, most notably cardiopulmonary bypass, members of the surgical or anesthesiology team withdraw one or more units of blood preoperatively and replace it with crystalloid or colloid solutions to produce a normovolemic, hemodiluted state. The blood is reinfused during or after the surgical procedure. The blood is stored at room temperature during this process, and the technique used must ensure sterility.

> **Acute normovolemic hemodilution:** A procedure whereby blood is removed before surgery and reinfused during or after surgery.

The units of blood removed from the patient must be labeled to indicate the patient's name, unique identifying number, and the date and hour of phlebotomy. The units may be stored in the operating room at room temperature (to preserve platelets) for no more than 8 hours or at 1° to 6° C for 24 hours.[1,2] Perioperative blood may not be used for transfusion for other patients.

If blood stored at room temperature for no more than 8 hours is not infused at the end of the operation, it can be stored in a monitored refrigerator. The units may not be stored for more than 24 hours if the arm was not adequately prepared before phlebotomy, or if this information is not known.

It is essential, even though the blood is being drawn and stored in the operating room, that the transfusion service be involved in establishing protocols for the monitoring of this procedure. If this is not the case, the medical director or his or her designee must ensure that the appropriate standards are being followed.

Intraoperative Salvage

In this procedure, blood-containing fluid is aspirated from the operative site, centrifuged or washed, and reinfused through a filter during the operative or postoperative period. **Intraoperative salvage** is most effective during surgical procedures in which relatively large amounts of blood (e.g., vascular procedures) pool in body cavities. This makes it relatively easy to aspirate the blood without introducing significant amounts of air, which can produce frothing and subsequent hemolysis of the blood. Many devices are currently available for intraoperative salvage of blood. The equipment and procedures selected must ensure that the blood collected is safely reinfused. Washing the blood before reinfusion removes fibrin, activated clotting factors, cellular debris, and other metabolites.

> **Intraoperative salvage:** The process of collecting blood-containing fluid from the surgical site. Blood thus collected can be reinfused with or without subsequent processing through a suitable filter.

Intraoperative blood units collected and processed under sterile conditions by a collection device that washes with 0.9% saline can be transfused immediately or stored at room temperature for 6 hours or at 1° to 6° C for 24 hours, provided that the refrigerated storage begins within 6 hours after collection of the unit began.

The units must be clearly labeled with the patient's first and last name, unique identifying number, date and time of the phlebotomy, expiration date, and a statement "for autologous use only."[2] The ABO type of the units must be determined and compared with the ABO type of the patient blood sample before the unit is issued. The transfusionist is responsible for determining, in writing, that all information identifying the blood unit with the intended recipient has been matched in the presence of the recipient.

Possible complications from the use of blood obtained by intraoperative salvage include hemolysis, disseminated intravascular coagulation, sepsis, and air embolism.

A written protocol should be established for the removal of blood by intraoperative salvage. The transfusion service should participate in the development of the protocol, which should then be approved and monitored by the hospital transfusion committee.

Postoperative Blood Salvage

Postoperative blood salvage: The process of collecting blood-containing fluid from a closed site such as chest tube drainage.

Postoperative blood salvage is considered the recovery of blood from a surgical site that may be reinfused into the patient with or without processing. Techniques available for postoperative blood salvage are usually of value only within the first 24 to 48 hours after surgery in patients actively bleeding into a closed site (e.g., chest cavity after cardiopulmonary bypass, joint cavity drainage). This procedure is contraindicated when there is evidence of infection or malignant tumor cells in the site from which the blood is being salvaged or when the rate of blood loss is less than 50 mL/hr. Blood is collected into a sterile plastic liner and labeled with the patient's first and last name, unique identifying number, and date and time of phlebotomy. It must be filtered (washing is optional) before it is returned to the patient. Blood must be reinfused within 6 hours after collection in order to minimize the proliferation of bacteria.[2] If the blood is removed from the patient's presence (e.g., to the blood bank for washing), the ABO type of the unit must be compared with the patient's ABO type before reinfusion. The transfusion service must have input into the development and implementation of the protocols to ensure adherence to standards of practice.

CHAPTER SUMMARY

1. The four main goals of transfusion therapy are to restore or maintain blood volume, oxygen-carrying capacity of the blood, hemostasis, and leukocyte function.
2. In component therapy, one unit of whole blood can be divided into a number of components so that many patients can benefit from the blood drawn from one volunteer blood donor. Table 14-1 reviews the indications and contraindications of the blood and blood components presented in this chapter.
3. A maximum surgical blood order schedule (MSBOS) reserves crossmatches for surgical procedures most likely to require blood transfusions. A type and screen is recommended for procedures that rarely require blood.
4. Inadequate posttransfusion platelet increments are most commonly associated with alloimmunization to

HLA. Transfusion of HLA-matched Platelets Pheresis may be indicated to improve the effectiveness of platelet transfusions. Inadequate posttransfusion platelet counts after infusion of HLA-matched platelets may be due to alloimmunization to platelet-specific antigens.

5. From 10% to 35% of hemophilia A patients make inhibitors to the Factor VIII molecule. Therapeutic responses to Factor VIII concentrate administration may no longer be seen, and alternative therapies may need to be initiated. Inhibitors may also be produced to the Factor IX molecule.
6. Acute normovolemic hemodilution, intraoperative salvage, and postoperative blood salvage decrease the transfusion of homologous blood. Each of these procedures has its own indications and contraindications.

REFERENCES

1. Triulzi DJ (ed): Blood Transfusion Therapy—A Physician's Handbook, 7th ed. Arlington, VA, American Association of Blood Banks, 2002.
2. Walker RH (ed): Technical Manual. Arlington, VA, American Association of Blood Banks, 2002.
3. Circular of Information for the Use of Human Blood and Blood Components. American Association of Blood Banks, American Blood Centers and American Red Cross, 2002.
4. Perioperative RBC transfusion consensus conference. JAMA 260:2700-2703, 1988.

5. Spence RK, Carson JA, Poses R, et al: Elective surgery without transfusion: Influence of preoperative hemoglobin level and blood loss on mortality. Am J Surg 159:320-324, 1990.

6. Zanjani ED, Ascensao JL: Erythropoietin. Transfusion 29:46-57, 1989.

7. Standards for Blood Banks and Transfusion Services, 22nd ed. Arlington, VA, American Association of Blood Banks, 2003.

8. Simpson MB: The clinical use of platelet preparations. In Summers SH, Smith DM, Agranenko VA (eds): Transfusion Therapy: Guidelines for Practice. Arlington, VA, American Association of Blood Banks, 1990.

9. NIH Consensus Conference: Platelet transfusion therapy. JAMA 257:1777-1780, 1987.

10. Evans CS: Alloimmunization and refractoriness to platelet transfusion. Lab Med 23:528-532, 1992.

11. Murphy MF, Waters AH: Platelet transfusions: The problem of refractoriness. Blood Rev 4:16-24, 1990.

12. Buchholz DH, Miripol J, Aster RH, et al: Ultraviolet irradiation of platelets (plts) to prevent recipient alloimmunization [abstract S91]. Transfusion 28:26S, 1988.

13. Menache D, Grossman BJ, Jackson CM: Antithrombin III: Physiology, deficiency, and replacement therapy. Transfusion 32:580-588, 1992.

14. Hillyer CD, Silberstein LE, Ness PM, et al: Blood Banking and Transfusion Medicine: Basic Principles and Practice. Philadelphia, Churchill Livingstone, 2003.

15. Nabi Biopharmaceuticals: WinRho SDF (online), www.nabi.com/winrho.html, 2003.

16. Oberman HA: Appropriate use of plasma and plasma derivatives. In Summers SH, Smith DM, Agranenko VA (eds): Transfusion Therapy: Guidelines for Practice. Arlington, VA, American Association of Blood Banks, 1990.

17. Mannucci PM: Desmopressin (DDAVP) in the treatment of bleeding disorders: The first 20 years. Blood 90:2515-2521, 1997.

18. Smith KJ: Factor IX concentrates: The new blood products and their properties. Transfus Med Rev 6:124-136, 1992.

19. Harmening DM: Clinical Hematology and Fundamentals of Hemostasis, 4th ed. Philadelphia, FA Davis, 1999.

Expert Opinion

BLOOD SUBSTITUTES 2004

Robert M. Winslow, MD

The techniques of collecting, crossmatching, and storing human blood for transfusion matured during and after World War II and have become part of the immense business of blood banking. However, since the discovery of the circulation of blood and the publication of William Harvey's classic book in 1628, alternatives to this practice have been sought. All manner of solutions have been tried, including wine, milk, and, more recently, hemoglobin solutions, perfluorocarbon emulsions, and liposome-encapsulated hemoglobin.[1]

The modern efforts at producing a "blood substitute" (really solutions that carry oxygen, or "red cell substitutes") were driven by the military up to the early 1980s: Any reduction in weight, volume, or elimination of crossmatching, and longer shelf-life, would be of tremendous value to the military, who would prefer to ship bullets than blood to a battlefield. Since the discovery that human immunodeficiency virus (HIV) (and other viruses) can be transmitted by transfusions, efforts to develop alternatives have intensified. Many millions of dollars have been spent by industry and government in recent years on research and development in this area. However, although several have been studied in phase III clinical trials in humans, and in spite of promising research results, blood substitutes are still not available to the clinician, and concern persists about their toxicity.[2]

Perfluorocarbons (PFCs) are relatively simple, inert materials (Teflon is an example) that have the unique ability to dissolve a large amount of oxygen. Because PFCs are inert, they do not react with any other materials, and therefore they are biologically safe. However, they are also immiscible with biologic fluids and must be emulsified with surfactants in order to be injected into the bloodstream. Emulsions that contain phospholipids and other materials have been used clinically (such as for hyperalimentation), but they may cause unpleasant side effects such as flulike symptoms. These may limit the volume of PFC emulsions that can be used in a patient. Nevertheless, one emulsion (Fluosol-DA) was approved by the Food and Drug Administration (FDA) for limited use in coronary angioplasty.[3] Newer emulsions that contain more PFC (and therefore more oxygen) have also been tested in humans, but to date have not been approved for clinical use. A significant limitation to PFC emulsions is that in order to carry amounts of oxygen similar to those carried by red cells or hemoglobin solutions, patients must breathe high concentrations of oxygen, and their lungs must allow inspired oxygen to enter the blood.

In the past several years, predominant efforts have been directed at developing red cell substitutes based on cell-free hemoglobin. Hemoglobin solutions would eliminate the dependence on oxygen breathing, which

Continued

limits PFC emulsions because hemoglobin binds oxygen chemically. Hemoglobin by itself, however, is not suitable for direct infusion into humans because it is rapidly cleared from the circulation, and can cause kidney damage. Hemoglobin must therefore be modified in some way to correct these problems. Some products use either outdated human red cells or cow blood as the starting material, and then chemically cross-link the hemoglobin with smaller molecules to prevent elimination from the circulation. Other products have used hemoglobin produced by human genes inserted into *Escherichia coli,* yeast, or transgenic pigs. Such molecules subsequently can be modified chemically, or genetic modifications can be introduced to eliminate the need for chemical modification. Some of these products have also been tested in human trials. However, while kidney toxicity, a concern with early products, has been largely eliminated, concern remains that cell-free hemoglobin may raise blood pressure due to vasoactivity that may limit large-scale use in humans.

In the course of studying the vasoactivity of one product manufactured for study by the U.S. Army,[4] a new paradigm has emerged that eliminates vasoactivity by the counterintuitive properties of high oxygen affinity and high viscosity.[5] Animal studies with a product that utilizes this new approach[6] have demonstrated the ability to "target" oxygen delivery to hypoxic tissue.[7] It is still early in the clinical development of this new product (called MP4), but trials have progressed successfully so far through phase II testing.

Should the new concept of targeted oxygen delivery be successfully translated into a clinical product, it will raise additional issues that will need to be confronted. For example, if such products are more effective in delivering oxygen to tissues than red blood cells, the meaning of hemoglobin and hematocrit measurements will need to be reconsidered. For example, the presence of 1 or 2 g/dL of plasma hemoglobin can oxygenate tissue with a reduction of hematocrit by about 10 percentage points,[8] thus permitting a lower hematocrit transfusion trigger.

The third general class of red cell substitutes is liposome-encapsulated hemoglobin (LEH).[9] These products combine liposome technology with hemoglobin purification and modification to produce an artificial red cell. Potentially, LEH could solve many of the problems caused by cell-free hemoglobin. However, liposome technology is not yet sufficiently developed to allow large volumes to be injected into humans. Liposomes are known to stimulate macrophages to produce cytokines and could interfere with normal functioning of the reticuloendothelial (macrophage-monocyte) system. Thus the recipient's immune status could be compromised. In addition, large-scale production of sterile liposomes has proven to be difficult, further limiting commercial development. At present, no LEH is in human clinical trials.

One of the by-products of the intense scrutiny of transfusion practices and research into blood substitutes is that we now understand much more about the physiology of blood transfusion. The "transfusion trigger," the hematocrit or hemoglobin concentration at which red cells are given, has been sharpened, and there is much closer monitoring of transfusion services in hospitals now. This attention has reduced the number of "frivolous" transfusions and has increased the number of autologous transfusions, both positive outcomes. These activities have also caused an evolution in our thinking about the way blood substitutes might be used when they reach the clinic. The concept that one would simply choose "artificial" over real blood for all transfusions is naive. As the clinical indications for blood transfusion are continually refined, so are the anticipated uses of blood substitutes. Thus certain types of solutions might be especially suited to coronary angioplasty, to priming heart-lung bypass pumps, for emergency blood replacement, or for surgical bleeding. Still others could be used to preserve organs for transplantation, and so on. It is likely that the blood bank of the future will provide an array of products—some natural, some synthetic—to be used for augmentation of oxygen transport. The clinician and blood banker of the future will need a solid understanding of the physiology underlying oxygen transport to tissues in order to use these different products in the most effective ways.

REFERENCES

1. Winslow R: Hemoglobin-based Red Cell Substitutes. Baltimore, Johns Hopkins University Press, 1992.
2. Winslow RM: Alternative oxygen therapeutics: Products, status of clinical trials, and future prospects. Curr Hematol Rep 2:503-510, 2003.
3. Robalino B, Marwick T, Lafont A, et al: Protection against ischemia during prolonged balloon inflation by distal coronary perfusion with use of an autoperfusion catheter or Fluosol. J Am Coll Cardiol 20:1378-1384, 1992.
4. Winslow RM: Alpha-crosslinked hemoglobin: Was failure predicted by preclinical testing? Vox Sang 79:1-20, 2000.
5. Winslow RM: Current status of blood substitute research: Towards a new paradigm. J Intern Med 253:508-517, 2003.

6. Vandegriff KD, Malavelli A, Wooldridge J, et al: MP4, a new nonvasoactive PEG-Hb conjugate. Transfusion 43:509-516, 2003.

7. Tsai AG, Vandegriff KD, Intaglietta M, Winslow RM: Targeted O_2 delivery by low-P50 hemoglobin: A new basis for O_2 therapeutics. Am J Physiol Heart Circ Physiol 285:H1411-H1419, 2003.

8. Drobin D, Kjellstrom BT, Malm E, et al: Hemodynamic response and oxygen transport in pigs resuscitated with maleimide-polyethylene glycol–modified hemoglobin (MP4). J Appl Physiol 96:1843-1853, 2004.

9. Rudolph AS, Rabinovici R, Feuerstein GZ: Red Blood Cell Substitutes: Basic Principles and Clinical Applications. New York, Marcel Dekker, 1998.

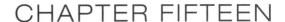

CHAPTER FIFTEEN

Adverse Effects of Blood Transfusion

Deborah T. Firestone and Christine Pitocco

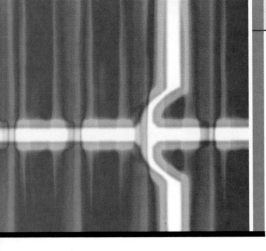

LEARNING OBJECTIVES

After reading and studying this chapter, the student should be able to:

1. Define the term transfusion reaction.
2. Describe the pathophysiology of immune hemolysis.
3. Describe the symptoms, management, and prevention of immune hemolytic transfusion reactions.
4. Describe the symptoms, management, and prevention of the following immune nonhemolytic transfusion reactions:
   Febrile
   Allergic
   Anaphylactic
   Transfusion-related acute lung injury
5. Describe the symptoms, management, and prevention of the following categories of nonimmune transfusion reactions:
   Bacterial contamination
   Circulatory overload
   Physical/chemical hemolysis
6. Describe the symptoms, management, and prevention of the following categories of immunologic delayed transfusion reactions:
   Delayed hemolytic
   Graft-versus-host disease
   Posttransfusion purpura
7. Describe the management and prevention of the following categories of nonimmunologic delayed transfusion reactions:
   Hemosiderosis
   Disease transmission
8. Identify steps that should be taken by the patient care staff when a hemolytic transfusion reaction is first suspected.
9. Discuss the performance and interpretation of the three steps that should be part of the preliminary laboratory investigation of any suspected hemolytic transfusion reaction.
10. Given the patient signs and symptoms and results of the preliminary investigation, determine which (if any) additional tests might be required to determine the cause and extent of transfusion-associated immune hemolysis.

OVERVIEW

Blood transfusion is a temporary form of therapy that lasts only as long as the life span of the blood or component transfused (e.g., red blood cells have an average life span of 120 days). The beneficial effect of each unit of blood or blood component transfused is accompanied by the possibility that the patient may experience an adverse reaction to the product transfused. It becomes the responsibility of the health care provider requesting the transfusion to determine whether the benefits outweigh the potential risks. The three leading causes of transfusion-related death reported between 1999 and 2001 by the Food and Drug Administration (FDA), Center for Biologics Evaluation and Research (CBER), were bacterial contamination, acute hemolytic transfusion reactions, and transfusion-related acute lung injury (TRALI). These three causes were reported to account for 42.4% of the 189 transfusion-related fatalities reported during this 3-year period.[1]

Any unexpected or unfavorable sign or symptom that occurs during or shortly after the transfusion of a unit of blood or one of its components should be considered to have been caused by the product until proven otherwise. It may be impossible to assess the severity of a **transfusion reaction** by the symptoms because a life-threatening (acute hemolytic) and relatively mild (nonhemolytic febrile) transfusion reaction may initially cause exactly the same symptoms (e.g., fever, chills). Therefore any adverse reaction to a unit of blood or one of its components should be considered a potentially life-threatening reaction until clinical observations and/or laboratory results establish otherwise.

Transfusion reactions may be acute or delayed. In acute transfusion reactions, clinical signs and symptoms occur during or within 24 hours after the completion of the transfusion. A delayed transfusion reaction may not be evident for days, weeks, months, or even years after the transfusion. Acute and delayed transfusion reactions are classified as immunologic (mediated by antibody-antigen reaction) or nonimmunologic (Fig. 15-1).

PATHOPHYSIOLOGY OF IMMUNE HEMOLYSIS

In vivo lysis of red blood cells can result from the interaction of complement components with the red cell membrane (i.e., **intravascular hemolysis**) (Fig. 15-2) or the removal of cells sensitized with IgG and/or complement by the reticuloendothelial system (i.e., **extravascular hemolysis**). Intravascular hemolysis refers to the destruction of cells in the vasculature, with free hemoglobin and red cell stroma released to the plasma. Intravascular hemolysis is most commonly due to antibodies in the ABO blood group system. However, anti-Kidd, anti-Vel, anti-Tj^a, and anti-Le^a can also activate complement, resulting in intravascular lysis of red cells. Whether or not the complement cascade will be activated depends on specific antibody/antigen characteristics such as antibody class, subclass, specificity, and titer and antigen density. Activation of the complement cascade results in the release of **anaphylatoxins** such as C3a and C5a that act on a variety of cells to cause the production and release of mediators such as **histamine** and **leukotrienes.** It is the local and systemic release of these mediators that act on mast cells to cause the release of the vasoactive substances **serotonin** and histamine, which mediate the clinical signs and symptoms of a transfusion reaction.

Transfusion reaction: Any adverse outcome associated with the infusion of blood or blood components.

Intravascular hemolysis: The destruction of transfused red cells within the vascular compartment due to either immunologic or nonimmunologic means, which is commonly associated with the transfusion of ABO-incompatible red cells.

Extravascular hemolysis: The premature removal of incompatible transfused red cells from the circulation by the phagocytic cells of the reticuloendothelial system (liver and spleen).

Anaphylatoxins: Substances that stimulate the release of mediators such as histamine from mast cells and basophils, resulting in the symptoms of immediate sensitivity independent of IgE.

Histamine: A substance produced from the amino acid histidine, the release of which results in increased gastric secretion, dilation of capillaries, and contraction of bronchial smooth muscle.

Leukotrienes: A series of compounds that function as regulators of allergic and inflammatory responses. They can cause bronchial constriction.

Serotonin: The chemical 5-hydroxytryptamine, which is a potent vasoconstrictor.

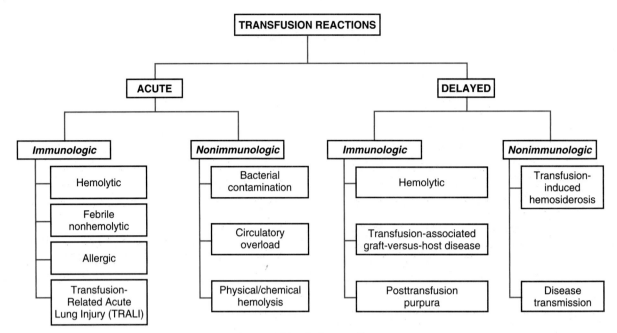

Fig 15-1 Transfusion reactions.

The complement cascade may proceed to completion with subsequent lysis of red cells if the quantity of incompatible cells exceeds the body's normal control mechanisms, or C3b bound to red cells may be engulfed by phagocytes bearing C3b receptors. Small amounts of hemoglobin can be bound by plasma haptoglobin. However, when the hemoglobin-binding capacity of haptoglobin is exceeded, **hemoglobinemia** occurs. The hallmark of an ABO-incompatible transfusion

Hemoglobinemia: The presence of free hemoglobin in the plasma.

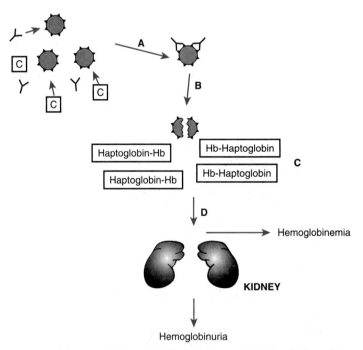

Fig. 15-2 Intravascular hemolysis. **A,** Complement attaches to the antigen-antibody complex on the red blood cells. **B,** Complement activation proceeds to the C9 stage with subsequent lysis of the red blood cell. **C,** Hemoglobin (Hb) is released from the red cell and can be bound by haptoglobin. **D,** If the amount of hemoglobin released exceeds the binding capacity of haptoglobin, hemoglobinemia and/or hemoglobinuria results.

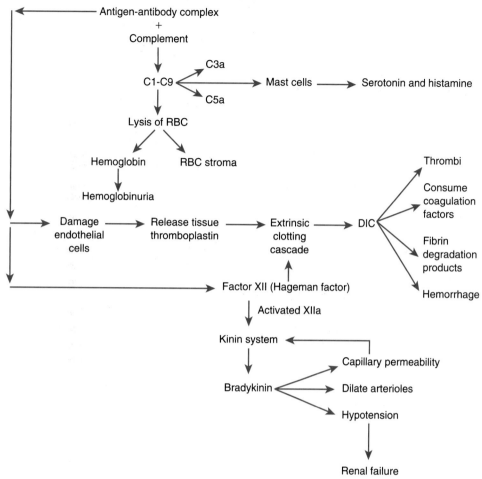

Fig. 15-3 Pathophysiology of intravascular hemolysis.

is hemoglobinemia, and if the renal threshold for hemoglobin is exceeded, **hemoglobinuria** will be present.[2] Fig. 15-3 reviews the pathophysiology of intravascular hemolysis.

Antigen-antibody complexes are also capable of activating the "intrinsic" coagulation cascade by acting on **Factor XII (Hageman factor),** which then becomes activated XIIa. Activated XII (XIIa) acts on the kinin system to produce **bradykinin,** which results in an increase in capillary permeability and dilation of arterioles, which ultimately leads to hypotension. This sequence of events may also increase the expression of tissue factor by leukocytes and endothelial cells, which can lead to the activation of the "extrinsic" coagulation cascade; its release is associated with disseminated intravascular coagulation (DIC). DIC may cause (1) formation of thrombi that can lodge in the liver, lungs, and kidneys; (2) consumption of coagulation factors and platelets; and (3) activation of the fibrinolytic system, leading to production of fibrin degradation products, all of which can lead to widespread oozing or uncontrolled bleeding. Another sequela of acute hemolytic transfusion reactions is renal failure, which is largely attributed to hypotension resulting in renal vasoconstriction, and formation of thrombi in the renal vasculature due to the deposition of antigen-antibody complexes.[2]

In extravascular hemolysis, red blood cells are removed from the circulation and destroyed by phagocytosis. Antibodies most commonly involved are anti-Jk[a], anti-Fy[a], and anti-K. Extravascular hemolysis is rarely as severe as that seen with intravascular hemolysis because complement activation usually is not complete (red

Hemoglobinuria: The presence of hemoglobin in the urine.

Factor XII/Hageman factor: A serine protease (molecular weight 80,000) in the intrinsic coagulation pathway. Factor XII activation during the process of immune hemolysis contributes to both intravascular coagulation and activation of the kinin system.

Bradykinin: A polypeptide substance capable of inducing hypotension, increasing the permeability of capillaries, and eliciting pain.

cells are coated with C3b), and cells are gradually removed and destroyed as they circulate through the liver and spleen. Signs and symptoms of extravascular hemolysis include fever and a developing anemia. Expected laboratory abnormalities are increased bilirubin levels and a positive direct antiglobulin test (DAT).

ACUTE IMMUNOLOGIC TRANSFUSION REACTIONS
Hemolytic Transfusion Reactions

An acute hemolytic transfusion reaction (AHTR) is most commonly defined as the hemolysis of donor red cells, within 24 hours of transfusion, by preformed alloantibodies in the recipient circulation. AHTRs are less commonly associated with the hemolysis of recipient red cells by transfused donor antibodies. Clerical errors (mislabeling blood or misidentification of patients) account for 80% of AHTRs.[1] Acute hemolytic transfusion reactions are rare (incidence of 1:38,000 to 1:70,000),[2] but when they do occur, they are one of the most dangerous transfusion reactions possible. Life-threatening acute hemolytic transfusion reactions are most commonly due to ABO-incompatible blood being transfused to a recipient with naturally occurring ABO alloantibodies (anti-A, anti-B, anti-A,B). Signs and symptoms of an acute intravascular hemolytic transfusion reaction may be manifested when as little as 10 to 15 mL of ABO-incompatible blood has been infused. Fever is the most common initial manifestation of an acute transfusion reaction and is frequently accompanied by chills. In the early stages of a hemolytic reaction, when signs and symptoms may be absent, the patient may have mild complaints such as a general sense of anxiety or uneasiness, as well as pain at the infusion site, back, and/or chest.[3] The most serious sequela of an acute intravascular hemolytic transfusion reaction is acute renal failure.[1] In unconscious or anesthetized patients, diffuse bleeding at the surgical site may be the first indication of intravascular hemolysis and may be accompanied by hemoglobinuria and hypotension.[2]

The risk of a fatal acute hemolytic transfusion reaction is approximately 1:160,000, and morbidity and mortality rates can be roughly correlated with the amount of incompatible blood transfused. It therefore becomes the transfusionist's responsibility to closely monitor the transfusion recipient for signs or complaints that would indicate that an adverse reaction is taking place. The earlier the reaction is noted and the transfusion discontinued, the less incompatible blood is infused.

Management

Early recognition of the clinical signs and symptoms of a hemolytic transfusion reaction, discontinuation of the existing transfusion, and preventing the transfusion of additional incompatible cells are the essential first steps to be taken in managing a hemolytic transfusion reaction.[3] The intravenous line should be kept open in the event that therapeutic intervention is necessary. A priority in these situations is cardiovascular support and prevention of renal failure. Adequate perfusion of the kidneys can be accomplished by transfusing fluids, primarily normal (0.9%) saline, and administering **diuretics** such as furosemide to increase adequate urine output.

The management of consumption coagulopathy, with its resultant DIC, is more complicated. The use of platelets, fresh-frozen plasma, and cryoprecipitate to replenish depleted coagulation factors and heparin to treat DIC is not universally accepted.[2,3] Because of the complexity of the symptoms, consultation with a specialist is recommended before initiating treatment.

Prevention

It is virtually impossible to prevent all acute hemolytic transfusion reactions. Pretransfusion compatibility testing is designed to decrease the probability of an acute hemolytic transfusion reaction by identifying existing alloantibodies and transfusing blood that is ABO, Rh, and crossmatch compatible with the recipient's serum. Hemolysis can still occur, even when a crossmatch is compatible, because of

Diuretics: Substances that increase urine output either by increasing the rate of glomerular filtration or by decreasing tubular reabsorption.

human error (the most common cause). Human error will never be eliminated, but it can be minimized by taking certain steps. The most common errors resulting in acute hemolytic transfusion reactions involve the misidentification of blood samples, donor units, and intended transfusion recipients.[2] Each transfusion service should have a written standard operating procedure manual that includes all steps to be followed from the collection to the distribution of all blood and blood components for transfusion. Careful adherence to every step of the transfusion process, from drawing the blood sample to administering the donor unit, is critical. It is the phlebotomist's responsibility to accurately identify the intended transfusion recipient and correctly label the tube of blood at the patient's bedside. Once the tube arrives in the blood bank, it is the technologist's job to make sure it is properly labeled and there are no discrepancies with the transfusion request. The patient's previous pretransfusion records (if any) are examined, and it then becomes the technologist's responsibility to perform, interpret, and document all pretransfusion tests using laboratory protocols that adhere to American Association of Blood Banks (AABB) standards of practice.[4] Appropriate protocol must be followed when blood is released from the blood bank to ensure that the correct donor unit is signed out of the blood bank for the correct recipient. The final check rests with the transfusionist, who must take all the necessary precautions to ensure that the intended transfusion recipient is correctly identified. This includes checking the name and number on the patient's armband against the same information on the compatibility slip or tag on the donor unit. New technologies that use computerized portable data terminals at the patient's bedside to identify patients, specimens, and blood components are under investigation.[1] It is essential that there be a mechanism in place for the training and assessment of all clinical, nursing, and laboratory personnel involved in the drawing, testing, and transfusion of blood and blood products.

Febrile Nonhemolytic Transfusion Reactions

Febrile nonhemolytic transfusion reactions (FNHTRs) are common and estimated to occur in 0.5% to 6% of all red cell transfusions[2] and up to 30% of platelet transfusions.[1] A febrile transfusion reaction is defined as a rise in temperature of greater than 1° C, which may be accompanied by chills and/or rigor. Symptoms may occur during the transfusion or not be manifested until 1 to 2 hours after its completion.[2] A diagnosis of a febrile nonhemolytic transfusion reaction is generally made by excluding other causes of fever (e.g., bacterial contamination of blood, acute hemolytic transfusion reaction, TRALI).

FNHTRs are thought to be due to a reaction between human leukocyte antigens (HLAs) and/or leukocyte-specific antigens on transfused lymphocytes, granulocytes, or platelets in the donor unit and antibodies in previously alloimmunized recipients.[5] Multiply transfused individuals and multiparous women represent the largest populations experiencing this type of transfusion reaction. It is not a routine part of transfusion reaction workups to identify these antibodies owing to the difficulty in demonstrating their presence in vitro. Febrile nonhemolytic transfusion reactions, especially those associated with platelet transfusions, may be caused by the infusion of biologic response modifiers, such as cytokines, that have accumulated in the platelet concentrate during storage.[2]

Management

Treatment is aimed at the prevention of FNHTRs or amelioration of the symptoms. Fever usually responds to **antipyretics.** Acetaminophen is preferred over aspirin because it does not affect platelet function.

Prevention

Febrile nonhemolytic transfusion reactions in susceptible populations can often be prevented by administering antipyretics before transfusion and transfusing leukocyte-

Febrile nonhemolytic transfusion reactions: Fever responses due to a reaction between HLAs and/or leukocyte antigens on donor white cells and antibodies in transfusion recipients. These reactions can be associated with the transfusion of any component containing residual donor white cells and can be reduced by transfusing leukocyte-reduced components.

Antipyretics: Agents that reduce fever.

reduced blood components.[5] Prestorage leukocyte reduction is recommended to prevent reactions that occur as a result of the accumulation of cytokines during storage.

Allergic Transfusion Reactions

Allergic reactions can be mild, moderate, or life-threatening in severity and are associated with the amount of plasma transfused.[3] From 1% to 5% of all blood transfusion recipients experience mild allergic reactions.[1] Generally, symptoms are mild and include localized **urticaria, erythema,** and itching. Fever or other adverse effects are usually not present. In some instances, there may be symptoms indicative of airway involvement such as hoarseness, wheezing, **dyspnea,** and substernal pain.[3]

Urticarial reactions are not well understood but are believed to be an allergic response between antibodies in the recipient's plasma and plasma proteins in donor blood.[1] There is usually not a specific identifiable antigen to which the patient is reacting.[3]

Management

When a patient experiences a mild urticarial transfusion reaction, the transfusion is stopped, intravenous access is maintained, and **antihistamines** are administered orally or intramuscularly. The transfusion can be restarted after symptoms have subsided, which generally takes 15 to 30 minutes. A detailed investigation is not warranted. More severe reactions would require the transfusion to be discontinued and a more aggressive treatment of symptoms (e.g., epinephrine, oxygen, intubation).

Prevention

Patients who experience recurrent urticarial reactions can be pretreated with antihistamines before transfusion. Washed red blood cells may be indicated for transfusion to a patient who experiences repeated severe urticarial reactions.

Anaphylactic Transfusion Reactions

Anaphylactic (or anaphylactoid) is the most severe form of an allergic transfusion reaction. These transfusion reactions are rare, but when they do occur, they can be life-threatening emergencies. Symptoms occur after the transfusion of only a few milliliters of blood or plasma and include skin flushing, nausea, abdominal cramps, vomiting, diarrhea, laryngeal edema, hypotension, shock, cardiac arrhythmia, cardiac arrest, and loss of consciousness. Fever is notably absent.

Anaphylactic transfusion reactions are sometimes associated with antibodies to IgA. Antibodies to IgA are common in the population (incidence of approximately 1 in 700 individuals), whereas the incidence of anaphylactic transfusion reactions is not (1:20,000 to 1:50,000).[2] This disparity lends credence to the supposition that there are other causative mediators for this type of reaction.[2]

Management

Immediate attention is focused on the clinical condition of the patient, and a diagnosis of anaphylactic transfusion reaction is generally made retrospectively. Treatment is directed toward aggressive management of the patient's symptoms and should include stopping the transfusion, keeping the line open with normal saline, treating hypotension, and administering **epinephrine** subcutaneously.

Prevention

IgA-deficient donors usually go unrecognized in the population unless they know of a family history or have had some laboratory test performed (e.g., immunoelectrophoresis) which indicates that they are IgA deficient. Individuals usually become aware of their IgA deficiency when they experience an anaphylactic transfusion reaction and laboratory tests reveal the presence of antibodies to IgA. Subsequent transfusions to IgA-deficient donors must lack IgA. IgA-deficient

---

Urticaria: Hives.

Erythema: Redness of the skin caused by capillary dilation.

Dyspnea: Shortness of breath.

Antihistamines: Agents that oppose the action of histamine and thus reduce the symptoms associated with histamine release, including increased gastric secretion, flushing of the skin, headache, hypotension, and constriction of bronchial smooth muscle.

Anaphylactic transfusion reactions: Severe immunologic responses to transfusion that are both rapid and life-threatening. Systemic anaphylaxis produces changes in circulation and bronchioles consistent with shock. Anaphylactic transfusion reactions cannot be predicted by routine pretransfusion testing.

Epinephrine: A hormone produced by the adrenal medulla that can be used as a vasoconstrictor and bronchiole dilator.

donors should be encouraged, when possible, to have their blood and/or plasma collected and stored for future autologous use. When this is not possible, red cells and platelets can be washed to remove the majority of plasma present. Currently, the only way to ensure that a plasma product lacks IgA is for the product to have been manufactured from blood drawn from an IgA-deficient donor. IgA-deficient plasma can be obtained from rare donor registries.

Transfusion-Related Acute Lung Injury

Transfusion-related acute lung injury (TRALI) should be suspected when a patient exhibits acute respiratory insufficiency and/or x-ray findings indicative of bilaterally symmetric **pulmonary edema** following a transfusion without evidence of cardiac failure or an alternative cause for the respiratory failure. This type of reaction is typically accompanied by chills, fever, and hypotension. Other symptoms can include dyspnea, cyanosis, tachycardia, and **hypoxemia**.[3] Symptoms generally appear within 1 to 2 hours of the completion of the transfusion.[2]

TRALI is most often associated with passively transfused antibodies to HLA or neutrophil antigens that react with the transfusion recipient's granulocytes. One or two antibodies have been identified in the donor blood of 89% of TRALI cases.[1] The reverse situation (granulocyte antibodies in a previously sensitized transfusion recipient react with granulocytes in transfused blood or plasma products) can also occur. The reaction between granulocyte antigens and antibodies initiates a sequence of events that leads to increased permeability of the pulmonary circulation with subsequent infiltration of high-protein fluid. A second mechanism set forth to explain the etiology of TRALI is the accumulation of reactive lipid products from donor cell membranes during storage, resulting in activation of neutrophils and subsequent damage to and leakage of capillary endothelium.[2] Components implicated in this type of transfusion reaction always contain plasma. Although the exact incidence rate is not known, it has been speculated to be as frequent as 1 in 5000 transfusions.[2]

Management

The transfusion must be stopped immediately and appropriate respiratory support administered. Although intravenous steroids are often used in the management of patients experiencing TRALI, they appear to have little if any value.[2] In most cases, symptoms resolve within 2 to 4 days following treatment.[2]

Prevention

It is not practical to perform widespread screening of donor plasma for leukoagglutinins or to eliminate those populations that most commonly form these antibodies (multiply transfused individuals and multiparous women) from the donor pool. It has been suggested that blood from donors known to have been implicated in TRALI previously not be used to manufacture plasma-containing components. However, there is no consensus on this because the initiating event in TRALI is a reaction between antibodies in donor plasma to recipient HLA or neutrophil antigens. It is unlikely that the same donor would be transfused to the same patient (unless it was a directed donor). It has been suggested that the accumulation of lipid mediators in components can be reduced by prestorage leukocyte reduction or shortening the shelf life of components (e.g., platelets). Once again, there is no consensus on this.[3]

ACUTE NONIMMUNOLOGIC TRANSFUSION REACTIONS
Bacterial Contamination

Bacterial contamination is believed to be the most common transfusion-related infectious source of morbidity and mortality.[6] Bacteria may be introduced into a unit of blood through skin contaminants during venipuncture or donors with

Transfusion-related acute lung injury: Pulmonary edema, not associated with cardiac failure, that is usually due to the transfusion of preformed donor leukoagglutinins in the plasma of blood components.

Pulmonary edema: An accumulation of fluid in the lungs.

Hypoxemia: Insufficient oxygenation of the blood.

asymptomatic bacteremia. Multiplication of bacteria may occur in blood and blood components stored at refrigerated temperatures but is more likely to occur in blood components stored at room temperature. An increase in bacterial contamination of platelets has been associated with an extension in the amount of time platelets are stored at room temperature and plastic bags with increased gas permeability.

Bacterial contamination of blood and blood products is rare, but the results can be life-threatening. Bacterial contamination of red cells is most often due to *Yersinia enterocolitica* followed by *Serratia liquifaciens,* whereas platelets are most often contaminated with *Staphylococcus* and *Enterobacteriaceae.*[6] The incidence of bacterial contamination of red cells has been estimated to be 1:31,000 with an overall fatality rate of 1:1,000,000.[3,7] The incidence of bacterial contamination in platelets may be as high as 1:700 for pooled random-donor platelet concentrates and 1:4000 for single-donor platelet concentrates.[3] In most cases, implicated units have been stored for 4 or 5 days and have bacterial counts in excess of 10^5 **CFU**/mL.[7]

Clinically, the patient may experience high fever, shock, hemoglobinuria, renal failure, and DIC. Transfusion of units with high bacterial counts may result in severe or fatal reactions, whereas transfusion recipients of units with low bacterial counts may manifest relatively mild symptoms such as fever and chills.[7]

Management

These transfusion reactions must be promptly recognized and treated in order to avoid a fatal outcome. The transfusion must be stopped immediately and intravenous antibiotics administered. Hypotension, if present, can be treated with fluids, including plasma expanders and **vasopressors** such as dopamine. If DIC occurs, appropriate therapy should be initiated.

If bacterial contamination is suspected, the unit should be visually examined for blood clots, hemolysis, or an unusual color. Bacterial contamination can be confirmed by a positive Gram stain but cannot be ruled out if the Gram stain is negative. The component, the patient's blood, and all intravenous solutions should be cultured for aerobic and anaerobic organisms at refrigerated, room, and body temperatures.

Prevention

Blood components are not routinely tested for the presence of bacteria immediately before transfusion. Prevention of bacterial contamination depends on strict adherence to established laboratory protocols for the drawing, preparation, storage, and release of blood and components. This includes a careful donor history, as well as aseptic treatment of the donor's arm before and during phlebotomy. Aseptic techniques should be maintained during the preparation of all blood components in order to decrease the number of skin bacteria that reach the blood unit.[7] Since contaminated organisms from the skin appear to be in the first 5 to 10 mL of blood drawn, it has been proposed that discarding this initial amount of blood drawn would reduce the incidence of bacterial contamination from the skin.[3] The storage conditions of blood and components should be properly maintained, and all blood and blood components need to be carefully examined before release from the blood bank. The current edition (twenty-second) of *Standards for Blood Banks and Transfusion Services* calls for blood banks and transfusion services to have a method to limit and detect bacterial contamination in all platelet components.[4]

Circulatory Overload

Acute pulmonary edema, caused by the inability of the circulatory system to handle an increased fluid volume, can occur in any patient who is transfused too rapidly.[1] Although the true frequency of this type of transfusion reaction is unknown because it is often not recognized and is rarely reported to the blood bank, it is believed to

CFU (Colony-forming units): Minimum number of cells on the surface of media that give rise to a visible colony of offspring.

Vasopressors: Substances that cause the contraction of the muscle fibers in capillaries and arteries, resulting in vasoconstriction and diminished blood flow.

be a common occurrence.[2] Susceptible populations are primarily the very young, the elderly, and patients with a small total blood volume or cardiopulmonary disease.[1] These individuals are unable to tolerate a rapid expansion of their blood volume and may experience **cyanosis, orthopnea,** hypertension, severe headache, difficulty breathing, or congestive heart failure during or soon after the transfusion.

Management

When transfusion-induced congestive heart failure is suspected, the transfusion may be stopped or continued very slowly and intravenous diuretics administered. The patient may be placed in an upright position and given oxygen to facilitate breathing. If symptoms are not relieved or if pulmonary edema exists, phlebotomy may be indicated.

Prevention

Transfusion-induced congestive heart failure can best be prevented by identifying susceptible patients and transfusing them with small aliquots of the most concentrated product available over a longer period of time. It is often advisable to divide a red cell unit into aliquots and transfuse one aliquot at a time, while storing the remaining aliquots between 1° and 6° C. Each aliquot should be infused within a 4-hour period, the maximum time allowed to infuse a unit, and subsequent aliquots can be administered as needed within a 24-hour period. It may be indicated, in certain situations, to administer diuretics before or during the transfusion.

Hemolysis due to Physical or Chemical Means

Nonimmune hemolysis of red cells due to physical or chemical means can occur through a number of mechanisms, including, but not limited to, the following: exposure to improper temperature during storage, during shipment, or before infusion (e.g., malfunctioning blood warmers); improper component preparation (e.g., inadequate deglycerolization of frozen cells); mechanical stress (e.g., roller pumps used in cardiopulmonary bypass surgery, infusion of blood through a small-bore needle); use of non–FDA-approved equipment (e.g., microwave oven); and administration or mixing of red cells with intravenous fluids other than 0.9% sodium chloride (normal saline) or other FDA-approved solutions.[3]

This type of situation is unique in that the blood, which is ABO, Rh, and crossmatch compatible with the patient, is hemolyzed before it is transfused to the patient. Asymptomatic hemoglobinuria is the most common initial symptom. Patients do not experience fever, chills, hypotension, or any other signs or symptoms that might accompany an immune hemolytic transfusion reaction or the infusion of bacterially contaminated blood.

Management

The transfusion should be discontinued and intravascular access maintained with normal saline. It is important that steps be taken to document the cause of the nonimmune hemolytic episode and rule out hemolysis due to other causes such as a hemolytic transfusion reaction. A diagnosis of nonimmune hemolysis due to physical or chemical means is usually one of exclusion.

Patients who receive lysed cells may be able to tolerate the free hemoglobin transfused and clear it from their system without much difficulty. On the other hand, the major reported complications of nonimmune hemolysis are cardiac arrhythmias due to hyperkalemia and renal failure, both of which would warrant appropriate medical treatment.[3]

Prevention

Hemolysis due to physical or chemical means can be prevented by adherence to the standard operating procedure established for the proper preparation, storage,

Cyanosis: Bluish discoloration of the skin due to decreased oxygen saturation of the blood.

Orthopnea: Difficulty breathing in any but an erect position.

and infusion of blood as set forth in the blood bank's procedure and policy manual. Written standards should state the acceptable temperature ranges for equipment used to store and warm blood. Only FDA-approved equipment should be used for this purpose. If the temperature is outside the acceptable range, the blood should not be used. Laboratory technologists should follow established protocols for the preparation of blood, and transfusionists should be properly educated and follow the institution's standard operating procedures for the administration of blood and components.

Summary 15-1 lists the acute adverse effects of transfusion.

DELAYED IMMUNOLOGIC TRANSFUSION REACTIONS
Hemolytic Transfusion Reactions

A **delayed hemolytic transfusion reaction** (DHTR), by definition, occurs at least 24 hours after transfusion of the implicated unit. Hemolysis is usually extravascular, and red cells are destroyed in the recipient's circulation by antibody produced as a result of an immune response induced by the transfusion. Although DHTRs may be the result of primary or secondary exposure to a red cell antigen, primary alloimmunization is rarely associated with hemolysis because the time needed for a primary immune response usually exceeds the normal life span of the transfused cells.

DHTRs are most commonly due to an anamnestic response (secondary exposure to a red cell antigen). In this situation, during pretransfusion testing, the patient has a negative antibody screen even though he or she has produced antibody as a result of previous exposure, either through pregnancy or transfusion, to a foreign red cell antigen and mounted an immune response. However, the titer of the antibody has subsided with time and is no longer at a detectable level in the serum. Exposure to the same antigen a second time may cause IgG antibody to reappear within hours or days of the transfusion. This subsequent exposure to the antigen produces an anamnestic antibody response resulting in increased production of IgG antibodies that are capable of reacting with any transfused cells present. Although antibodies against antigens in the Rh (most commonly c, E, and C), Kidd (Jk), Duffy (Fy), and Kell (K) groups have been associated with DHTRs, anti-Jk^a is often implicated.[5]

In most cases, anamnestic production of antibody does not result in hemolysis, hence the term **delayed serologic transfusion reaction** (DSTR).[2] However, red cell destruction does occur in some patients. Patients are generally asymptomatic, and hemolysis may only be noted by a decline in the patient's hemoglobin that is more rapid than usual or the absence of the expected rise in hemoglobin. Fever, the most common initial symptom, may be accompanied by mild jaundice. Hemoglobinuria may occasionally be noted, and renal failure is rare. There is usually a delay of between 3 days to 2 weeks between the transfusion and onset of symptoms.[5]

A delayed transfusion reaction can be diagnosed through serologic findings in patients who manifest no clinical symptoms. The DAT is generally negative but may be positive 3 to 7 days after transfusion and show a mixed-field pattern of agglutination. The patient's IgG antibody reacts only with the corresponding antigen on transfused, not patient, cells. If the implicated antibody is capable of activating the complement cascade, complement (C3d) may also be present on the red blood cells. Antibody may or may not be detected in the serum. If the sample is drawn too early in the immune response, when the antibody titer is still low, all available antibody may be attached to donor red blood cells. It is only when the antibody titer increases and is bound to all available antigen sites on transfused donor cells that unbound antibody is detectable in the recipient's serum. Incompatible crossmatches may be noted in subsequent requests for transfusions if

Delayed hemolytic transfusion reaction: Accelerated destruction of transfused red cells usually associated with an anamnestic antibody response to alloantigen(s) on donor red cells. These reactions may not be recognized for days or weeks after transfusion. Because delayed reactions are often asymptomatic, many may go unreported.

Delayed serologic transfusion reaction: Delayed reaction associated with the production of red blood cell alloantibodies after transfusion in which there is no clinical evidence of hemolysis.

Primary and secondary immune responses are discussed in Chapter 2.

Summary 15-1

Acute Adverse Effects of Transfusion

IMMUNOLOGIC

Hemolytic Transfusion Reactions

Estimated risk per unit transfused: 1:38,000 to 1:70,000

Mediators: complement-mediated lysis of ABO-incompatible red cells

Signs/symptoms: fever, chills, anxiety, hypotension, diffuse bleeding, hemoglobinemia, hemoglobinuria, acute renal failure

Management/prevention: decrease opportunities for error, treat acute renal failure and DIC

Febrile Nonhemolytic Transfusion Reactions

Estimated risk per unit transfused: 1:17 to 1:200 (red blood cells); 1:3 to 1:100 (platelets)

Mediators: antibodies to lymphocytes, granulocytes, or platelets

Signs/symptoms: fever, chills

Management/prevention: antipyretics, leukocyte depletion

Allergic Transfusion Reactions

Estimated risk per unit transfused: 1:33 to 1:100 (mild); 1:20,000 to 1:50,000 (anaphylactic)

Mediators: antibodies to plasma proteins (mild reactions), antibodies to IgA (anaphylactic reactions)

Signs/symptoms: urticaria, erythema, itching; anaphylaxis

Management/prevention: antihistamines; treat symptoms, transfuse IgA-deficient component

Transfusion-Related Acute Lung Injury

Estimated risk per unit transfused: 1:5000 to 1:190,000

Mediators: donor/recipient white blood cell antibodies

Signs/symptoms: fever, chills, dyspnea, cyanosis, tachycardia, hypotension, hypoxemia, noncardiogenic pulmonary edema

Management/prevention: vigorous respiratory support

NONIMMUNOLOGIC

Bacterial Contamination

Estimated risk per unit transfused: 1:31,000 (red blood cells); 1:700 (pooled random-donor platelet concentrates); 1:4000 (single-donor platelet concentrates)

Mediators: endotoxins produced by gram-negative bacteria

Signs/symptoms: fever, shock, hemoglobinuria, DIC, renal failure

Management/prevention: intravenous antibiotics, treat hypotension and DIC

Circulatory Overload

Estimated risk per unit transfused: common

Mediators: fluid volume

Signs/symptoms: cyanosis, orthopnea, hypertension, severe headache, difficulty breathing, congestive heart failure

Management/prevention: administer subsequent transfusions slowly and in small volumes

Physical/Chemical Hemolysis

Estimated risk per unit transfused: rare

Mediators: exogenous destruction of red blood cells

Signs/symptoms: hemoglobinuria

Management/prevention: document and rule out hemolysis due to other causes the donor unit contains the antigen for which the recipient has the corresponding antibody.

Management

Treatment is rarely necessary because clinical problems associated with DHTRs are uncommon. The presence of a previously undetected red cell alloantibody in a patient manifesting hemolysis, coupled with identification of the corresponding antigen from one or more of the transfused units, supports a diagnosis of DHTR.

When a DAT becomes positive on a recently transfused patient, an elution should be performed and the antibody identified. When the DAT is positive and the indirect antiglobulin test is negative or unequivocal, the eluate may be used to crossmatch additional units for the patient. Subsequent blood products transfused should be antigen negative for the patient's corresponding antibody.

Prevention

It is impossible to prevent a DHTR due to primary alloimmunization because when a patient receives a blood transfusion, any red cell antigen transfused that the patient lacks is potentially immunogenic. There is no unequivocal way to prevent a DHTR due to an anamnestic antibody response, but blood bank technologists can take certain steps to minimize the possibility. It is important to check a patient's previous hospital record for evidence of alloimmunization. If a patient had a positive antibody screen previously, even though it may currently be negative, antigen-negative blood must be crossmatched. Specimens for compatibility testing on patients who have been pregnant or transfused within the past 3 months must be no more than 72 hours old. This allows for the detection of rapidly developing antibodies capable of causing decreased survival of transfused red blood cells. These antibodies could be missed if a specimen was not representative of the patient's current immunologic status. AABB Standards mandate that permanent records be kept of patients with clinically significant antibodies and that records be reviewed before red cells are transfused.[2]

Transfusion-Associated Graft-versus-Host Disease

Transfusion-associated graft-versus-host disease (TA-GVHD) results from the transfusion of immunologically competent lymphocytes into an immunologically incompetent host. The engrafted lymphocytes mount an immunologic response against the recipient's tissue, resulting in **pancytopenia** with bleeding and infectious complications. Symptoms usually appear within 12 days of transfusion. TA-GVHD is rare but it is fatal in approximately 90% of affected patients.[2]

The risk for an individual to develop TA-GVHD depends on whether the recipient is immunocompromised (and the degree to which the recipient is immunocompromised), the degree of HLA similarity between the transfusion donor and recipient, and the number of transfused T lymphocytes capable of multiplying and engrafting. Examples of specific populations at risk include, but are not limited to, recipients of cellular components from blood relatives, immunocompromised recipients of hematopoietic progenitor cell or organ transplants, patients with congenital cellular immunodeficiencies, fetuses receiving intrauterine transfusion, and neonates undergoing exchange transfusion.

A diagnosis of TA-GVHD is generally made postmortem. Lymphocytes of both the donor and host, as well as skin fibroblasts of the host, can be HLA typed to document that donor lymphocytes were engrafted. In addition, the presence of clinical signs and symptoms associated with TA-GVHD in a susceptible host also help confirm the diagnosis.

Management

TA-GVHD usually does not respond to most treatment regimens.

Transfusion-associated graft-versus-host disease: Proliferation of immunologically competent donor cells in an immunocompromised recipient. Also at risk are individuals who receive blood and components from blood relatives. Such reactions can be avoided by irradiation of blood and components that contain white cells.

Pancytopenia: Decreased numbers of all blood cell lines.

Prevention

The key to preventing TA-GVHD is to avoid transfusing immunologically competent lymphocytes to populations at risk of developing the disease. All blood and blood components, with the exception of fresh-frozen plasma and cryoprecipitate, contain a sufficient number of lymphocytes to initiate GVHD in a susceptible recipient. The simplest way to reduce the risk of TA-GVHD is irradiation of all blood components before infusion in order to inactivate lymphocytes. A minimum radiation dose of 2500 cGy is targeted to the midline of the component and a minimum of 1500 cGy to other parts of the component.[2] Irradiation inactivates T lymphocytes and does not have an adverse effect on the other humoral and cellular components of the blood.[2]

Posttransfusion Purpura

Posttransfusion purpura (PTP) is rare and most commonly occurs in women in their sixth or seventh decade of life. The majority of cases involve patients whose platelets are Pl[A1]-antigen negative who become alloimmunized, through previous pregnancy or transfusion, to make the corresponding antibody (anti-Pl[A1]). Approximately 5 to 10 days following transfusion of a product containing platelets, the patient experiences a sudden onset of severe thrombocytopenia (platelet count less than 10,000/μL). The thrombocytopenic episode is due to the destruction of both the transfused Pl[A1]-positive platelets and the patient's Pl[A1]-negative platelets. The mechanism for the destruction of the patient's autologous platelets is not fully understood. It has been speculated that Pl[A1]-positive platelets may release Pl[A1] antigen that is then adsorbed onto the patient's Pl[A1]-negative platelets, making them a target for the preexisting anti-Pl[A1] antibodies. Another theory is that transfusion of Pl[A1]-positive platelets initiates production of a platelet autoantibody, as well as the alloantibody.[8]

> **Posttransfusion purpura:** Red discoloration of the skin caused by hemorrhage resulting from immune destruction of transfused platelets by antiplatelet antibodies in the recipient.

Management

The diagnosis of PTP should be made as soon as possible because deaths from cerebral hemorrhage have been reported. Treatment regimens have included corticosteroids (the role of which is controversial) and plasma exchange therapy, both of which are now being supplanted by intravenous immunoglobulin (IVIG) therapy. IVIG appears to block the antibody-mediated clearance of target cells.[3] The efficacy of treatment regimens is difficult to gauge because the thrombocytopenic episode is generally self-limiting.

DELAYED NONIMMUNOLOGIC TRANSFUSION REACTIONS
Transfusion-Induced Hemosiderosis

The daily excretion rate of iron in nonbleeding patients is 1 mg.[5] Each unit of blood contains approximately 250 mg of iron complexed with hemoglobin. **Hemosiderosis** is not a problem for most transfusion recipients but may be dangerous for the chronically transfused (e.g., patients with beta-thalassemia major, congenital hemolytic anemias, or aplastic anemia). Complications arise when excess iron is not removed but deposited in the liver, heart, and endocrine glands, causing the eventual failure of those organs.

> **Hemosiderosis:** Deposition of iron in tissues and organs, which may result from the long-term administration of blood to patients with chronic anemia.
>
> **Neocytes:** A population of relatively young red cells. Larger and less dense younger red cells can be separated from older red cells that are smaller and more dense by differential centrifugation techniques. During automated cell washing, the young cells are pushed out of the bag earlier and collected for transfusion.
>
> **Desferoxamine:** An investigative drug (ICL670) that functions as a chelator of iron. It has been shown to be effective in the treatment of iron overload in multiply transfused patients.

Management

In susceptible populations (e.g., patients with hemoglobinopathies) management can be geared toward reducing the frequency of transfusion, as well as reducing iron stores in the body (without a concomitant decrease in hemoglobin). Transfusing **neocytes** would prolong the interval between transfusions, thus decreasing the amount of iron a patient would receive within a given time frame. Infusing an iron-chelating agent such as **desferoxamine** would reduce the accumulation of iron deposits within the body. Desferoxamine is administered nightly through a subcutaneous pump, a difficult process that can result in poor patient compliance.[2]

Summary 15-2 lists the delayed adverse effects of transfusion.

Disease Transmission

The transmission of disease by blood components has been a topic of intense investigation by researchers in the past decade. It has long been known that certain infections can be transmitted through blood transfusions. The discovery that the deadly virus responsible for the acquired immunodeficiency syndrome (AIDS) could be transmitted through blood transfusion, coupled with the public's increasing concern over the safety of the blood supply, has placed increasing demands on the blood banking community to develop more sensitive and specific assays for screening blood. Advances in infectious disease testing continue to improve the safety of the nation's blood supply. (See the section on donor testing for more information on infectious disease testing of donor blood.)

Hepatitis

The transmission of **hepatitis A virus** through blood transfusions is extremely rare because the period of viremia is very short and there is no carrier state. Testing for serologic markers indicative of infection with **hepatitis B virus** (HBV) and **hepatitis C virus** (HCV) has significantly reduced the risk of transmission of these diseases through blood transfusion. In addition to the extensive medical

Hepatitis: Inflammation of the liver.

Hepatitis A virus: Virus that is generally transmitted by the fecal-oral route; transmission by transfusion is extremely rare.

Hepatitis B virus: Virus that is transmitted by transfusion, but the incidence has decreased with the advent of sensitive donor screening for the surface antigen (HbsAg) and antibody to core antigen (anti-HBc).

Hepatitis C virus: Before the viral genome was discovered, this disease was referred to as non-A, non-B (NANB) hepatitis. The implementation of nucleic acid testing in 1999 has decreased the incidence of transfusion-transmitted infection.

Summary 15-2

Delayed Adverse Effects of Transfusion

IMMUNOLOGIC
Delayed Hemolytic Transfusion Reactions

Estimated risk per unit transfused: 1:5000 to 1:11,000
Mediators: IgG antibodies
Signs/symptoms: shortened red cell survival, decreased hemoglobin, fever, jaundice, hemoglobinuria
Management/prevention: antigen-negative blood for subsequent transfusions

Transfusion–Associated Graft-versus-Host Disease

Estimated risk per unit transfused: rare
Mediators: viable donor lymphocytes
Signs/symptoms: fever, skin rash, anorexia, nausea, vomiting, diarrhea, pancytopenia
Management/prevention: gamma irradiation of cellular components

Posttransfusion Purpura

Estimated risk per unit transfused: rare
Mediators: platelet-specific antibodies
Signs/symptoms: thrombocytopenia, clinical bleeding
Management/prevention: intravenous immunoglobulins

NONIMMUNOLOGIC
Transfusion-Induced Hemosiderosis

Estimated risk per unit transfused: is essentially inevitable after transfusion of 100 units
Mediator: iron overload
Signs/symptoms: subclinical to organ failure
Management/prevention: decrease frequency of transfusions, neocytes, iron chelation therapy

history obtained on each donor to assess his or her risk for HBV and HCV infection (see section on donor selection for more information), units are currently tested for hepatitis B surface antigen (HBsAg) and antibodies to hepatitis B core antigen (anti-HBc) and hepatitis C virus (anti-HCV). Donors who indicate a potential risk factor for hepatitis as part of their medical history are not allowed to donate, and donations with repeatedly reactive screening test results for HBsAg, anti-HBc, and anti-HCV are not used for transfusion. This, coupled with the implementation of nucleic acid screening assays for hepatitis C virus by blood centers in 1999, has decreased the estimated risk per unit transfused for hepatitis B to 1:63,000 and hepatitis C to 1:1,600,000.[6] The **hepatitis D virus** can be transmitted through blood transfusion but is capable of producing disease only when the hepatitis B virus is also present. The risk of acquiring hepatitis D from a blood supply screened for hepatitis B is low.

Hepatitis D virus: Capable of causing disease only in the presence of HBV. Screening of blood for HBV results in a low risk of transfusion-associated hepatitis D infection.

Human Immunodeficiency Virus

All blood components are capable of transmitting human immunodeficiency virus type 1 **(HIV-1)**. Transmission of this disease has been markedly reduced since the introduction, in 1985, of an immunologic assay for anti–HIV-1. In addition, donors at risk for contracting AIDS are excluded from donating blood.

HIV-1/2, HTLV-I/II: Viruses that have been documented to be transmitted by blood transfusion.

Research is being directed toward the development of more sensitive assays for the detection of HIV-1 antigen and antibody. This will decrease transmission of the disease by the small number of blood donors who are unaware that they have been exposed to the virus and have not yet seroconverted or have low levels of antibodies that are below the sensitivity level of existing tests.

Human immunodeficiency virus type 2 **(HIV-2)** is endemic in West Africa and much rarer elsewhere. It appears to be transmitted the same way as HIV-1 and has similar clinical manifestations. The prevalence of HIV-2 infection in the United States appears to be rare, with West Africans more likely to be infected than natives of the United States.[9]

Since 1985, blood centers have been screening donor blood for antibodies to HIV-1 and HIV-2. The introduction of the screening test for the HIV-1 antigen (p24) in 1996 reduced the window period from 22 to 16 days. In 1999, the major blood collecting organizations implemented HIV nucleic acid testing on an investigational basis, which is estimated to have further reduced the window period to 10 days. The estimated risk for HIV-1 and HIV-2 per unit transfused is 1:1,900,000.[6]

Human T-cell Lymphotropic Virus

Human T-cell lymphotropic virus type I **(HTLV-I)** is a retrovirus associated with adult T-cell leukemia/lymphoma. The disease is endemic in southern Japan, certain Pacific islands, sub-Saharan Africa, and the Caribbean basin.[6] Human T-cell lymphotropic virus type II **(HTLV-II)** is also a human retrovirus that exhibits a high degree of nucleic acid homology with HTLV-I. A high prevalence has been reported in Native American populations and intravenous drug users in the United States.[6] Donor screening for HTLV-I was implemented in 1988, and, despite the cross-reactivity of HTLV-II with viral lysates from HTLV-I, it was estimated that this screening test missed approximately 50% of HTLV-II infections. A combined screening test for HTLV-I/II was introduced in 1998, and the current estimated risk per unit transfused for HTLV-I/II is 1:641,000.[6]

Cytomegalovirus

Cytomegalovirus (CMV) is transmitted by viable leukocytes in transfused blood. Populations at risk of contracting severe CMV infections include premature low birth weight neonates born to seronegative mothers, recipients of intrauterine transfusions, and seronegative recipients of organ, marrow, or peripheral blood progenitor cell transplants.[6]

Cytomegalovirus: A virus transmitted by the viable leukocytes in blood components, which is of special concern when transfusing immunocompromised recipients. Leukodepletion of components and the transfusion of CMV-negative blood are methods of reducing risk.

The supply of blood from donors who are CMV negative for transfusion to populations at risk is limited. Leukocyte-reduced components ($\leq 5 \times 10^6$ leukocytes per component) have been shown to reduce, if not prevent, posttransfusion CMV infections in certain high-risk populations.[6]

Although the overall prevalence rate for CMV antibodies in the population is between 40% and 90%, only a small percentage (less than 1%) of these units are capable of transmitting the virus.[10]

Malaria

The transmission of the **malaria** parasite through blood transfusion is rare (0 to 5 per million). There is no effective screening test for the detection of this parasite, but donors at high risk of acquiring and therefore transmitting the disease (e.g., travelers to areas endemic for malaria, donors who emigrated from a malarial area within the past 3 years) are deferred from donating blood for a prescribed period of time.

Babesiosis

Babesiosis is generally caused by the species *Babesia microti,* a protozoan parasite of rodents, and is transmitted through the bite of the *Ixodes scapularis* tick. Babesiosis is characterized by fever, malaise, and hemolytic anemia and may be mistaken for malaria because of the similarity in symptoms. The rodent and tick vectors for the babesia parasite are prevalent along the coastal areas of the northeastern United States. In the past 20 years, there have been approximately two dozen reported cases of transfusion-associated babesiosis in the United States.[1] No serologic assay is available to identify blood donors infected with babesiosis, so prevention relies on excluding donors at risk of having contracted the disease.

Syphilis

It is rare for **syphilis** to be transmitted through a blood transfusion. For this to occur, the blood would have to be drawn during the brief period of spirochetemia and organisms would have to be viable at the time of transfusion. The causative organism of syphilis, *T. pallidum,* does not ordinarily survive for longer than 72 hours at 1° to 6° C, so only components stored at room temperature or transfused promptly after collection have any risk of transmitting the disease. AABB Standards no longer require that serologic tests for syphilis be performed on donor blood. However, syphilis screening tests are required by the FDA.

This is by no means a comprehensive list of all infectious agents that are transmitted by blood transfusions, as the number and variety of new ones continue to increase. Other transfusion-associated agents include, but are not limited to, the following: Chagas' disease, variant Creutzfeldt-Jakob disease (vCJD) (a rare, degenerative, and fatal nervous system disorder), SEN-V, and West Nile virus. The growing number of cases of vCJD in Europe has resulted in new FDA deferral policies for potential blood donors. SEN-V is a virus related to hepatitis, and although there are currently no blood tests to detect the virus, studies indicate that multiply transfused patients have higher rates of infection with SEN-V than non-transfused patients.[1] The West Nile virus (WNV) was first recognized in 1999; humans are infected through the bite of an infected mosquito. Cases of possible transmission of WNV via transfusion have been reported.[11] With each new agent discovered, the blood banking community will be challenged to optimize the safety of the blood supply.

There are a variety of methods currently available, or under investigation, to improve the safety of the blood supply. Solvent/detergent treatment of plasma is effective against lipid-enveloped viruses such as HCV, HBV, HTLV-I and II, and WNV.[1] It was initially licensed in 1985 for use in the manufacture of factor VIII concentrate and although licensed by the FDA, is not currently available in the

---

Malaria/babesiosis: Protozoan diseases transmitted by transfusion. Both are rare, and no donor testing is available.

Syphilis: A sexually transmitted disease that is rarely transmitted by the transfusion of blood that has been stored more than 72 hours. Serologic testing for syphilis is performed on donor blood.

United States.[12] A psoralen, combined with ultraviolet A (UVA) light, has been shown to inhibit the replication of viruses such as HIV and HCV in platelets and plasma.[11,12] This process is currently undergoing clinical trials in the United States.[6] A combination of heat treatment, solvent/detergent treatment, and purification steps with monoclonal antibodies has been used in the manufacture of factor concentrates to provide a product with a lower risk of transmitting disease than cryoprecipitated antihemophilic factor from individual blood donors.[6]

INVESTIGATION OF SUSPECTED TRANSFUSION REACTIONS

The responsibility for recognizing the signs and symptoms of a potential transfusion reaction generally lies with the individual attending to the patient; this individual may be a nurse, physician, or other member of the health care team. The institution's patient care manual should clearly specify what actions should be taken in the event of a suspected transfusion reaction.

1. If a transfusion reaction is suspected, the transfusion should be stopped. This limits the amount of blood or blood component infused and minimizes the potential adverse effects.
2. The intravenous line should be kept open with normal saline while the patient is evaluated in order to ascertain if a transfusion reaction occurred.
3. All labels, forms, and patient identification should be checked at the patient's bedside to determine if the patient received the intended component.
4. The suspected transfusion reaction should be reported to the transfusion service and the patient's physician.
5. If, after initial evaluation, it is determined that the patient has experienced either a mild allergic or circulatory overload transfusion reaction, the transfusion service does not need to evaluate postreaction blood samples from the patient. If signs and symptoms are indicative of a reaction other than mild allergic or circulatory overload, postreaction blood samples should be sent to the laboratory for evaluation.[2]
6. Requested blood samples (EDTA and clot tube), discontinued bag of blood or component, administration set without the intravenous needle, attached intravenous solutions, and all related forms and labels should be sent to the blood bank as soon as possible. Care must be taken to avoid mechanical hemolysis when drawing the posttransfusion blood sample.
7. Other blood samples are sent to the blood bank for evaluation of acute hemolysis as requested by the blood bank medical director or patient's physician.

The blood bank or transfusion service shall have a manual that specifies the policies, processes, and procedures to be followed in the evaluation of a suspected transfusion-related complication. The clinical signs and symptoms the patient experiences as part of a transfusion reaction may be unique to a particular type of reaction or shared by many.

When a patient experiences an acute transfusion reaction, all possible causes must be considered before making a diagnosis and initiating the appropriate therapy. The possibility of an acute hemolytic transfusion reaction should always be considered and then ruled out.

Preliminary Investigation

A suggested preliminary outline for the laboratory investigation of a suspected acute hemolytic transfusion reaction includes the following steps.

Clerical Check

Examine all blood container labels and prereaction patient records for clerical errors. Administration of a unit of donor blood to the wrong patient is one of the most common causes of death and serious morbidity in transfused patients. It is imperative that all labels and records attached to the donor bag, prereaction records relevant to the donor unit and intended transfusion recipient, and records relating to the issue and transfusion of the donor unit be carefully examined for errors. If a discrepancy is found, the patient's physician or other responsible health care professional should be notified. A thorough search must then be conducted to determine if other patient samples or donor units have been misidentified or issued to the wrong recipient. Finally, every step of the transfusion process, from the drawing of the intended transfusion recipient's blood to the actual transfusion, needs to be carefully traced in order to determine where, how, and why the error was made.

Visual Inspection for Free Hemoglobin

Inspect the postreaction serum or plasma sample for hemolysis. If the serum or plasma appears hemolyzed, compare it with the prereaction sample if it is available. Pink or red discoloration of the serum or plasma in a postreaction sample may indicate the presence of free hemoglobin from the intravascular destruction of donor red blood cells. Intravascular hemolysis of as little as 5 to 10 mL of red cells can result in hemoglobinemia that is visible to the naked eye.[2] The amount of hemoglobin released is proportional to the volume of donor red blood cells destroyed.

When the destruction of the donor red blood cells is extravascular and the hemolytic process less acute, the patient's serum or plasma may be icteric after a few hours. Icterus is usually maximal 5 to 7 hours after red blood cells have been destroyed, so it is advisable to draw a second sample at that time.

If the postreaction serum or plasma sample appears abnormal, compare it with the prereaction sample, if available. Discoloration in the postreaction sample only is indicative of a hemolytic process.

Direct Antiglobulin Test

Perform a direct antiglobulin test (DAT) on a postreaction sample. An EDTA sample is preferable to a clot tube for a DAT because in addition to supplying an adequate amount of anticoagulated cells, a positive DAT result with anti-C3d on cells from an EDTA tube can only be due to in vivo activation of the complement cascade, whereas in a clot tube it could be due to in vitro activation of the complement cascade. If the DAT on the postreaction sample is positive, perform a DAT on a prereaction sample, if available.

The DAT may be positive if incompatible cells are not immediately destroyed or removed from the circulation. Care should be taken to look for mixed-field agglutination because the transfused cells, rather than the recipient's cells, are affected. Antibody-and/or complement-coated cells may be rapidly destroyed, which would result in a negative DAT if the postreaction blood sample was drawn several hours after a suspected reaction. A postreaction sample for a DAT should therefore be drawn as soon as possible following the report of the suspected hemolytic transfusion reaction.

A positive DAT result on a postreaction sample and a negative result on a prereaction sample indicates an antigen-antibody incompatibility that occurred as a result of the transfusion. A positive DAT on a postreaction sample, as well as a prereaction sample, does not provide evidence for detecting IgG on transfused cells.

Repeat ABO Testing

Because the most common and often most serious cause of acute hemolytic transfusion reactions is associated with the transfusion of incompatible ABO red blood cells, a repeat ABO typing has been added to the AABB Standards as a requirement for the initial testing of any suspected hemolytic event.[4]

Interpretation of Preliminary Tests for a Suspected Hemolytic Transfusion Reaction

If no clerical error has occurred, the postreaction serum or plasma is not pink or red, the DAT on the postreaction sample is negative, and the ABO type of the donor cells are correct, a hemolytic transfusion reaction (especially due to ABO incompatibility) is highly unlikely. Once an acute hemolytic transfusion reaction has been ruled out, other potential causes for the patient's signs and/or symptoms can be explored.

The presence of discoloration and/or a positive DAT on a postreaction sample indicates that hemolysis has probably occurred. However, it is important to note that if hemolysis occurs during transfusion without the patient experiencing any signs or symptoms of an acute hemolytic transfusion reaction, nonimmunologic causes of hemolysis should be explored.

Follow-Up Testing

If the preliminary laboratory tests outlined previously suggest a hemolytic process, additional laboratory tests may be required to substantiate the cause and extent of the hemolysis and follow the clinical condition of the patient. The procedure manual must contain specific instructions outlining the extent of the laboratory testing to be performed.

The following laboratory tests may be helpful to include when investigating an acute hemolytic transfusion reaction.

Antibody Detection Tests

Perform antibody detection tests for clinically significant antibodies on the recipient's pretransfusion and posttransfusion samples, as well as donor blood from an attached segment or the unit. It may be advisable to use enhancement techniques (polyethylene glycol, extended incubation time, gel, enzymes) when testing the prereaction sample if routine methods yield negative or inconclusive results.[2,13]

Observations

Antibody screen on pretransfusion sample: negative
Antibody screen on posttransfusion sample: positive

Possible causes

Delayed hemolytic transfusion reaction, sample identification error, or passive transfer of antibody from a recently transfused unit
The antibody should be identified, and red cells from transfused donor units should be tested for the corresponding antigen. All subsequent blood transfused to the recipient should be negative for the corresponding antigen; if an antibody is detected in the donor's blood that was not previously recorded, it should be identified, records should be examined to determine how the discrepancy occurred, and the patient's pretransfusion blood sample should be phenotyped for the corresponding antigen.

Observations

Initial antibody screen on pretransfusion sample: negative
Repeat antibody screen on pretransfusion sample: positive
Antibody screen on posttransfusion sample: positive

Possible cause

Error made in pretransfusion testing
The antibody should be identified, records should be examined to determine how the discrepancy occurred, and donor units should be phenotyped for the corresponding antigen.

Crossmatching Tests

Perform compatibility tests of the recipient's pretransfusion and posttransfusion samples with donor blood from a segment still attached to the unit or a sample of red blood cells from the bag.

Observations

Donor cells + pretransfusion serum: compatible
Donor cells + posttransfusion serum: incompatible

Possible causes

Delayed hemolytic transfusion reaction, wrong patient sample used, wrong patient sample drawn, antibody against low-incidence antigen that might have been missed by an immediate-spin or computer crossmatch in pretransfusion testing if the antibody screen was negative

Observations

Donor cells + pretransfusion serum: incompatible
Donor cells + posttransfusion serum: incompatible

Possible causes

Error occurred in pretransfusion testing, wrong patient sample used

Observation for Hemolysis

Examine the blood remaining in the unit and the administration tubing for hemolysis.

Observation

Hemolysis in administration tubing, not donor bag

Possible cause

Blood was hemolyzed after it left the bag before it was transfused to the patient
  This could have happened if the administration tubing was used for the infusion of a solution that was incompatible with the blood or the blood hemolyzed when passed through a blood warmer whose temperature was above the acceptable range.

Observation

Hemolysis in administration tubing and donor bag

Possible cause

Blood was hemolyzed in the bag
  This could happen for a number of reasons, including, but not limited to, the following: red cells have been diluted with an incompatible solution, bacterial contamination, or other physical/chemical causes of hemolysis.

Detection of Urine Hemoglobin or Metabolites

The test for hemoglobin should be performed on the supernatant of a centrifuged sample of a fresh specimen of urine collected after transfusion. Hemolysis of red blood cells results in the presence of hemoglobin in the urine. The presence of intact red blood cells (hematuria) is indicative of hemorrhage into the urinary tract, not hemolysis. If the urine sample was collected days after the reaction, it may be advisable to test for hemosiderin.

Monitoring DAT and Antibody Detection Tests

Perform DAT and antibody detection tests on specimens obtained at intervals after the reaction. In an anamnestic antibody response, antibody may initially only be detectable on red cells and not in the serum until all available antigen sites on donor red cells have been bound by antibody.

Monitoring Hemoglobin and Hematocrit

This should be performed on a regular basis in order to determine if the expected posttransfusion increase (1 to 1.5 g/dL hemoglobin and 3% to 5% hematocrit per unit)[2] was seen.

Serum Bilirubin Determinations

Peak levels of bilirubin, a by-product of red cell destruction, occur 5 to 7 hours after transfusion and disappear within 24 hours if kidney function is normal.

Gram Stains/Cultures

Gram stain the recipient's supernatant plasma for bacteria and culture the contents of the blood bag. The presence of bacteria in the recipient's plasma and/or the blood bag confirms the diagnosis of a transfusion reaction due to bacterial contamination of the blood. A positive unit culture coupled with a negative patient culture (or no patient culture) is presumptive evidence of bacterial contamination. A positive culture on the patient and a negative culture on the unit does not provide sufficient evidence to support a diagnosis of bacterial contamination.[13] The unit should also be examined for abnormal appearance (clots) and discoloration (brownish, opaque, muddy, purple), both of which may be indicative of bacterial contamination.

Serum Haptoglobin

Measure serum haptoglobin in the recipient's pretransfusion and posttransfusion samples. The normal ranges of haptoglobin levels are variable, so posttransfusion levels are best evaluated in comparison with pretransfusion levels. Serum haptoglobin levels are rarely of value when investigating acute hemolytic transfusion reactions and are most beneficial when demonstrating subtle or chronic hemolysis. Haptoglobin can rapidly regenerate when depleted, so if measurements are made several days after a hemolytic episode, normal levels may already have been restored.

Delayed transfusion reactions should be investigated to the extent necessary to identify the cause of the reaction. It may not be necessary to perform all of the tests needed as part of an acute transfusion reaction workup. The recipient's pretransfusion samples are required to be kept for only 7 days. If symptoms of a delayed hemolytic transfusion reaction are experienced after this period of time, a pretransfusion sample of the recipient's blood may not be available for analysis.

The blood bank physician must evaluate all work performed as part of a transfusion reaction workup, and interpretation of all tests must be recorded in the patient's chart. If the evidence suggests a hemolytic reaction or bacterial contamination, the patient's physician must be immediately notified. Results and interpretations of all tests performed, as well as the cause of the reaction, must be recorded in the blood bank and be available if the patient requires subsequent transfusions. Records must be kept in the blood bank for a minimum of 5 years. Records of patients who have had transfusion complications or evidence of alloimmunization should be held indefinitely.[2]

Reporting Transfusion Reactions

The blood bank or transfusion service shall have a process in place that clearly stipulates each step that needs to be taken when reporting transfusion reactions. When suspected cases of transfusion-transmitted diseases (e.g., hepatitis, AIDS) have been confirmed, the blood collecting facility shall be notified immediately, and thereafter in writing, of the suspected transfusion infection. Notification should also be given of any other serious complication that occurs and is suspected to be due to a quality of the donor or blood component.[4]

Fatalities that occur as a direct result of a blood transfusion must be reported within 24 hours to the Director, Office of Compliance, Center for Biologics Evaluation and Research, Food and Drug Administration and in writing, within 7 days.[2]

CHAPTER SUMMARY

1. A transfusion reaction is defined as an adverse reaction to any unit of blood or blood component transfused. Transfusion reactions can be acute (occurring during the transfusion or within 24 hours after its completion) or delayed (occurring at least 24 hours after transfusion, but can be days, weeks, months, or years later) and can be classified as immunologic (mediated by antibody-antigen reactions) or nonimmunologic in origin.

2. The red cell destruction manifested in acute hemolytic transfusion reactions can be intravascular or extravascular. Intravascular destruction of red blood cells is most commonly due to an ABO incompatibility, which then activates the complement cascade. In extravascular hemolysis, red blood cells are removed from the circulation and destroyed by phagocytosis in the liver and spleen.

3. The most common acute immune transfusion reactions are febrile nonhemolytic transfusion reactions (FNHTRs) and mild allergic reactions. Fever is the initial symptom of FNHTRs, and allergic reactions are manifested by urticaria, itching, and erythema. Other immune transfusion reactions include life-threatening anaphylactic transfusion reactions and transfusion-related acute lung injury (TRALI). Bacterial contamination, circulatory overload, and hemolysis due to physical/chemical means are examples of acute nonimmune transfusion reactions.

4. Delayed transfusion reactions can also be immunologic or nonimmunologic in origin. Delayed hemolytic transfusion reactions are most commonly due to anamnestic exposure to red cell antigens. Symptoms include fever, decline in hemoglobin and hematocrit, and mild jaundice, and medical intervention is rarely necessary. Two other examples of immunologic

delayed transfusion reactions are transfusion-associated graft-versus-host disease (TA-GVHD) and posttransfusion purpura. TA-GVHD results from the transfusion of immunologically competent T lymphocytes to an immunologically incompetent host. In posttransfusion purpura, transfused PI^{A1}-positive platelets, as well as the patient's own PI^{A1}-negative platelets, are destroyed by the patient's anti-PI^{A1}.

5. Nonimmunologic causes of delayed transfusion reactions include transfusion hemosiderosis and disease transmission.

6. In cases of suspected transfusion reactions, the transfusion should be stopped and the intravenous line kept open with saline. A clerical check should be performed at the bedside and the transfusion service notified. Requested blood samples, discontinued blood or component bag, administration set, intravenous solutions, and related forms and labels must be sent to the blood bank. Other samples are sent as requested.

7. Preliminary investigation in the blood bank of suspected transfusion reactions includes a clerical check, visual inspection of pretransfusion and postreaction samples for hemolysis, and a DAT on pretransfusion and posttransfusion samples. If preliminary tests show no hemolysis, further tests need not be performed. If the results of preliminary tests suggest that a hemolytic process occurred, additional laboratory tests (e.g., repeat ABO and Rh typing, repeat compatibility testing) are required. Results and interpretations of all laboratory tests performed must be kept in the blood bank for a minimum of 5 years.

8. Fatalities that occur as a result of blood transfusion must be reported within 24 hours to the Food and Drug Administration.

REFERENCES

1. Goodman C, Chan S, Collins P, et al: Ensuring blood safety and availability in the US: Technological advances, costs, and challenges to payment—final report. Transfusion 43(Suppl):3S-44S, Aug 2003.

2. Noninfectious complications of blood transfusion and transfusion-transmitted diseases. In Bresher ME (ed): Technical Manual. Bethesda, MD, American Association of Blood Banks, 2002.

3. Davenport, RD: Management of transfusion reactions. In Mintz PD (ed): Transfusion Therapy: Clinical Principles and Practice. Bethesda, MD, American Association of Blood Banks, 1999.

4. American Association of Blood Banks (AABB): Standards for Blood Banks and Transfusion Services, 22nd ed. Bethesda, MD, American Association of Blood Banks, 2003.

5. Perrotta PL, Snyder EL: Non-infectious complications of transfusion therapy. Blood Rev 15:69-83, 2001.

6. Transfusion-transmitted diseases. In Brecher ME (ed): Technical Manual. Bethesda, MD, American Association of Blood Banks, 2002.

7. Smith LA, Wright-Kanuth MS: Bacterial contamination of blood components. Clin Lab Sci 16:230-238, 2003.

8. Waters AH: Post-transfusion purpura. Blood Rev 3:83-87, 1989.

9. O'Brien TR, George JR, Holmberg SD: Human immunodeficiency virus type 2 infection in the United States. Epidemiology, diagnosis and public health implications. JAMA 267:2775-2779, 1992.

10. Lamberson HV, Dock NL: Prevention of transfusion-transmitted cytomegalovirus infection. Transfusion 32:196-198, 1992.

11. Wright-Kanuth M, Smith LA: Transfusion risks: Transmission of viral, bacterial, or parasitic agents. Clin Lab Sci 16:221-229, 2003.

12. Fricke W, Kouides P: Viral safety of plasma products. Lab Med 34:667-671, 2003.

13. Davenport R: Guidelines for the Laboratory Evaluation of Transfusion Reactions. Bethesda, MD, American Association of Blood Banks, 2003.

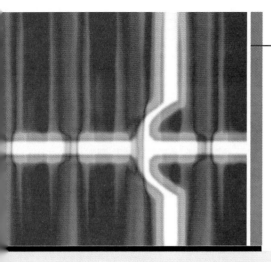

Clinical Considerations

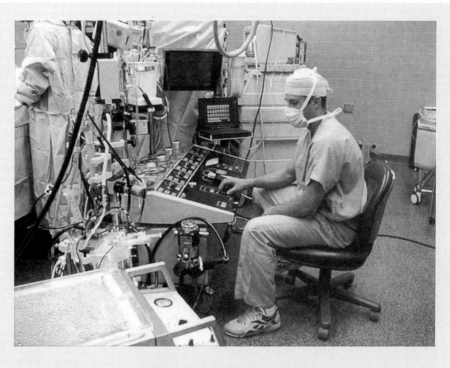

The practice of transfusion medicine involves the treatment of a wide variety of clinical conditions. Some patients may present unique serologic and/or clinical problems for the blood bank, including massive transfusion and/or excessively rapid transfusion, recipients whose clinical status alters their tolerance to transfusion products, patients who have difficult serologic problems, patients who require special component processing, and patients with altered immune function. This can result in the need for alterations in the standard pretransfusion testing protocols (e.g., use of maternal serum for infants), additional patient monitoring (e.g., laboratory testing), modifications in blood components and products (e.g., irradiation), and other novel approaches to therapy (e.g., therapeutic phlebotomy). These patients can also have unique serologic problems such as the mixed cell populations seen after hematopoietic progenitor cell (HPC) transplant.

Massive transfusions are associated with a number of adverse physiologic consequences. In addition, the nature of the injury or the underlying disease of the massively transfused patient can further complicate the clinical picture. Infants, because of their size and other physiologic factors, constitute another population requiring specialized approaches to pretransfusion testing and component therapy. Other special populations include patients with end-stage liver disease, burn patients, and those needing interventions such as therapeutic pheresis or therapeutic phlebotomy.

The transplantation of hematopoietic stem/progenitor cells has advanced from research limited to a few sites to a common medical procedure. Sources of HPCs include the bone marrow, cord blood, peripheral blood, and fetal liver. Many diseases are currently treated with HPC transplantation, and research is focused on the potential for HPC transplantation in a broad array of malignant and nonmalignant disorders. HPC transplantation requires the involvement of the blood center and the transfusion service, as well as component transfusion support before and after transplant.

Dealing with these patients requires specialized techniques and knowledge. In these special instances, there is an urgent need for open communication between the blood bank staff and the clinician. In cases in which standard protocols or procedures are altered, careful documentation is essential. These patients provide a special challenge to the blood banking professional.

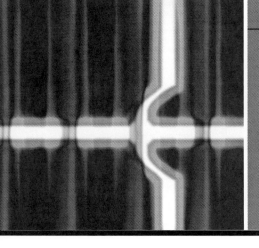

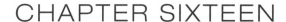

CHAPTER SIXTEEN

Hemolytic Disease of the Fetus and Newborn

Patricia L. Strohm

LEARNING OBJECTIVES

After reading and studying this chapter, the student should be able to:

1. Define *hemolytic disease of the newborn* (HDN).
2. List three types of HDN based on antibody specificity.
3. Briefly discuss other clinical conditions that can be associated with newborn hemolysis or jaundice.
4. List two conditions associated with maternal immunization that can cause the destruction of other (non–red cell) lines in the fetus or newborn.
5. Define the following terms:
   Hydrops fetalis
   Icterus gravis neonatorum
   Kernicterus
6. State three criteria that are necessary for HDN to develop.
7. Discuss the pathophysiology of HDN, differentiating between the disease course in utero and postpartum.
8. Describe the routine prenatal testing necessary to diagnose, monitor, and treat HDN.
9. List which testing and patient information is critical to the treatment of HDN once the disease has been detected.
10. Describe the cordocentesis procedure.
11. Describe the titration procedure and discuss variables that must be controlled to ensure the accuracy and reproducibility of the procedure.
12. Interpret titer results and suggest clinical implications of the findings.
13. Define *critical titer* and discuss how this value is determined.
14. Describe the amniocentesis procedure.
15. Discuss the procedure used to analyze amniotic fluid for bilirubin and L/S ratios.
16. Identify factors that can affect the accuracy of amniotic fluid analysis results.
17. Describe the intrauterine transfusion procedures: intraperitoneal and intravascular.
18. When provided with the ABO and Rh group of the mother and the fetus and the identity of the maternal antibody(ies), select the appropriate blood for intrauterine transfusion.
19. Discuss AABB Standards with regard to the selection of blood for intrauterine transfusion.
20. Discuss the interpretation of cord blood hemoglobin and bilirubin levels in the early postpartum period.

21. Describe the exchange transfusion procedure.
22. Applying AABB Standards, select appropriate blood for exchange transfusion.
23. Briefly discuss the use of simple transfusion of red cells for the correction of neonatal anemia.
24. Compare and contrast ABO-HDN with HDN associated with other blood group alloantibodies.
25. Describe the use of RhIG in the prevention of HDN due to anti-D.
26. Describe methods for screening and quantitation of fetal-maternal bleeds.
27. Given the fetal cell count per 1000 adult cells in a Kleihauer-Betke test, calculate the number of 300 μg doses of RhIG that should be administered to prevent maternal alloimmunization.
28. Discuss factors that can cause false-positive results in the Kleihauer-Betke stain.

OVERVIEW

Commonly known only as **hemolytic disease of the newborn** (HDN), this disease affects the fetus and is capable of causing in utero death. Fetal red blood cells leak into the maternal circulation, causing production of unexpected antibody, directed against one or more "foreign" antigens found on the fetal red cells. The IgG component of the antibody then crosses the placenta into the fetal circulation, causing destruction of the fetal red cells. This can result in varying degrees of anemia. The most severely affected fetus may develop cardiac failure, edema, and potentially death. The term *hemolytic disease of the newborn* developed because early treatment was limited to preterm delivery and treatment of the newborn; no techniques were available to reach the fetus and initiate treatment before delivery.

Later developments included recognition of the cause of the disease, methods to determine severity, early delivery of the infant, exchange transfusions, intrauterine transfusion, and finally prevention of the most common cause of severe disease: anti-D (Summary 16-1).

HDN involves alloimmunization of the mother to a red cell antigen (or antigens) found on the fetal red cells, and this is the primary focus of this chapter. Red cell alloimmunization is commonly divided into three types based on antibody specificity: (1) ABO; (2) Rh, anti-D alone or in combination (anti-CD, anti-DE, anti-CDE); and (3) other alloantibodies. In addition, mothers with warm autoimmune hemolytic anemia or IgG antibody directed against drugs that could be

Hemolytic disease of the newborn: A disease characterized by the destruction of fetal/newborn red cells resulting from the placental transfer of maternal alloantibody.

Summary 16-1

Landmarks in Treatment of Hemolytic Disease of the Newborn

1940–1941 Recognition of $Rh_o(D)$ antigen/antibody
1947–1951 Exchange transfusion
1952–1955 Preterm delivery
1956–1961 Amniocentesis and Liley graph
1963: Intraperitoneal Intrauterine transfusion
1968: Introduction of postdelivery RhIG
1984: Antenatal use of RhIG
1988: Intravascular intrauterine transfusion

Glucose-6-phosphate dehydrogenase (G6PD) deficiency: A deficiency of an enzyme in the pentose pathway associated with hepatomegaly, hypoglycemia, acidosis, decreased serum haptoglobin, and failure to thrive.

Thalassemia: An inherited anemia caused by the production of abnormal hemoglobin molecules.

Hereditary spherocytosis: An inherited disorder characterized by hemolysis, spherocytosis, anemia, jaundice, and splenomegaly.

Idiopathic thrombocytopenic purpura: Abnormally low numbers of circulating platelets of unknown origin.

Hydrops fetalis: A clinical condition in infants characterized by cardiac insufficiency with resultant edema and respiratory distress.

Icterus gravis neonatorum: Jaundice of the newborn resulting from accelerated red cell destruction.

Kernicterus: A grave condition resulting from the passage of bilirubin into the brain and spinal cord.

Extramedullary erythropoiesis: Production of red cells outside of the bone marrow.

Hepatosplenomegaly: Enlargement of the liver and spleen.

Erythroblastosis fetalis: A synonym for hemolytic disease of the newborn. The hemolytic disease is associated with anemia, jaundice, splenomegaly, edema, and the presence of immature red cells in the circulation (erythroblasts).

administered to the infant can cause very similar laboratory and clinical findings. Other causes of fetal or newborn hemolysis, associated anemia and hydrops, and/or jaundice include the following:

1. Genetic red cell membrane or enzyme deficiencies such as **glucose-6-phosphate dehydrogenase (G6PD) deficiency, thalassemia, hereditary spherocytosis,** and disorders of hemoglobin synthesis.[1,2]
2. Acquired defects of the red cells secondary to infections such as rubella, cytomegalovirus, human B19 parvovirus, and others.[1-5]
3. Prematurity and physiologic jaundice due to insufficient production of glucuronyl transferases.[6]

Mothers may also be immunized to cells other than red cells, such as platelets and granulocytes. The presence of maternal platelet alloantibody, or platelet autoantibody such as in **idiopathic thrombocytopenic purpura** cases, can cause severe bleeding in the fetus or newborn, which must be recognized and treated. Neutropenia in the newborn is more commonly related to sepsis than to alloimmunization of the mother, but it remains a possibility that is difficult if not impossible to prove.

Hemolysis caused by maternal red cell alloimmunization was recognized as early as the 1600s, and its various findings such as **hydrops fetalis, icterus gravis neonatorum,** and **kernicterus** were described in detail in the late 1890s and 1900s. Each was thought to define a distinct disease. Diamond and colleagues[7] showed that they are all aspects of the same condition, which is also characterized by hemolytic anemia, **extramedullary erythropoiesis, hepatosplenomegaly,** and an outpouring of nucleated red cells termed **erythroblastosis fetalis.** Levine and Stetson[8] first suggested fetal-maternal blood group incompatibility to explain the findings. It took the discovery of anti-Rh, later called anti-Rho or anti-D, by Landsteiner and Weiner,[9] as well as the findings of Levine and colleagues[10] recognizing the immunization process of the mother by the fetal red cells, to clarify the cause of the disease. Subsequently, many other blood group antigens have been found that are capable of causing varying degrees of severity of the same disease. Many of the known antigens were first described following delivery of an affected infant.

Anti-D is normally used as the model to describe this condition because historically it caused the most severe disease in the greatest number of women. However, with the advent of Rh immune globulin (RhIG), the number of cases has dramatically declined and the importance of other alloantibodies capable of causing the same disease has risen. The numbers of non-D alloantibodies found, excluding ABO, appear to be increasing.[11] This may be due to increased numbers of transfusions causing alloimmunization or to increased screening of Rh-positive mothers, often previously ignored.

Since the discovery of Rh-HDN in 1940, methods of treatment for the infant and then the fetus have been developed. These were followed by the introduction of RhIG for postpartum and then antepartum administration, which reduced the incidence of HDN due to anti-D from 13% to 0.2%,[12] a truly amazing medical advance.

Unfortunately, anti-D and other alloantibodies continue to cause the disease, and the blood bank, other laboratories, and physicians must continue to identify and treat these cases as they appear. Continuous communication and cooperation between the physician and the laboratory are mandatory to coordinate findings and plan interventions.

The disease has the following three prerequisites, which define the testing needed to recognize the disease and recommend treatment:

1. The mother must lack the antigen and be exposed to it by pregnancy or transfusion.
2. The fetus must have the antigen (inherited from the father) and the antigen must be well developed in utero.
3. The mother must produce IgG antibody of sufficient titer.

The severity of the disease can vary from mild (subclinical), requiring no treatment, to severe, requiring intervention as early as 18 to 20 weeks of gestational age.

It is theoretically possible that essentially all women could be immunized to some antigen the fetus possesses and the mother lacks, given the number of antigens known to exist. Fortunately, the actual proportion sensitized is only 10% to 15%, owing to such factors as variations in antigenic strength, ability to respond, number of exposures to the antigen(s), and other reasons (see next section).[13]

PATHOPHYSIOLOGY

The fertilized egg enters the uterine cavity and implants itself on the uterine wall. The placenta, the organ through which the fetus acquires all nutrients and excretes all wastes, forms the implantation point. The fetal blood vessels form the umbilical cord connecting the developing fetus to the placenta (Fig. 16-1). Within the placenta the fetal blood passes into many small villi (treelike structures containing fetal capillaries) separated from the maternal blood supply (a tiny pocket or sac of blood) by a thin membrane. This membrane allows passage of oxygen, nutrients, and waste product molecules. Larger molecules and intact cells do not cross the intact membrane (Fig. 16-2). This membrane can be ruptured relatively easily, because it is only about two cells thick. Implantation may be incomplete or the placenta malformed, or abdominal trauma (blows to the abdominal area, auto accidents, falls, amniocentesis) may damage the placental membranes, causing the rupture of one or more of the villi or intravillous spaces. This can allow fetal cells to cross into the maternal circulation (termed **fetal-maternal hemorrhage**) during the pregnancy, exposing the mother to "foreign" fetal antigens. The reverse type of bleed, mother to fetus, is possible but less likely to happen owing to the relatively higher pressures on the fetal side of the membrane. More commonly exposure occurs when the placenta shears off or separates from the uterine wall at delivery[11] (Fig. 16-3). This disrupts the fetal circulation in the villi, allowing more fetal cells to enter the maternal circulation.

Fetal red cells are formed as early as 2 to 3 weeks of gestational age, and by 9 weeks red cell production is well established in the liver and beginning in the bone marrow spaces. Most blood group antigens are well developed and fully expressed as early as 10 to 12 weeks; exceptions include ABO, I, P_1, Lewis, Cartwright, and others.[13-16] When the fetus has inherited paternal genes coding for production of antigens that the mother lacks, the potential for HDN exists.

Passage of fetal red cells into the maternal circulation allows recognition by the mother's **reticuloendothelial (RE) system** of the "foreign" red cells. Primary sensitization involves recognition of the foreign antigen, processing by the

Fetal-maternal hemorrhage: The passage of red cells from the maternal to the fetal circulation as a result of placental trauma or at delivery.

Reticuloendothelial (RE) system: A system of phagocytic cells in the liver, spleen, and bone marrow that are involved in the destruction of antibody-coated cells in disorders such as hemolytic disease of the newborn. The RE system is discussed in detail in Chapter 2.

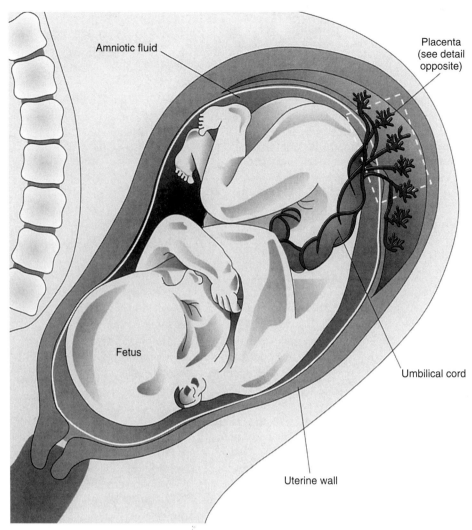

Fig. 16-1 Pregnancy: the fetus and placenta. *(From Blood Group Antigens and Antibodies as Applied to Hemolytic Disease of the Newborn. Ortho Diagnostics Systems, Inc., Raritan, NJ, 1968.)*

Responders: Individuals who produce antibody when stimulated by foreign antigen.

lymphocytes, and finally antibody production in those women who are **responders.** The ability to respond and produce antibody is likely an inherited characteristic.[13] It is affected by the dose (volume) of antigen presented, the phenotype (the fetal red cells are always heterozygous for causative antigen), the ability of the antigen to cause a response, how often the antigen is presented (multiple small bleeds versus one major bleed), and whether fetal cells are ABO compatible with the maternal serum.[13]

The time factor in primary sensitization and the fact that only IgG antibody can cross the placenta are the major reasons why severe HDN is rare in the first pregnancy. Succeeding antigen-positive pregnancies are at far greater risk. Major fetal-maternal bleeds usually occur at delivery. Thus the **primary immune response** occurs after the first delivery of an antigen-positive child. During the second or succeeding antigen-positive pregnancies, even very small leaks of fetal red cells can cause a **secondary (anamnestic) antibody response** in the mother.

Primary immune response: The characteristics of the immune response to the first or primary antigen presentation.

Secondary (anamnestic) antibody response: The characteristics of the immune response to a second or subsequent exposure to a specific antigen. This response varies from the primary response with regard to time, titer, antibody class, and antibody affinity and avidity.

These IgG antibodies cross the placental barrier, enter the fetal circulation, and attach to the specific antigen on the fetal red cells. The red cells are then removed by the Fc receptors of the macrophages within the fetal spleen and liver. The bilirubin (indirect fraction) produced by the degradation of the hemoglobin is excreted via the placenta to the maternal circulation, where it is converted to the water-soluble form (direct fraction) and excreted by the mother (Fig. 16-4).

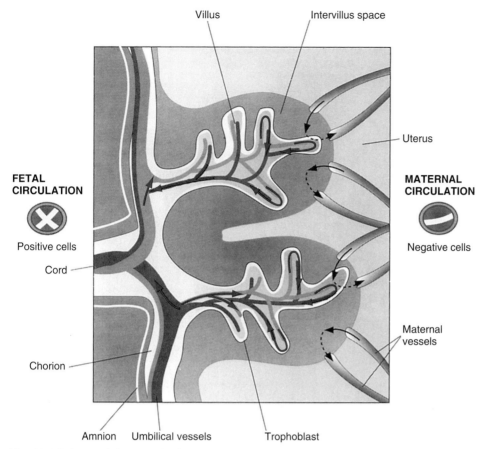

Fig. 16-2 Scheme of placental circulation. *Arrows* depict separate routes of fetal and maternal circulations within the placenta. *Dotted lines* represent oxygen, nutrient, and waste exchange through the placental barrier. *(From Blood Group Antigens and Antibodies as Applied to Hemolytic Disease of the Newborn. Ortho Diagnostics Systems, Inc., Raritan, NJ, 1968.)*

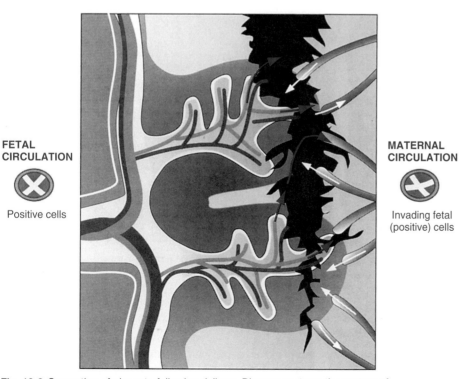

Fig. 16-3 Separation of placenta following delivery. Diagram portrays the rupture of placental vessels (villi) and connective tissue, allowing escape of fetal blood cells. *(From Blood Group Antigens and Antibodies as Applied to Hemolytic Disease of the Newborn. Ortho Diagnostics Systems, Inc., Raritan, NJ, 1968.)*

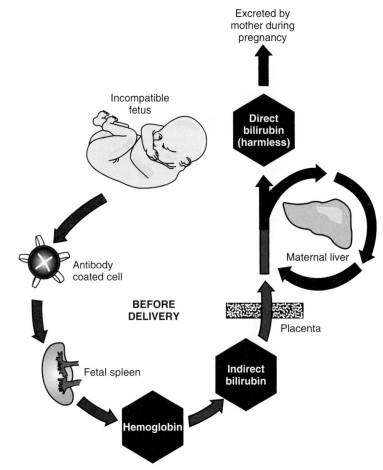

Fig. 16-4 Metabolism of bilirubin antepartum. Bilirubin produced in the fetal spleen passes via the placenta to the maternal circulation and to the mother's liver, where it is converted to excretable direct bilirubin. *(From Blood Group Antigens and Antibodies as Applied to Hemolytic Disease of the Newborn. Ortho Diagnostics Systems, Inc., Raritan, NJ, 1968.)*

Hypoxia: Insufficient delivery of oxygen to the tissues.

Portal hypertension: Increased pressure in the portal vein, which delivers blood to the liver. This is commonly due to some obstruction of blood flow through the liver.

Ascites: An accumulation of fluid in the peritoneal cavity, often associated with obstruction of the portal vein.

Hepatocellular damage: Damage to cells of the liver.

Hypoalbuminemia: Decreased serum albumin levels.

Edema: A general term for the accumulation of fluid in the tissues.

As the level of maternal IgG antibody increases, the fetus becomes more anemic owing to increased red cell destruction. Erythropoiesis (red cell production) is increased, and more immature red cells are released into the fetal circulation (erythroblastosis fetalis). As the demand for red cells increases, both the liver and spleen again begin to produce red cells (extramedullary erythropoiesis). Both organs become enlarged (hepatosplenomegaly) as a result of the need to produce red cells and the need to remove the damaged (antibody-coated) red cells.

Progressive anemia causes tissue **hypoxia.** This in turn triggers increased cardiac output and fluid and salt retention by the kidneys. The hepatic involvement leads to **portal hypertension** with development of **ascites, hepatocellular damage** producing **hypoalbuminemia,** and generalized **edema** (hydrops fetalis).[11]

At birth the infants are anemic but *not* jaundiced. Up until birth, the bilirubin has been processed and excreted by the mother's liver. After birth the infant must process bilirubin by itself (Fig. 16-5). The infant liver usually cannot process the bilirubin adequately owing to lack of sufficient levels of glucuronyl transferase to convert indirect to direct bilirubin, and jaundice develops (icterus gravis neonatorum).[17] Indirect bilirubin is normally bound to albumin within the circulation. When the level of bilirubin exceeds the binding capacity of the albumin, it builds up in the body tissues and may cross the blood-brain barrier, precipitating within the basal ganglion and causing permanent brain damage (kernicterus).

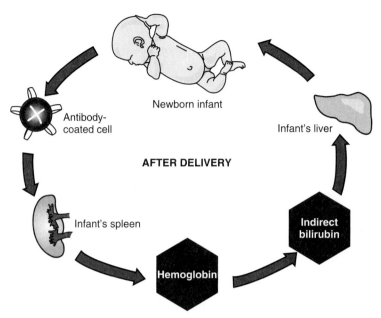

Fig. 16-5 Metabolism of bilirubin following delivery. The liver of the neonate does not produce enough glucuronyl transferase and cannot convert all the bilirubin to an excretable form. Consequently, bilirubin accumulates in tissues, causing jaundice and brain tissue damage. *(From Blood Group Antigens and Antibodies as Applied to Hemolytic Disease of the Newborn. Ortho Diagnostics Systems, Inc., Raritan, NJ, 1968.)*

Treatment can be instituted either **antepartum** or **postpartum.** Antepartum treatment focuses on the anemia and involves early delivery if gestational age and lung development allow or **intrauterine transfusions** (IUTs), either intraperitoneal or intravascular. Postpartum treatment focuses on the bilirubin levels and only secondarily on the anemia and involves exchange transfusions. The decision about the type of intervention and the timing relies on laboratory test results and clinical findings.

Antepartum: Before delivery.

Postpartum: After delivery.

Intrauterine transfusion: Treatment of fetal anemia by the transfusion of blood to the fetus. Blood can be infused into the peritoneal cavity, from which it is absorbed by the fetus, or can be administered directly into the umbilical vein.

PRENATAL TESTING OF THE MOTHER
Initial Testing

Initial testing is usually ordered during the first prenatal visit and includes ABO grouping, Rh typing including weak D (D^u), and antibody screening. The initial ABO grouping is a blood bank routine but yields little or no information concerning the potential for ABO-HDN. In fact, no good laboratory tests are available to predict ABO-HDN even though we are often asked to do so[16] (see section on ABO-HDN). Determination of the D and weak D (D^u) status of the mother determines the need for antepartum RhIG administration and helps clarify the weak D(D^u) findings at delivery.

The **antibody screening** serves to detect most red cell alloantibodies the mother may have circulating in her serum, both IgM and IgG. Anti-Le^a and anti-I are commonly found IgM antibodies, but they do not cross the placenta or cause HDN. The antibody screening does not detect all alloantibodies such as those directed against low-frequency antigens and other antigens not represented on the antibody screening cells and therefore is not totally foolproof. HDN can develop whenever IgG antibody is formed and is detected either by appropriate monitoring by the physician in charge of the case or at, or immediately following, delivery. Antibody screening is routinely repeated at about 28 weeks of gestational age on Rh-D and weak D (D^u) negative mothers before or concomitant with the administration of RhIG. Unfortunately, Rh-positive mothers are often not tested

Refer to Chapter 11 for a discussion of the **antibody screening** procedure.

again until delivery, when they sometimes are found to have had undetected alloantibody production during the pregnancy and an affected infant. Fortunately, unless the antibody is formed as part of secondary response (recall of previously stimulated antibody) rather than initial stimulation, the infant is not severely affected but may only require treatment such as **phototherapy**[17] or even, more rarely, **exchange transfusions.**

One note of caution: If a weak anti-D is detected in the Rh-negative mother, check her history very carefully to determine if she has received antepartum RhIG for any reason such as an amniocentesis done early in pregnancy for genetic reasons or for abdominal trauma from a fall or auto accident. These women should receive repeat doses of RhIG at 12-week intervals until delivery, and thus anti-D, which has been passively administered, may be detected at 28 weeks or at delivery. In these cases, additional RhIG is required if the baby is Rh positive (see section on RhIG).

Identification

Once an antibody has been detected in the prenatal patient, it must be identified. The *specificity* of the antibody determines its clinical significance to the fetus as well as to the mother. As noted earlier, antibodies such as I, P_1, Sd^a, Lewis, Chido, Rodgers, Lutheran, and Cartwright seldom cause HDN due to either the presence of soluble antigen in the fetal circulation or depressed development of the antigen on the fetal and newborn red cells.

Ig Class

The Ig class of the antibody determines whether an antibody is IgM or IgG. Certain antibodies known to occur without red cell stimulation, such as anti-M, anti-E, and anti-S, must be investigated using **dithiothreitol (DTT)** or **2-mercaptoethanol (2-ME),** which cleave the disulfide bonds within each antibody structure. The IgM agglutinating activity is removed. IgG antibody is still detectable and can be titered, assuming that care is taken in the testing phases. The IgG portion of the antibody is capable of causing HDN, and the antibody must be proven to be totally IgM to be ignored. Repeat testing every 6 weeks is strongly recommended to ensure that the antibody remains totally IgM.

Determining the **IgG subclass** (IgG1, IgG2, IgG3, or IgG4) can, to some degree, determine the clinical significance of the antibody. All IgG antibodies cross the placenta. IgG1 and IgG3 are the most clinically significant because they are able to cause sensitized red cells to adhere to the Fc receptors on macrophages, with possible hemolysis resulting.[18,19] IgG1 antibody crosses the placenta much earlier, potentially resulting in more red cell destruction in utero and therefore lower cord hemoglobin levels at birth. Antibodies of class IgG3 cross the placenta in lesser quantity during pregnancy and do not reach the levels of IgG1 in the fetal circulation, resulting in lower levels of fetal red cell destruction and higher cord hemoglobin levels at birth. However, the rate of bilirubin rise due to increased red cell destruction after birth is much higher, reflecting the higher potential for hemolysis by this subclass.[14,19] Although subclassifying the IgG antibody can furnish useful information, conflicting results in various studies plus difficulty in doing the testing have limited its use.[18]

Maternal History

Maternal history is of importance to the outcome and timing of intervention. Women with previously affected infants usually have equally or more severely affected infants in the succeeding antigen-positive pregnancy, so intervention may be necessary at an earlier gestational age.[11] A history of previous transfusions may have sensitized the woman or caused overt production of alloantibody(ies), but their importance will depend on the specificity and fetal antigen status.

Phototherapy: The use of light to degrade bilirubin in mildly jaundiced infants.

Exchange transfusion: The simultaneous withdrawal of blood and infusion of compatible donor blood to infants with hemolytic disease of the newborn. The procedure removes antigen-positive cells, provides cells that are compatible with maternal antibodies, decreases bilirubin levels, and corrects anemia.

Dithiothreitol (DTT), 2-mercaptoethanol (2-ME): Dithiothreitol (DTT) is a potent reducing agent that cleaves the intersubunit disulfide bonds of IgM molecules, thereby abolishing both agglutinating and complement-binding properties of the molecule. 2-Mercaptoethanol can also be used for this purpose. It is important to remember that DTT inactivates antigens in the Kell system. Refer to Chapter 12 for a discussion of DTT techniques. Refer to Chapter 2 for a discussion of immunoglobulin structure and function.

Ig subclass: Heavy chain structural differences that result in distinctive functional differences in the Ig class. IgG, for example, has four distinctive subclasses. Refer to Chapter 2 for a discussion of Ig structure and function.

Inheritance

Testing of the father (not necessarily the husband of the mother) of the fetus is essential. This often involves some delicate questioning of the mother and on occasion the involved man. In laboratories that specialize in prenatal testing, this is often the role of the technologist. In most cases except D, the zygosity of the father can be determined and the probability of the fetus possessing the antigen determined. In the case of D, the most probable genotype can be predicted.

If the father lacks the antigen entirely and the presence of the alloantibody can be explained by prior pregnancies by another consort and/or transfusions, the woman can be released to normal prenatal care. Otherwise, the only concern is transfusion for the mother if she requires blood at delivery. If the father is unavailable or unwilling to be tested, the assumption is made that the fetus is antigen positive until proven otherwise. Of note is the increase of in vitro fertilization, which raises the issue of the blood types of the egg and/or sperm donor, and therefore the fetal antigen status, when the woman who is carrying the fetus has alloantibody(ies).[20]

Testing the Fetus

Many advances have been made in determining the fetal blood type using several different approaches with varying degrees of risk to the mother and/or the fetus, including **amniocentesis, chorionic villi** sampling, and **cordocentesis**. The former two procedures yield cellular material allowing for genetic testing using polymerase chain reaction (PCR) amplification methods and the latter a fetal blood sample for serologic determination of antigen type, as well as other important parameters (see later sections). All of these approaches are invasive, carry an inherent risk for spontaneous miscarriage, and/or have potential for increasing the antibody titer and specificities.[17] This could lead to increased severity of the disease should the fetus prove positive for the antigen(s) in question.

Most recently, progress has been made in obtaining fetal DNA (rather than fetal cells) from maternal plasma using PCR amplification test methods.[21] Expertise in testing and interpretation and careful controls are required.[22] Controls should include maternal and paternal blood samples run in parallel. However, fetal DNA may not be present or detectable in every instance. The advantage is that it is noninvasive.

Amniocentesis: The aspiration of fluid from the sac surrounding the fetus (amniotic sac).

Chorionic villi: A branching, vascular process of the embryonic membrane forming part of the placenta.

Cordocentesis: The technique of obtaining blood from the umbilical cord vein.

ASSESSING RISK TO FETUS/INFANT
Titration

Although **titer** results are held in low regard by some physicians, standardized reproducible titers do give information on the probable severity of HDN. The major need is for each institution to use one standard method and correlate its titer results with the actual outcomes, that is, the clinical condition of the infant at birth. Titrations are most valuable in the pregnancy when the antibody is first detected. Studies done early in the pregnancy establish a baseline value for comparison and assess the potential need for more invasive procedures.[22] Serial twofold dilutions of the maternal serum are tested against a single-source red cell suspension that possesses the antigen.[17] Variables can include the following:

1. Choice of test cell: homozygous versus heterozygous; or R_2R_2 versus R_1R_1 versus R_oR_o for anti-D, anti-CD, anti-DE, or anti-CDE. The same test cell should be used throughout a given pregnancy. Therefore using cells freshly drawn from a walking donor are best for each antibody titer done. In the case of low-frequency antigens or multiple antibody, possibly the best choice is the father if he is ABO compatible with the maternal serum.
2. Media: saline, albumin, low ionic strength solution, and antiglobulin give different answers.

Titer: The highest dilution at which agglutination can be detected. Titration procedures in antibody identification are discussed in Chapter 12. Titers of maternal antibody are used as indicators of the course and severity of hemolytic disease of the newborn.

3. Temperature and time of incubation.
4. Techniques: single pipette, change pipette with each tube, automatic pipette, volume of serum or dilution to be tested, and percentage of test cells and their suspending media.

Variables can be controlled reasonably well, especially when a single donor's cells are used rather than commercial panel or screening cells. The intertechnologist reliability is the hardest to control. By using a check-off in which a new technologist duplicates the procedure, variation can be controlled. A second control is also required. The previous serum sample is repeated when the new sample is titered. Comparisons of both samples show whether the amount of circulating antibody is increasing, stable, or falling. Titers are repeated every 4 weeks to detect any changes. Some physicians prefer to perform them every 2 weeks in the third trimester.

A rising titer usually indicates maternal response to stimulus from antigen-positive fetal cells leaking across the placenta. On occasion, maternal antibody increases even though the infant is shown to lack the antigen. The reason for these findings is not known. When titers are high at the beginning of a pregnancy owing to preformed antibody, changes are difficult to detect and have much less meaning because critical titer levels usually have been exceeded.

A **critical titer** is defined as that titer at or below which there have been no stillbirths or severely affected infants. This value should be established by each laboratory using its own titer values and evaluating an infant's cord hemoglobin levels and clinical condition at and immediately following delivery. Even then some antibodies are so rare that there are not enough investigated cases on which to rely. In these instances, 32 is often a good titer value to work with for the majority of antibodies. This seems to be a reliable method and one often used in the reported literature.[15,16,22-25] In women with previously affected infants, lower values, as low as 8, may be used to indicate when further intervention is needed. This is especially true of anti-K because it has been reported to inhibit growth of K+ erythroid progenitor cells.[22]

Even when a titer is established as a reliable tool, problems remain. An increase of only one tube or a score of less than 10 is usually caused by one of the previously discussed procedural variables. Stable titers below the critical level usually indicate an antigen-negative infant, and further, more invasive intervention is not indicated. Low titers that increase two tubes (score of 10) indicate a good probability of an antigen-positive child who could be affected. Until critical levels are reached, however, more invasive procedures should not be performed, primarily because of the risks involved, such as the following:

1. Risk of immunization and/or increase in maternal antibody titer if fetal cells gain direct access to maternal circulation owing to placental damage.
2. Injury to the fetus: usually minor scratches, but direct puncture could cause injury or fetal death.
3. Damage to the placenta or umbilical cord, premature labor, rupture of the membrane of the sac, hematoma in placenta or cord, overt hemorrhage, and/or infection.

Amniocentesis

Amniocentesis, developed in 1956 but not applied to HDN until 1961, involves insertion of a needle through the mother's abdominal wall, penetration of the amniotic sac, and withdrawal of a small amount of fluid for analysis. The positions of the fetus and the placenta are determined by **ultrasonography** so that damage to either by the needle can be avoided. This procedure is normally used for genetic counseling, bilirubin level determinations (ΔOD450), and **fetal lung maturity** studies.

Initially amniocentesis was the most accurate predictor of the fetal condition. Amniotic fluid is produced by the fetal gastrointestinal tract, lungs, kidneys, and

Critical titer: That titer at or below which no severely affected infants or stillbirths have been reported. This value is determined by data from the institution. If no data are available, a titer of 32 is often used as a benchmark.

Ultrasonography: Using high-frequency, inaudible sound (approximately 20,000 cycles per second) to produce an image of an organ or tissue based on the fact that ultrasound waves move at different velocities in tissues of differing elasticity and density.

Fetal lung maturity: A measure of the ability to inflate alveolar spaces and allow oxygen transport to red blood cells, which is related to the production of pulmonary surfactant (lipids). Lung maturity is often monitored using the lecithin/sphingomyelin (L/S) ratio. Other tests for fetal lung maturity include phosphatidylglycerol.

amniotic membrane. The volume of fluid increases steadily up to 36 to 37 weeks of gestational age and then remains relatively stable. Conditions in which too little or too much fluid is produced usually are linked to fetal kidney problems. The fetus is constantly swallowing and inhaling the fluid throughout the pregnancy. The fetus is totally surrounded and floats within the fluid; therefore the fluid contains cells of various origins.

Because of the cells present, it is possible to do genetic determinations by culturing the cells found in the fluid. However, the testing cannot be done before gestational age of 12 weeks, when enough fluid is present to culture and sufficient time is available (10 days to 4 weeks) to obtain results. Cordocentesis, direct sampling of fetal blood from the umbilical cord, allows 48-hour culture reports of chromosome analysis but must wait until gestational age of 16 to 18 weeks, when the vessels are large enough to visualize and enter (see following section).[2,26]

Amniocentesis to evaluate HDN is typically done at gestational age of 18 to 20 weeks, when medical intervention is feasible. Treatment, when indicated, usually consists of either intravascular or intraperitoneal transfusions. Amniocentesis has similar risk factors (miscarriage or fetal loss[26]) to those associated with cordocentesis but is technically easier and the placenta can be avoided more easily. Therefore, after titration studies, it is used as the second tool to evaluate HDN. The amount of bilirubin found in the amniotic fluid relates reasonably well with the amount of red cell destruction occurring in the fetus. Both chemical and spectrophotometric analyses have been used to determine the amount of bilirubin pigment in the fluid. Spectrophotometry is currently the accepted method used in conjunction with Liley's[27] graphs, which relate optical density of the fluid at 450 nm to fetal hemoglobin levels when delivery is within 7 to 10 days. These graphs have been modified to extend them to earlier gestational age as experience has grown with evaluating younger fetuses (Fig. 16-6). It should be noted that bilirubin values obtained by chemical means are not usable on the Liley graph, which was designed for ΔOD450 values.

Normally a scanning spectrophotometer is used to measure the light absorbance of the fluid over a range from around 300 nm to 600 to 650 nm. Normal fluids from unsensitized women have a smooth curve from 650 nm to 315 nm. Remember that a normal level of bilirubin is found in amniotic fluid owing to routine destruction of "old" red cells. In HDN cases, an elevation in the amount present forms a peak at 450 nm, the point at which bilirubin pigment's light absorbance is maximum. The difference or change at 450 nm is the ΔOD450 value. An extrapolated "normal" line is drawn, usually between 375 nm and 525 nm, and the height (change or Δ) in absorbance at 450 nm is calculated (Fig. 16-7). This value is then plotted against gestational age of the fetus on a Liley graph, which is a semilog graph, to predict the probable severity of disease at that moment in time. Predictions correlate well with cord hemoglobin levels if delivery or intervention occurs within 1 week. Note that the dividing lines angle downward as gestational age increases (see Fig. 16-6). This is primarily a dilutional effect as the volume of fluid increases with gestational age.

Single-point values above 0.3 require immediate intervention, IUT if gestational age is less than 32 weeks and delivery if gestational age is greater than 32 weeks and fetal lung maturity has been demonstrated. Values below this require repeat testing to establish a trend that is predictive. Sharp increases in zone II or into zone III usually require immediate intervention. The presence of plateaus or identical values over increasing gestational age is a danger sign, usually requiring weekly or more frequent repeat testing to evaluate the fetal condition. Decreasing values may indicate an antigen-negative fetus or a mildly affected antigen-positive fetus and allow greater intervals between tests, but unless they decrease sharply into the lower portion of zone I the infant may still be clinically affected by HDN and require exchange transfusion after delivery.

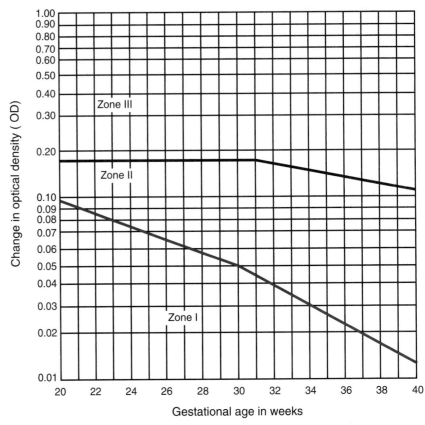

Fig. 16-6 Liley graph (modified). *(From Buck SA: Hemolytic disease of the newborn. In Harmening D (ed): Modern Blood Banking and Transfusion Practice, 2nd ed. Philadelphia, FA Davis, 1989, p 323.)*

L/S ratio: Levels of two phospholipid surfactants found in the amniotic fluid. As the fetal lung matures, the lecithin levels increase and the sphingomyelin remains constant. An L/S ratio of greater than 2.0 is a good predictor of fetal lung maturity.

Kleihauer-Betke stain: A technique used to quantitate fetal-maternal hemorrhage based on the fact that fetal hemoglobin is resistant to acid elution, whereas adult hemoglobin is not. Estimates of fetal bleed are made from counts of fetal cells per 1000 adult cells in a sample of maternal blood.

Meconium: The first stool produced by a newborn.

Vernix: The deposit that covers the fetus during intrauterine life.

Several factors associated with amniotic fluid analysis can affect test results:[28]

1. Turbidity: This can usually be solved by high-speed centrifugation as long as the sample is not to be used to determine fetal lung maturity because the rupture of cells in the fluid can affect the lecithin/sphingomyelin **(L/S) ratios.**

2. Blood: The presence of a few red cells rarely affects results. If more than 5% of the sample is red cells, two problems are created: Hemoglobin peaks on the scan at 580, 540, and 415 nm, which obscure and falsely elevate the $\Delta OD450$, and the contamination with serum bilirubin can also falsely elevate the findings. Maternal blood with normal serum bilirubin levels only marginally affects the value, but fetal blood with its increased bilirubin levels invalidates the results. To determine the source of the blood (mother or fetus), a **Kleihauer–Betke stain** or related tests are used. This stain is based on the fact that adult hemoglobin (A) elutes easily from the red cells in an acid environment, whereas fetal hemoglobin (F, the primary type found in the fetal circulation) resists elution. If the cells are fetal in origin, the remaining red cells can be typed or otherwise tested if not previously done during cordocentesis. Clearance of blood usually takes between 1 and 2 weeks. Blood in the amniotic fluid can be due to placental damage during the procedure, fetal injury from the needle, or antepartum bleeding.

3. **Meconium:** This substance is a green, viscous, semisolid material usually found in the fetal intestine consisting of mucopolysaccharide, squamous cells, fetal hair, **vernix,** and cholesterol. Meconium imparts a green color to the fluid and has an absorbance between 415 and 405 nm on scan. The presence of this pigment invalidates the test, often completely obscuring

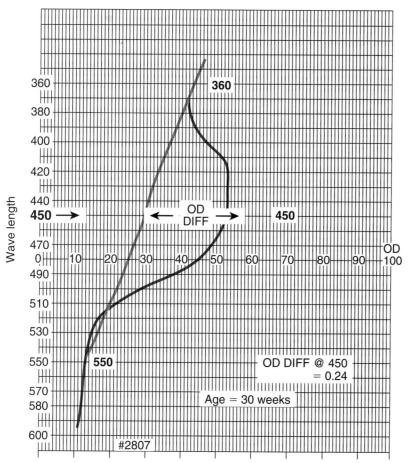

Fig. 16-7 Spectral scan of bilirubin in amniotic fluid. *(From Buck SA: Hemolytic disease of the newborn. In Harmening D (ed): Modern Blood Banking and Transfusion Practice, 2nd ed. Philadelphia, FA Davis, 1989, p 322.)*

the 450 nm peak. When present late in pregnancy, it usually indicates fetal distress and should be immediately reported to the physician. It is occasionally seen early in pregnancy, but the significance of this finding is unknown. Meconium is usually cleared from the fluid in 2 to 3 weeks.

4. Light: Visible light and ultraviolet light degrade bilirubin. Exposure of the fluid to winter sunlight results in half the bilirubin being degraded within 12 to 18 minutes. Fluorescent light degrades the bilirubin by one half in about 10 hours. Therefore amniotic fluid is immediately placed in amber glass or plastic containers at collection and protected from all light exposure until the scan is complete.

5. Dilution: Usually **polyhydramnios** can easily be noted on ultrasound examination and gives false-low values. This can be overcome by using cordocentesis (see next section).

> **Polyhydramnios:** An excessive amount of amniotic fluid.

6. Other fluids: Ascitic fluid from the fetal abdomen or urine from the fetus or mother may, rarely, be obtained by accident. Urine has a distinctive curve, and creatinine values on urine greatly exceed amniotic fluid values. Ascitic fluid has much deeper pigmentation than amniotic fluid. The use of real-time ultrasonography to guide the amniocentesis has essentially eliminated these problems.

7. Multiple sacs: In multiple pregnancies, great care must be taken by the physician to obtain fluid from each sac so that each infant is evaluated separately, because marked differences between infants may occur.

One final note is that titer studies and repeat antibody identifications should be continued following amniocentesis or cordocentesis procedures. New antibodies can be initiated by the procedures and titer levels can rise significantly. The physician needs to be warned of these possible sequelae.

Percutaneous Umbilical Blood Sampling or Cordocentesis

If indicated by titer or amniotic fluid ΔOD450 values, direct sampling of the fetal blood can be done to determine antigen type and hemoglobin level. A description of the technique and indications for the procedure are available elsewhere.[2,3,26] Before performing percutaneous umbilical blood sampling (PUBS), a donor blood unit should be prepared and ready for transfusion so treatment can be immediate and fetal risk lessened.[17] The collected blood sample is assessed for purity (to ensure that it is fetal blood) by any of several methods. One method is to test the sample on an automated cell counter, which produces a histogram of the mean corpuscular volume. Fetal cells measure in the 118 to 135 fL range, and distinct differences from maternal mean corpuscular volume, can be seen as a mixed population. Other methods (such as the **Apt test**[29]) are available but destroy the sample.

After determining purity, the same sample can be typed for ABO, Rh, or other implicated antigens, and a direct antiglobulin test (DAT) can be performed if indicated. Very rarely, heavily antibody-coated red cells give false-negative reactions, especially in the Rh system when protein-fortified antisera are used. Use of chemically modified antisera or saline-reactive (usually IgM antibody) reagents yields the correct type. Given the maternal antibody identification and the presence of a positive DAT, it can readily be inferred that the fetus is antigen positive. If the fetus is proven to be antigen negative, no further testing needs to be done on the mother. If the fetus is antigen positive, the same sample can be used to determine the fetal hemoglobin, which may have already been accomplished if purity was measured on the cell counter. If significant anemia is present, intervention is an intrauterine transfusion. If no significant anemia is present, follow-up is done with serial amniocentesis for ΔOD450 and ultrasound evaluations.

INTERVENTION
Intrauterine Transfusion

The objective of an IUT is to treat the fetal anemia. Bilirubinemia is not a problem in utero. After IUT, the transfused antigen-negative donor red cells survive normally, ensuring good oxygenation of the fetal tissues. Tissue hypoxia is reduced and the excess fluid accumulation starts to clear, decreasing the possibility of heart failure. Fetal red cell production is suppressed, so less destruction occurs. With the reduced red cell production and destruction, the liver and spleen gradually return to normal size.

Before 32 weeks and/or when the fetal lung is not mature enough to handle oxygen transportation, IUTs are used to treat the anemia. Intraperitoneal IUTs were introduced by Liley[30] in 1963. They involve the placement of a needle and catheter into the peritoneal space of the fetus, with infusion of packed red cells directly into that space. The necessary volumes are based on gestational age and estimated blood volume.[28] Because the fetal hemoglobin is not known, the volume administered and the timing for future transfusions is based on experience and ΔOD450 values. One rule of thumb used is (gestational age − 20) × 10 = mL of donor red cells required.

Example

A 24-week fetus:

$$24 - 20 = 4 \times 10 = 40 \text{ mL}$$

Fetal absorption of the red cells occurs via the lymphatic duct. Absorption is about 10% to 12% per day but can be more variable if the fetus is hydropic with

Apt test: Mix one part bloody fluid with five parts water. Supernatant must be pink to proceed. Mix five parts supernatant with one part 1% (0.25 N) NaOH. Centrifuge 2 minutes. Pink = fetal blood. Yellow/brown = maternal blood. Adult hemoglobin is less resistant to alkali denaturation than is fetal hemoglobin and is converted to alkaline globin hematin.

ascites.[11] The IUT is repeated at 2- to 3-week intervals to compensate for fetal growth and concomitant increase in blood volume and O_2 transport needs. Early IUTs may be slightly closer together than later ones, because initially there is continuing fetal red cell destruction, which lessens as more donor cells, resistant to destruction, are administered. Expertise in doing intraperitoneal IUTs needs to be maintained because intravascular transfusion is not always possible owing to maternal size, placental placement, and/or fetal size and position.

Intravascular transfusions are the preferred method because the infusion is directly into the umbilical vein. Also, the volume of blood needed can be precisely determined using the pretransfusion hemoglobin, the donor blood hemoglobin, the desired posttransfusion hemoglobin, and the estimated fetoplacental blood volume.[26,31] Volumes of transfused red cells can vary from 20 to 175 mL based on these parameters. Fetal red cell destruction is estimated at 0.3 g/dL (3 g/L) per day, so future transfusions can be planned to maintain the hemoglobin level at 10 g/dL (100 g/L). Once initiated, transfusions are continued until delivery. Other conditions that have been treated with IUTs include parvovirus infections, large fetal-maternal hemorrhage, and α-thalassemia.[17]

Regardless of the type of procedure planned, the availability of a fetal blood sample to determine the fetal ABO group and Rh type may allow use of blood other than group O Rh negative. However, most centers continue to use group O negative unless the parents are adamant about using maternal blood or a directed donor or the antibody specificity necessitates Rh-positive red cells. Certain requirements remain regardless of the source of the blood:[17,32]

1. The red cells must be negative for the antigen(s) corresponding to the specific antibody(ies), including ABO, found in the maternal serum *and* crossmatch compatible with maternal serum.

2. Donors should be group O or the same group as the maternal and fetal blood group (e.g., mother and fetus are both group A). The blood must be Rh negative if the child is negative or the antibody is anti-D. Rh-positive blood may be used if it is compatible with the mother's antibody(ies) and the baby is Rh positive.

3. **CMV-negative blood** is required by most neonatologists to prevent infection/reinfection of the infant.[24] Red blood cells leukocyte reduced by filtration are an acceptable substitute in most cases.

4. Blood must be irradiated to prevent **graft–versus–host disease** because the fetus is considered to be immunologically "naive." All subsequent blood and cellular components transfused in the neonatal period must also be irradiated.

5. Frozen/deglycerolized or fresh (less than 7 days of age) washed packed red cells, with hematocrit of 80% to 90%, should be used. Blood with hematocrit above 90% is too thick to infuse, and mechanical damage to the cells may occur when they are forced through the small-bore catheter. Fresh washed cells have better oxygen transport, lower K^+ levels, and no plasma or anticoagulant, and the high hematocrit lessens the chance of volume overload.

6. Blood should be negative for hemoglobin S to prevent the donor blood from sickling in the low oxygen tensions found in the fetal circulation.

7. If maternal red cells are used, they must be washed or frozen/deglycerolized to remove antibody-containing plasma.

8. The father and his direct relatives should not be donors for IUT, exchange, or simple transfusions because they possess the antigen and possibly other undetected antigens to which the mother may have produced antibody, especially **HLA** antibodies that are not detectable by routine red cell testing and probably would not be detected by compatibility testing.[33]

CMV-negative blood: Negative for the antibody to the cytomegalovirus (CMV). CMV-negative blood is preferred for immunocompromised recipients to decrease the risk of infection. Low risk of CMV transmission can also be accomplished by leukocyte reduction (less than 5×10^6 white blood cells).

Graft-versus-host disease (GVHD): The pathologic condition that develops when immunocompetent cells from a donor engraft in a recipient and recognize the recipient tissues as foreign. GVHD is further discussed in Chapter 8.

HLA: Human leukocyte antigen.

Early Delivery

Mild to moderate HDN can now be accurately determined using amniotic fluid analysis and/or PUBS. This obviates the necessity for early delivery with its attendant risks of respiratory distress syndrome.[13] Technical expertise in IUTs allows even the severely affected infant to deliver nearer term rather than at 30 to 34 weeks. The L/S ratio and detection of phosphatidyl glycerol indicate that the lungs are mature and ready to inflate and transport O_2. However, greater gestational development is now possible. Again, exchange transfusions are used as needed postpartum.

IMMEDIATE POSTPARTUM PERIOD

Hemoglobin and bilirubin values obtained from the cord blood best define the extent of disease and the need and urgency of intervention (normal cord blood hemoglobin range is 13 to 19 g/dL, 130 to 190 g/L). Venous or heel-stick hemoglobin values vary widely (range, 14 to 22 g/dL, 140 to 220 g/L), primarily owing to the presence or absence and volume of placental blood "transfused" to the infant at delivery. The volume can vary from less than 75 mL to 125 mL, depending on the position of the infant during delivery (above or below the placenta) and the time when the cord is clamped. This makes it more difficult to determine the need for exchange versus simple transfusions.[1,13]

The concern after birth is primarily hyperbilirubinemia and secondarily the degree of anemia, especially if intrauterine transfusions have been done. The rate of rise in the bilirubin level, the degree of anemia, and other factors are used to establish the need for and timing of exchange transfusion.

A cord hemoglobin above 14 g/dL (140 g/L) indicates mild to no disease. There may be clinical or laboratory evidence of HDN, such as a positive DAT or slight elevation of bilirubin, but these usually do not require intervention. A cord hemoglobin of 11 to 14 g/dL (110 to 140 g/L) indicates mild to moderate disease with possible intervention if bilirubin rises dramatically and the possibility of kernicterus arises. A cord hemoglobin of less than 11 g/dL (110 g/L) usually requires immediate exchange transfusion. Falsely elevated cord hemoglobin can occur as a result of maternal-fetal bleeds or twin-twin bleeds, and differential diagnosis is imperative. This may require Kleihauer-Betke stains or serologic testing to detect mixed populations of red cells.

Exchange Transfusion

The ABO group and Rh type of the infant's red cells must be determined.[32] Remember that red cells heavily coated with maternal antibody may have false-negative reactions, especially Rh typing. The reverse (serum) grouping is not required because any antibody present is of maternal origin. Cord blood or heel-stick samples are acceptable for testing. DATs are not required. If not previously done, they can be diagnostic. Two other potential problems should also be mentioned. Cord blood can be contaminated with **Wharton's jelly,** a clear mucoid substance that supports the umbilical vessels within the cord. This substance can produce rouleaux-type agglutination and false-positive cell typing results. It can be avoided by careful washing (six to eight times) of the cord cells before testing.

If the fetus has received one or more IUTs, it may be difficult or virtually impossible to determine the true ABO and Rh owing to the large number of transfused red cells. Remember that the purpose of the IUT is to shut down the fetal red cell production to reduce destruction; if it is done correctly, the majority of circulating red cells can and should be donor red cells. In these cases, reliance is placed on the original red cell sample obtained before the first IUT. Also, the same blood group is used for exchange that was used for the IUT. Mixed cell populations can be seen in twin-twin transfusions and must be recognized when present.

The choice of blood is usually group O whole blood if the infant is group O or group O red cells with group-specific or group AB plasma for the non-O

Wharton's jelly: A gelatinous substance from the umbilical cord that is rich in hyaluronic acid. This substance can contaminate cord blood specimens and interfere with serologic testing.

infant. Donor red cells must be group specific or compatible with the infant *and* compatible with the maternal ABO antibodies (Table 16-1).[17,32]

AABB Standards require testing for anti-A and/or anti-B using the antiglobulin test and the neonate's serum if other than group O red cells are transfused.[32] This can be obviated by the use of maternal serum for crossmatching, because the mother is the source of the circulating antibody. Future non-O transfusions require antiglobulin testing for the appropriate ABO antibody, as well as compatibility testing of the specific antigen-negative unit; both requirements can, of course, be accomplished in a single crossmatch of the specific unit using neonate serum/plasma. Once the ABO or other unexpected antibodies become undetectable in the infant's serum (requires testing with A1 and/or B cells and antigen-positive group O reagent cells), transfusions can be administered without further crossmatches or other testing during the current admission (see following discussion of antibody screening).

If the plasma of the selected red cell unit is incompatible with the infant's red cells, all plasma must be removed and group AB plasma substituted. On occasion, albumin is substituted for some of the plasma volume to aid in bilirubin binding and removal during the exchange transfusion or is administered before the exchange. Because an exchange transfusion may temporarily lower clotting factor levels, it is not recommended to substitute albumin as the sole diluent of the red cells. Unless the neonate's platelet count is well below normal, supplemental platelet transfusions are not usually needed even though the unit being administered has few, if any, viable platelets. The reconstituted unit should have a hematocrit of 50% or greater, the exact figure being determined by the physician.

Antibody screening and crossmatching are required using either the maternal serum or infant serum when unexpected antibodies are present.[32] Usually maternal serum is used initially for both identification and crossmatching because it is in greater supply. Crossmatches using either sample are required until the antibody is no longer detectable in the infant serum.[32] Obviously, if you use the mother's serum as long as possible, frozen aliquots from time of delivery are acceptable, but you will not know when the antibody is gone from the infant circulation.

If the infant is discharged and readmitted, all testing must be repeated using a new infant blood sample.[32] If no antibody is detected and group O blood is used, no further testing is required.

Eluates are not done unless the mother is unavailable and infant serum is insufficient or too weakly reactive to use for identification and/or crossmatching.

In addition to the ABO group selection outlined previously, the Rh type of the unit must be selected. Rh-negative blood is transfused if the infant is Rh negative and/or if the unexpected antibody is anti-D. Rh-positive units may be used if the infant is Rh positive and the unit is negative for any antigens to which the

TABLE 16-1 ABO Group of Donor Red Cells for Exchange Transfusions*		
Infant's Group	Mother's Group	Donor Red Cells
O	O, A, B	O
A	O, B	O
	A, AB	A, O
B	O, A	O
	B, AB	B, O
AB	A	A, O
	B	B, O
	AB	AB, A, B, O

*Choice of donor cells is listed in order of preference.

mother has made a clinically significant antibody, if that antibody is detectable in the infant's serum/plasma. Irradiation is not required for donor units, other than units from blood relatives, when used for exchange transfusion. It is required for infants who have received IUTs.[32] It is recommended in any exchange transfusion as an added precaution.[33]

The unit selected is usually less than 3 days old, but units up to 7 days old have been used, as have frozen/deglycerolized units, appropriately reconstituted. CPD or CPDA-1 is a common anticoagulant. Heparin is no longer used. Adsol washed or packed cells are acceptable, but some neonatologists prefer not to use them.[17,33] CMV-negative and/or leukocyte-reduced units are recommended for all neonates by many but are not required. It is recommended that the units be negative for hemoglobin S.[17]

A "double volume" exchange is usually requested and is 80% to 90% effective in removing red cells and 25% to 35% effective in removing bilirubin.[34] Exchange transfusion removes the sensitized red cells, maternal circulating antibody, and some of the bilirubin. Most of the bilirubin is in the extracellular space, and rebound occurs as this bilirubin is returned to the circulation. Repeat bilirubin determinations are needed every 4 to 6 hours until the values stabilize and start to fall, indicating that the infant's liver enzymes are functioning.

It is of note that in recent years the use of IUTs has allowed fetal delivery at later gestational age, resulting in larger infants. It may not be possible to provide the calculated blood volume for a "double volume" exchange with one unit of red cells and one unit of plasma. Consultations with the perinatalogists are mandatory to avoid extra donor exposures to meet a "calculated" volume.

Owing to continued low-level infant red cell production, the hemoglobin is monitored over several weeks to ensure appropriate hemoglobin levels in the infant. Even normal newborns have a drop in hemoglobin production following delivery,[1] and this delay in production is more pronounced in the transfused infant.

As a special note, when no donor blood compatible with the maternal antibody is available (multiple antibodies present or one directed against a high-frequency antigen) *and* exchange transfusion is required *immediately,* incompatible blood can be used and is effective. Although repeat exchange transfusion may be needed in these cases, it is far better to use incompatible blood than to have brain damage because of a delay in transfusion. It should be noted that exchange or simple transfusions can be required for other reasons than alloimmunization or autoimmunization of the mother against her child's red cell antigens, such as (1) fetal-maternal bleeding at any time during the pregnancy with or without immunization of the mother, (2) twin-twin bleeds, (3) obstetric problems such as placenta previa, (4) congenital hemoglobinopathy, (5) impaired production of red cells for various reasons, and (6) human B19 parvovirus infection with hydrops fetalis.[1] Any of these can lead to a lower than normal cord hemoglobin level, as can a clotted cord blood sample.

Simple Transfusions

Small aliquot transfusions of red cells only are used to correct anemia caused by the original HDN, laboratory testing (iatrogenic blood loss), or other reasons. The requirements for selection of blood are the same as those outlined for exchange transfusions. The major problems with simple transfusions are related to how the donor blood is collected and administered. Many of these transfusions are from CPDA-1 quadruple blood packs, allowing for the separation of five aliquots using an inverted gravity-sedimented method. The red cells are allowed to drain into the individual attached satellite packs in the needed volumes and can be subdivided from there if more than one order is received at a time. This allows four sterile aliquots before the original pack must be entered, and a 24-hour outdate is required. Many neonatologists accept units over 5 days old, especially if they can receive aliquots from a single-donor unit for a given infant. Sterile docking devices allow the attachment of additional transfer packs, thus removing the need to enter the main blood unit. Individual hospital transfusion services must set up their own policies with the input of the neonatologists.

ABO-HDN

ABO-HDN (the most common form of the disease) is distinctly different from other forms of HDN. It is usually a subclinical condition even though antibody may be found on the red cells or in the cord/infant serum. The infant's course is usually benign, requiring no treatment. Mild disease (some degree of hemolysis) can be successfully treated with phototherapy. Moderate to severe disease has been seen, on rare occasions, with some infants requiring exchange transfusion.

An excellent discussion of ABO-HDN can be found elsewhere.[16] A brief summary of the differences and possible reasons follows.[16,34] Clinical findings include the following: (1) the first child can be affected; (2) the DAT is negative or only weakly positive; (3) the cord hemoglobin is usually normal; (4) the cord bilirubin is normal, rising between 24 and 48 hours if at all; and (5) spherocytes are present in the peripheral blood.

Some of the reasons for the decreased degree of hemolysis, even though high levels of IgG antibody are present in the maternal serum, include (1) the presence of soluble A and/or B substances in the fetal circulation, (2) the presence of A and/or B substances in the placental and fetal tissues, and (3) the diminished strength of the A and B antigens on the fetal and infant red cells.

ABO-HDN is more common in group O mothers with group A infants. However, group B infants of group O or A (particularly A_2) mothers occasionally are affected. Of note is that ABO-HDN is two to six times more common in blacks than in whites, and the cause of the more severe disease is anti-B rather than anti-A.[13]

Owing to the variability of findings in ABO-HDN, postnatal workups should be limited to infants showing clinical jaundice or anemia rather than testing cord bloods of all infants born of group O mothers or all cord bloods regardless of maternal blood type, which has been advocated in the past. In the vast majority of cases no treatment is necessary, in some phototherapy may be needed, and in very rare cases simple or exchange transfusion may be required. Each case needs to be evaluated and worked up individually. As previously stated, no good investigative tools are available to predict ABO-HDN in the antepartum period.

PREVENTION

Only one form of HDN currently can be prevented with appropriate administration of **Rh immune globulin (RhIG):** HDN due to anti-D. Various suggestions such as limiting transfusions in females under age 50 or at minimum matching the units for K:1 and c, the two antigens causing the majority of non-D HDN and the more severe disease, have not been followed in the vast majority of transfusion services. ABO-HDN is impossible to prevent, because the antibodies occur in the mother no matter what measures are taken.

Rh Immune Globulin

RhIG consists of concentrated, purified anti-D gamma globulin preparation obtained from hyperimmunized donors. The method of preparation and purification produces a product that does not transmit viral infection.[11,17] The drug is administered intramuscularly, and it acts as an immunosuppressant in the nonsensitized Rh-negative recipient exposed to red cells containing the D antigen. The exact mechanism of action to prevent immunization is unknown but is postulated to be a blocking mechanism of the Fc receptor sites.[11,34] Because the mother is not

Rh immune globulin (RhIG): A solution of gamma globulin containing anti-D. A 300 μg dose of RhIG, if administered within 72 hours of delivery, protects against alloimmunization of the mother to the D antigen of the fetus. Each vial of 300 μg of RhIG protects against 30 mL of fetal whole blood or 15 mL of packed cells.

sensitized, a subsequent Rh-positive pregnancy is unaffected. It has been shown that 300 μg of RhIG prevents sensitization to 15 mL of Rh-positive red cells or 30 mL of whole blood. That is about 20 μg/mL of red blood cells for protection from sensitization.

The first widespread use started in 1968 with a 300 μg dose given postpartum (within 72 hours of delivery) to Rh-negative, D and weak D (D^u) women who delivered a D or weak D (D^u) positive or untyped infant, or 50 μg following a first-trimester abortion. The incidence of sensitization to the D antigen was reduced by 98%, but a residual 2% to 3% of women were still being sensitized. Antepartum use (introduced in 1984) of the 300 μg dose in Rh-negative women at 28 to 32 weeks, preferably 28 weeks, was shown to reduce the risk to 0.2%.[11] Other possibilities for exposure include amniocentesis, transplacental fetal-maternal bleeds due to any of several reasons previously mentioned, and administration of Rh-positive blood products in emergency situations. See Table 16-2 for a suggested RhIG administration protocol. Amniocentesis done very early in pregnancy (12 to 16 weeks) for genetic testing or other reasons requires a repeat administration of RhIG within 12 weeks. The timing is related to the half-life of the circulating passive antibody and the need to maintain levels adequate for protection when the possibility of another bleed increases as the pregnancy progresses.[11,12,17] Inadvertent or emergency administration of Rh-positive blood products such as platelets or even packed cell or whole blood components to Rh-negative unsensitized women of childbearing age should be considered individually and the appropriate dose of RhIG administered if it is deemed useful and if Rh-negative blood is available for any needed subsequent treatment.

The use of RhIG in the woman proven to be weak D (Du) positive remains controversial, because the potential for the mosaic weak D (D^u) to make alloanti-D exists.[13,17,22,32,35,36] The major problem is to determine if the woman is truly weak D (D^u) positive or has had a large fetal bleed causing a false-positive test. Unless records exist proving that she is weak D (D^u) positive before pregnancy

TABLE 16-2 Rh Immune Globulin Administration Recommendations	
Abortions: spontaneous or induced	
First trimester	50 μg
After first trimester	300 μg
Full-term delivery of Rh-positive infant	300 μg*
Stillbirth (unless fetus proves to be Rh negative)	300 μg*
Amniocentesis	
Genetic: 12 to 16 weeks followed by	
Additional dose(s) every 12 weeks	300 μg
Final dose at delivery, if infant is Rh positive	300 μg
Second or third trimester	300 μg
Possible second dose in 12 weeks or at delivery if infant is Rh positive	300 μg*
Transplacental fetal-maternal hemorrhages	300 μg*
Threatened abortion, external cephalic version, antepartum hemorrhage, maternal abdominal trauma	
Possible repeat dose if not delivered within or near 12 weeks	
Antepartum prophylactic about 28 weeks	300 μg
Must be followed by second dose at delivery if infant is Rh positive	

*Maternal whole blood sample **must** be evaluated for possible excessive fetal-maternal hemorrhage (greater than 30 mL fetal whole blood). Calculate appropriate dosage based on quantitative measure of the volume of bleed.

and/or within the first trimester, proof must be obtained by testing the sample for the presence of Rh-positive fetal red cells. Administration of RhIG does not hurt a weak D (D^u) positive mother and therefore should be given if desired by the physician or patient. (The maximum volume of red cells that would be destroyed is 15 mL.) A larger than normal fetal bleed must be identified and the appropriate volume of RhIG given to prevent sensitization.[32]

Given the number of situations in which antepartum RhIG may have been administered, occasions arise when the mother has a weak anti-D present at delivery. A rare baby may have a positive DAT owing to anti-D if the mother has received multiple doses of RhIG, but the clinical course is benign and requires no treatment.[11,12] Unless it can absolutely be proven that she is producing her own anti-D (the antibody is IgM, titer is greater than 32), testing for an excessive fetal bleed and administration of RhIG must be done.[32] Administration of RhIG to a sensitized woman does not hurt her, and nonadministration when indicated could cause sensitization and subsequent affected infants. Therefore the recommendation is as follows: When in doubt, administer at least one dose and test for the need for more than one dose of RhIG.

SCREENING FOR FETAL-MATERNAL BLEEDS

A blood sample is obtained after delivery or other event suspected to have caused a fetal-maternal bleed such as amniocentesis, abortion, or auto accident. The initial screening is done, usually by a **Rosette test,** using this postevent sample of maternal (Rh-negative) blood. A suspension of these red cells is treated with anti-D, which reacts with any Rh-positive cells present (due to a fetal bleed/leak). These Rh-positive cells become coated with anti-D and then are washed to remove unattached antibody. Known D-positive test cells are added, which attach to the anti-D, forming obvious rosettes on microscopic examination of the cell suspension. This test is not reliable when the infant/fetus or mother is weak D (D^u) positive. The rosetting test is a qualitative test, and when it is positive a quantitative test is necessary to determine the actual volume of Rh-positive fetal cells in the maternal circulation. This is usually done by a Kleihauer-Betke stain or a modification of it. This stain uses a monolayer blood film or smear of the red cells being tested. The cells are fixed using alcohol. An acid buffer is used to elute or remove hemoglobin A or adult hemoglobin because it is more soluble than hemoglobin F, the predominant hemoglobin in fetal red cells. The slide is then counterstained, usually with eosin. Cells containing hemoglobin F stain darkly whereas hemoglobin A cells appear as **ghost cells.** The cells are then counted to determine the ratio of fetal to adult cells. The most common formula for determining the volume of the fetal bleed is as follows (where 5000 is an estimate of the maternal blood volume):

> Number of fetal cells/1000 adult cells $\times$ 5000 = mL of fetal whole blood

The answer is then divided by 30 (the volume of Rh-positive whole blood for which one vial of RhIG protects) to determine the number of vials of RhIG to be given to the Rh-negative, unsensitized mother. The stain is also used to determine the volume of fetal bleed in other situations than when RhIG is required, such as a stillbirth in which the cause is unknown.

Problems exist with the stain that may cause false-positive results: (1) faulty technique: hemoglobin F elutes if left too long in the eluting solution; (2) fetuses do produce some hemoglobin A, so cells are missed; (3) genetic hemoglobinopathies, such as persistence of fetal hemoglobin, thalassemia, and sickle cell trait or disease; and (4) pregnancy: 10% to 25% of pregnant women produce elevated levels of hemoglobin F between 10 and 32 weeks of gestation.[13,16,17,37-39] Some women still have elevated levels at term.[13,37] All of these conditions produce elevated levels of fetal hemoglobin in the maternal circulation and can cause

Rosette test: A screening test for fetal-maternal hemorrhage. The test is based on the principle that Rh-positive fetal cells coated with anti-D form rosettes with Rh-positive indicator cells, thus making them distinguishable from the Rh-negative maternal cell population.

Ghost cells: Cells that appear pale and unstained.

difficulties in interpretation of the stain. Experience and testing of known problem blood films make recognition of the differences between the findings in these conditions and a true fetal bleed possible. Occasionally cells appear to be totally fetal but may not be, and the slide becomes uninterpretable.

Several formulas have been developed that increase the number of vials of RhIG to compensate for possible errors in this testing.[17,38] The increased numbers seem prudent in those few instances in which multiple vials are required. It should be noted that one vial should be given even if no fetal cells are detected in the testing.

OTHER CAUSES OF HEMOLYTIC DISEASE AND DISEASES OF SIMILAR ETIOLOGY

Maternal Warm Autoimmune Hemolytic Anemia

Although it is a rare event, maternal warm autoimmune hemolytic anemia can cause hemolysis in the fetus/infant due to transplacental passage of IgG antibody. Although normally the fetus is only mildly affected, severe disease has been reported.[40,41] The severity of the disease in the fetus/infant appears to be directly related to the severity in the mother. Appropriate treatment of the mother and timely assessment of the fetus should be made using the same criteria as with alloimmunization.

Maternal Alloimmunization to Platelets

The antigen involved is usually PLA1, although other specificities have been implicated.[29,42] The process of immunization is the same as in HDN. The antibody produced crosses the placenta, causing thrombocytopenia in the infant. Although it is similar to HDN, there are differences. The first child can be affected. Once it is known, future pregnancies can be monitored and some of the complications eliminated for subsequent children. The father can be typed for the antigen, as can the fetus using cordocentesis. If the fetus is found to be antigen positive and/or thrombocytopenic, treatment can be instituted. Transfusion can be initiated using either the mother's washed platelets or platelets from an antigen-negative maternal sibling or known donor. The life span of these platelets is extremely limited, however, requiring weekly transfusions. Normally this procedure is reserved for the period immediately before and/or after delivery. One treatment being tried is the administration of intravenous immune gamma globulin to the mother.[42] This appears to block the destruction in the fetus, and platelet counts are increased. This reduces the possibility of fetal bleeding, particularly intracranial hemorrhage, during the pregnancy and increases the probability of delivering a viable healthy infant. Delivery is usually carefully planned for around 37 weeks by cesarean section. Maternal platelets are obtained in advance by apheresis and are available for immediate transfusion once the plasma is removed. In emergency situations in which maternal or antigen-negative platelets are not available, random platelets should be used. The response, although temporary, may be adequate. Once the initial thrombocytopenia resolves, there are no further problems.

Maternal Autoimmune Thrombocytopenia

In this disorder maternal autoantibody can cross the placenta and affect the fetal platelets. There is no good correlation between maternal platelet count and fetal platelet count. Obtaining a fetal count by cordocentesis poses a problem if the mother has a very low count herself. If the count can be determined and the fetus is thrombocytopenic, therapy is instituted for the mother, usually with intravenous immune globulin and/or steroids. The count is repeated in 3 weeks, but if the count remains low, therapy is usually discontinued and the pregnancy is followed by ultrasound evaluations until about 37 weeks. If a fetal platelet count can be obtained at that time, it is highly predictive of the neonatal counts; if it is less than 50,000, delivery is normally by cesarean section. Treatment of the infant can then be instituted.

CHAPTER SUMMARY

1. Hemolytic disease of the newborn and fetus is caused whenever the fetus inherits a red cell antigen from the father that the mother lacks. The maternal immune system then recognizes the antigen as foreign and produces IgG antibody directed against the specific antigen. This antibody must be produced in high enough titer to cross the placenta and affect the fetal red cells.

2. ABO-HDN is the most common form of the disease, but no antepartum tests can accurately predict severity of the disease. Indeed, the direct antiglobulin test (DAT) is often negative, although mild hemolysis and jaundice may develop. This makes it difficult to differentiate ABO-HDN from physiologic jaundice seen in some term and many preterm infants.

3. Rh HDN, caused by anti-D alone or in combination, causes the most severe form of the disease. HDN due to anti-D can be prevented with appropriate administration of RhIG.

4. Virtually all other IgG alloantibodies can cause HDN, with anti-c and anti-K1 causing the most severe cases. Some antibodies are known to cause no hemolysis or very little hemolysis owing to soluble substances in the fetal serum/plasma or few antigen sites on the fetal red cells. These include ABO, I, P_1, Lewis, Lutheran, Chido, Rodgers, and Cartwright blood group antibodies. The specificity of the antibody is therefore of prime importance.

5. Methods of determining timing and need for intervention include maternal history, paternal zygosity for the antigen(s), titration studies on maternal serum, and amniocentesis. Cordocentesis can assist when the father is heterozygous or unavailable.

6. Elevations in bilirubin pigments in the amniotic fluid and/or defined anemia by cordocentesis determine intervention by direct red cell transfusions to the fetus in utero, either intravascularly or intraperitoneally. Bilirubinemia alone does not affect the fetus because the mother clears the pigment without damage to the fetus. Anemia is the primary problem for the fetus.

7. Once fetal lung maturity is reached (usually at 32 to 34 weeks of gestational age), the fetus can be delivered and exchange transfusions used to treat bilirubinemia in addition to the anemia. Bilirubinemia is the primary danger after delivery rather than anemia, although that is also closely monitored.

8. Blood used for IUTs or exchange transfusions is carefully selected to protect the infant and provide the best possible product for the problem being treated. Certain testing is required of all units administered, although in emergencies certain requirements can be ignored.

9. Prevention of Rho(D) immunization is possible by appropriate detection of fetal-maternal bleeds during and following a pregnancy. The testing must be carefully interpreted owing to various complications found in the staining procedure commonly used.

10. Prevention of other (non-D) alloimmunization to red cells is not currently possible.

11. Other autoantibodies and alloantibodies directed against red cells or against other cells such as platelets can endanger the fetus and must be recognized and treated appropriately.

REFERENCES

1. Luban NLC: Physiology of normal and premature infants. In Luban NLC, Keating LJ (eds): Hemotherapy of the Infant and Premature. Arlington, VA, American Association of Blood Banks, 1983.
2. Sacher RA, Falchuk SC: Percutaneous umbilical blood sampling. Crit Rev Clin Lab Sci 28:19-35, 1990.
3. Ludomirski A: The anemic fetus–direct access to the fetal circulation for diagnosis and treatment. In Kennedy MS, Wilson S, Kelton JG (eds): Perinatal Transfusion Medicine.
Arlington, VA, American Association of Blood Banks, 1990.
4. Kevy SV, Fosburg M, Wolfe L: The use of platelets, plasma and plasma derivatives in the newborn. In Luban NLC, Keating LJ (eds): Hemotherapy of the Infant and Premature. Arlington, VA, American Association of Blood Banks, 1983.
5. Peters MT, Nicolaides KH: Cordocentesis for the diagnosis and treatment of human fetal parvovirus infection. Obstet Gynecol 75:501-504, 1990.

6. Greenberg J, Sacher RA: Exchange transfusion in the newborn. In Luban NLC, Keating LJ (eds): Hemotherapy of the Infant and Premature. Arlington, VA, American Association of Blood Banks, 1983.

7. Diamond LK, Blackfan KD, Baty JM: Erythroblastosis fetalis and its association with universal edema of the fetus, icterus gravis neonatorum and anemia of the newborn. J Pediatr 1:269-309, 1932.

8. Levine P, Stetson RE: An unusual case of intragroup agglutination. JAMA 113:126-127, 1939.

9. Landsteiner K, Weiner AS: An agglutinable factor in human blood recognized by immune sera for rhesus blood. Proc Soc Exp Biol Med 43:223, 1940.

10. Levine P, Burnham L, Katzin EM, Vogel P: The role of isoimmunization in the pathogenesis of erythroblastosis fetalis. Am J Obstet Gynecol 42:925-937, 1941.

11. Bowman JM: Historical overview: Hemolytic disease of the fetus and newborn. In Kennedy MS, Wilson SM, Kelton JG (eds): Perinatal Transfusion Medicine. Arlington, VA, American Association of Blood Banks, 1990.

12. Bowman JM: Suppression of Rh isoimmunization: A review. Obstet Gynecol 52:385-393, 1978.

13. Mollison PL: Blood Transfusion in Clinical Medicine, 7th ed. Oxford, Blackwell Scientific, 1983.

14. Kline WE: Chemistry of blood group antigens and antibodies in hemolytic disease of the newborn. In Bell CA (ed): A Seminar on Perinatal Blood Banking. Arlington, VA, American Association of Blood Banks, 1978.

15. Nossaman JK: Laboratory evaluation of the immunized patient. In Tregallas WM, Wallas CH (eds): Prenatal and Perinatal Immunohematology. Chicago, American Association of Blood Banks, 1981.

16. Vengelen-Tyler V: The serologic investigation of hemolytic disease caused by antibodies other than anti-D. In Garratty G (ed): Hemolytic Disease of the Newborn. Arlington, VA, American Association of Blood Banks, 1984.

17. Brecher ME (ed): Technical Manual of the American Association of Blood Banks, 14th ed. Bethesda, MD, American Association of Blood Banks, 2003.

18. Nelson JM, Carlson DE: New developments in antenatal diagnosis and treatment—hemolytic disease of the newborn/fetus and other disorders. In Kennedy MS, Wilson S, Kelton JG (eds): Perinatal Transfusion Medicine. Arlington, VA, American Association of Blood Banks, 1990.

19. Garratty G: Factors affecting the pathogenicity of red cell auto- and alloantibodies. In Nance SJ (ed): Immune Destruction of Red Blood Cells. Arlington, VA, American Association of Blood Banks, 1989.

20. Mair DC, Scofield TL: HDN in a mother undergoing in vitro fertilization with donor ova (letter). Transfusion 43:288-289, 2003.

21. Finning KM, Martin PG, Soothill PW, Avent ND: Prediction of fetal D status from maternal plasma: Introduction of a new noninvasive fetal RHD genotyping service. Transfusion 42:1079-1085, 2002.

22. Judd WJ: Practice guidelines for prenatal and perinatal immunohematology, revisited. Transfusion 41:1445-1452, 2001.

23. Caine ME, Mueller-Heubach E: Kell sensitization in pregnancy. Am J Obstet Gynecol 154:85-90, 1986.

24. Wenk RE, Goldstein P, Felix JK: Alloimmunization of hr'(c), hemolytic disease of newborns, and perinatal management. Obstet Gynecol 76:623-626, 1986.

25. Wenk RE, Goldstein P, Felix JK: Kell alloimmunization, hemolytic disease of the newborn, and perinatal management. Obstet Gynecol 66:473-476, 1985.

26. Foley MR, Sonek J, O'Shaughnessy R: Cordocentesis: Cracking the diagnostic and therapeutic barrier between fetus and physician. Ob/Gyn Rep 1:152-166, 1989.

27. Liley AW: Liquor amnii analysis in the management of the pregnancy complicated by rhesus sensitization. Am J Obstet Gynecol 82:1359-1370, 1961.

28. Queenan JT: Modern Management of the Rh Problem, 2nd ed. Hagerstown, MD, Harper & Row, 1977.

29. Gabbe SG, Niebyl JR, Simpson JL (eds): Obstetrics: Normal and Problem Pregnancies. Edinburgh, Churchill-Livingstone, 1986.

30. Liley AW: Intrauterine transfusion of fetus in haemolytic disease. BMJ 2:1107-1109, 1963.

31. Nicolaides KH, Clewell WH, Mibashan RS, et al: Fetal haemoglobin measurement in the assessment of red cell isoimmunisation. Lancet 1:1073-1075, 1988.

32. Fridey JL (ed): Standards for Blood Banks and Transfusion Services, 22nd ed. Bethesda, MD, American Association of Blood Banks, 2003.

33. Luban NLC, DePalma L: Special considerations in blood transfusion during the perinatal period. In Kennedy MS, Wilson S, Kelton JG (eds): Perinatal Transfusion Medicine. Arlington, VA, American Association of Blood Banks, 1990.

34. Buck SA: Hemolytic disease of the newborn. In Harmening D (ed): Modern Blood Banking and Transfusion Practice, 2nd ed. Philadelphia, FA Davis, 1989.

35. American College of Obstetrics and Gynecology: Prevention of Rho(D) isoimmunization. Technical Bulletin 79, Aug 1984.

36. Konugres A, Polesky H, Walker R: Rh immune globulin and the Rh positive, Du variant mother. Transfusion 22:76-77, 1982.

37. Pembrey ME, Weatherall DJ, Clegg JG: Maternal synthesis of hemoglobin F in pregnancy. Lancet 1:1350-1355, 1973.

38. Sebring ES: Fetomaternal hemorrhage—incidence and methods of detection and quantitation. In Garratty G (ed): Hemolytic Disease of the Newborn. Arlington, VA, American Association of Blood Banks, 1984.

39. Sebring ES, Polesky HF: Fetomaternal hemorrhage: Incidence, risk factors, time of occurrence, and clinical effects. Transfusion 30:333-338, 1990.

40. Lawe JE: Successful exchange transfusion of an infant for AIHA developing late in mother's pregnancy. Transfusion 22:66-69, 1982.

41. Sokol RJ, Hewitt S, Stamps B: Erythrocyte autoantibodies, autoimmune haemolysis and pregnancy. Vox Sang 43:169-176, 1982.

42. Strauss RG: Perinatal platelet and granulocyte transfusions. In Kennedy MS, Wilson S, Lelton JG (eds): Perinatal Transfusion Medicine. Arlington, VA, American Association of Blood Banks, 1990.

FURTHER READING

Bowman John: Thirty-five years of Rh prophylaxis. Transfusion 43:1661-1666, 2003.

Frigoletto RD, Jewett JF, Konugres AA (eds): Rh Hemolytic Disease: New Strategy for Eradication. Boston, GK Hall Medical Publishers, 1982.

Issitt PD, Anstee DJ: Applied Blood Group Serology, 4th ed. Montgomery Scientific Publications, Durham, NC, 1998.

Kennedy MS, Wilson SM, Kelton JG (eds): Perinatal Transfusion Medicine. Arlington, VA, American Association of Blood Banks, 1990.

Rossi EC, Simon TL, Moss GS, Gould SA (eds): Principles of Transfusion Medicine, 2nd ed. Baltimore, Williams & Wilkins, 1996.

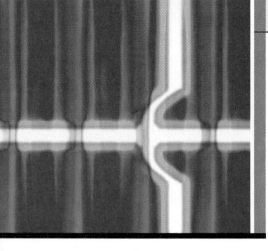

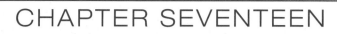
CHAPTER SEVENTEEN

Transfusion Issues in Selected Patient Populations

Sally V. Rudmann and Kathy K. Nicol

CHAPTER OUTLINE

LEARNING OBJECTIVES

After reading and studying this chapter, the student should be able to:

1. Define the term hemorrhagic shock.
2. Briefly describe the four classes of shock.
3. State three common definitions for massive transfusion.
4. List the three goals in the patient management of massive blood loss.
5. Describe the physiologic responses to rapid blood loss.
6. Discuss options for fluid replacement in hemorrhagic shock.
7. Briefly describe current practice with regard to the use of "transfusion triggers."
8. Briefly discuss four general categories of negative outcomes associated with massive transfusion.
9. Discuss the use of whole blood versus red blood cells and "fresh" versus "nonfresh" blood in the treatment of massive transfusion.
10. List indications for the use of fresh frozen plasma, cryoprecipitate, and platelets in the treatment of the massively transfused patient.
11. Discuss the physiologic consequences of hypothermia and strategies used to avoid it in massive transfusion.
12. Describe the AABB Standards for blood-warming devices.
13. Discuss the issues surrounding the emergency release of blood and components.
14. Define autologous transfusion and briefly state how it can be useful in the treatment of massive blood loss.
15. Describe the AABB Standards relating to autologous salvage.
16. Discuss the rationale for and against the use of microaggregate filters in massive transfusion.
17. Define the term therapeutic plasma exchange (TPE).
18. Describe the general principles of therapeutic plasma exchange in disease.
19. List three types of selective plasma exchange procedures.
20. Discuss the ASFA/AABB categories for therapeutic pheresis.
21. Briefly describe four general categories of disorders in which plasma exchange may be useful as a therapeutic tool.
22. Describe a specific example of one disease in each category listed in objective 21.
23. Define therapeutic cytapheresis and indicate two disorders in which it is useful as a therapeutic tool.
24. Briefly describe the use of therapeutic phlebotomy in the treatment of polycythemia.

25. Briefly discuss four disorders associated with thermal injury.

26. List two treatment goals associated with burn resuscitation.

27. Discuss the indications for blood component therapy in burn patients.

28. List six functions of the liver.

29. Discuss four conditions associated with liver disease that have implications for transfusion therapy.

30. Describe the hemostatic disorders associated with liver transplant.

31. Discuss the criteria for selection of suitable components for liver transplant patients.

32. Describe one protocol that could be followed when antigen-negative units are not available in sufficient numbers to meet the transfusion needs of a liver transplant recipient.

33. List five physiologic differences between neonates and adults that may affect transfusion therapy decisions.

34. Describe the hematologic variables in the neonatal period that affect transfusion therapy decisions.

35. Describe the indications for transfusion, technical issues, and pretransfusion testing requirements for both simple and exchange transfusions.

36. Given the blood volume, donor hemoglobin, pretransfusion hemoglobin, and desired posttransfusion hemoglobin, calculate the volume necessary for direct transfusion to a neonate.

37. List three methods that are used to provide small aliquots of blood for infant transfusion.

38. Discuss the use of additive solution blood for the transfusion of neonates.

39. Describe current practice standards for pretransfusion testing during the neonatal period.

40. Define exchange transfusion and extracorporeal membrane oxygenation (ECMO).

41. State the approximate amount of blood replaced during a single- and a double-volume exchange transfusion.

42. List the criteria used for the selection of blood for exchange transfusion and ECMO.

43. Briefly state the indications for the use of fresh frozen plasma, platelets, and granulocytes in infants.

Transfusion therapy can be associated with unique problems in patients with various clinical conditions. This chapter introduces the reader to selected clinical settings that affect decisions regarding transfusion support. The chapter includes a discussion of massive transfusion, therapeutic hemapheresis and therapeutic phlebotomy, transfusion in burn patients, transfusion in liver disease, and transfusion to infants and children.

It is not within the scope of this text to provide an all-inclusive review of transfusion therapy. This chapter provides an overview of some of the more common categories of transfusion recipients for the clinical laboratory scientist and other blood bank practitioners. The interested reader can find additional information by referring to the suggested readings.

MASSIVE TRANSFUSION
Hemorrhagic Shock

Initial symptoms associated with acute blood loss generally appear after a loss of 15% to 20% of the **blood volume.** A more severe consequence of blood loss, **hemorrhagic shock,** is associated with larger volume blood losses and is the most common cause of shock in injured patients.[1] Shock, a syndrome associated with circulatory collapse and insufficient tissue perfusion, has grave consequences if left untreated.[2,3] Shock can be categorized into four classes based on severity.[1] These classes are differentiated based on patient vital signs, mental status, and estimated bleed. There is a rough correlation between the class and the type of surgical and fluid replacement strategies necessary for survival (Table 17-1).

Blood loss, however, can be difficult to estimate. Extensive blood loss, such as that associated with fractures of the femur or pelvis, can be invisible, making an underestimate more probable, whereas other bleeding, such as that associated with open wounds, is more obvious and can lead to an overestimate of loss. The complex presentation of the massively bleeding patient makes it imperative that no one single variable, patient symptom, physical sign, or laboratory value be used as the sole predictor for treatment decisions. Previous reliance on a transfusion trigger of 10 g/dL has been generally abandoned. Research has clearly shown that oxygen consumption, within a certain range, is not correlated with hemoglobin level. Likewise, experience with surgical **hemodilution** has demonstrated that patients can deliver adequate oxygen to tissues at significantly lower hemoglobin values.[4-6]

Despite the fact that administration of blood and blood products is a central feature of the treatment regimen for trauma victims at risk for hemorrhagic shock, concerns regarding the adequacy of the blood supply and risks associated with transfusion require careful assessment of the relative risk-benefit ratio. These issues, in addition to recent concerns about the association of transfusion with increased

Blood volume: Approximately 75 mL/kg (about 10 units in a 70 kg adult).

Hemorrhagic shock: Serious derangement of the circulatory system resulting from the loss of fluid of sufficient quantity to overcome the ability of the vasculature to compensate by vessel constriction. Symptoms of shock include hypotension, coldness of the skin, tachycardia, and insufficient tissue perfusion. Immediate resuscitation is aimed at the restoration of volume.

Hemodilution (acute normovolemic hemodilution): A perioperative procedure whereby blood is drawn from a patient immediately before surgery and volume is replaced by fluids such as normal saline. Blood is held for reinfusion at the end of the procedure or earlier if indicated.

TABLE 17-1 Classification Scheme for Hemorrhagic Shock*				
	Class I	Class II	Class III	Class IV
Blood loss (mL)	Up to 750	750-1500	1500-2000	> 2000
Blood loss (% blood volume)	Up to 15%	15%-30%	30%-40%	> 40%
Pulse rate	< 100	> 100	> 120	> 140
Blood pressure	Normal	Normal	Decreased	Decreased
Pulse pressure (mm Hg)	Normal to increased	Decreased	Decreased	Decreased
Respiratory rate	14-20	20-30	30-40	> 35
Urine output (mL/hr)	> 30	20-30	5-15	Negligible
CNS/mental status	Slightly anxious	Mildly anxious	Anxious, confused	Confused, lethargic
Fluid replacement (3:1 rule)	Crystalloid	Crystalloid	Crystalloid and blood	Crystalloid and blood

Adapted with permission from Advanced Trauma Life Support Program for Doctors. Chicago, American College of Surgeons, 1997, p 98.
*For a 70-kg man.

risk for infectious complications and the possible contribution of transfusion-associated cytokine precursors in posttraumatic systemic inflammation, have led to a more judicious approach to transfusion in acute trauma.[4,7]

In most cases, treatment of patients who experience excessive blood loss involves the transfusion of blood and blood components. Therapy is aimed at the replacement of oxygen-carrying capacity, lost fluid, and coagulation proteins and platelets. Whereas all transfusions have potential adverse reactions, the transfusion of massive amounts of stored blood is associated with some unique physiologic consequences.

Definition of Massive Transfusion

Although there is no universally accepted definition for the term massive transfusion, the following formulistic definitions, which take into account both the amount and the rate of blood loss, are useful. By definition, massive transfusion is often described as the replacement of one or more blood volume(s) (10 to 12 units) within a 24-hour period, the replacement of 50% of the blood volume within 3 hours,[7-13] or the loss of 1.5 mL of blood per kilogram of body weight per minute for at least 20 minutes.[14] Massive transfusion can also be expressed in terms of the need for red cell replacement (4 units in 4 hours with continued bleeding) or sufficient bleeding to warrant plasma and/or platelet replacement.[13] Using the **calculations that apply to exchange transfusions,** the transfusion of one blood volume is approximately equivalent to a two-thirds exchange.[4,10,12] Thus the patient who has rapidly lost one blood volume is left with approximately one third of his or her own blood remaining in circulation. After a loss of two to three blood volumes, less than 15% of the residual blood remains.[12] Massive blood loss can occur in a variety of clinical settings—some anticipated, such as cardiac surgery and liver transplant, and others unexpected, such as massive trauma. In both cases, patient management is similar and involves the following three steps: recognition, resuscitation, and blood component transfusion.[12]

Physiologic Response to Blood Loss
Oxygen Delivery

The initial physiologic response to acute anemia is an increase in cardiac output accomplished by an increase in stroke volume, increased heart rate, or both.[15] The ability of the heart to respond is limited by the ability of the myocardium to extract sufficient oxygen, which is accomplished by dilation of the coronary arteries. A diseased heart may be compromised in its ability to compensate for acute anemia, and increased demands may precipitate cardiac ischemia. Another compensatory mechanism for acute anemia takes place in the tissues through the recruitment of additional capillaries or increased flow through existing beds. When anemia is chronic, these other compensatory mechanisms are supplemented by increased levels of 2,3-diphosphoglycerate (2,3-DPG) resulting in a shift to the right in the **oxygen dissociation curve** favoring the release of oxygen in the tissues (off-loading).[7]

Volume

In blood loss, the body attempts to correct the decrease in intravascular fluid volume by shifting fluid and protein from the extravascular spaces into the vasculature. This physiologic response, transcapillary refill, takes place during the first few hours after hemorrhage, resulting in a restoration of blood volume and in the dilution of the circulating red cells, resulting in normovolemic anemia. This shift of fluids results in a temporary decrease in the patient's hemoglobin and hematocrit, which may not accurately reflect the magnitude of the blood loss. This, in addition to large-volume fluid resuscitation, makes early laboratory parameters difficult to interpret.[7,8,16]

Calculations that apply to exchange transfusions: After the transfusion of one blood volume, approximately 65% to 75% of the patient's blood has been replaced with donor blood. For a complete discussion of the mathematical models used in plasma exchange and exchange transfusion refer to Weinstein R: Basic principles of therapeutic blood exchange. In McLeod BC, Price TH, Weinstein R (eds): Apheresis: Principles and Practice, 2nd ed, Bethesda, MD, American Association of Blood Banks, 2003.

Oxygen dissociation curve: A graph representing the relationship between pO_2 and oxygen saturation. A shift to the right favors the release of O_2 at a given pO_2 facilitating the off-loading of O_2 in the tissues. A shift to the left favors the binding of O_2 to hemoglobin.

Early shifts of fluid into the vasculature result in hematologic values that may decrease hemoglobin and hematocrit, thereby overestimating the magnitude of the bleed. This is intensified by the massive administration of fluid during shock therapy.

Mediator Release

Hemorrhage, especially if complicated by infection, triggers a number of cascades, including the coagulation cascade, the complement cascade, and the fibrinolytic system. A number of cell types are activated with the subsequent release of biologic mediators. Among these substances, oxygen radicals, proteases, prostaglandins, interleukins, and tissue necrosis factor are implicated in damage to the endothelium and activation of disseminated intravascular coagulation. These, in addition to a number of other causes such as dilution and delayed synthesis of coagulation proteins, contribute to the complex multifactorial hemostatic dysfunction that is frequently associated with acute blood loss and massive transfusion.

Treatment of Massive Blood Loss
Volume Replacement

Treatment of massive hemorrhage centers on the urgent need for the replacement of volume. Volume replacement is generally more important than red cell replacement in the treatment of shock. Immediate resuscitation is generally accomplished by the administration of crystalloids such as lactated Ringer's solution and saline. Fluid resuscitation may be sufficient for some patients who by definition fall into class I and II shock.[16,17] Other patients may respond only transiently or may be totally unresponsive to fluid resuscitation, as in class III and IV shock. These patients usually require surgical intervention and the administration of crossmatch-compatible or type-compatible, uncrossmatched blood. In the case of a class IV shock victim, unresponsiveness to resuscitation may require immediate release of O-negative, uncrossmatched blood.[7] Whereas some physicians believe that colloids (e.g., albumin, dextran) have no clinical advantage in early resuscitation, there is a continuing dispute regarding the appropriate choice of resuscitation fluids (**crystalloid** versus **colloid**).[8] It is clear that for any given volume replacement goal, less colloid need be administered. However, colloid therapy is associated with increased cost and the possibility of allergic reaction. Most data indicate that the choice of fluid does not clearly affect the outcome.[17] Data clearly support the fact that fresh frozen plasma (FFP) is not indicated for volume replacement owing to the risk of transfusion-transmitted infection and the availability of other suitable fluids.[8] Once oxygenation is ensured, the top priorities in the management of the massively transfused patient are the reversal of hypotension and the prevention of hypothermia. Extended periods of **hypoperfusion** and **hypothermia** are associated with most of the complications of massive transfusion.[7,16]

Red Blood Cell Transfusion and Transfusion "Triggers"

The decision of whether or not to transfuse red cell products is complex. Hemoglobin-based transfusion triggers may not be accurate measures of blood loss, and can either underpredict or overpredict actual transfusion needs. The earlier practice of transfusion to maintain a hematocrit of 30% (hemoglobin of 10 g/dL) is not supported by most recent research. Normovolemic resting patients with normal cardiopulmonary function can tolerate hemoglobin levels as low as 5 g/dL without evidence of tissue hypoxia.[5] In general, patients with hemoglobin levels greater than 10 g/dL rarely need red cell transfusions whereas those with hemoglobin levels below 7 g/dL frequently require transfusion.[6] It is more difficult to predict the transfusion needs of those who fall between 7 and 10 g/dL. The decision to transfuse is more rationally made by consideration of the hemoglobin within the context of the overall patient condition and the severity of ongoing blood loss. Hemoglobin alone provides insufficient data for a decision to or not to transfuse.

The use of **intraoperative salvage** and reinfusion has become a useful adjunct to allogeneic transfusion. Advantages of autologous salvage include blood conser-

---

Crystalloid/colloid: Crystalloids, which are solutions of anions and cations, are both isotonic and isosmotic with plasma. When administered, these fluids can equilibrate between the vascular and extravascular compartments. Colloids, because of their oncotic properties, stay within the vascular compartment. For this reason less colloid needs to be administered to achieve the same increase in volume.

Hypoperfusion: Inadequate supply of blood to an organ or tissue.

Hypothermia: Decreased body temperature (core temperature less than 35° C).

Intraoperative salvage: The collection of blood-containing fluid from the surgical field for processing and reinfusion.

vation and decreased risk of infectious complications.[7] Other blood conservation strategies include the administration of recombinant human erythropoietin (rHuEPO), preoperative autologous donation (PAD), perioperative hemodilution, and the use of blood-loss reduction drugs such as desmopressin, antifibrinolytic agents, and/or fibrin glue.[6] There are sufficient research data to demonstrate the effectiveness of these interventions in reducing the overall reliance on allogeneic transfusion in selected patient populations.

Treatment of Coagulopathy

After resuscitation has been achieved and oxygen delivery needs satisfied, there is often a requirement for plasma products and platelet administration to achieve hemostasis in massively transfused patients. A detailed discussion of these treatment options follows. A schematic representation of transfusion/treatment decisions can be found in Table 17-2.

Adverse Consequences of Massive Transfusion
Overview

The transfusion of massive amounts of stored blood can result in a number of adverse clinical consequences[12,18] (see Summary 17-1). Despite a large body of literature on the topic of massive transfusion, data do not always clearly differentiate between the effects of the patient's injury or illness and the transfusions themselves. Because most massively transfused patients have hypovolemia, hypothermia, **acidosis, hyperkalemia,** extensive wounds, tissue destruction, impaired immunologic defenses, and **hypoperfusion injury,** it is difficult to measure transfusion outcomes.[10] Despite these confounding circumstances, the literature presents some consistent findings regarding the dangers of massive transfusion. These adverse consequences stem, in part, from the fact that refrigerator-stored red blood cells (RBCs) and whole blood undergo changes during storage **(storage lesion)** and, in addition, contain significant concentrations of anticoagulant/preservative solution.[10] Compared with fresh blood, stored blood is relatively **hypernatremic, hypoglycemic, hyperammonemic,** and **hyperphosphatemic.**[10,19,20] In general, most of the negative outcomes of massive transfusion can be divided into four categories: the effect of dilution, the impact of the transfusion of anticoagulant/preservative solutions, the effect of products of blood storage lesion, and the impact of the rapid infusion of cold blood (see Summary 17-2). The dangers associated with massive

Acidosis: An increase in the hydrogen ion concentration (decreased pH), which can result from the accumulation of acid substances or the loss of buffering capability.

Hyperkalemia: Elevated levels of potassium in the blood, which can result from the transfusion of large amounts of potassium in units of stored bank blood.

Hypoperfusion injury: Tissue/organ injury resulting from inadequate blood flow.

Storage lesion: Changes that occur in banked blood over the storage period, including decreases in adenosine triphosphate and 2,3-DPG and increased potassium.

Hypernatremia: Increased blood sodium.

Hypoglycemia: Decreased blood glucose.

Hyperammonemia: Excess ammonia in the blood.

Hyperphosphatemia: An excess of phosphate in the blood.

TABLE 17-2 Massive Bleeding: Guide to Transfusion Therapy Decisions

Hypovolemic Shock	Inadequate O$_2$ Delivery	Moderate Coagulopathy	Increasing Risk of Hemorrhage	Severe Coagulopathy
>25%-30% blood loss	Hemoglobin < 6 g/dL or 6-10 g/dL with clinical signs of hypoxia	Coagulation factors ≤ 30% PT/aPTT ≥ 1.5 × normal	**Moderate Thrombocytopenia** Platelets ≤ 100 × 10^6/µL PT/aPTT ≥ 1.5 × normal	Coagulation factors ≤ 15% Fibrinogen ≤ 1.0 g/L PT/aPTT ≥ 1.8 × normal **Severe Thrombocytopenia** Platelets ≤ 50 × 10^6/µL

1. **Restore Blood Volume:** Crystalloid or colloid
2. **Maintain Tissue O$_2$:** Red blood cells or whole blood (1 unit will raise hemoglobin by 1 g/dL)
3. **Achieve Hemostasis:** Fresh frozen plasma (dose: 1 unit/10-20 kg) and/or cryoprecipitate (dose: 2 mL/kg)
4. **Reverse Thrombocytopenia:** Platelets (dose: 1 unit/10 kg) (each unit should raise the platelet count by 5000-10,000/µL)

Summary 17-1

Some Possible Adverse Physiologic Consequences of Massive Transfusion

ADVERSE CONSEQUENCE	CONTRIBUTING FACTORS
Coagulopathy	Dilution, shock, DIC, hypothermia
Decreased O_2 delivery to tissues	Reduced 2,3-DPG levels—shift to left in O_2 dissociation curve
Acid-base imbalance	Acidic pH of stored blood, metabolic acidosis from hypovolemia
Citrate toxicity	Component of anticoagulant/preservative solutions
Hypothermia	Administration of cold components and fluids
Immunosuppression	Mechanism unclear
Potassium overload	Potassium levels in stored red cell products
Hypocalcemia and/or hypomagnesemia	Citrate in anticoagulant/preservative solutions
Respiratory distress	Microaggregates in stored blood

Summary 17-2

Categories of Adverse Outcomes of Massive Transfusion

Effects of products of storage lesion
Impact of rapid infusion of cold blood and fluids
Effect of dilution
Impact of anticoagulant/preservative solutions

transfusion are related to either the quantity of blood infused (e.g., dilutional coagulopathy) or the rate of infusion (e.g., citrate toxicity).[10]

Coagulopathy

Trauma patients may exhibit hemostatic abnormalities due to a number of factors, some related to the trauma, for example, disseminated intravascular coagulation, and some related to transfusion and fluid administration, for example, dilution of platelets and coagulation factors and/or hypothermia.[4,12]

In extended transfusion settings in which large quantities (measured in blood volumes) are transfused, the patient's own blood becomes increasingly diluted by the stored blood. Stored blood that is more than 7 days old is depleted of functional platelets and granulocytes and has minimal quantities of the labile coagulation Factors V and VIII. This may result in dilutional thrombocytopenia or dilutional coagulopathy.[21] Diffuse bleeding, often associated with massive transfusion, continues to be attributed, at least in part, to the dilutional effects of transfusion. Diffuse bleeding associated with thrombocytopenia is the most common hemostatic abnormality associated with massive transfusion.[4] Abundant scientific evidence indicates that diffuse bleeding is multifactorial and can be correlated with decreased tissue perfusion, as well as transfusion-related dilution. Bleeding has been strongly correlated with the extent/duration of hypotension. Patients with severe hypotension for more than 1 hour are at increased risk for severe coagulopathies. These data support the theory that coagulopathy can be associated with insufficient transfusion, as well as with too much.[16,22]

Coagulopathy can also be associated with hypothermia subsequent to the rapid administration of cold fluids, shock, and thermal regulatory dysfunction.

As a patient's blood is lost and "diluted" with stored bank blood, platelet numbers and labile coagulation factors are lost, resulting in a hemostatic dysfunction. Because hemostatic dysfunction is also associated with hypoperfusion and hypotension, it is difficult to determine whether the hemostatic abnormality is due to excessive or inadequate transfusion.

Hypothermia has been associated with increased platelet sequestration and decreased clotting factor activity. In these cases, diffuse bleeding may be associated with normal coagulation testing values run at 37° C. In such cases, hypothermia should be considered as a contributing factor and rewarming of the patient may be a more prudent course of action than the administration of platelets and/or fresh frozen plasma.[7]

The decision to replace coagulation proteins and platelets in the bleeding, massively transfused patient is based on both the patient's clinical status and laboratory measures of hemostasis. There is general agreement that the routine replacement of clotting factors and platelets is not justified, and this practice has been generally discontinued.[12,16,22-24] Some laboratory values have been found to be fairly good predictors of microvascular bleeding and therefore useful for identifying those patients who might benefit from the administration of platelets and fresh frozen plasma. Although mild elevations in the prothrombin time (PT) and activated partial thromboplastin time (aPTT) are not strongly correlated with bleeding, a PT and an aPTT of greater than 1.5 to 1.8 times the control value have been reported to be highly predictive of microvascular bleeding. A platelet count of 50×10^9/L or below and a fibrinogen level of less than 0.5 g/L were also shown to be highly predictive. These data have led to the following recommendations: administration of platelets to bleeding patients with platelet counts of less than 100×10^9/L, prophylactic administration of platelets to patients with a platelet count of less than 50×10^9/L, and administration of FFP or cryoprecipitate to patients with a fibrinogen of 0.8 g/L or less.[7,12,25] The American Society of Anesthesiologists has recommended similar "critical values" as indicators of high risk for microvascular bleeding: platelet counts of less than 50×10^9/L, PT and/or aPTT values of greater than 1.5 times normal control, coagulation factor levels of less than 30%, and fibrinogen concentrations less than 0.8 to 1.0 g/L.[26] The American College of Surgeons and the American Association of Blood Banks (AABB) *Technical Manual* both recommend that the transfusion of blood and components should be guided by the following laboratory tests: PT, aPTT, platelet count, and fibrinogen.[1,27] Refer to Table 17-2 for a flow diagram of elements that affect transfusion decisions.

Components of Anticoagulant/Preservative Solutions

Components of the anticoagulant/preservative solutions may also result in adverse consequences in massive transfusion. This is particularly true for neonatal patients. Included in this category of adverse reactions are citrate toxicity, potassium toxicity, acid-base imbalances, and hyperinsulinemia.

Citrate Toxicity

Anticoagulant/preservative solutions used for blood collection and storage contain sodium citrate. Because citrate resides in the plasma, risk of toxicity is associated with those components that have the largest plasma volumes such as FFP and Platelets.[4] Because of the action of the anticoagulant chelating agents, transfused blood has no ionized calcium and has excess quantities of citrate, which could potentially bind the serum calcium and magnesium of the recipient.[10,28] Citrate levels of currently licensed anticoagulant/preservative solutions are outlined in Table 17-3. Currently, AS-3 Red Blood Cells deliver the highest quantity of citrate per unit.[28] The component infused, the nature of the anticoagulant/preservative, the size of the recipient, and the rate and duration of infusion are all important variables in estimating the risk of citrate toxicity. Citrate load following transfusion is difficult to predict accurately owing to the many variables associated with administration, distribution, metabolism, and excretion. Rapid administration of blood and components can, under some circumstances, exceed the ability of the body to remove citrate.[28] Normal serum citrate levels are approximately 1 mg/dL (0.25 mmol/L), but these may reach 100 mg/dL (25.0 mmol/L) in massive transfusion. Although hypocalcemia is rarely found in transfused adults, it may pose

It is important to remember that stored bank blood differs substantially from the patient's own blood. These differences are due to the relatively large volume of anticoagulant/preservative solution present in bank blood and to the effects of storage on the product. These changes are of greatest concern when large volumes of blood are infused or when the recipient is less capable of metabolizing and excreting these substances.

Agents such as citrate prevent coagulation by chelating calcium. Transfused citrate is available to bind serum calcium and magnesium of the recipient and can potentially result in hypocalcemia in the massively transfused recipient.

TABLE 17-3 Content of Current Anticoagulant/Preservative and Additive Solutions

	ANTICOAGULANT/PRESERVATIVE SOLUTIONS (mg)			ADDITIVE SOLUTIONS (mg)		
	CPD	CP2D	CPDA-1	AS-1	AS-3	AS-5
Shelf life (days)	21	21	35	42	42	42
Sodium citrate	1660	1660	1660	0	588	0
Citric acid	188	188	188	0	42	0
Dextrose	1610	3220	2010	2200	1100	900
Dibasic sodium phosphate	140	140	140	0	276	0
Adenine	0	0	17.3	27	30	30
Mannitol	0	0	0	750	0	525
Sodium chloride	0	0	0	900	410	877

Hyperinsulinemia: Excess insulin in the blood.

Hypoglycemia: Low blood glucose.

a risk to individuals with liver dysfunction or other impairments that might influence citrate catabolism, such as perfusion, body temperature, acid-base balance, and glomerular filtration rate.[9,10] There have been reports of arrhythmias and acute myocardial failure after the rapid administration of citrated blood.[8] Although most patients who undergo massive transfusion do not require calcium supplementation, in some cases such treatment is critical. If calcium levels become critically low, it can be administered as calcium gluconate or calcium chloride.[9,16] Treatment with supplemental calcium carries significant risk and should be carefully monitored.[1] Excessive calcium replacement has been associated with cardiac arrest.[28]

Hyperinsulinemia

Transfused blood may carry a significant glucose load, which may result in **hyperinsulinemia.** On completion of the transfusion, this may result in **hypoglycemia.**[10] This is of particular concern in the transfusion of the neonate.

Acid-Base Imbalances

Transfusion of anticoagulant/preservative solutions that contain the products of storage lesion can result in clinically significant acid-base imbalances.[29,30] Severely ill patients may also have a significant metabolic acidosis at the onset of the transfusion.[10,16] Although acid-base imbalances are commonly associated with massive transfusion, the exact role of transfusion is not always clear.[8] Early in massive transfusion, metabolic acidosis is a common finding and can be fatal if not corrected. Generally, the acidosis reverses with cessation of hemorrhage and improved tissue perfusion. However, if hemorrhage cannot be controlled, the condition should be treated. Treatment with exogenous alkali may also carry significant risk because an alkaline pH increases the affinity of hemoglobin for oxygen and can depress ventilation. Such consequences must be carefully weighed in the treatment of the severely compromised patient.[10] As transfusion continues, metabolic alkalosis can be seen in conjunction with hypokalemia. This changing acid-base profile can be explained by the fact that transfused blood contains citrate and lactate, which are both acidic and can contribute to acidosis. These products are metabolized to bicarbonate, leading to a subsequent metabolic alkalosis. In alkalosis, intracellular hydrogen ions are exchanged for extracellular potassium in an attempt to neutralize the base, and hypokalemia may result.[8,10]

Other Adverse Effects

The massive transfusion of bank blood greater than 7 days old results in lower red cell concentrations of 2,3-DPG, with a resultant shift to the left of the oxygen dissociation curve.[19] Although the 2,3-DPG levels return to normal within 24 hours after transfusion, this reduction in the delivery of oxygen may hinder tissue perfusion in the already compromised massively transfused patient.[8,10] Cytokine-induced tissue damage may also result in part from the administration of stored blood that contains significant numbers of leukocytes.[12]

A more recently identified adverse effect of transfusion is immunosuppression. In the massively transfused patient, a loss of resistance to infection is a leading cause of death. This immunosuppressive effect was originally noted in kidney transplant recipients, who had more successful engraftment if previously transfused (the opposite of what was expected). Posttransfusion immunosuppression has been documented in some patients with solid tumors, although data are conflicting.[3,22] The possible association between transfusion and immunosuppression requires additional research data but could prove to be a significant adverse outcome in the massively transfused patient.

In a study published in 1999, researchers reported leukopenia as an adverse consequence of massive transfusion. In this study, all 23 of the study population who received greater than 50 units of blood became leukopenic (less than 4.0×10^9) during the first day after massive transfusion. The mechanism and significance of transfusion-associated leukopenia are not clear.[30]

Transfusion Issues

Red Blood Cells versus Whole Blood and "Fresh" Versus "Nonfresh"

Replacement of oxygen-carrying capacity in acute blood loss can be accomplished by the infusion of either Red Blood Cells or Whole Blood.[8,23] Whole Blood, which is not readily available from most blood centers, is generally reserved for patients who are actively bleeding and have sustained a blood loss in excess of 25% of their blood volume and are at risk for hemorrhagic shock. Administration of Red Blood Cells in conjunction with crystalloids and/or colloids is also suitable for massively transfused patients.[1,17,23]

The definition of "fresh" Whole Blood varies by institution, ranging from blood less than 24 hours old to blood administered within 5 to 7 days of collection. The debate continues regarding the use of fresh blood, especially those units less than 24 hours old. Some argue that the use of fresh Whole Blood is optimum for massive transfusion because it offers both optimally functional red blood cells and volume simultaneously with the administration of functional coagulation proteins.[12,25] Disadvantages of fresh Whole Blood usage include the inability to complete all infectious disease testing and the less efficient use of a single donation. Although some authors suggest that Whole Blood and fresh Whole Blood may have some advantages, there is evidence that use of component therapy is effective in the treatment of massively bleeding patients.[12,25,30] Advantages and disadvantages of Whole Blood compared with Red Blood Cells are outlined in Table 17-4.

Transfusion of Platelets

In bleeding patients, Platelet administration may be necessary to offset the thrombocytopenia associated with massive transfusion. Dilutional thrombocytopenia has

TABLE 17-4 Advantages and Disadvantages of Whole Blood versus Red Blood Cells	
Whole Blood	Red Blood Cells
Provides both O_2-carrying capacity and volume	Provides O_2 carrying capacity in less volume
Flows easily	May flow slowly without dilution
Must transfuse type specific	May transfuse type specific or type compatible
Other components cannot be prepared from the donation	Other components can be prepared from the donation
Contains a significant quantity of anticoagulant preservative	Much of the anticoagulant/preservative solution is removed
Plasma contains the products of storage lesion	Products of storage lesion may be removed with plasma

Petechiae: Small purplish spots on the skin due to pinpoint hemorrhages often associated with platelet dysfunctional states.

been associated with excessive bleeding and **petechiae** in the gut and urinary tract, mucosal bleeding, wound bleeding, and bleeding from cannula sites.[9,12] Thrombocytopenia may be further aggravated by platelet consumption, preexisting platelet dysfunction, and/or hypothermia. Unless the platelet count falls below a critical value, most practitioners, however, do not recommend the use of prophylactic Platelet therapy in the absence of clinical bleeding.[8,12] Research suggests that it is very difficult to drive the platelet count below 50×10^9/L in a patient with a functional marrow; however, bleeding patients with platelet counts below 50 to 100×10^9/L may benefit from administration of Platelets.[3,22] Ten platelet concentrates contain as much as 500 mL of plasma and therefore may also provide a source of labile coagulation factors assuming that they are administered early in the storage period.[23] Room temperature storage of Platelets will reduce the activity of Factors V and VIII:C.

Transfusion of Fresh Frozen Plasma and/or Cryoprecipitated AHF

FFP is rarely indicated in persons who are massively transfused and who have mild to moderately prolonged coagulation screening values (less than 1.5 to 1.8 times control).[1,8,9,12,17] A National Institutes of Health Consensus Report discouraged the prophylactic use of FFP in massive transfusion. Before this report, routine administration of Platelets and FFP was common practice in large-volume transfusion.[31] On the other hand, researchers have shown that patients with transfusion volumes in excess of two blood volumes may experience significant dilutional changes in coagulation proteins (less than 30%), especially when resuscitation is accomplished using Red Blood Cells and large volumes of crystalloid solutions. In such cases, especially in patients with hepatic dysfunction, transfusion with FFP has been recommended.[12,21] A suggested trigger for the transfusion of FFP is when the PT and aPTT exceed 1.5 to 1.8 times the upper limit of normal in conjunction with clinical evidence of coagulopathy.[12,16,25]

Fibrinogen is the first of the coagulation factors to be adversely affected by dilution in massive transfusion and is proportional to the amount of hemodilution. After 1.5 blood volumes have been replaced, fibrinogen levels may fall to critical levels (less than 1.0 g/L) with resultant bleeding. Both FFP and cryoprecipitate are sources of fibrinogen. Cryoprecipitate, because of its smaller volume, can be thawed and made available more readily to control blood loss associated with hypofibrinogenemia.[12]

Other Components/Derivatives

Prothrombin complex concentrate (PCC) or recombinant Factor VIIa (rVIIa) have been shown to be effective in reducing blood loss in patients with liver dysfunction or vitamin K deficiency (PCC) and in hemophiliacs with Factor VIII inhibitors, intraabdominal bleeding with DIC, and liver transplantation (rVIIa).[12,14]

Blood/Fluid Warming

The massive transfusion of cold blood and/or fluids has been associated with hypothermia and subsequent cardiac arrhythmias and cardiac arrest. In addition, hypothermia is associated with many of the adverse reactions of massive transfusion. Hypothermia leads to a general decrease in metabolic rate.[32] The cold patient theoretically cannot metabolize citrate or lactate,[10,16,17] regenerate 2,3-DPG,[10] or metabolize drugs[17,32] as efficiently as the normothermic patient. Hypothermia also contributes to acidosis and hypoperfusion;[10,32] results in increased release of intracellular potassium, decreased red cell deformability, impaired platelet function,[3] and increased blood viscosity;[17] and has been associated with impaired hemostatic function.[10,32] Summary 17-3 lists the physiologic consequences associated with hypothermia. Interventions aimed at correcting hypothermia have been generally successful.[10] The risk of transfusion-associated hypothermia can be reduced by the

Summary 17-3

Clinical Features Associated with Hypothermia

Decreased metabolism of citrate and lactate
Decreased ability to regenerate 2,3-DPG
Platelet dysfunction
Impaired drug metabolism
Increased blood viscosity
Impaired hemostatic function
Acidosis
Hypoperfusion
Cardiac arrhythmias

use of an in-line blood warmer. Instruments are available for this purpose and allow for the rapid and carefully controlled warming of blood during infusion.[8,32] The AABB Standards require that blood be warmed during passage through the closed transfusion set and should not reach temperatures above 38° C. Blood warmers must have an audible warning system that indicates unacceptable temperatures.[33] Other strategies used to prevent hypothermia during resuscitation and massive transfusion include the use of fluid warmers, mixing blood with warmed saline, and increasing the temperature in surgical suites.[10,16]

Emergency Release

When selecting blood for massive transfusion, the blood bank is often faced with inadequate quantities of type-specific blood. When other than type-specific Red Blood Cells must be transfused, the red cells of the donor must be ABO compatible with the serum of the recipient (type compatible). In the case of whole blood transfusion, only the same type as the recipient (type specific) can be administered. In addition, donor red cells should be negative for any antigen that corresponds to a clinically significant antibody in the serum of the recipient. Unless it is not available, Rh-negative Red Blood Cells should be given to Rh-negative recipients. If it is not available, Rh-positive Red Blood Cells can be given to an unimmunized Rh-negative recipient. Special care is taken to avoid transfusion of Rh-positive blood to Rh-negative women of childbearing age. Rh-positive blood, however, should not be withheld in cases of life-threatening emergency.[27,33,34]

In the emergency setting, it may not be feasible to wait for the completion of pretransfusion testing before releasing blood or components. In these situations, it is important to carefully document the need for the urgent release of blood and deviations from the customary testing protocols.[33,34] Blood bank records should contain a signed order from the physician stating the reason for emergency release, and blood must be clearly labeled indicating that the pretransfusion compatibility testing has not been completed.[33] If the ABO type of the recipient has not been determined, O-negative Red Blood Cells are customarily selected.[3,8,33,35] O-positive blood is equally safe and can be selected in the event of a shortage of O-negative units. Subsequent to the release of the units, compatibility testing should be completed as soon as possible. In no cases should previous records alone be used as the source of ABO typing for the selection of blood.[27,33] Emergency situations should not be seen as sufficient rationale for noncompliance with strict procedures for the positive identification of the recipient, complete specimen labeling, and careful adherence to all identification protocols and procedures.[33]

Pretransfusion testing can be abbreviated or eliminated when there is sufficient reason to believe that delay in transfusion would risk life or limb.

Autotransfusion

Autologous blood is potentially the safest option in emergency transfusion. Blood from thoracic drainage and from the abdominal cavity (as long as the gastrointestinal tract is intact) is considered adequately "clean" for transfusion. Such blood-containing fluids can be reinfused with or without additional processing. Autologous blood carries no risk of immunologic incompatibility or disease transmission, but there is increased risk of contamination and possible deleterious effects associated with the infusion of microemboli and cellular debris.[3] Blood collected perioperatively or posttraumatically should not be transfused to other patients. Methods must ensure that the reinfusion is safe and aseptic and that adequate procedures are in place to properly identify the donor-recipient. Written procedures must be maintained, which include the investigation of adverse reactions, and a program of quality assurance must be in place. There must be a documented process to ensure that perioperative products are handled in such a way to limit deterioration and prevent damage.[36] It is imperative that, as with all blood transfusions, extreme caution be used to ensure a safe and efficacious blood product and to carefully identify the donor-recipient.

Components such as platelet gel, fibrin sealant, apheresis RBCs, and cryoprecipitate may be prepared from blood salvaged perioperatively. Such processes, which involve the manipulation of Whole Blood, require periodic quality control. Programs should have documentation of acceptable levels of factors in the components that they prepare and transfuse.[36]

Use of Filters

All blood must be infused using a sterile blood infusion set with a standard 170 μm blood filter. The use of microaggregate filters (less than 170 μm) in massive transfusion is a more controversial issue. Microaggregates, composed of nonviable granulocytes, platelets, and fibrin, form during the first few days of blood storage, increasing in size and number throughout the storage period. Microaggregates range in size from 20 to 200 μm, but the majority are less than 50 μm in diameter.[37] Microaggregate filters are either screen filters that remove particles by physical blockage or depth filters that adsorb particles. Although reports have linked microaggregate particles in stored blood with acute respiratory distress syndrome, there is no consistent evidence of a causal relationship. The use of microaggregate filters in massive transfusion is not well supported by empirical data, and their routine use is not indicated.[8,10,16,17,37] As with any filter capable of removing leukocytes, microaggregate filters should not be used when transfusing granulocytes.[33] Such filters may be contraindicated if they delay transfusion in exsanguinating patients.

THERAPEUTIC HEMAPHERESIS AND THERAPEUTIC PHLEBOTOMY
Therapeutic Plasmapheresis or Plasma Exchange

Plasma exchange (therapeutic plasmapheresis [TPE]) has been used to treat patients with a wide range of diseases/conditions. Plasma exchange is defined as the removal of pathologic plasma components and the replacement of lost volume with fluids such as normal plasma, crystalloids, or colloids. The goal of plasma exchange is the reduction in the concentration of the pathologic substance and/or the replacement of some missing factor, thus improving the course of the disease.[8,27,38,39] Plasma exchange has been used in a wide variety of clinical states to remove a substance that is either a normal component of plasma, such as low-density lipoprotein (LDL) cholesterol, or a disease-related component, such as abnormal paraproteins, antibodies, or immune complexes.[40]

Early manual plasmapheresis procedures involved the removal of whole blood, off-line centrifugation, and subsequent reinfusion of the red cell fraction. Such procedures were used widely for commercial harvesting of plasma, as well as in therapeutic settings. With the advent of disposable, closed plastic bag systems and the development of more sophisticated technology, the process of plasma exchange became safer and more efficient, as well as more sensitive[41] (Fig. 17-1). Plasma

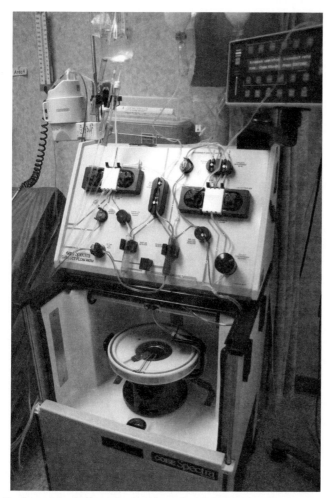

Fig. 17-1 Equipment for therapeutic plasma exchange (TPE) with centrifuge bowl exposed.

exchange, although often effective at removing the targeted pathologic substance, also removes normal plasma components, and it is for this reason that much current research in plasma exchange is aimed at the investigation of methods that facilitate the removal of the specific components involved in the pathophysiology of the disease with minimal loss of normal plasma constituents.[38] In some instances, selective removal of plasma components can be achieved by physiochemical methods such as filtration or cryofiltration and by more specific techniques such as adsorption. Because target molecules often have molecular weights over 100,000 (larger than albumin), they can be effectively removed from plasma by various ultrafiltration procedures.[42,43] On the other hand, selective removal can sometimes be accomplished by adsorption and immunoadsorption. In these techniques, a specific ligand is tightly bound to a matrix through which the plasma is passed. Ligands can be relatively nonspecific, such as charcoal, or can be highly specific, such as monoclonal antibody.[38] The offending plasma solute adheres to the ligand and is thereby removed from the plasma, which is then returned to the patient.

Plasma exchange has proven useful in a number of diseases (Summary 17-4). The process, however, is aimed at the alleviation of symptoms associated with the accumulation of a plasma solute and does not alter the course of the disease. Generally, plasma exchange is accompanied by other therapies, such as chemotherapy in paraproteinemias, in order to extend remission.[40] Efficacy of these procedures is enhanced if the disease factor is contained predominantly in the

Summary 17-4

Selected Conditions for which Plasma Exchange is Indicated

Hematologic Diseases
Myeloma/paraproteins/hyperviscosity
Thrombotic thrombocytopenic purpura
Coagulation factor inhibitors

Renal and Metabolic Diseases
Rapidly progressing glomerulonephritis
Familial hypercholesterolemia
Renal transplant rejection

Autoimmune and Rheumatic Diseases
Rheumatoid arthritis
Cryoglobulinemia
Idiopathic thrombocytopenic purpura

Neurologic Disorders
Guillain-Barré syndrome
Myasthenia gravis
Lambert-Eaton syndrome

From McLeod BC: Introduction to the third special issue: Clinical applications of therapeutic apheresis. J Clin Apheresis 15:1-5, 2000.

intravascular compartment and the rate of accumulation is relatively slow.[39] For example, plasma exchange is more effective in removing IgM, which is predominantly an intravascular protein, than IgG, which has a larger extravascular pool.[40]

Plasma Exchange in Selected Disorders
Thrombotic Microangiopathies: Thrombotic Thrombocytopenic Purpura and Hemolytic Uremic Syndrome

Plasma exchange has proven to be a useful tool in the treatment of thrombotic thrombocytopenic purpura (TTP), a microangiopathic disorder. Platelet microthrombi found in primary TTP are generally associated with the presence of large multimers of von Willebrand factor resulting from a deficiency of a von Willebrand cleaving protein, a metaloprotease (MP), found in normal plasma.[41,44] Secondary TTP is associated with an IgG antibody against this MP.[45] TTP is characterized by hemolytic anemia, thrombocytopenia, fever, neurologic disorders, renal insufficiency and can progress to acute renal failure.[44-49] Plasma from TTP patients activates normal platelets, and this activation has been shown to be neutralized by the addition of normal plasma. These findings have led to the use of plasma exchange in this disorder.[40] FFP or FFP Cryoprecipitate Reduced is generally used as the replacement fluid in TTP patients; it is believed that these fluids supply the missing protease.[41,44,49] When used in combination with antiplatelet therapy and dialysis, plasma exchange has been reported to dramatically improve survival rates. Platelet transfusions in these patients are contraindicated and have been associated with delayed recovery and decreased survival rates.[45,46,49,50-52] The use of plasmapheresis in TTP is an example of how therapeutic apheresis is used for the replacement of a "missing" factor (in this case a protease) rather than the removal of a pathologic substance (such as an abnormal paraprotein). The AABB and the American Society for Apheresis (ASFA) have categorized plasma exchange as a category I therapy (standard therapy) for TTP (Table 17-5).[53]

TABLE 17-5 ASFA and AABB Categories of Indications for Therapeutic Apheresis

Category	Definition
I	Standard first-line or adjunctive therapy; well supported by research and clinical data
II	Generally accepted as a secondary therapy
III	Not clearly indicated due to conflicting or insufficient data; used only when conventional therapies fail
IV	Not indicated except in approved research protocols

From Smith JW, Weinstein R, Hillyer KL: Therapeutic apheresis: A summary of the current indication categories endorsed by the AABB and the American Society for Apheresis. Transfusion 43(6):820-822, 2003.

Hemolytic uremic syndrome (HUS) is characterized by similar clinical symptoms and histopathology; however, the etiology of the disorder differs from that of TTP.[44,49] Because of inclusive data and inconsistent findings, the 2003 AABB/ASFA category for treatment of HUS is category III. Applications in this category are reserved for life-or-death, last-ditch efforts rather than standard therapy (category I) or routine adjunctive therapy (category II) (see Table 17-5).[53]

Neurologic Disorders

Plasma exchange has been clinically useful in patients with a number of neurologic disorders with similar autoimmune characteristics, such as myasthenia gravis, Guillain-Barré syndrome, and multiple sclerosis.[40,54,55] Plasma exchange is especially useful in myasthenia gravis, a disease of the neuromuscular junction. Myasthenia gravis patients have been shown to have an autoantibody that binds to acetylcholine receptors on the postsynaptic membrane. Complement fixation has been demonstrated and may have a role in receptor destruction.[55] In these patients, plasma exchange, with or without the concurrent administration of immunosuppressive therapy, has resulted in lowered levels of circulating antibody and clinical improvement.[38-41,56,57] One major advantage of plasma exchange in these patients is the rapid clinical response (as early as two 3 to 4 L exchanges), which could prove life saving in patients with respiratory failure.[41] Therapeutic plasma exchange is considered standard therapy in myasthenia gravis (category I) (see Table 17-5).[53]

Acute inflammatory demyelinating polyradiculoneuropathy (AIDP), or Guillain-Barré syndrome, is now considered to be the most frequently occurring paralytic disorder (2 cases in 100,000 persons). The disease course can vary from mild neurologic symptoms to severe, life-threatening forms that require ventilatory support. Two thirds of affected patients suffer from persistent neurologic defects and as many as 1 in 20 die from complications of the disease.[55] The pathophysiology of the disease is associated with activation of both the cellular and humoral immune mechanisms. Excess T-cell activation noted in these patients is considered to be a secondary consequence of an initial antibody attack on myelin.[55] Therapeutic plasma exchange with or without concurrent intravenous immunoglobulin therapy has been shown to be effective in AIDP. AIDP is classified as a category I indication for TPE (see Table 17-5).[53]

Dysproteinemias

Plasma exchange has also proven successful in the treatment of patients with various dysproteinemias.[45,58,59] Dysproteinemias are disorders characterized by circulating monoclonal or polyclonal paraproteins. Included in this category of disorders are multiple myeloma, macroglobulinemia, cryoglobulinemia, pyroglobulinemia, and connective tissue disease. The accumulation of a paraprotein is associated with hyperviscosity, hypervolemia, bleeding, and renal failure. Of these, hyperviscosity is a major cause of the clinical symptoms associated with these diseases such as headache, dizziness, and visual and cardiac disturbances.[40,58,60-63] Because the relationship between plasma viscosity and paraprotein concentration is exponential, the removal of even small quantities by plasma exchange results in a dramatic reduction of viscosity, with a subsequent reduction in associated clinical symptoms.[45,60,64,65] Multiple myeloma when complicated by renal failure has a poor prognosis. In these cases, TPE is an effective way to remove accumulated light chains. Clinical trials have demonstrated reversal of kidney failure in a significant number of patients treated with TPE, and it is considered a category II indication in these patients (see Table 17-5).[53]

Renal Disease

Plasma exchange has proven useful as a clinical tool in renal diseases of immune origin, such as rapidly progressive glomerulonephritis (RPGN) and renal transplant rejection. RPGN is associated with deteriorating renal function over a rather short period and includes Goodpasture's syndrome and Wegener's granulomatosis.[66] Goodpasture's syndrome is characterized by autoimmune damage to lung and glomerular tissue and is associated with significant mortality and morbidity rates. Plasma exchange in conjunction with immunosuppressive therapy has resulted in substantial clinical improvement,[40,41,66] and it is considered a category I indication.

Plasma exchange has also been used in an attempt to prolong renal allograft survival. Outcomes have been variable, and the role of plasma exchange in these patients remains uncertain.[40,66] Currently, plasma exchange in renal allograft is category IV (see Table 17-5).[53]

Hypercholesterolemia

Plasma exchange has been successful in the treatment of patients with familial hypercholesterolemia that cannot be controlled by the usual protocols of diet and medication. The disorder is characterized by decreased number of LDL receptors in the liver. As a result, LDL is not removed from the blood, resulting in the accumulation of LDL cholesterol and lipoprotein (a) (Lpa) with subsequent premature atherosclerosis.[66] This condition is associated with significant morbidity and mortality rates in the third decade of life. Selective removal of LDL has been accomplished by the use of immunoadsorption columns and hollow-fiber membrane filters.[38,40,66,67] Removal of LDL cholesterol by TPE or selective adsorption, along with adjunctive therapy aimed at decreasing production of LDL, has been generally successful in reducing LDL and preventing associated clinical problems. Recently, a device for selective removal of LDL has been approved by the FDA.[68] Familial hypercholesterolemia is a category I indication for selective adsorption and a category II indication for TPE[53,66] (see Table 17-5).

Technical Considerations in Plasma Exchange

During plasma exchange, plasma is removed while replacement fluid is infused. Fig. 17-2 is a schematic diagram of the plasma exchange process. Calculations that estimate the efficacy of plasma exchange are based on the assumptions that the blood volume does not change, that the toxic substance is not mobilized from the extravascular spaces, that production remains at a steady state, and that the rate of synthesis and the rate of catabolism are balanced.[27,60,69] The efficiency of substance removal decreases progressively during exchange. Generally, exchange is limited to one plasma volume (40 mL plasma per kilogram of body weight). In some cases, multiple plasma volumes may be exchanged to maximize the removal of the target substance. Such procedures are lengthy and less efficient. In early phases of plasma exchange, crystalloid solutions may be used for volume replacement. Later in the procedure, colloids, such as albumin, are generally indicated to avoid an excessive drop in colloid oncotic pressure. In high-volume exchanges, FFP may be indicated to avoid dilutional coagulopathy.[27,60] However, the use of FFP, except in TTP where it provides a missing substance, is controversial.[41]

Therapeutic Cytapheresis

Therapeutic cytapheresis involves the removal of specific cellular components from the patient's circulation. Cytapheresis can involve the removal of leukocytes (leukapheresis), red cells (erythropheresis), and platelets (plateletpheresis). The goal of therapeutic cytapheresis is to decrease the hemorrhagic and thrombotic complications associated with abnormally high concentrations of cellular elements[70] (Summary 17-5). Candidates for therapeutic cytapheresis generally have platelet counts in excess of 500×10^9/L or white cell numbers of 100,000/μL or more. Data suggest that complications in these patients are due to abnormal circulating cells such as white blood cells from a malignant clone, activated platelets, or leukocytes with abnormal adhesion characteristics.[71] Therapeutic cytapheresis may be successful in these disorders by two mechanisms: (1) the reduction of cell number and (2) the selective removal of abnormal cells.

Therapeutic leukapheresis has been used as a treatment modality in patients with both acute myelocytic leukemia (AML) and chronic myelocytic leukemia (CML). Patients whose white counts exceed 100,000/μL may experience leukostasis with subsequent vaso-occlusion, which can result in fatal pulmonary or cardiac collapse or cerebrovascular insufficiency.[39,71] Leukapheresis has been useful in achieving rapid cytoreduction in these patients and is more rapid than cytotoxic therapy.[41]

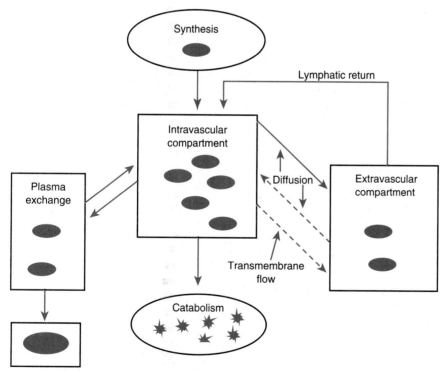

Fig. 17-2 A diagram of the dynamic interaction between intravascular and vascular spaces during plasma exchange. The effectiveness of plasma exchange is affected by the distribution of the substance in extravascular versus intravascular spaces, the rate at which the substance equilibrates between compartments, and the impact of substance removal on rates of synthesis and catabolism. *(Modified with permission from Weinstein R: Basic principles of therapeutic blood exchange. In McLeod BC, Price TH, Weinstein R [eds]: Apheresis Principles and Practice, 2nd ed. Bethesda, MD, American Association of Blood Banks, 2003.)*

Summary 17-5

Selected Conditions for which Therapeutic Cytapheresis is Indicated

PLATELETPHERESIS (THROMBOCYTAPHERESIS)
Thrombocytosis (thrombotic or hemorrhagic)

LEUKOCYTAPHERESIS
Leukemia (with hyperleukocytosis)
Cutaneous T-cell lymphoma
Hairy cell leukemia

ERYTHROCYTAPHERESIS
Sickle cell anemia (with vaso-occlusion)

LYMPHOCYTAPHERESIS
Rheumatoid arthritis

Sources: Brecher ME (ed): AABB Technical Manual, 14th ed. Bethesda, MD, American Association of Blood Banks, 2002; Barth WF: Viscosity of serum in relationship to serum globulins. In Sunderman FW, Sunderman FW Jr (eds): Serum Proteins and the Dysproteinemias. Philadelphia, JB Lippincott, 1964; McLeod BC: Introduction to the third special issue: Clinical applications of therapeutic apheresis. J Clin Apheresis 15:1-5, 2000.

Plateletpheresis and erythropheresis are used less frequently but may be of use in the immediate reduction of platelet number or the removal of abnormal red cells.[27,39] Plateletpheresis has been shown to provide control of symptoms in patients with symptomatic thrombocytosis, but does not have a role in long-term management of myeloproliferative diseases.[71,72] Disorders of platelet function may also respond to plateletpheresis, perhaps due to the selective removal of larger, more dense dysfunctional platelets.[41] Therapeutic plateletpheresis provides rapid reduction in platelet number. Because there is no correlation between platelet count and development of symptoms, efficacy is generally determined by observations of change in the clinical status of the patient. The most common application of erythropheresis has been in sickle cell anemia patients. This disease has a high incidence in the United States (more than 50,000 cases) and is associated with high morbidity and mortality rates because of vaso-occlusion during crisis.[70]

Relatively new applications of cytapheresis include the harvesting of normal cell populations followed by ex vivo manipulation and reinfusion. For example, it has been demonstrated that lymphocytes, if harvested and cultured in the presence of lymphokines such as interleukin-2 (IL-2) and T-cell growth factor, develop antitumor activity. These lymphokine-activated killer cells (LAK cells) represented early attempts at immunomodulation by the infusion of modified autologous or allogeneic cells. This relatively new area of inquiry is known as "adaptive immunotherapy."[41]

Cytapheresis also provides a mechanism for the selective harvesting of peripheral blood progenitor cells (PBPCs), which can be used for marrow reconstitution after myeloablative therapy in patients with acute myelogenous leukemia and other hematopoietic disorders.[41]

Standards of Practice

The AABB Standards require that therapeutic plasmapheresis, plasma exchange, and cytapheresis include a written request by the patient's physician, who is responsible for carrying out the procedure.[33] The blood bank or transfusion service must maintain a written procedure for all methods, including the operation of any equipment used. As with all blood bank procedures, these must show evidence of periodic review, and update if indicated. Blood bank records should include the patient's identification, the type of procedure, the nature and volume of components removed and infused, any adverse reactions, and medication administered (if any). Written informed consent should be obtained from the patient before the pheresis procedure. The patient should be made aware of the procedure, its benefits and limitations, and any possible adverse reactions and should be given the opportunity to ask questions.[33]

Therapeutic Phlebotomy

Therapeutic phlebotomy is the removal of red cells from a patient for some medical indication. The removal of red cells can be useful in the reduction of blood viscosity, which, in turn, may facilitate organ perfusion and decrease the probability of thrombosis. In addition, withdrawal of red cells can be used to reduce hemoglobin in patients with iron overload and thus prevent iron-associated organ damage.

Red cell volume is the major contributor to blood viscosity. It is well established that increases in hematocrit above 50% raise viscosity, thereby increasing resistance to blood flow. It is generally recommended that phlebotomy be used to maintain a hematocrit of 45% or less.[73] Therapeutic phlebotomy has been useful in decreasing blood viscosity in patients with both primary and secondary **polycythemia**. The procedure is generally safe for most patients.

Therapeutic phlebotomy requires the written request of the patient's physician. With the exception of units from patients with **hemochromacytosis**, blood collected by therapeutic phlebotomy may not be used for allogeneic transfusion and must be discarded. If blood from hemochromacytosis patients is used, it must meet all standards for allogeneic transfusion.[33]

TRANSFUSION IN BURN PATIENTS
An Overview of Thermal Injury

The extent of injury in burns depends on the temperature of the source, the duration of contact, and the conductivity of the involved tissue. Injury results from the transfer of heat from some exogenous source and, depending on the depth and extent of the burn, can result in skin damage, vascular injury, and metabolic dysfunction.

Skin Injury

Skin provides a barrier to microorganisms and limits the loss of body heat and water. In burns these protective functions of the skin are lost. Water loss in intact skin is estimated to be approximately 15 mL/m^2/hr. In full-thickness burns (third-degree burns), fluid loss can increase to as much as 200 mL/m^2/hr. This increase in loss of body water results in hypertonic dehydration. Burns also compromise the ability of the skin barrier to prevent infection.[74]

Vascular Injury

A serious consequence of burns is the loss of vascular integrity with an associated increase in capillary permeability. Increased capillary permeability extends to areas remote from the site of burn injury. As a result, fluid and protein escape from the vasculature, with a subsequent decrease in blood volume and accumulation of fluid in interstitial spaces resulting in edema. Fluid can also be lost into the skin, in which case it appears as blisters or exudate.[74,75] In contrast to normal skin water loss, the fluid lost from burns contains variable amounts of protein and electrolytes and is similar to plasma. The protein content of this fluid is highest during the first 24 hours after the burn. Most fluid is lost from the vasculature in the first 24 hours, after which remote capillary permeability normalizes and interstitial fluid gradually

Polycythemia: An increase in red cell mass that may be a primary disorder (polycythemia vera) or a secondary response to sustained hypoxia.

Hemochromacytosis: A disease characterized by the deposition of hemosiderin in parenchymal cells. Acquired and secondary forms of the disease exist.

The depth of burns is expressed as first-, second-, and third-degree burns (from least to most severe). Third-degree burns are also known as full-thickness burns.

returns from the vascular space. The loss of fluid in burn victims has physiologic consequences similar to acute blood loss and results in hypoperfusion, shock, and diminished kidney function.[74] The loss of plasma can result in hemoconcentration and increased blood viscosity, which can further exacerbate this hypoperfusion.[74-76]

Red Cell Destruction

Red cell loss in burns is difficult to estimate; however, as with other consequences of thermal injury, the loss of red cells correlates with the extent of the injury. Blood loss can be expressed as a percent of blood volume based on the percent of surface burns. Each 1% of burn corresponds to a 2.6% blood loss for adults and a 3.4% loss for children.[77] Red cell loss can result from direct hemolysis of blood by heat, entrapment in occluded vessels, removal of heat-modified red cells by the reticuloendothelial system, and/or burn-related gastrointestinal bleeding. Blood loss is further complicated by a decrease in erythropoiesis, which has been associated with burn injury.[74,76] Research evidence suggests that decreased RBC production is associated with a circulating inhibitor that inhibits erythropoiesis but not granulopoiesis.[77,78]

In addition to blood loss related to the physiology of burns, surgical excision and grafting are associated with major blood loss, as much as three liters for larger excisions.[79-82] The combined effect of these is significant decreases in red cell mass and oxygen-carrying capacity.

Infection

After initial resuscitation to restore volume and tissue perfusion, burn patients are left with open skin wounds. Infection is the most common cause of morbidity and mortality in burn patients.[83,84] Mortality is frequently associated with pneumonia and sepsis by *Pseudomonas aeruginosa* and other microorganisms. The probability of wound infection is increased because burn patients demonstrate a burn-related defect in white cell phagocytic activity and serum opsonic activity.[83] This defect may be due in part to a deficiency in fibronectin, a plasma cryoglobulin that has **opsonic activity** and mediates the clearance of microorganisms by the reticuloendothelial system. Fibronectin depletion is maximal at 12 hours following burn, and the magnitude of the deficiency is related to the severity of the burn. A secondary depletion of fibronectin has been associated with infection.[74]

Therapy in Burn Patients
Initial Replacement of Volume

As in the hemorrhaging patient, the initial treatment in the therapy of burn patients is aimed at reversing hypovolemia and hypoperfusion. This generally involves the infusion of large volumes of crystalloids. Shock in burn patients is a gradual process and may be masked by the general constriction of blood vessels in the **splanchnic** area and skin, which maintains blood pressure but may seriously compromise organ perfusion, especially to the kidney.[75] Burn shock has a complex etiology characterized by both hypovolemic and cellular shock complicated by burn edema and large-volume fluid shifts between the vascular and extravascular compartments. Changes in vascular permeability associated with thermal injury are associated with the release of multiple mediators, including histamine, bradykinin, vasoactive amines, platelet release products, components of complement activation, prostaglandins, and leukotrienes. Release of these mediators has been linked with either increased capillary permeability or microvascular hydrostatic pressure. The microvascular changes associated with this complex interaction result in disruption of normal capillary barriers between the intravascular and interstitial compartments with a resultant depletion of plasma volume.[85] Thermal injury is also associated with a change in cell transmembrane potential and a subsequent increase in intracellular sodium concentrations. Without adequate resuscitation this progressively deteriorates, leading to cell death.[85]

Opsonic activity: Refers to the presence of substances in the serum that potentiate the phagocytosis of particles by macrophages and neutrophils.

Splanchnic: Refers to the large organs in any of the body cavities.

It has been estimated that patients can recover from burns of 15% or less body surface area without transfusion. If the burn area exceeds 15%, resuscitation should begin immediately to avert irreversible shock. Dosages can be calculated using the extent of the burn and the body weight as variables. Victims with extensive full-thickness burns may need immense volumes to achieve resuscitation (for example, a 70 kg adult with a 50% body surface burn could require 7 to 14 L during the first 24 hours).[74] Controversy exists regarding the use of colloids and Whole Blood in early resuscitation.[86] Colloid administered in the first 24 hours is lost as a result of the increased capillary permeability. During the second 24 hours, improvement may be seen after colloid administration owing to the reversal of capillary damage.[74] Whole Blood administration during early resuscitation has been reported to be superior to other fluid therapies by some researchers who reported improvement in anemia, oncotic pressure, acid-base balance, oxygenation, hemodynamics, and myocardial function and protection from bacterial infection after administration of Whole Blood.[87] Risks of transfusion, such as transfusion-transmitted viral infection, must be weighed against the benefits of Whole Blood in resuscitation.

Red Cell and Blood Component Therapy

Red Blood Cells are generally not administered during the first 24 hours after the burn because the loss of plasma results in hemoconcentration and increased viscosity. Although some centers have successfully managed special patients with severe burns without blood, Red Blood Cells are frequently necessary after initial fluid resuscitation to treat anemia resulting from red cell loss, surgical blood loss, and gastrointestinal bleeding.[74,87] Granulocyte transfusion may be useful in the treatment of burn-related sepsis in cases in which leukocyte function is impaired and sepsis is refractory to antibiotic therapy. The efficacy of this therapy in burn patients has not been documented. The demand for Granulocytes as a treatment for overwhelming infection has been diminishing. Cryoprecipitated AHF may be useful in burn patients as a source of fibronectin. It has been demonstrated that the infusion of Cryoprecipitated AHF is associated with a reversal of the opsonic defect for a period of 24 hours after infusion. This has been associated with improvement in pulmonary function, limb blood flow, and oxygen consumption.[74]

Contraindications to Transfusion in Burns

Data have suggested that blood transfusion may carry a risk of immunosuppression. Because infection is the most serious complication of thermal injury, evidence of increased infection associated with transfusion is a significant finding. In a study of 594 burn patients, Graves and colleagues[88] have reported a relationship between number of units transfused and infectious morbidity that is independent of age and extent of burn. These data are consistent with those in areas of tissue transplant rejection and tumor metastases, which support the immunosuppressive effect of transfusion. Additional data are necessary to further substantiate this in patients with thermal injury. Growing concern over the risk of transfusion has resulted in a more conservative approach to transfusion in burn patients, transfusing only when the hematocrit falls below 25% or 30% in critically ill patients or those with cardiovascular disease.[79,80] Intraoperative salvage has been demonstrated to safely reduce the requirement for red cell transfusion during burn excision.[82]

TRANSFUSION IN LIVER DISEASE AND LIVER TRANSPLANTATION
Physiology

The liver is the largest intraabdominal organ of the body and receives 20% of the cardiac output.[74,89] The liver's blood is supplied by the hepatic artery and the portal vein. Contact between liver cells (hepatocytes) and the blood takes place in the permeable capillaries of the liver known as sinusoids. The liver has a number of complex functions, including the formation of bile, carbohydrate storage, gluconeogenesis, reduction and conjugation of steroid hormones, detoxification, production of plasma proteins such as albumin and coagulation proteins, inactivation of ammonia (urea formation), and the production of cholesterol, triglycerides, fatty acids, and glycogen.[2,89] Liver function is maintained so long as the hepatocyte function is preserved and blood flow is adequate. Hepatocellular damage without a concurrent derangement in blood flow can be reversed through cellular regeneration. Cellular damage associated with diminished blood flow results in a more severe pathology. In cirrhosis, for example, hepatic cells are destroyed and replaced by fibrous scar tissue that compromises hepatic circulation. Cirrhosis can result from alcoholism, drugs and toxins, heavy metal poisoning, metabolic disorders, viral hepatitis, and congestive heart failure. Of these, alcoholism and viral infection are the most common causes.[2,74] Liver disease can result in an impairment of any of the liver functions, which can lead to a complex clinical picture. Some of the outcomes of liver disease affect transfusion decisions, and these are emphasized in this discussion.

Liver Disease: Implications for Transfusion
Portal Hypertension

The accumulation of scar tissue in the liver is associated with diminished blood flow. Some of the blood flow is rerouted through **collateral venous circulation.** This, in turn, results in a decreased supply of nutrients to the liver, compromising liver metabolic function, and interferes with the ability of the liver to excrete wastes. Diminished blood flow also results in a chronic elevation of portal venous pressure known as portal hypertension. An increased pressure can result in engorgement of the spleen with associated splenic enlargement. The resulting hypersplenism results in the premature removal of platelets and leukocytes from the circulation and can result in a significant thrombocytopenia. Another sequela of portal hypertension is the development of **esophageal varices** and related gastrointestinal bleeding. Diminished blood flow is also associated with the accumulation of fluid in the interstitium (edema) and in the abdominal cavity (ascites). These fluid shifts result mainly from the decreased production of albumin by the liver and the increased portal venous pressure.

Effects of Massive Transfusion

For a number of reasons, patients with end-stage liver disease frequently receive large-volume transfusions and are at risk for the toxic effects associated with the infusion of large quantities of anticoagulant/preservative solution and blood storage lesion products. A frequent complication of liver disease is hepatorenal syndrome or hepatic nephropathy. The syndrome is characterized by decreased renal blood flow associated with renal vascular constriction.[2] These patients are unable to effectively excrete potassium and are at greater risk for transfusion-associated hyperkalemia and associated cardiac dysfunction.[90] Massively transfused patients with liver dysfunction also experience as much as a 20-fold increase in citrate, with a concomitant decrease in serum calcium and associated decreases in cardiac function. As a result, patients with end-stage liver disease are at greater risk for transfusion-related hyperkalemia, hypocalcemia, and acidosis. These patients also develop a perioperative alkalosis, probably associated with the quantity of citrate infused.[91] Because citrate metabolism is positively correlated with body core temperature, hypocalcemia may be further exacerbated by the hypothermia that is associated with large-volume resuscitation with crystalloids and bank blood.

Hemostatic Abnormalities
Coagulation Factor Deficiencies

Patients with liver disease have a number of hemostatic abnormalities that may contribute to an increased tendency to bleed (Summary 17-6). Because all of the

Collateral circulation: Secondary side branching of the circulatory system that carries blood from areas otherwise occluded.

Esophageal varices: Enlarged veins or arteries in the esophagus that tend to rupture and bleed.

Summary 17-6

Factors Contributing to Hemostatic Disorders in Liver Disease

Thrombocytopenia
Platelet dysfunction
Decreased synthesis of coagulation proteins
Dysfibrinogenemia
Hyperfibrinolysis

coagulation proteins are formed in the liver, severe liver disease is associated with a multiple factor deficiency (early depletion of Factors II, VII, IX, and X followed by a general depression in all coagulation protein synthesis) that cannot be corrected by the administration of vitamin K. Factor VIII is generally normal or increased in liver disease patients,[74,92] which may reflect an increased synthesis of the molecule at a site other than the liver.[93] Because Factor VII has the shortest half-life (2 to 6 hours), it can be depleted to a greater extent than other factors, resulting in a prolonged PT. The aPTT is less affected but is prolonged in severe disease.[27,93,94] Decreased synthesis of coagulation factors correlates with the extent of hepatocellular damage. The PT is a relatively accurate predictor of the severity of the disease, and a PT of 1.5 times normal is an indicator of severe disease and a poor prognosis.[74,95]

Fibrinolysis

Liver disease is also associated with increased fibrinolytic activity due, at least in part, to a decreased clearance of fibrin(ogen) degradation products and fibrinolytic activators, as well as a decreased synthesis of fibrinolytic inhibitors. Abnormal synthesis of fibrinogen molecules has also been reported to be associated with liver disease.[93]

Thrombocytopenia

The tendency to bleed is further complicated by the thrombocytopenia that is secondary to splenomegaly,[93] reduced levels of thrombopoietin,[93] and other factors such as the direct toxic effect of alcohol on platelets and coexisting immune thrombocytopenia.[27,93,94] Because liver patients are often massively transfused, these hemostatic defects can be complicated by the dilutional coagulopathy and dilutional thrombocytopenia associated with the massive administration of stored bank blood. Along with significant prolongation of the PT, these patients may exhibit prolonged bleeding times and thrombin times as much as two times the normal value.[94]

Blood Loss

Patients with liver disease are prone to blood loss related to the development of esophageal varices. Such bleeding can be extensive and difficult to control. In addition, patients with liver disease may require invasive procedures, which further increase the risk of blood loss. Patients may bleed as a result of liver biopsy procedures, and large blood losses are frequently associated with surgical resection of the liver and liver transplantation procedures.[16,91,92,96,97]

Hematologic Disorders

In addition to the effect of blood loss, a number of factors can result in anemia in liver disease, including toxic effects of alcohol on the bone marrow, nutritional deficiencies, and the effect of infectious agents. Severe end-stage liver disease can be associated with hemolytic anemia. In this syndrome lipids accumulate on the red cell membranes, resulting in the production of target cells and bizarre-shaped spur cells that have a decreased survival. Viral hepatitis has been associated with a secondary aplastic anemia that can be fatal if left untreated.

Transfusion Therapy in Liver Disease
Red Cells

Liver disease patients frequently need Red Blood Cell transfusion to replace oxygen-carrying capacity lost as a result of hemorrhage, decreased red cell production, and/or decreased survival. Because liver disease is frequently associated with nutritional deficiencies (such as iron and folate), it is important to correct these inadequacies before the initiation of Red Blood Cell transfusion. In addition, because the anemia of liver disease is generally associated with hypervolemia and accumulation of fluids in the tissues, Red Blood Cell rather than Whole Blood transfusion is the treatment of choice.[27] If, however, the patient requires both oxygen-carrying capacity and volume, as in massive blood loss, Whole Blood may be the component of choice. The plasma in Whole Blood, although deficient in labile coagulation Factors V and VIII, is a source of other coagulation factors for the liver patient.[74]

Treatment of Hemostatic Deficiencies

Patients with liver disease have impairments in clotting and fibrinolysis along with reduced platelet number and function.[93] Because of their decreased coagulation factor activities, liver patients are also at increased risk for dilutional coagulopathy resulting from the administration of red blood cells.[98] Current therapies available for these patients include vitamin K, Cryoprecipitated AHF, exchange plasmapheresis, FFP, and Platelet transfusions.[98] Vitamin K can be used to increase the production of coagulation proteins due to vitamin K deficiency associated with biliary obstruction and malnutrition, but is not effective in reversing the coagulopathy associated with parenchymal disease. In the latter case, FFP is appropriate replacement therapy. Laboratory assessment of bleeding risk is difficult in liver patients. Studies attempting to correlate PT results with risk of hemorrhage in liver patients have not been successful.[93,99] Despite this, FFP is often used before invasive procedures in liver disease patients when the PT reaches greater than 1.5 to 1.8 times the midpoint of the normal range.[93] Large quantities of plasma (12 to 20 mL/kg) given within 8 to 12 hours of the procedure are generally required to correct the PT in liver disease patients.[98] The inability of standard doses of FFP to provide the anticipated benefit may be due in part to the fact that the transfused proteins are rapidly equilibrated between the vascular and the ascitic fluid.[94] Exchange plasmapheresis may be indicated in patients whose coagulopathy is not corrected by administration of FFP.

Cryoprecipitated AHF may be useful in the correction of hypofibrinogenemia. Generally the goal is to maintain fibrinogen concentrations of 1.0 mg/L. Prothrombin complex concentrates are contraindicated because of the risk of thrombosis and DIC in these patients.[93,95] Bleeding in liver disease must be carefully assessed owing to the complex causes, which may include any or all of the following: local disruption of blood vessels, platelet dysfunction and thrombocytopenia, fibrinolytic activity, dysfibrinogenemia, DIC, and nutritional deficiencies.

Platelet transfusion may be indicated to correct the thrombocytopenia (platelet counts less than $50 \times 10^9/L$) and thrombocytopathy, but Platelet transfusions frequently result in a less than optimal posttransfusion increment owing to sequestration of transfused platelets in the spleen. Platelet function may improve with the administration of 1-deamino-8-d-arginine **vasopressin (DDAVP)**.[98]

Accelerated fibrinolytic activity may not be controlled by the administration of FFP alone, and the use of antifibrinolytic agents may be useful in these patients,[9,27,94] but the use of such agents carries an increased risk of thrombosis.[93]

Vasopressin (DDAVP): A synthetic form of vasopressin useful in the treatment of hemostatic disorders due to its ability to release stores of high molecular weight von Willebrand factor (vWF) with a subsequent increase in Factor VIII. Because of the function of vWF in platelet adhesion and formation of the platelet plug, DDAVP has also been used in a variety of platelet disorders.

Blood and Component Therapy in Liver Transplantation
Overview

Although there have been a number of nonsurgical approaches attempted in patients with liver failure, liver transplantation is currently considered to be the best alternative for irreversible acute liver failure, as well as selected patients with chronic liver disease with and without cirrhosis in both adult and pediatric populations.[100] The blood bank plays an important role in the support of the patient requiring liver transplant. Patients undergoing liver transplantation are generally in end-stage hepatic failure. They are at high risk for excessive bleeding owing to the presence of preexisting hemorrhagic disorders (such as esophageal varices), technical factors associated with the surgery (such as the length of the procedure), and disease-associated hemostatic dysfunctions (such as multiple coagulation deficiencies and thrombocytopenia). In addition, the removal of the diseased liver during the procedure leaves the patient ahepatic for some time, which further complicates the coagulopathy. This phase is associated with a disproportionate decrease in Factors VIII and V, along with decreases in fibrinogen and increased evidence of fibrinolysis. The period continues until approximately 30 to 60 minutes after donor liver revascularization and is the most difficult one in which to maintain hemostasis. During this period, fibrinolysis is common, caused by a sudden release of tissue plasminogen activator (tPA) complicated by the inability of the liver to metabolize tPA.[99] The postoperative period is often associated with a hypercoagulable state, perhaps owing to the slow recovery of normal levels of anticoagulant proteins such as antithrombin III and proteins C and S after surgery. These factors further increase the demand for transfusion support.[92]

Estimates of Component Demand

Although blood usage in liver transplantation has decreased over the past decade, liver transplant patients can be expected to require 10 to 20 units of red cells, 15 or more units of FFP, and 10 or more doses of platelets during the procedure and in the immediate postoperative period.[99,101] Occasional patients may require ultramassive transfusions (multiple blood volumes) resulting in excessive demands on the transfusion service.[99] The blood bank must see to it that a sufficient inventory is on hand at the time of the surgery. Efficient communication must be maintained between the blood bank and the surgical team during and after the procedure. Periodic laboratory monitoring of hemoglobin, platelet count, PT, aPTT, and fibrinogen is recommended to monitor the coagulation status. Bedside monitoring of the whole blood clotting time using **thromboelastography (TEG)** can be used to supplement other coagulation tests.[101]

Institutions performing intraoperative salvage may require fewer units of homologous blood. In some cases, up to one third of the patient's transfusion needs can be met using shed blood.[101,102] Predeposit autologous donations can be made in a subset of liver patients, such as those with **amyloidosis,** who have fairly good hematologic function.[102]

Rapid infusion devices are commonly used in liver transplant procedures. Such devices make use of sterile reservoirs into which banked blood, salvaged blood, plasma, and fluids can be added. Blood and components along with crystalloids and colloids are passed through appropriate high-capacity filters, a roller pump, and a blood/fluid warming device. Such devices can allow for the delivery of blood and fluids at rates of 5 L/min or more.[99]

Component Selection

In early phases of the procedure, the use of Whole Blood may be the optimal strategy because the product provides necessary volume support, oxygen-carrying capacity, and stable coagulation factor, while subsequently reducing donor exposure and simplifying the transfusion management. During the ahepatic phase, due

Thromboelastography (TEG): A mechanical-electrical whole blood clotting system that measures the kinetics of clot formation and the strength and dissolution of the clot.

Amyloidosis: A group of conditions associated with the deposition of insoluble proteins (amyloids) in organs and tissues resulting in organ dysfunction.

CMV-safe (CMV risk–reduced) blood: Blood that carries minimal risk of CMV infection, including blood from CMV-seronegative donors or blood that has been leukocyte reduced (less than 5×10^6 leukocytes).

to the cessation of the production of coagulation factors and enhanced risk of fibrinolysis, additional component support is generally required. FFP and/or Cryoprecipitated AHF along with Red Blood Cells are generally indicated. Some studies have compared the use of Whole Blood throughout liver transplant procedures, demonstrating it to be as effective as conventional component therapy in the prevention of coagulopathy.[103]

Owing to the high posttransfusion rate of cytomegalovirus (CMV) infection in liver transplant patients, **CMV-safe (CMV risk–reduced) blood** should be used for CMV-seronegative recipients of CMV-negative organs. In the case of CMV-positive recipients or those receiving a CMV-positive graft, CMV-safe blood is not necessary.[101,102,104,105]

The decision to use leukocyte-reduced blood components in liver transplant patients to achieve a reduced risk of CMV infection and human leukocyte antigen (HLA) alloimmunization is complicated by the fact that the transfusion of blood containing lymphocytes has been shown to confer an immunosuppressive effect with a subsequent improvement in graft survival. On the opposite side of the argument is the fact that leukocytes present in blood and components may result in the development of HLA antibodies in the recipient, which could result in allograft rejection.[102,104]

Serologic Problems

It has been reported that significant numbers of liver transplant patients have serologic problems such as positive direct antiglobulin tests (DATs) and alloantibodies before surgery. This further complicates the pretransfusion evaluation of these patients. It has been reported that significant red cell alloantibodies are present in 6% of liver transplant patients.[104] Given the large transfusion demands of these patients, sufficient numbers of antigen-negative units are frequently not available to meet the patient's requirements. Protocols for switching from antigen-negative to antigen-positive units generally call for the use of antigen-negative units at the beginning of the surgery (first 5 to 10 units), switching to unscreened units for the middle of the case, and reverting to antigen-negative units at the end of the procedure (last 5 to 10 units).[102,104] Protocols of this nature require careful estimates of blood usage, patient status, and blood and component inventory. Successful implementation of such a strategy requires close communication between the surgical team and the transfusion service.

ABO and Rh Compatibility

Except in situations in which organs are not available, liver should be ABO compatible with the recipient. Due to the shortage of organs, ABO major mismatch allografts are used in as many as 6% of adult and 2% of pediatric cases.[104] Although hyperacute rejection is not common in liver transplants with ABO major mismatches, acute graft failure occurs in a large proportion of these cases. Methods to reduce rejection include plasmapheresis to reduce the titer of ABO isoagglutinins and splenectomy.[104]

Passenger lymphocytes transplanted with the organ may continue to survive and function in the recipient.[99,104] Transplanted B lymphocytes may continue to actively produce antibodies that they produced in the donor. The production of donor-derived ABO red cell antibodies has been reported in recipients who have received ABO-incompatible livers most commonly when O organs are transplanted into group A_1 recipients.[99,101] In these cases, donor-derived antibodies generally appear in 1 to 2 weeks and can persist for up to 6 months. Donor-derived ABO antibodies can result in a positive DAT and/or overt hemolysis in the recipient. During this period, blood selected for transfusion should be compatible both with the recipient and with the donor-derived antibody(ies).[101] Antibodies to other blood group antigens such as $Rh_o(D)$ can be produced in a similar manner.[101]

Type-specific Red Blood Cells and FFP are generally used, if available, for group O and group A recipients. Group B recipients who require large quantities of blood are usually switched to group O Red Blood Cells, whereas group AB recipients are generally switched to group A in an effort to conserve the inventory of group O cells. The general rule, as with all massive transfusion, is to switch the RBCs first followed by FFP and to reverse this order when switching back to the patient's type.[99] Unless not available, Rh-negative red cells are generally preferred for Rh-negative women of childbearing age who have no preformed anti-D. In massive transfusion, strict adherence to this guideline may not be feasible.[99,102] In cases in which D-negative liver transplant patients are exposed to the D antigen through transfusion, the incidence of anti-D production has been reported to be less frequent than in other patients.[99]

As in other situations, the transfusion of massive quantities of blood can result in a number of metabolic complications. These consequences of massive transfusion are addressed in more detail in preceding sections of this chapter.

TRANSFUSION DURING THE NEONATAL PERIOD
Physiologic Differences between Newborns and Adults

Infants have significant physiologic differences from older children and adults. Because of this, transfusion to children, especially during the neonatal period, provides unique problems. Summary 17-7 lists some of the physiologic characteristics of newborns that can affect transfusion decision making. The most obvious of these differences is the small size of newborns, especially preterm or **low birth weight** infants. In addition, children have hematologic values that differ from those of adults and demonstrate significant fluctuations in these reference ranges during the first year of life.[106] Newborns also have better cardiovascular adaptive capacity and withstand volume expansion better than adults. These factors may result in differing indications for transfusion in this population.[8,107] The volume of blood to be transfused in infants should be carefully calculated because blood volume not only varies with body weight but the blood volume per kilogram of body weight also varies with age.

The relative immaturity of the newborn's immune system places the newborn at a greater susceptibility to transfusion-transmitted infection, most importantly to CMV.[108,109] Immunity in the newborn is primarily provided by passive antibodies acquired from the mother.[110] For the most part these are protective, except in hemolytic disease of the newborn (HDN) and neonatal autoimmune thrombocytopenia (NAIT), where the antibodies are directed against either the fetal red cells or platelets. This is also the reason why there are few alloantibodies encountered in

Low birth weight: Infants weighing less than 1500 g.

A complete discussion of hemolytic disease of the newborn can be found in Chapter 16.

Refer to Chapter 15 for a more complete discussion of adverse reactions to transfusion.

Summary 17-7

Characteristics of Newborn Infants that Affect Transfusion Therapy Decisions

Small size
Physiologic anemia
Iatrogenic blood loss
O_2 affinity of fetal hemoglobin
Immature immune system
Presence of maternal alloantibodies
Variations in blood volume with age
Shortened red cell survival
Decreased erythropoiesis
Cardiovascular adaptive capacity
Immature coagulation factors

infants compared to adults. Production of antibodies generally can be seen by 4 to 6 months of age. Typical adverse reactions are rarely seen in infants, with febrile reactions most commonly reported.[111] Transfusion-associated graft-versus-host disease (TA-GVHD) may be a concern, especially in low birth weight infants and those with an immunodeficiency. The products of red cell storage lesion (i.e., potassium) and concentration of substances found in the preservative-anticoagulant solutions (i.e., dextrose, adenine, or citrate) may also have adverse affects on ill neonates.

Hematologic Values in the Newborn Period

The postpartum hemoglobin values in newborns generally peak the day after birth, at which time the hemoglobin is approximately 5% greater than at birth.[107] This is followed by a progressive decline in hemoglobin, which begins on the second or third day of life. The first 6 to 12 weeks of life are characterized by a **physiologic anemia,** which is more severe in the preterm infant.[8,107,112] Multiple factors produce a diminished red cell mass in infants, predominantly erythropoietin production, growth of the infant, and volume of fetal hemoglobin. The magnitude of the hemoglobin fall is inversely proportional to gestational age.[107] Fetal hemoglobin production is the greatest in the last weeks of gestation, so premature infants have a lower hemoglobin, and also a lower nadir hemoglobin as a result of physiologic anemia.[112] Generally, the lowest hemoglobin is found between 3 and 18 months of age. The mean hemoglobin value of term infants at 8 weeks is approximately 11 g/dL (110 g/L) and frequently falls as low as 9 g/dL (90 g/L). Infants of low birth weight may have hemoglobin nadirs far below this level (7 to 8 g/dL), which occur earlier and tend to last longer.[113] In addition, most of the hemoglobin in newborns is fetal hemoglobin, which has a higher affinity for oxygen than does adult hemoglobin. The newborn, therefore, has a leftward shift of the oxygen dissociation curve, with a resultant decrease in the efficiency of oxygen delivery to the tissues.[8,107] Although these physiologic conditions are well tolerated by the normal infant, they can add to the difficulty of managing the seriously ill newborn.[114] Many other reasons for neonatal anemia exist, including hemorrhage, hemolysis (enzyme or red cell membrane defects), and aplasia. Coagulation complications may also play a role in the frequency of transfusions.

Direct/Simple Transfusion in the Newborn
Indications

Survival of exceedingly premature infants has been made possible by advanced technology. Newborns, especially those of low birth weight, may require substantial transfusion support during the first few months of life.[115,116] Infants weighing 1250 g or less at birth most likely need transfusion. The efficacy of direct transfusion for anemic infants in cardiorespiratory collapse has been established.[113] Reports exist stating that neonates with severe pulmonary/cardiac disease should be maintained at 13 g/dL. The use of red cell booster transfusion in the healthy, anemic infant is more controversial but has been reported effective for infants with low hemoglobin values associated with recurrent apnea, poor weight gain, or the combination of dyspnea, tachycardia, and failure to thrive.[113,117-120]

In this population anemia is often associated with **iatrogenic blood loss** from laboratory sampling. Procedures to minimize the collection of samples and repeat testing decrease the need for red cell replacement. It has been suggested that withdrawal of blood for laboratory testing be carefully monitored and that replacement be considered when the blood loss exceeds 10% of the infant's calculated blood volume.[27]

Technical Considerations

Transfusion dosages should be calculated using the blood volume of the child. Highest blood volumes are seen in early infancy (80 to 90 mL/kg) and decrease to adult levels (70 to 75 mL/kg) by approximately 1 year of age. Blood volumes of

Physiologic anemia: The progressive fall in hemoglobin during the first 3 to 18 months of life.

Iatrogenic blood loss: Because the sampling of blood for laboratory procedures is the major factor leading to the need for transfusion in low birth weight infants, every attempt is made to reduce the quantity and frequency of blood drawing from these patients. Pediatric institutions use microsamples whenever feasible.

preterm infants can reach 100 to 105 mL/kg. The typical transfusing dose is 10 to 15 mL/kg of body weight. The formula for the calculation of the amount of blood for direct red cell transfusion is as follows:[107]

$$\text{Volume of RBCs} = \text{Blood volume} \times (\text{Posttransfusion hemoglobin} - \\ \text{Pretransfusion hemoglobin})/\text{Donor hemoglobin}$$

In children, the transfusion of 3 mL of packed cells per kilogram of body weight raises the hemoglobin by 1 g/dL.[107]

Vascular access can be a challenge in infants. In the neonatal period access can usually be achieved through the umbilical vein and arteries.[107,113] After this period, a vein must be located that is large enough to accommodate a 23- or 25-gauge needle or catheter. Short infusion sets with minimal dead space are useful in infant transfusion. Such sets must be equipped with a standard 170 μm blood filter.

Because infants usually require small aliquots of blood rather than whole units, a number of approaches have been developed to provide the most suitable product while minimizing donor exposure and waste. Techniques to provide these small transfusion quantities include multiple packs, multiportion systems, frozen aliquots, half-unit donations, and sterile connection devices[121] (Fig. 17-3). The use of dedicated red cell units has resulted in reduced donor exposure.[27,122]

Plastic blood drawing packs with a main collection bag and three integrally connected satellite bags allow for the sterile separation of four aliquots of blood with the same outdate as the original unit (Fig. 17-4). These small aliquots can be further divided into smaller quantities with a potential of two or four aliquots from each pack (a total of 8 to 16 aliquots) with 24-hour outdates. These units are easily obtained from the collection facility, and are ideal for those institutions with a low-volume infant transfusion program. Sterile connection devices allow for direct aliquoting into either a smaller (transfer) bag or syringe (Fig. 17-5), while maintaining the original outdate of the primary unit. These may be more practical for a larger-volume infant transfusion service. As with all blood components, these aliquots must be fully labeled (Fig. 17-6), and it must be possible to trace any aliquot from donation to final disposition.[27,33]

Alternatively, a single unit of red cells can be adjusted to a suitable hematocrit (by using either physiologic saline, albumin, or FFP) and can be sampled through an injection site coupler into a labeled syringe or bag. Aseptic techniques must be used at all times, and the risk of contamination is greater using this procedure. As with all open systems, this unit of blood outdates 24 hours after entry.[33] This approach is useful in a setting where multiple infants require small transfusions and the demand is predictable.

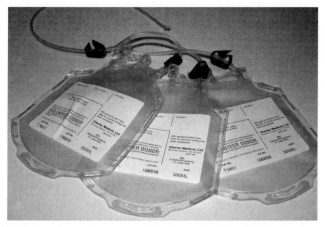

Fig. 17-3 Plastic transfer packs connected by integral tubing allowing for the sterile transfer of aliquots of blood and components.

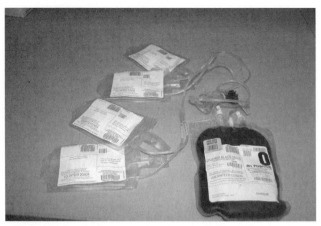

Fig. 17-4 A "quad pack" consists of a main donor collection bag with three attached transfer packs for sterile transfer of small aliquots.

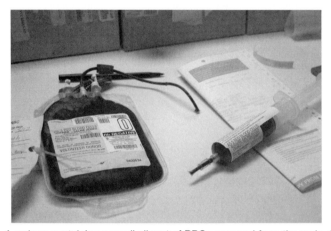

Fig. 17-5 A syringe containing a small aliquot of RBCs removed from the main donor bag using a sterile docking device. This method allows for the use of a dedicated unit for a patient, thereby limiting donor exposure.

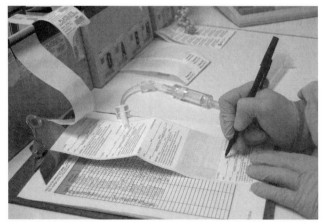

Fig. 17-6 Labeling process for component aliquots to ensure proper identification.

Other techniques for provision of small aliquots for infant transfusion include the subdivision of red cells after glycerolization but before freezing. Aliquots can be thawed as needed. This is an expensive technique but does provide blood that is high in **2,3-DPG** and has minimal amounts of protein, citrate, and potassium.

Units of less than 450 mL can be drawn for infant transfusion. This approach permits the inclusion of low-weight individuals (less than 110 lb) into the donor pool. In these instances, a calculated amount of anticoagulant is removed from the main bag and a reduced volume of whole blood collected.[27]

Differing opinions remain concerning the safety of different additive solutions to be used for neonates. The additional quantities of adenine, dextrose, and mannitol present in these units may be harmful to seriously ill neonates. However, in a review of the use of additive solution (AS) red cells in neonatal transfusions, Luban and colleagues[123,124] recommended that AS red cells pose no significant risk in small-volume transfusion (less than 10 mL/kg), and Goodstein and colleagues[125] reported that the blood glucose changes were less in infants transfused with AS red cells (compared to CPD red cells). Occasionally potassium due to storage lesion is questioned (0.05 mEq/mL), but this should not be a concern in small-volume transfusions (5 to 10 mL/kg) because the daily requirement of K^+ is usually greater than the bioavailable potassium. Additive solutions may be removed by saline washing in infants with severe renal or hepatic insufficiency and in selective massive transfusion settings.[27,123-125]

2,3-DPG: Adequate levels of 2,3-DPG facilitate the off-loading of oxygen to the tissues.

If less than 300 mL of blood is drawn, the anticoagulant/preservative must be reduced proportionally.

Pretransfusion Testing

Pretransfusion testing for the neonatal patient should include ABO forward typing and Rh typing. ABO reverse typing is not routinely performed because most antibodies present in the newborn are of maternal origin, including ABO antibodies.[126,127] Reverse grouping may be omitted during the neonatal period. Repeat ABO and Rh typing on additional specimens can be omitted for the duration of the hospital stay within the neonatal period (first 4 months of life).[33]

A red cell transfusion to a neonate is unlikely to result in alloimmunization. However, if other than group O cells are selected for transfusion, the infant's serum must be tested as appropriate for the presence of anti-A and/or anti B.[33] Initial testing may also include the antihuman globulin test (direct Coombs' test). If negative, this test need not be repeated during the remainder of the hospital admission. If the test is positive for anti-A and/or anti-B, compatible red cells must be transfused. An initial test (antibody screen) must be performed to detect unexpected red cell antibodies, using the serum of the mother and/or newborn. If negative, the test does not have to be repeated for any single admission during the neonatal period. If positive, blood should be selected that is negative for the antigen that corresponds to the antibody detected.[27,33]

Exchange Transfusion/Extracorporeal Membrane Oxygenation
Technical Considerations

Exchange transfusion, ranging from partial to double volume, can be used for the correction of severe bilirubinemia and anemia associated with hemolytic disease of the newborn (removing unconjugated bilirubin, antibody-coated red cells, and maternal antibodies).[27,107,128] In addition, it has been widely used for infants with a variety of serious diseases such as DIC, acute respiratory distress syndrome, and sepsis.[27]

A single-volume exchange replaces approximately 65% to 75% of the blood volume, and a double-volume exchange (approximately one unit of blood) replaces approximately 85% to 90%.[107,128] Generally, the size of the aliquot of blood removed at one time is 5% to 10% (5 mL/kg or 5% of volume replaced over 2 to 4 minutes); two methods/techniques are used: isovolemic (simultaneous) and discontinuous. The decision regarding the size of the exchange and the aliquot to be withdrawn varies with the clinical condition of the neonate (there is no documented benefit of greater than two volume exchanges). Exchange transfusion is not without risk to the infant, and careful thought should be given to the risk versus the benefits of the procedure.[129-131] Depending on exchange volume, coagulation factors may need to be replaced. Thrombocytopenia typically is not an issue unless preexisting thrombocytopenia exists. Citrate-phosphate-dextrose is the most common anticoagulant used in exchange transfusion; therefore infant calcium and magnesium levels should be monitored during large-volume exchange. Calcium gluconate can be administered prophylactically during extended exchange procedures.[107] In addition, high glucose levels in anticoagulants may result in hyperinsulinemia and subsequent hypoglycemia on completion of the transfusion.

Extracorporeal membrane oxygenation (ECMO), a modified cardiopulmonary bypass process, could be considered a "massive" transfusion situation in a neonate. It is initiated to provide "rest" to either the heart (following open heart surgery) or lungs (sepsis, aspiration, or diaphragmatic hernia). This process results in qualitative and quantitative platelet anomalies and often other associated coagulation abnormalities.[132,133]

Selection of Blood for Exchange Transfusion or ECMO

Relatively fresh blood is recommended for exchange transfusion.[128] Most centers supply blood that is 5 to 7 days old or less. Low birth weight infants (less than 1200 g) should receive blood that is CMV negative and irradiated to prevent GVHD.[8,27,33,107] Irradiation is strongly recommended when donor units are drawn from blood relatives. In addition, blood for exchange should be negative for hemoglobin S and, unless administration is extremely slow, should be warmed to 37° C during infusion. Having a warmed product helps to reduce the risk of a coagulopathy, cardiac arrhythmia, or significant hemolysis. A number of blood warming devices are available for such purposes.[8,19,27]

Selection of blood for exchange transfusion in cases in which maternal alloantibody is directed toward antigens on the infant's red cells (hemolytic disease of the newborn) should be compatible with the mother's serum. Crossmatching may be done using the mother's serum if available. Maternal serum is often available in larger quantities and usually has the highest concentration of offending antibody. If maternal serum is not available, an eluate from the infant's cells provides a source of those antibodies implicated in the disease process. Because the ABO groups of the infant and mother frequently are not the same, O cells are commonly used for exchange transfusion or ECMO. The units need be Rh negative only when the infant is Rh negative or the maternal serum contains anti-D.[27]

Non–Red Cell Components
Fresh Frozen Plasma

FFP provides an excellent source of both stable and labile coagulation factors for neonatal transfusion. Indications for the use of FFP in neonates are similar to those in adults. Premature neonates are at a higher risk of a hemorrhagic diathesis due to low levels of the vitamin K–dependent coagulation factors (Factors II, VII, IX, and X), which are produced in the liver. Left untreated, this condition can result in life-threatening gastrointestinal and central nervous system hemorrhage. Fifty percent of functional coagulation factor is all that is necessary for adequate hemostasis. In an emergency, FFP can be used to replace deficiencies of Factor VIII or XI if recombinant factors are unavailable. If an infant possesses less than 1% activity, a dose of 20 to 25 mL/kg usually will result in correction. The standard dose is

10 mL/kg, which is adequate in most circumstances.[27] FFP has also been used as a source of cholesterol supplementation in infants with Smith-Lemli-Opitz syndrome (a disorder caused by an inborn error of cholesterol metabolism)[134] and Hunter's syndrome.[135]

FFP has similar risks of infectious disease, including human immunodeficiency virus (HIV). SD-plasma, a solvent-detergent treated plasma product used in Europe, has minimal risk of enveloped viruses (hepatitis B virus, hepatitis C virus, and HIV). Most leukocytes are disrupted during the freeze-thaw process; however, small numbers of viable lymphocytes have been recovered. CMV has not been shown to be transmitted, and it remains questionable as to the need for irradiation because TA-GVHD has not been reported. FFP can be divided into small-volume units after thawing. Thawed FFP must be administered within 24 hours after thawing.[33]

Platelet Transfusion

The normal range of platelet counts in newborns is similar to that in adults. Counts lower than $100 \times 100^9/L$ may require intervention, especially if the infant requires mechanical ventilation or is on ECMO. Generally, however, spontaneous hemorrhage is not seen in infants until the platelet count falls below $10 \times 10^9/L$, and they are relatively stable down to a platelet count of $50 \times 10^9/L$.[27] If administered in a dose of 5 to 10 mL/kg, either platelet apheresis or whole blood–derived platelet concentrates should raise the platelet count of an average term infant by $50 \times 10^9/L$ to $100 \times 10^9/L$. The process of aliquoting from an apheresis product is similar to red cells, and thus provides the benefit of reduced donor exposure. Both products are available in a prestorage leukocyte-reduced form to minimize the risk of CMV; however, platelet concentrates are typically more readily available and cost less. As with adults, 1-hour and 24-hour posttransfusion platelet counts can be done to assess efficacy. Platelets should be group compatible because the infusion of incompatible plasma is less well tolerated in infants than in adults (a 10 mL/kg dose is 10 mL/kg of incompatible plasma).[27,33] The routine reduction of platelet volume for infants by means of additional centrifugation steps is both unnecessary and unwise, unless a specific reason exists to do so.[107]

Granulocyte Transfusion

The white blood cell count in newborns is typically elevated during the first hours after birth, thought to be due to the stress of delivery. Circulating neutrophils have a half-life of approximately 8 hours, and premature neonates' neutrophils have lower functional activity. The storage pool of neutrophils in the neonatal marrow is reduced compared to adults, and in a septic situation it may be rapidly exhausted, resulting in neutropenia. In the clinical situation of sepsis, with a neutropenic (absolute neutrophil count less than $3000/\mu L$) febrile neonate, unresponsive to antibiotics, a granulocyte product may be warranted.[136] In neonate, either a buffy-coat preparation or a leukapheresis product may be used. These products usually have a significant amount of red cell "contamination," thus requiring ABO/Rh compatibility. If the neonate meets criteria for "CMV low risk," it must be seronegative because these products cannot be leukocyte reduced, and due to the significant number of lymphocytes the product requires irradiation. The short half-life of neutrophils prompts urgent use of the product on availability, and the typical "dose" is one product per day for several days, usually 5 days. With the large number of white blood cells being administered, caution during the infusion is necessary. This is especially required if the patient is receiving **amphotericin B** because an acute respiratory distress reaction could result due to neutrophil degranulation.[107,137-139]

Amphotericin B: An antifungal agent used for patients with progressing, potentially fatal fungal infections.

CHAPTER SUMMARY

1. Massive transfusion, neonatal transfusion, therapeutic pheresis and phlebotomy, burns, and liver disease are examples of conditions that present unique transfusion problems.

2. Massive blood loss of 35% to 40% of the blood volume is associated with hemorrhagic shock and requires immediate resuscitation followed by blood component support.

3. The treatment of massive blood loss centers on the replacement of volume, the correction of hypoperfusion, and the maintenance of normal body temperature.

4. Adverse consequences of massive transfusion are generally due to the effect of dilution, the transfusion of anticoagulant/preservative solutions, the infusion of storage lesion products, and the impact of the infusion of cold blood.

5. Adverse reactions to massive transfusion include dilutional coagulopathy, citrate toxicity, hyperinsulinemia, and acid-base imbalances.

6. Massive hemorrhage may require the transfusion of whole blood or red blood cells, platelets, and fresh frozen plasma.

7. Blood warming is generally indicated when massive quantities of cold blood are to be administered.

8. It may be necessary to release blood before the completion of pretransfusion testing when a delay in transfusion would risk life or limb.

9. Salvaged autologous blood provides the safest alternative for transfusion in massive blood loss.

10. All blood and components must be infused using a standard blood filter. The use of microaggregate filters in massive transfusion is controversial.

11. Neonates have hematologic and physiologic variables that differ from those of adults, including size, blood volume/body weight, fluctuations in hemoglobin, oxygen dissociation curve, cardiovascular adaptive capacity, ability to produce blood group alloantibodies, susceptibility to infection, and graft-versus-host disease.

12. Infants weighing less than 1500 g at birth are classified as low birth weight babies.

13. The most common cause of neonatal transfusion is the loss of blood for laboratory testing.

14. A number of techniques are used to obtain small aliquots for infant transfusion, including multiple packs, multiportion sampling, frozen aliquots, and half-unit donations.

15. Controversy exists regarding the use of additive solution blood in neonates.

16. Special standards for neonatal pretransfusion testing limit the number of times such testing needs to be repeated during the neonatal period for any given hospital admission.

17. Partial exchange transfusions are useful for reducing red cell mass and correcting anemia in patients who cannot tolerate additional volume.

18. Exchange transfusions are the treatment of choice for the reduction of bilirubinemia and treatment of anemia in infants with hemolytic disease of the newborn.

19. Exchange transfusions are associated with many of the same risks as adult massive transfusion.

20. Blood for exchange transfusion should be relatively fresh, CMV negative, irradiated, negative for hemoglobin S, and compatible with the mother's serum.

21. FFP and platelets may be indicated in neonatal transfusion therapy.

22. Plasma exchange is useful in a number of diseases and is generally used to remove an offending substance from the blood, with subsequent replacement of lost fluid with plasma, colloids, or crystalloids.

23. Plasma exchange has therapeutic value in thrombotic thrombocytopenic purpura, neurologic disorders (e.g., myasthenia gravis), dysprotein-emias (e.g., multiple myeloma), renal disease (e.g., Goodpasture syndrome), and hypercholes-terolemia.

24. The efficacy of plasma exchange requires that the toxic substance is not mobilized from extravascular spaces, that the blood volume does not change, and that the rate of production remains the same.

25. Therapeutic cytapheresis involves the removal of cellular components (red cells, leukocytes, or platelets) to reduce symptoms in disorders such as sickle cell anemia.

26. Therapeutic phlebotomy is the removal of patient blood for some medical indication such as polycythemia.

27. Burn injury involves the transfer of heat from an exogenous source and can result in skin damage, vascular injury, and metabolic dysfunction.

28. The amount of burn injury depends on both the depth and the extent of the burn.

29. Thermal injury can involve loss of water from the skin, increased vascular permeability, direct or indirect red cell destruction, and infection.

30. Burns are treated much like acute hemorrhage with initial volume replacement to prevent shock followed by blood component support.

31. Owing to the many functions of the liver, liver disease is a complex clinical picture.

32. Factors associated with liver disease that have transfusion implications include portal hypertension, massive transfusion, hemostatic abnormalities, potential for blood loss, and hematologic abnormalities.

33. Patients with end-stage hepatic disease may need red cells to replace oxygen-carrying capacity lost from increased red cell destruction, decreased marrow production, and blood loss.

34. Treatment of hemostatic disorders in liver disease may require transfusion with FFP (for multiple coagulation deficiencies) and platelets (to correct thrombocytopenia). Prothrombin complexes are contraindicated owing to the risk of thrombosis and DIC in liver disease patients.

35. Bleeding in liver disease can have multiple causes, including local disruption of vessels, platelet dysfunction and thrombocytopenia, fibrinolytic activity, DIC, and nutritional deficiencies.

36. Blood transfusion therapy has an important role in liver transplantation, especially during the ahepatic phase.

REFERENCES

1. American College of Surgeons: Advanced trauma life support: Program for doctors, 6th ed. Chicago, American College of Surgeons, 1997.
2. Berner JJ: Effects of Diseases on Laboratory Tests. Philadelphia, JB Lippincott, 1983.
3. Hamilton SM: The use of blood in resuscitation of the trauma patient. Can J Surg 36:21-27, 1993.
4. Spence RK, Jeter EK, Mintz PD: Transfusion in surgery and trauma. In Mintz PD (ed): Transfusion Therapy: Clinical Principles and Practice. Bethesda, MD, American Association of Blood Banks, 1999.
5. Weiskopf RB, Viele MK, Feiner J, et al: Human cardiovascular and metabolic response to acute, severe isovolemic anemia. JAMA 279(3):217-221, 1998.
6. Toy P: Red blood cell transfusion and the transfusion trigger, including the surgical setting. In Hillyer CD, Silberstein LE, Ness PM, Anderson KC (eds): Blood Banking and Transfusion Medicine: Basic Principles and Practice. Philadelphia, Churchill Livingstone, 2003.
7. Davis KA, Gamelli RL: Transfusion therapy in the care of trauma and burn patients. In Simon TL, Dzik WH, Snyder EL, et al (eds): Rossi's Principles of Transfusion Medicine, 3rd ed. Philadelphia, Lippincott Williams & Wilkins, 2002.
8. Heustis DW, Bove JR, Case J: Practical Blood Transfusion, 4th ed. Boston, Little, Brown & Co, 1988.
9. Mollison PL, Engelfriet CP, Contreras M: Blood Transfusion in Clinical Medicine, 8th ed. Oxford, Blackwell Scientific, 1987.
10. Collins JA, Knudson MM: Metabolic effects of massive transfusion. In Rossi EC, Simon TL, Moss SG (eds): Principles of Transfusion Medicine. Baltimore, Williams & Wilkins, 1991.
11. Jones J, Engelfriet CP: Massive blood replacement. Vox Sang 77:239-250, 1999.
12. Erber WN: Massive blood transfusion in the elective surgical setting. Trans Apheresis Sci 27:83-92, 2002.
13. Hellstern P, Haubelt H: Indications for plasma in massive transfusion. Thromb Res 107:S19-22, 2002.
14. Blauhut B: Indications for prothrombin complex concentrates in massive transfusions. Thromb Res 95:S63-69, 1999.
15. Tuman KJ: Tissue oxygen delivery. The physiology of anemia. Anesthesiol Clin North Am 8(3):451-469, 1990.
16. Donaldson MDJ, Seaman MJ, Park GR: Massive blood transfusion. Br J Anaesth 69:621-630, 1992.
17. Nolan TE, Gallup DG: Massive transfusion: A current review. Obstet Gynecol Surv 46:289-295, 1991.
18. Sohmer PR, Scott RL: Massive transfusion. Clin Lab Med 2:21-24, 1982.
19. Moroff G, Dende D: Characterization of biochemical changes occurring during storage of red cells. Transfusion 23:484-489, 1983.
20. Moore GL, Peck CC, Sohmer PR, Zuck TF: Some properties of blood stored in anticoagulant CPDA-1 solution: A brief summary. Transfusion 21:135-137, 1981.
21. Phillips TF, Soulier G, Wilson RF: Outcome of massive transfusion exceeding two blood volumes in trauma and emergency surgery. J Trauma 27:903-910, 1987.
22. Collins JA: Recent developments in the area of massive transfusion. World J Surg 11:75-81, 1987.
23. Triulzi DJ (ed): Blood Transfusion Therapy: A Physician's Handbook, 7th ed. Bethesda, MD, American Association of Blood Banks, 2002.
24. Hewitt PE, Machin SJ: Massive blood transfusion. BMJ 300:107-109, 1990.
25. Ciavarella D, Reed RL, Counts RB, et al: Clotting factor levels and the risk of diffuse microvascular bleeding in the massively transfused patient. Br J Haematol 67:365-368, 1987.
26. American Society of Anesthesiologists Task Force on Blood Component Therapy: Practice guidelines for blood component therapy. Anesthesiology 84:732-747, 1996.
27. Brecher ME (ed): AABB Technical Manual, 14th ed. Bethesda, MD, American Association of Blood Banks, 2002.
28. Dzik WH, Kirkley SA: Citrate toxicity during massive blood transfusion. Transfus Med Rev 2:76-94, 1988.
29. Wilson RF, Binkley LE, Sabo FM, et al: Electrolyte and acid-base changes with massive blood transfusion. Am Surg 58:535-544, 1992.
30. Hakala P, Hiippala S, Syrjala M: Massive blood transfusion exceeding 50 units of plasma poor red cells or whole blood: The survival rate and occurrence of leukopenia and acidosis. Injury 30:619-622, 1999.
31. NIH Consensus Conference: Fresh frozen plasma indications and risks. JAMA 253:551-553, 1985.
32. Iserson KV, Huestis DW: Blood warming: Current applications and techniques. Transfusion 31:558-571, 1991.

33. Fridey JL: Standards for Blood Banks and Transfusion Services, 22nd ed. Bethesda, MD, American Association of Blood Banks, 2002.

34. Labadie LL: Transfusion therapy in the emergency department. Emerg Med Clin North Am 11:379-406, 1993.

35. Harrison CR, Sawyer PR: Special issues in transfusion medicine. Clin Lab Med 12:743-757, 1992.

36. Guidance for Standards for Perioperative Autologous Blood Collection and Administration. Bethesda, MD, American Association of Blood Banks, 2002.

37. Snyder EL, Bookbinder M: Role of microaggregate blood filtration in clinical medicine. Transfusion 23:460-470, 1983.

38. Klein HG: Plasma exchange in the future: Innovations and new indications. In Rossi EC, Simon TL, Moss GS (eds): Principles of Transfusion Medicine. Baltimore, Williams & Wilkins, 1991.

39. Sacher RA, Ruma TA: Therapeutic hemapheresis. In Henry JB (ed): Clinical Diagnosis and Management by Laboratory Methods, 17th ed. Philadelphia, WB Saunders, 1984.

40. Sloand EM, Klein HG: Therapeutic apheresis. In Westphal RG, Kasprisin DO (eds): Current Status of Hemapheresis: Indications, Technology and Complications. Arlington, VA, American Association of Blood Banks, 1987.

41. Quillen K, Berkman EM: Introduction to therapeutic apheresis. In McLeod BC, Price TH, Weinstein R (eds): Apheresis: Principles and Practice, 2nd ed. Bethesda, MD, American Association of Blood Banks, 2003.

42. Valbonesi M: Cascade filtration in the management of paraproteinemic and immune complex disease. In Lysaght MJ, Gurland H (eds): Plasma Separation and Plasma Fractionation: Current Status and Future Directions. Basel, Karger, 1983.

43. Malchesky PS, Asanuma Y, Zawicki I, et al: On-line separation of macromolecules by membrane filtration with cryogelation. Artif Organs 4:205-207, 1980.

44. Bosch T, Wender T: Extracorporeal plasma treatment in thrombotic thrombocytopenic purpura and hemolytic uremic syndrome: A review. Ther Apher 5(3):182-185, 2001.

45. Grima KM: Therapeutic apheresis in hematological and oncological diseases. J Clin Apheresis 15:28-52, 2000.

46. Rossi EC: Plasma exchange in thrombotic microangiopathies. In Rossi EC, Simon TL, Moss GS (eds): Principles of Transfusion Medicine. Baltimore, Williams & Wilkins, 1991.

47. Siddiqui FA, Lian ECY: Novel platelet-agglutinating protein from a thrombotic thrombocytopenic purpura plasma. J Clin Invest 76:1330-1337, 1985.

48. Andreoli TE, Carpenter CCJ, Plum F, Smith LH (eds): Cecil Essentials of Medicine. Philadelphia, WB Saunders, 1986.

49. Moake JL: Mechanisms of disease: Thrombotic microangiopathies. N Engl J Med 347(8):589-600, 2002.

50. Harkness DR, Byrnes JJ, Lian ECY, et al: Hazard of platelet transfusion in thrombotic thrombocytopenic purpura. JAMA 246:1931-1933, 1981.

51. Gottschall JL, Pisciotta AV, Darin J, et al: Thrombotic thrombocytopenic purpura: Experience with whole blood exchange transfusion. Semin Thromb Hemost 7:25-32, 1981.

52. Schwartz ML, Brenner W: Severe preeclampsia with persistent postpartum hemolysis and thrombocytopenia treated by plasmapheresis. Obstet Gynecol 65:S53-55, 1985.

53. Smith JW, Weinstein R, Hillyer KL: Therapeutic apheresis: A summary of the current indication categories endorsed by the AABB and the American Society for Apheresis. Transfusion 43(6):820-822, 2003.

54. Khatri BO, Dau PC: Plasma exchange in neurological disorders. In Rossi EC, Simon TL, Moss GS (eds): Principles of Transfusion Medicine. Baltimore, Williams & Wilkins, 1991.

55. Weinstein R. Therapeutic apheresis in neurological disorders. J Clin Apheresis 15:74-128, 2000.

56. Dau PC: Plasmapheresis therapy in myasthenia gravis. Muscle Nerve 3:468-482, 1980.

57. Dau PC, Lindstrom JM, Cassel CK, et al: Plasmapheresis and immunosuppressive drug therapy in myasthenia gravis. N Engl J Med 297:1134-1140, 1977.

58. Hemapheresis survey results: News briefs. American Association of Blood Banks 11(5), 1988.

59. Kelly JJ, Adelman LS, Berkman E, Bhan I: Polyneuropathies associated with IgM monoclonal gammopathies. Arch Neurol 45:1355-1359, 1988.

60. Berkman EM: Plasma exchange in the dysproteinemias. In Rossi EC, Simon TL, Moss GS (eds): Principles of Transfusion Medicine. Baltimore, Williams & Wilkins, 1991.

61. Beck JR, Quinn BM, Meier FA, Rawnsley HM: Hyperviscosity syndrome in paraproteinemia. Transfusion 22:51-53, 1982.

62. McGrath MA, Penny R: Paraproteinemia. J Clin Invest 58:1155-1162, 1976.

63. Russell JA, Powles RL: The relationship between serum viscosity, hypervolemia and clinical manifestations associated with circulating paraprotein. Br J Haematol 39:163-175, 1978.

64. Barth WF: Viscosity of serum in relationship to serum globulins. In Sunderman FW, Sunderman FW Jr (eds): Serum Proteins and the Dysproteinemias. Philadelphia, JB Lippincott, 1964.

65. Pinching AJ, Peters DK: Remission of myasthenia gravis following plasma-exchange. Lancet 12:1373-1376, 1976.

66. Winters JL, Pineda AA, McLeod BC, Grima KM: Therapeutic apheresis in renal and metabolic diseases. J Clin Apheresis 15:53-73, 2000.

67. Leitman SF, Smith JW, Gregg RE: Homozygous familial hypercholesterolemia. Transfusion 29:341-346, 1989.

68. McLeod BC: Introduction to the third special issue: Clinical applications of therapeutic apheresis. J Clin Apheresis 15:1-5, 2000.

69. Weinstein R: Basic principles of therapeutic blood exchange. In McLeod BC, Price TH, Weinstein R (eds): Apheresis: Principles and Practice, 2nd ed. Bethesda, MD, American Association of Blood Banks, 2003.

70. Peetoom F: Therapeutic cytapheresis. In Westphal RG, Kasprisin DO (eds): Current Status of Hemapheresis: Indications, Technology and Complications. Arlington, VA, American Association of Blood Banks, 1987.

71. Hester J: Therapeutic cell depletion. In McLeod BC, Price TH, Weinstein R (eds): Apheresis: Principles and Practice, 2nd ed. Bethesda, MD, American Association of Blood Banks, 2003.

72. Taft EG: Treatment by thrombocytapheresis. In MacPherson JL, Kasprisin DO (eds): Therapeutic Hemapheresis, vol II. Boca Raton, FL, CRC Press, 1985.

73. Eisenstaedt RS: Therapeutic phlebotomy. In Rossi EC, Simon TL, Moss GS (eds): Principles of Transfusion Medicine. Baltimore, Williams & Wilkins, 1991.

74. Ness PM: Transfusion therapy of patients with liver disease, burns and neurosurgery. In Umlas J, Silvergleid AJ (eds): Transfusion for the Patient with Selected Clinical Problems. Arlington, VA, American Association of Blood Banks, 1982.

75. Muir IFK, Barclay TL, Settle JAD: Burns and Their Treatment, 3rd ed. London, Butterworths, 1987.

76. Guo A, Sheng Z, Wang D, et al: The use of blood in burn shock. J Burn Care Rehabil 10:226-240, 1989.

77. Budny PG, Regan PJ, Roberts AHN: The estimation of blood loss during burn surgery. Burns 19:134-137, 1993.

78. Wallner SF, Vautrin R: The anemia of thermal injury: Mechanism of inhibition of erythropoiesis. Proc Soc Exp Biol Med 181:144-150, 1986.

79. Mann R, Heimbach DM, Engrav LH, Foy H: Changes in transfusion practices in burn patients. J Trauma 37(2): 220-222, 1994.

80. Sittig KM, Deitch EA: Blood transfusions: For the thermally injured or for the doctor? J Trauma 37(3):369-372, 1994.

81. Housinger TA, Lang D, Warden GD: A prospective study of blood loss with excisional therapy in pediatric patients. J Trauma 34(2):262-263, 1993.

82. Jeng JC, Boyd TM, Jablonski KA, et al: Intraoperative blood salvage in excisional burn surgery: An analysis of yield, bacteriology and inflammatory mediators. J Burn Care Rehabil 19(4):305-311, 1998.

83. Ono Y, Kunii O, Kanegasaki S: Defect of opsonophagocytic function in burned patients: Reversal by transfusion of normal plasma or by cell wall–active antibiotics. Antibiot Chemother 44:115-119, 1991.

84. Peterson VM, Robinson WA: Hematologic changes in burn patients. In Boseick JA (ed): The Art and Science of Burn Care. Rockville, MD, Aspen, 1987.

85. American Burn Association: Practice guidelines for burn care. J Burn Care Rehabil (Suppl), Apr 2001.

86. Murison MSC, Laitung JKG, Pigott RW: Effectiveness of burn resuscitation using two different formulae. Burns 17:484-489, 1991.

87. Schlagentueit S, Snelling CFT, Germann E, et al: Major burns managed without blood or blood products. J Burn Care Rehabil 11:214-220, 1990.

88. Graves TA, Cioffi WG, Mason AD: Relationship of transfusion and infection in a burn population. J Trauma 29:948-952, 1989.

89. Ganong WF: Review of Medical Physiology, 11th ed. Los Altos, CA, Lange Medical, 1983.

90. Ellis R, Bieston JT, Witherington SS, et al: Liver transplantation: Effect of washing bank blood in

91. Marquez J, Martin D, Virji MA, et al: Cardiovascular depression secondary to ionic hypocalcemia during hepatic transplantation in humans. Am J Anesthesiol 65:457-461, 1986.

92. Nusbacher J: Blood transfusion support in liver transplantation. Transfus Med Rev 5:207-213, 1991.

93. Alving B: Transfusion of the patient with acquired coagulation defects. In Hillyer CD, Silberstein LE, Ness PM, Anderson KC (eds): Blood Banking and Transfusion Medicine. Philadelphia, Churchill Livingstone, 2003.

94. Thompson AR: Acquired and complex coagulation factor disorders. In Rossi EC, Simon TL, Moss GS (eds): Principles of Transfusion Medicine. Baltimore, Williams & Wilkins, 1991.

95. Counts RB: Acquired bleeding disorders. In Menitove JE, McCarthy LJ (eds): Hemostatic Disorders and the Blood Bank. Arlington, VA, American Association of Blood Banks, 1984.

96. Lambert CJ, Meydrech EF, Scott-Conner CE: Major hepatic resection: A 10-year experience with emphasis on special problems. Am J Gastroenterol 85:786-790, 1990.

97. Rouch DA, Thistlethwaite LL, Emond JC, et al: Effect of massive transfusion during liver transplantation on rejection and infection. Transplant Proc 20:1135-1137, 1988.

98. Toy P: Plasma transfusion and alternatives. In. Simon TL, Dzik WH, Snyder EL, et al (eds): Rossi's Principles of Transfusion Medicine. Philadelphia, Lippincott Williams & Wilkins, 2002.

99. Dzik W: Solid organ transplantation. In Petz LD, Swisher SN, Kleinman S, et al (eds): Clinical Practice of Transfusion Medicine, 3rd ed. New York, Churchill Livingstone, 1996.

100. Abecassis M, Blei AT, Flamm S, Fryer JP: Liver transplantation. In Stuart FP, Abecassis M, Kaufman DB (eds): Organ Transplantation. Landes Bioscience, 2000, Georgetown, Tex.

101. Ramsey G: Transfusion therapy in solid organ transplantation. In Simon TL, Dzik WH, Snyder EL, et al (eds): Rossi's Principles of Transfusion Medicine. Philadelphia, Lippincott Williams & Wilkins, 2002.

102. Ramsey G, Mintz P: Transfusion in solid organ transplantation. In Mintz PD (ed): Transfusion Therapy: Clinical Principles and Practice. Bethesda, MD, American Association of Blood Banks, 1999.

103. Laine E, Steadman R, Calhoun L, et al: Comparison of RBCs and FFP with whole blood during liver transplant surgery. Transfusion 43:322-327, 2002.

104. Triulzi DJ: Transfusion Support in Solid-Organ Transplantation. Transfusion Medicine Update, Institute for Transfusion Medicine, April 2001, www.itxm.org/TMU2001/

105. Smith DM, Lipton KS: Leukocyte reduction for the prevention of transfusion-transmitted cytomegalovirus (TT-CMV). American Association of Blood Banks, Association Bulletin #97-2, April 23, 1997.

106. Gray JM: The use of blood components in fetal and neonatal medicine. In Umlas J, Silvergold AJ (eds): Transfusion for the Patient with Selected Clinical Problems. Arlington, VA, American Association of Blood Banks, 1982.

107. Strauss RG: Neonatal red blood cell, platelet, plasma, and neutrophil transfusions. In Simon TL, Dzik WH, Snyder EL, et al (eds): Rossi's Principles of Transfusion Medicine. Philadelphia, Lippincott Williams & Wilkins, 2001.

108. Grossman BJ, Smetana DR, Slade BA: Neonatal pretransfusion testing for cytomegalovirus antibody. Transfusion 29:830-831, 1989.

109. Gunter KC: Transfusion-transmitted cytomegalovirus: The part-time pathogen. Pediatr Pathol Lab Med 15:515-534, 1995.

110. Landor M: Maternal-fetal transfer of immunoglobulins. Ann Allergy Asthma Immunol 74:279-283, 1995.

111. Boo NY, Chan BH: Blood transfusion reactions in Malaysian newborn infants. Med J Malaysia 53:358-364, 1998.

112. Salsbury DC: Anemia of prematurity. Neonatal Netw 20: 13-20, 2001.

113. Strauss RG: Current issues in neonatal transfusions. Vox Sang 51:1-9, 1986.

114. Dame C, Juul SE: The switch from fetal to adult erythropoiesis. Clin Perinatol 27:507-526, 2000.

115. Widness JA, Seward VJ, Kromer IJ, et al: Changing patterns of red cell transfusion in very low birth weight infants. J Pediatr 129:680-687, 1996.

116. Alagappan A, Shattuck KE, Malloy MH: Impact of transfusion guidelines on neonatal transfusions. J Perinatol 18:92-97, 1998.

117. Strauss RG: Blood banking issues pertaining to neonatal red blood cell transfusions. Transfus Sci 21:7-19, 1999.

118. Radhakrishnan KM, Chakravarthi S, Pushkala S, et al: Component therapy. Indian J Pediatr 70:661-666, 2003.

119. Levy GJ, Strauss RG, Hume H, et al: National survey of neonatal transfusion practices: I. Red blood cell therapy. Pediatrics 91:523-529, 1993.

120. Hume H, Blanchette V, Strauss RG, et al: A survey of Canadian neonatal blood transfusion practices. Transfus Sci 18:71-80, 1997.

121. Donowitz DG, Turner RB, Searcy MAM, et al: The high rate of blood donor exposure for critically ill neonates. Infect Control Hosp Epidemiol 10:509-510, 1989.

122. Strauss RG, Burmeister LF, Johnson K, et al: AS-1 red cells for neonatal transfusions: A randomized trial assessing donor exposure and safety. Transfusion 36: 873-878, 1996.

123. Luban NLC, Strauss RG, Hume HA: Commentary on the safety of red cells preserved in extended-storage media for neonatal transfusions. Transfusion 31:229-235, 1991.

124. Strauss RG, Burmeister LF, Johnson K, et al: Feasibility and safety of AS-3 red blood cells for neonatal transfusions. J Pediatr 136:215-219, 2000.

125. Goodstein MH, Herman JH, Smith JF, et al: Metabolic consequences in very low birth weight infants transfused with older AS-1 preserved erythrocytes. Pediatr Pathol Lab Med 18:173-185, 1999.

126. Brugnoni D, Airo P, Graf D, et al: Ineffective expression of CD40 ligand on cord blood T cells may contribute to poor immunoglobulin production in the newborn. Eur J Immunol 24:1919-1924, 1994.

127. Rondini G, Chirico G: Hematopoietic growth factor levels in term and preterm infants. Curr Opin Hematol 6:192-197, 1999.

128. DePalma L, Luban NLC: Blood component therapy in the neonatal period: Guidelines and recommendations. Semin Perinatol 14:403-415, 1990.

129. Batton DG, Maisels MJ, Shulman G: Serum potassium changes following packed red cell transfusions in newborn infants. Transfusion 23:163-164, 1983.

130. Ratcliff JM, Elliot MJ, Wyse RKH, et al: The metabolic load of stored blood: Implications for major transfusions in infants. Arch Dis Child 61:1208-1214, 1986.

131. Sasidharan P, Heimler R: Alterations in pulmonary mechanics after transfusion in anemic preterm infants. Crit Care Med 18:1360-1362, 1990.

132. Zavadil DP, Stammers AH, Willett LD, et al: Hematological abnormalities in neonatal patients treated with extracorporeal membrane oxygenation (ECMO). J Extra Corporeal Technol 30:83-90, 1998.

133. Robinson TM, Kickler TS, Walker LK, et al: Effect of extracorporeal membrane oxygenation on platelets in newborns. Crit Care Med 21:1029-1034, 1993.

134. Irons MB, Nores J, Stewart TL, et al: Antenatal therapy of Smith-Lemli-Opitz syndrome. Fetal Diagn Ther 14:133-137, 1999.

135. Yatziv S, Statter M, Abeliuk P, et al: A therapeutic trial of fresh frozen plasma infusions over a period of 22 months in two siblings with Hunter's syndrome. Isr J Med Sci 11: 802-808, 1975.

136. Christensen RD, Rothstein G, Anstall HB, et al: Granulocyte transfusions in neonates with bacterial infection, neutropenia, and depletion of mature marrow neutrophils. Pediatrics 70: 1-6, 1982.

137. Dutcher JP, Kendall J, Norris D, et al: Granulocyte transfusion therapy and amphotericin B: Adverse reactions? Am J Hematol 31:102-108, 1989.

138. Illerhaus G, Wirth K, Dwenger A, et al: Treatment and prophylaxis of severe infections in neutropenic patients by granulocyte transfusions. Ann Hematol 5:273-281, 2002.

139. Menitove JE, Abrams RA: Granulocyte transfusions in neutropenic patients. Crit Rev Oncol Hematol 7:89-113, 1987.

FURTHER READINGS

Anderson KC, Ness PM (eds): Scientific Basis of Transfusion Medicine: Implications for Clinical Practice. Philadelphia, WB Saunders, 2000.

Herman JH, Manno CS (eds): Pediatric Transfusion Therapy. Bethesda, MD, American Association of Blood Banks, 2002.

Hillyer CD, Silberstein LE, Ness PM, Anderson KC (eds): Blood Banking and Transfusion Medicine: Basic Principles and Practice. Philadelphia, Churchill Livingstone, 2003.

Issitt PD, Anstee DJ: Applied Blood Group Serology, 4th ed. Durham, NC, Montgomery Scientific Press, 1999.

McLeod BC, Price TH, Weinstein R (eds): Apheresis: Principles and Practice, 2nd ed. Bethesda, MD, American Association of Blood Banks, 2003.

Mintz PD (ed): Transfusion Therapy: Clinical Principles and Practice. Bethesda, MD, American Association of Blood Banks, 1999.

Popovsky MA (ed). Transfusion Reactions, 2nd ed. Bethesda, MD, American Association of Blood Banks, 2001.

Simon T, Dzik WH, Snyder EL, et al (eds): Rossi's Principles of Transfusion Medicine, 3rd ed. Philadelphia, Lippincott Williams & Wilkins, 2002.

Vamvakas EC, Blajchman MA (eds): Immunomodulatory Effects of Blood Transfusion. Bethesda, MD, American Association of Blood Banks, 1999.

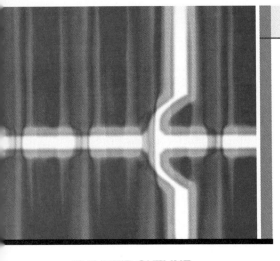

CHAPTER EIGHTEEN

Autoimmune and Drug-Induced Immune Hemolytic Anemias

Susan L. Wilkinson

LEARNING OBJECTIVES

After reading and studying this chapter, the student should be able to:

1. List four categories of autoimmune hemolytic anemia.
2. Briefly describe what information should be gathered before the initiation of a serologic investigation of a positive DAT.
3. State the approximate frequencies of the various types of immune hemolytic anemia and describe the usual serologic findings associated with each, that is, presence of IgG or C3 and reactivity of eluates.
4. Describe the common clinical and laboratory findings for autoimmune hemolytic anemia.
5. Briefly describe the treatment strategies used with autoimmune hemolytic anemia patients.
6. Discuss strategies for solving the serologic problems associated with warm autoimmune hemolytic anemia, including the resolution of ABO and Rh typing discrepancies and the detection and identification of alloantibodies.
7. Interpret serologic results in cases of warm autoimmune hemolytic anemia and select appropriate blood for transfusion if indicated.
8. Discuss strategies for solving the serologic problems associated with cold agglutinin syndrome and select appropriate blood for transfusion if indicated.
9. Describe the four categories or mechanisms for drug-induced immune hemolytic anemia.
10. For each category of drug-induced immune hemolysis, describe the common pattern of serologic characteristics.

OVERVIEW

Autoantibodies can be produced to a variety of self-antigens following a failure in the self–non-self discrimination mechanism of the immune system. Autoantibodies in warm autoimmune hemolytic anemia (WAIHA), cold agglutinin syndrome (CAS), paroxysmal cold hemoglobinuria (PCH), mixed-type autoimmune hemolytic anemia (cold and warm autoantibodies), and drug-induced immune antibodies may be responsible for decreased red cell survival and acquired immune hemolytic anemia. These immune manifestations may also present serologic challenges to the clinical laboratory scientist. The finding of a positive direct antiglobulin test (DAT) may be the first piece of serologic evidence to signal the presence of autoantibodies or, more rarely, drug-induced immune antibodies. Although the predictive value of a positive DAT is low (0.29%) if applied to all patients, its predictive value is considerably better (83%) when used to test the red cells of patients with hemolytic anemia.[1,2] As reported, between 1 and 9 of every 1000 blood donors may demonstrate a positive DAT without clinical manifestations of immune-mediated hemolysis.[3] Additionally, the incidence of a positive DAT in hospital patients has been reported to range from 1% to 15%.[3,4] Serologically, many of these donors and patients are indistinguishable from those with WAIHA. Additionally, some patients with immune hemolytic anemia have a negative DAT.[4,5] Whether autoantibodies are responsible for decreased red cell survival or not, their presence can affect pretransfusion testing. Before beginning any serologic studies, the following clinical information should be gathered:

1. Is there evidence of hemolysis? A positive DAT does not always mean the presence of immune hemolysis. The presence of hemolysis necessitates a serologic evaluation. However, if there is no hemolysis or shortened red cell survival in the patient, the serologic evaluation becomes less urgent.

2. What is the transfusion history of the patient and, if female, the pregnancy history? As will be seen, one of the more critical serologic evaluations is determining the possible presence of clinically significant alloantibodies in addition to autoantibody. Transfusion history may make a difference in the type of adsorption studies selected. Additionally, the simultaneous presence of alloantibody in a recently transfused individual with a positive DAT may represent a delayed hemolytic transfusion reaction or early alloantibody production.

3. What is the patient's diagnosis? This can provide extremely useful information in the assessment of autoantibodies. For example, certain disease states such as systemic lupus erythematosus (SLE) are associated with a high incidence of secondary WAIHA. In other patients, including those with infectious mononucleosis, CAS may be seen secondarily.

4. What medication is the patient taking? Certain drugs, including the cephalosporins and penicillins, are associated with a positive DAT. Drug information is also important when evaluating a nonreactive eluate.

AUTOIMMUNE HEMOLYTIC ANEMIAS

General Characteristics of the Immune Hemolytic Anemias

Several studies have reported the incidence of the various kinds of immune hemolytic anemia cases referred for evaluation[4-9] (Table 18-1). The most common

TABLE 18-1 Incidence of Various Kinds of Immune Hemolytic Anemias

Type	Percent of Cases
Warm autoimmune hemolytic anemia	60%[6]-70%[4]
Cold agglutinin syndrome	16%[4]-32%[7]
Mixed-type autoimmune hemolytic anemia	7%[6]-8%[8]
Paroxysmal cold hemoglobinuria	Rare to 2%[4]; described more frequently in children[9]
Drug-induced immune hemolytic anemia	12%[4]-18%[7]

type of autoimmune hemolytic anemia is WAIHA (60% to 70%), followed by CAS (16% to 32%). Drug-induced immune hemolytic anemia is the next most frequent (12% to 18%). Mixed-type autoimmune hemolytic anemia, which demonstrates characteristics of both WAIHA and CAS, is uncommon (7% to 8%), as is PCH (2%). PCH has, however, been reported more frequently in children.[9] Serologic findings within a specific type of autoimmune hemolytic anemia and drug-induced immune hemolytic anemia, for the most part, demonstrate common characteristics. These common characteristics include the immunoglobulin or protein found on the red cell, serum reactivity/nonreactivity and immunoglobulin class, and eluate reactivity/nonreactivity. These characteristics are summarized in Table 18-2.[4,5,7-10]

General Clinical and Laboratory Findings

Clinical findings in WAIHA can be highly variable, although most patients with a chronic form of the disease have fatigue, pallor, palpitations, mild jaundice, and shortness of breath. In the occasional patient with acute hemolysis, hemoglobinemia, hemoglobinuria, and profound anemia may be present. Moderate splenomegaly is usually noted. The most noted laboratory finding in WAIHA is a positive DAT, which will be described in greater detail. Peripheral blood smears may show microspherocytes, **polychromasia**, and, on occasion, fragmented and nucleated red cells. The reticulocyte count is usually elevated, as is **unconjugated bilirubin.** Serum **haptoglobin** levels are reduced or absent.

Clinical manifestations in chronic CAS often parallel those seen with chronic anemia, as described previously for WAIHA. Patients may experience rare episodes of acute hemolysis following cold exposure and demonstrate hemoglobinemia and hemoglobinuria. Patients may note acrocyanosis of their distal extremities, nose, ears, and chin following cold exposure. **Raynaud's phenomenon** has been reported.

In acute CAS secondary to infection with *Mycoplasma pneumoniae* or infectious mononucleosis, the hemolysis can be quite severe although the disease resolves fairly rapidly. The DAT is positive, as is the antibody screen. Peripheral blood smears demonstrate polychromasia, and the reticulocyte count is usually elevated. **Autoagglutination** of red cells may lead to errors in calculating red cell indices on automated cell counters. Similar findings are noted for PCH, although on occasion, shaking chills, back and leg pain, and abdominal cramps are associated with hemolytic episodes that include hemoglobinuria.

Clinical features in the drug-induced immune hemolytic anemias can be consistent with those of chronic or acute anemia. The DAT is consistently positive. Serologic findings are discussed in more detail in later sections of this chapter.

Treatment of Autoimmune Hemolytic Anemias

In WAIHA, most patients show marked improvement following treatment with **prednisone.** On occasion, to increase oxygen-carrying capacity, transfusion therapy may be required before treatment with prednisone has begun to decrease

Polychromasia (polychromatophilia): The bluish color of young erythrocytes in Wright-stained blood smears. These young cells are shown to be reticulocytes when stained with supravital stains.

Bilirubin (unconjugated): A breakdown product of hemoglobin. The unconjugated form is the lipid-soluble form that circulates, bound to serum proteins, en route to the liver, where it is conjugated.

Haptoglobin: A plasma glycoprotein that binds irreversibly to free hemoglobin and is removed from the circulation by the cells of the reticuloendothelial system.

Raynaud syndrome: Pallor and cyanosis of the extremities (especially the fingers) during exposure to the cold. The syndrome is secondary to a number of diseases, including cold agglutinin syndrome.

CAS can be associated with spontaneous agglutination of red cells in vitro, especially when blood specimens are stored at room temperature or below. These agglutinated cells can result in a number of errors in automated hematology cell-counting equipment, including artificially low red blood cell counts and macrocytosis, which result in calculated errors in red cell indices and hematocrit values. Agglutinins are generally visible if the tube is inverted. This error can be frequently overcome by warming the tube to 37° C or by replacing plasma with an equal volume of prewarmed (37° C) physiologic (0.9%) saline.

Prednisone: A synthetic corticosteroid used as an antiinflammatory agent.

TABLE 18-2 Characteristic Findings in Autoimmune Hemolytic Anemia and Drug-Induced Immune Antibodies

	DAT			
	IgG	C3	Serum	Eluate
Warm autoimmune hemolytic anemia			57% present with IgG warm autoantibody	IgG and reactive with normal cells
24%[7]-67%[4]	+	+		
20%[4]-66%[7]	+	0		
7%[7]-13%[4]	0	+		
Cold agglutinin syndrome	0	+	IgM autoantibody always present	Nonreactive
Mixed-type autoimmune hemolytic anemia	+	+	IgG warm autoantibody present	IgG and reactive
Paroxysmal cold hemoglobinuria	0	+	IgG biphasic hemolysin detectable	Nonreactive
Drug-induced immune hemolytic anemia				
Drug adsorption (penicillin type and drug dependent)	+	(+)	IgG antibody in serum and eluate reactive only with drug-sensitized red cells	
Immune complex (non-penicillin type and drug dependent)	(+)	+	Antibody may demonstrate reactivity in the presence of drug	Nonreactive
Membrane modification (nonimmunologic adsorption of protein)	+	+	Nonreactive	Nonreactive
Drug-induced autoimmune hemolytic anemia (methyldopa, procainamide, etc. and drug independent)	+	(+)	IgG warm autoantibody may be present	IgG and reactive with normal red cells

(+), Occasionally positive.

hemolysis and stabilize the patient. In those few patients who fail to respond to prednisone, splenectomy may be required. Cytotoxic drugs, including **azathioprine,** may be required when prednisone and splenectomy fail to correct the hemolytic process.

In most patients with CAS or PCH, anemia is mild, the disease is self-limiting, and treatment is largely symptomatic. Patients are advised to keep warm. Prednisone and splenectomy are generally ineffective, but, on occasion, cytotoxic drugs including **chlorambucil** or **cyclophosphamide** may be indicated. Transfusion therapy may be indicated for patients whose cardiovascular or cerebrovascular systems are compromised by the degree of anemia. Transfusion of the cells through a **blood-warming device** may be considered.

For drug-induced immune hemolytic anemias, treatment should always begin by discontinuing the drug. Other treatment may include the need for transfusion therapy if insufficient oxygen delivery is a concern.

WARM AUTOIMMUNE HEMOLYTIC ANEMIA
Warm Autoantibodies

The warm autoantibodies found in WAIHA are predominantly IgG immunoglobulins that react optimally at 37° C. Cases have been described with IgA and IgM autoantibodies, either in conjunction with IgG or, rarely, alone. As shown in Table 18-1, most cases of acquired autoimmune hemolytic anemia are found in this

Azathioprine: An immunosuppressive antimetabolite drug used to reduce disease symptoms in autoimmune disorders and to extend allograft survival in transplantation.

Chlorambucil, cyclophosphamide: Alkylating agents with antineoplastic activity. Because hypothermia is associated with many adverse clinical consequences, the use of blood-warming devices is recommended whenever a patient receives large-volume transfusions of stored bank blood. Refer to Chapters 11, 14, and 17 for additional information on this topic.

Blood-warming device: Blood warming is important in CAS to avoid reducing body temperature to the optimal temperature of reactivity of the cold autoantibody implicated in the disease.

category. WAIHA may manifest as a primary or idiopathic disease but also as a secondary disease in patients with lymphoma, SLE, and chronic lymphocytic leukemia. As stated previously, blood donors and hospital patients without hemolysis may have serologic characteristics that are indistinguishable from the serology of those with WAIHA.[3]

Direct Antiglobulin Test

In almost all cases of WAIHA, the DAT is positive when red cells are tested with polyspecific antiglobulin sera. When monospecific tests using anti-IgG and anti-C3d are performed, three categories, as shown in Table 18-2, are possible. In one study, the majority of cases of WAIHA demonstrated both IgG and C3d on the patients' red cells.[4] However, in an additional study, IgG only was noted more frequently.[7] Red cells with C3d only were found least frequently.

Rare cases of WAIHA manifest with a negative DAT.[4] These cases may be due to levels of IgG on the red cell that are below those detectable with conventional antiglobulin reagents. A negative DAT may also be seen when low-affinity IgG autoantibodies are washed from the cell surface in preparation of cells for the DAT. Last, IgA or IgM autoantibodies may initially result in a negative DAT due to routine reagents lacking these specificities. Additional strategies that have been used to evaluate these rare cases and prove unique immunoglobulin classes and levels are outlined by Petz and Garratty.[4]

Red Cell Typings

If **high-protein Rh-typing reagents** are used, warm autoantibody–sensitized red cells may cause positive results in the Rh control test, due to spontaneous agglutination in the presence of certain potentiators. Under these circumstances, low-protein Rh-typing reagents usually facilitate an accurate Rh typing. With the widespread use of IgM monoclonal Rh reagents that are low in protein and lack potentiators, false-positive Rh-typing results are now rarely encountered. However, exceptional red cell samples with large amounts of autoantibody may cause false-positive results when monoclonal Rh-typing reagents are used. On very rare occasions, ABO forward typings may also demonstrate spontaneous agglutination and give false-positive results, suggesting a group AB individual. In such cases, ABO reverse typings may not agree with the ABO forward typing. Certain chemicals can be used to remove IgG from the red cell surface, allowing for successful antigen typings. EDTA-glycine and **chloroquine diphosphate** can be used to dissociate antigen-antibody complexes from the patient's red cells, facilitating blood grouping results.[11,12] See Petz and Garratty[4] for detailed methods on the use of these chemicals.

Other red cell antigen typings can be performed on DAT-positive cells with the additional monoclonal reagents that are now available. These include, in addition to Rh reagents, Kell and Kidd system antisera. This information may be of value when performing allogeneic adsorptions (see discussion later in this chapter).

Serum Studies

In the event that transfusion therapy is needed for a patient with WAIHA, adequate assessment of the patient's serum for the presence and type of antibody is essential. An approach to this assessment is shown in Fig. 18-1. If the antibody screen is negative, additional studies with the patient's serum are not indicated. However, if the antibody screen is positive, antibody identification studies to determine the presence of **alloantibody, autoantibody, or alloantibody plus autoantibody** must be performed.

Alloantibody

If the antibody screen is positive and antibody identification studies indicate the presence of clinically significant alloantibody without autoantibody, the procedure

---

High-protein Rh-typing reagents: Although they have been almost completely replaced by monoclonal reagents, it is useful to note that "tube and slide anti-D" are high-protein reagents that can cause spontaneous agglutination of antibody-coated cells, resulting in a potentially false-positive D typing. A manufacturer's Rh control is run with these reagents to detect such coated cells. If the Rh control is positive, the anti-D typing cannot be interpreted.

Chloroquine diphosphate: Cells with a positive DAT also give false-positive results in any antigen typing test that involves the indirect antiglobulin phase of testing (e.g., anti-K). Chloroquine dissociates IgG from red cells without damaging the cell membrane. Cells thus treated can be used for antigen typing at the indirect antiglobulin phase of testing. This technique is particularly useful for phenotyping red cells of patients with warm autoantibody–coated red cells.

Alloantibody, autoantibody, or alloantibody plus autoantibody: The serum of an untransfused patient with WAIHA may have any of the following serologic combinations: no antibody in the serum and autoantibody in the eluate; autoantibody in the serum and the eluate; autoantibody and alloantibody in the serum and autoantibody in the eluate; or alloantibody only in the serum and autoantibody in the eluate. If the patient has been transfused, the serologic picture can be further complicated by the possible presence of alloantibody in the eluate (transfused cells) along with autoantibody.

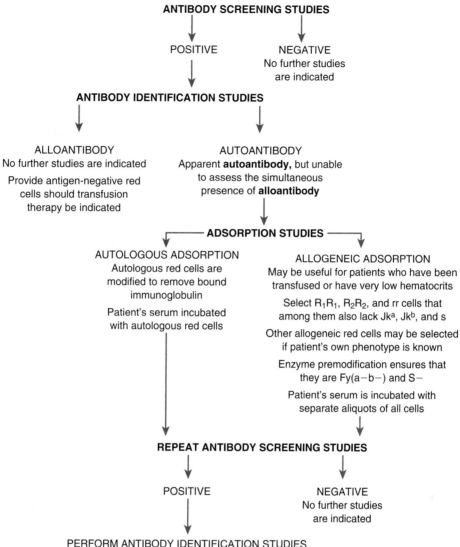

Fig. 18-1 Assessment of serum studies in warm autoimmune hemolytic anemia.

to identify appropriate units for transfusion is similar to that used for a patient without evidence of autoimmune disease. Following identification of the alloantibodies, antigen-negative units are selected for crossmatch and eventual administration. Even in the presence of minimal amounts of free serum autoantibody, alloantibody specificity(ies) may be readily apparent.

Autoantibody

Because autoantibody is directed toward antigens present on the patient's own red cells, free serum autoantibody may not be detected initially. However, as red cell antigen sites become saturated, free serum autoantibody is demonstrable in the patient's serum. Approximately 57% of patients with WAIHA have free serum autoantibody reacting by the indirect antiglobulin method when routine antibody screening studies are performed.[4] This finding is most significant in the patient who has been previously transfused or pregnant, because this is the patient at risk to produce clinically significant alloantibodies that would react also by the indirect antiglobulin test. Depending on the amount of free serum autoantibody, the presence of clinically significant alloantibody may be masked by autoantibody and therefore not readily demonstrable.

Adsorption Studies

If antibody identification studies demonstrate consistent and strong reactivity with all reagent red cells at the antiglobulin phase of testing, additional studies must be performed to determine if this is alloantibody, autoantibody, or a combination of alloantibody and autoantibody. The most appropriate course of action is to perform **adsorption studies** using the patient's serum and either autologous or allogeneic red cells. This is also summarized in Fig. 18-1.

A number of studies have used adsorption techniques to document the presence of alloantibodies when autoantibodies were also present. Wallhermfechtel and colleagues[13] retrospectively evaluated the practice of performing allogeneic adsorption studies to detect clinically significant alloantibodies in the serum of 125 patients with warm autoantibodies. Nineteen (15.2%) of the patients had clinically significant alloantibodies in their serum, with a total of 38 antibody specificities among the 19 patients. Sixteen of the 38 antibodies were not apparent until allogeneic adsorption studies were performed. In another study by Laine and Beattie,[14] 38% of cases studied demonstrated clinically significant alloantibody following autologous or allogeneic adsorption studies. In a study by James and colleagues,[15] 32% of patients exhibited significant alloantibody in addition to serum autoantibody. Sokol and colleagues[7] detected alloantibodies in only 14% of their patients with WAIHA, but these patients had previously received blood that was matched for the Rh and K antigens, likely reducing the risk of alloimmunization. Issitt and colleagues[16] detected alloantibodies in 43% of sera following alloadsorption, and Leger and Garratty[17] detected alloantibodies in 40% of sera using low ionic strength solutions, but 47% of sera using polyethylene glycol (PEG). These studies all confirm the importance of evaluating the sera of patients with WAIHA for alloantibodies, especially when transfusion therapy is required. Of additional interest is the study by Shirey and co-workers[18] in which antigen-matched donor blood was provided for patients with warm autoimmune hemolytic anemia. During the length of the study, no patients produced additional alloantibodies.

Autologous Adsorption

If the patient has not been transfused recently and if the red cell volume is sufficient, autologous adsorption is the method of choice when evaluating serum for the detection of alloantibody in the presence of free serum autoantibody. Initially, amounts of bound immunoglobulin are removed from the patient's red cells in order to optimize the autoadsorption procedure. In some procedures, the patient's red cells are also enzyme premodified to enhance the interaction of autoantibody with its antigen. Red cells are then incubated with the patient's serum. In general, it is often more efficacious to pretreat two aliquots of the patient's red cells and autoadsorb the serum twice. At least six different methods have been described for the autoadsorption of warm autoantibodies: 56° C **elution** with enzyme premodification,[19] ZZAP (dithiothreitol and cysteine-activated papain),[20] chloroquine diphosphate,[11] citric acid,[21] EDTA/acid,[12] and PEG.[22] ZZAP and PEG are the two most widely used methods, and in at least one study comparing both methods, similar results were noted.[17] For detailed procedures on these methods, consult the *Technical Manual*[23] and *Methods in Immunohematology*.[24]

Adsorption: The removal of antibody(ies) from the serum onto cells positive for the corresponding antigen(s) (the opposite of an elution). Adsorptions can be autologous or allogeneic and can remove autoantibody, alloantibody, or both. It is important to recall that a transfused patient has more than one population of red cells (self and donor[s]) for up to 4 months after transfusion. Care must be taken when interpreting testing performed using red cells from these patients. Antigen typing, for example, performed using a specimen of blood drawn following transfusion, does not provide accurate information regarding the phenotype of the patient because of the presence of "foreign" donor cells.

Elution: The process by which bound antibody is removed from red cells and captured in a fluid medium for further testing (e.g., antibody identification).

Following autoadsorption, an antibody screen should be performed with the autoadsorbed serum. If no reactivity is noted, units of blood for transfusion should be selected and pretransfusion testing completed for the patient. If reactivity in the antibody screen is noted, antibody identification studies should be performed. If alloantibody is identified, antigen-negative units are selected and pretransfusion testing is completed for the patient.

Reactivity in the antibody screen following autoadsorption may also indicate unsuccessful removal of all autoantibody. In some cases, two autoadsorptions are not adequate to remove all autoantibody. In addition, other autoantibodies do not bind to the patient's red cells because the method selected for autoadsorption has denatured antigens on the red cells, rendering them incapable of adsorbing the corresponding autoantibody. For example, auto-En^a has been reported to be the causative antibody in WAIHA. If pretreatment of the patient's red cells for autoadsorption uses proteolytic enzymes, the En^a trypsin-sensitive (TS) and En^a ficin-sensitive (FS) sites on glycophorin A are destroyed. If the autoanti-En^a is directed to one or both of these sites, autoantibody remains unadsorbed in the patient's serum. Similar findings can also be expected if the autoantibody has specificity in the Kell or LW blood group systems when ZZAP is used in the preparation of the patient's red cells for autoadsorption. Possible interpretations following autoadsorption are summarized in Fig. 18-1.

Allogeneic Adsorption

If the patient has been transfused recently or if the hematocrit is extremely low, allogeneic adsorption should be used to determine if clinically significant alloantibodies are present with warm autoantibodies. Usually, three different allogeneic blood samples are used in this procedure because of the blood group antigens they lack.[23,24] Generally, red cells from K−, R_1R_1, R_2R_2, and rr individuals are used. In addition, one of the cells should lack Jk^a and another cell, Jk^b. One cell should be s−. If the cells are to be enzyme premodified, which is suggested to enhance the interaction of autoantibody with antigen, all cells are functionally Fy(a−b−) and S−. If for some reason enzyme-premodified cells are not indicated, as in the suspected presence of autoanti-En^{a}FS, it is necessary to ensure that the Fy^a, Fy^b, and S antigens are each absent from at least one of the three allogeneic samples.

With the ability to test DAT-positive red cells for Rh, Kell, and Kidd system antigens using monoclonal reagents, it may be possible to use one or two selected allogeneic blood samples to facilitate adsorption of autoantibody. For example, if the patient is D+, C+, E−, c+, e+, K−, and Jk(a+b+) and our adsorbing cells are enzyme premodified, we only need to ensure that we select an adsorbing cell that is E−, K−, and s− (typing not done) to identify alloantibodies that this particular patient could produce.

Testing of the allogeneic adsorbed serum is as described for testing autologous adsorbed serum and is also summarized in Fig. 18-1.

Selection of Blood for Transfusion

Although it is clear that red cells for transfusion should lack antigens to serum alloantibodies, it is less clear how to select blood for transfusion in the presence of autoantibodies. Data are conflicting as to whether donor units compatible with patient autoantibody survive longer.[4,5,25]

If it is the local practice to select donor units lacking antigens to simple autoantibody specificities (e.g., autoanti-D, autoanti-c, autoanti-e), one must be sure that those cells do not stimulate alloantibody production in the recipient. For example, one should not use D-positive, e-negative cells to transfuse a D-negative patient with autoanti-e, because alloanti-D will most likely be produced. If autoantibody specificity is directed to more complex, high-incidence antigens such as anti-U, anti-LW, or anti-Rh29, it is difficult to consider the use of antigen-negative cells because these rare units of blood should be reserved for individuals who produce the respective alloantibodies. Johnson and co-workers[26] have published a most interesting case in which rare M^k homozygote red cells were required for transfusion in the presence autoanti-Pr. Transfusion in patients with WAIHA should be avoided whenever possible because the majority of patients can be managed successfully without red cell transfusions.

Elution and Autoantibody Specificity

The removal and testing of warm autoantibody from the patient's red cells can support the overall serologic and clinical findings in WAIHA. In the preparation of eluates from the red cells of patients with WAIHA, elution methods including digitonin-acid or glycine-HCl and those that use organic solvents (xylene, methylene chloride) are suitable.[24] Methods including 56° C heat or freeze-thaw methods are generally ineffective for warm autoantibodies.[10] The specificities of autoantibodies recovered from red cells of patients with warm autoantibodies are often directed to various portions of the Rh protein, although this may not be apparent unless rare D-deletion or Rh_{null} red cells are available for testing. Autoantibodies defining common Rh antigens, including D, C, E, c, and e, have been reported, along with numerous other specificities outside the Rh blood group system, which include anti-A, anti-B, anti-En[a], anti-Ge, anti-I[T], anti-Jk[a], anti-K1, anti-K4, anti-K5, anti-K13, anti-Lan, anti-LW[a], anti-N, anti-Sc1, anti-U, anti-Wr[b], anti-Di[b], anti-Vel, and anti-Xg[a].[4,5,10,23] Many of these same autoantibody specificities have also been reported in individuals without evidence of increased red cell destruction.[4,5]

It is important to remember that the specificity of these autoantibodies has little bearing on the transfusion management of patients requiring blood, or on the approach the clinician takes regarding treatment of the patient. However, it is important to know whether autoantibody recovered from the patient's red cells is reactive with normal red cells. Certain drugs, including penicillin and immune globulin, and diseases causing hypergammaglobulinemia can cause a strongly positive DAT due to IgG.[27-29] In these situations, an eluate is nonreactive. Based on these findings, the practice of routinely performing a complete antibody identification panel using the eluate recovered from patients with a positive DAT is not recommended. Instead, determination of eluate reactivity with normal red cells that should include no more than the antibody screening cells provides optimal and useful serologic information.

COLD AGGLUTININ SYNDROME AND PAROXYSMAL COLD HEMOGLOBINURIA
Cold Autoantibodies

Cold-reactive autoantibodies may be pathologic, causing cold agglutinin syndrome (CAS), which accounts for 16% to 32% of all cases of acquired immune hemolytic anemia. Paroxysmal cold hemoglobinuria (PCH) accounts for approximately 2% of all cases of acquired hemolytic anemia, although it has been reported more frequently in children (see Table 18-1).[4,7,9] CAS can occur as an idiopathic disease but is often associated secondarily with a number of infectious diseases, including *Mycoplasma pneumoniae* infection and infectious mononucleosis. PCH may rarely be idiopathic. It is most frequently associated with transient infections and is more appropriately categorized as Donath-Landsteiner hemolytic anemia.[30]

Harmless cold autoantibodies are much more frequent than those that cause immune red cell destruction. Although differences may exist relative to the clonal origin of harmless and pathologic cold autoantibodies, the most striking serologic difference in these autoantibodies is their **thermal range** of reactivity.[4,5,25,31] Antibodies causing disease usually bind to red cell antigens at temperatures between 30° and 32° C. Blood in the peripheral circulation (toes, fingers, nose) can fall to this temperature, facilitating antibody attachment followed by complement

Thermal range: The temperature range in which an antibody binds with its corresponding antigen. Thermal ranges are important predictors of the clinical significance of a blood group antibody. Cold autoantibodies can activate complement in vitro, especially in specimens that are stored at 4° C. To avoid this in vitro phenomenon, specimens can be collected in tubes containing chelating agents such as EDTA. In these specimens, calcium is bound and therefore complement cannot be fixed to red cells.

activation and red cell hemolysis as temperature increases to 37° C. Harmless autoantibodies may bind with antigen at room temperature but more frequently do not bind with antigen until temperatures are as low as 4° C. Other characteristics of pathologic and nonpathologic cold autoantibodies are listed in Table 18-3.

The immunoglobulin class of cold autoantibodies is most frequently IgM, although IgA and IgG cold autoantibodies have been reported.[4,5,25] The causative autoantibody of PCH is always IgG and is characterized by biphasic or bithermic hemolysis. This term is used because the autoantibody binds to red cells at low temperatures and then causes hemolysis via the activation of complement as the blood is warmed to 37° C. The antibody behavior serves as the basis for the Donath-Landsteiner test, used to identify patients with PCH.[23,24]

Direct Antiglobulin Test

The cells of patients with CAS and PCH are sensitized with C3d (see Table 18-2). Occasionally, harmless cold autoantibodies may bind to red cells in vitro, causing a false-positive DAT. Because this can occur, EDTA samples for direct antiglobulin testing on patients suspected of CAS should be collected and maintained at 37° C before testing is performed.[4,5,23]

Red Cell Typings

Potent cold autoantibodies may cause spontaneous agglutination of the patient's red cells, resulting in both ABO and Rh typing problems. Although collection and maintenance of samples at 37° C before testing may alleviate such problems, additional intervention may be required. **Thiol reagents,** including dithiothreitol and 2-mercaptoethanol, can be used to directly treat the patient's red cells, abolishing autoagglutination and permitting an accurate forward ABO and Rh typing.[23,24,32]

Thiol reagents: Substances that cleave the disulfide bonds of IgM antibodies, abolishing the ability of the molecule to agglutinate or bind complement.

Serum Studies

Unlike warm autoantibodies, cold autoantibodies nearly always are demonstrable in the serum. The specificity of autoantibodies in CAS most commonly includes anti-I, followed by anti-i and anti-IH.[4,5,25] Less commonly, autoantibodies specific for Pr and other glycoprotein antigens have been reported. In PCH, the autoantibody specificity is most commonly anti-P, although examples of anti-I, anti-i, and anti-Pr have also been reported.

As with warm autoantibodies, cold autoantibodies may present serologic problems if transfusion therapy is indicated. In performing antibody studies, cold autoantibodies may mask the presence of clinically significant alloantibodies, particularly if the autoantibody is capable of activating complement in vitro and if the antiglobulin reagent used in the laboratory contains both anti-IgG and anti-C3. This serologic problem is usually resolvable if anti-IgG–only reagents are used.

TABLE 18-3 Characteristics of Pathologic and Harmless Cold Antibodies

Characteristics	Pathologic Cold Autoantibodies	Harmless Cold Autoantibodies
Immunoglobulin class	IgM and rarely IgA or IgG	IgM
Thermal range	30° to 37° C	4° to 22° C
Specificity	Usually anti-I and rarely anti-i, anti-IH, or anti-Pr	Usually anti-I
Titer	Usually >1000 at 4° C in cold agglutinin syndrome. In mixed type autoimmune hemolytic anemia, the titer at 4° C may be <64	Usually <64 at 4° C
Clonal origin	Monoclonal in chronic disease	Polyclonal
Reactivity enhanced with albumin	Usually	Not usually

On occasion, however, cold autoantibodies may be so potent that binding to the erythrocyte is irreversible, causing spontaneous agglutination of cells at the antiglobulin phase of testing, even though anti-IgG–only reagents are used. Prewarming of serum and red cells to 37° C, followed with an antiglobulin procedure that avoids temperatures below 37° C, may alleviate such problems. In other patients, adsorption procedures are needed before transfusion therapy is possible.

Adsorption Studies
Autologous

Adsorption studies include the use of autologous cells or allogeneic cells. If the patient has not been transfused recently, autoadsorption is the method of choice. In this procedure, it is helpful to premodify the patient's red cells with proteolytic enzymes before adsorption at 4° C.[4,5,25,31] Results must be carefully interpreted because certain antigens to which cold autoantibodies are directed (e.g., Pr specificities) are denatured during the enzyme premodification step, preventing the adsorption of autoantibodies with these specificities. Repeat autoadsorption studies with unmodified red cells should remove such autoantibodies. Following adsorption with the patient's red cells, antibody screening studies should be performed to evaluate the presence of potential alloantibody. If antibody screening tests are positive, antibody identification studies should be performed. Tests with autoadsorbed serum may also be useful to resolve ABO reverse grouping discrepancies.

Allogeneic

If adsorption studies are indicated in a recently transfused individual, allogeneic adsorption may be attempted. Cells should be selected as described in the section for warm autoantibodies. Enzyme premodification of the selected red cells facilitates the process, but, again, consideration must be given to unexpected findings and Pr-related specificities. Following adsorption, antibody screening studies should be performed.

Elution and Autoantibody Specificity

In CAS or PCH, elution studies are not indicated because only C3d is present on the red cells. Elution may be indicated following transfusion when clinical findings suggest a delayed transfusion reaction in addition to cold autoantibodies.

MIXED-TYPE AUTOIMMUNE HEMOLYTIC ANEMIA

Mixed-type autoimmune hemolytic anemia (AIHA) has serologic features of both WAIHA and CAS. Patients with mixed-type AIHA account for approximately 8% of all cases of immune hemolytic anemia.[4,5,33] Most patients have severe hemolysis.[8] Like WAIHA and CAS, this form of immune hemolytic anemia may be primary or secondary to another disease process. Specificities for the warm autoantibody component appear to be similar to those described for WAIHA, although one report suggests that these autoantibodies define a unique antigenic determinant.[34] The specificities of the cold autoantibodies appear to be identical to those seen in CAS.

Direct Antiglobulin Test

Both IgG and C3d are usually detected on the patient's red cells. The IgG (and perhaps some C3d) is the result of IgG warm autoantibodies, whereas the majority of C3d is the result of complement activation initiated by the IgM cold autoantibodies.

Serum and Elution Studies

Both IgG warm autoantibodies and IgM cold autoantibodies are usually present in the patient's serum. Of interest is the finding that the cold autoantibodies, although of high thermal range (up to 37° C), have titers generally less than 64 when tested at 4° C.[8] If transfusion therapy is needed, evaluation of the patient's serum includes autologous and/or allogeneic adsorption. Procedures generally include those discussed previously for autoantibodies seen in WAIHA and CAS. If elution studies are performed, the eluate is reactive with normal red cells because of the warm-reactive autoantibody.

DRUG-INDUCED IMMUNE HEMOLYTIC ANEMIAS

Drug-induced immune antibodies may result in decreased red cell survival and may complicate pretransfusion testing. Drug-induced immune antibodies may be directed against the drug or one of its metabolites or against intrinsic red cell antigens. Serologic problems that arise because of drug-induced antibodies are resolved more quickly if an accurate drug history is obtained. Discontinuation of the drug in question generally mitigates the serologic findings, although this may take several weeks. As expected, discontinuation of the drug alleviates any hemolysis as well.

Four different mechanisms have been associated with a drug-related positive DAT, and these are summarized in Table 18-2. These include the following: drug adsorption or penicillin-type drug-dependent mechanism; immune complex or non-penicillin–type drug-dependent mechanism; membrane modification or non-immunologic adsorption of protein mechanism; and drug-induced autoimmune hemolytic anemia or drug-independent autoantibodies mechanism. It is important to remember that, even in the presence of a positive DAT, hemolysis may be absent. A list of some drugs associated with a positive DAT that may have caused red cell destruction is found in Summary 18-1. Proposed mechanisms are also shown.

Although this chapter defines four mechanisms for drug-induced immune hemolytic anemias, these distinctions are neither clear nor precise. Immune complexes, to date, have never been isolated from cases in which this has been proposed as the mechanism for red cell destruction or a positive DAT. Because of this, there is support to categorize these types of drug-induced cases as drug-dependent cases, although quite distinct from the penicillin-type drug-dependent mechanism.[4,35,36] To complicate matters further, a number of cases of drug-induced immune hemolytic anemias have been described where multiple mechanisms were demonstrable.[37-45] These are summarized in Table 18-4. As can be seen, these cases involved immune complex, drug adsorption, and drug-induced autoimmune hemolytic anemia. Nevertheless, as described by Petz and Garratty,[4] these categories are still useful when describing the serologic events that may be encountered in patients taking certain drugs and the hemolytic episodes that may occur.

Drug Adsorption or Penicillin-Type Drug-Dependent Mechanism

For this type of drug-dependent mechanism, the drug or one of its metabolites is adsorbed to the surface of the red cell. If antibodies to the drug are produced, they can then attach to the drug on the surface of the red cell, resulting in a positive DAT. This is shown in Fig. 18-2.[4] Drugs known to cause a positive DAT that may increase red cell destruction include the penicillins and cephalosporins.[4,5]

Approximately 3% of all patients receiving high-dose intravenous penicillin develop a positive DAT via this mechanism. But only a very small percentage of these patients develop immune hemolysis.[4] Most often, only IgG is detectable on the red cells, although C3, in addition to IgG, has been reported. Unless alloantibodies are concomitantly present, routine antibody screening tests are nonreactive.

If elution studies are performed, the eluate is nonreactive with normal red cells. Penicillin-sensitized red cells must be prepared in vitro and then tested with the eluate in order to demonstrate reactivity and specificity.[4] Antibodies to the drug are also present in the patient's serum, and these, like antibody recovered from an elution procedure, are demonstrable only when the serum is tested with penicillin-sensitized red cells. Procedures for the preparation of drug-sensitized red cells are

SUMMARY 18-1

Some Drugs Associated with a Positive DAT and Probable Red Cell Destruction

DRUG ADSORPTION OR PENICILLIN-TYPE DRUG-DEPENDENT MECHANISM

Penicillin G	Erythromycin
Methicillin	Carbromal
Nafcillin	Cefazolin
Tetracycline	Cefamandole
Cephalothin	

MEMBRANE MODIFICATION OR NONIMMUNOLOGIC ADSORPTION OF PROTEIN

Cephalothin	Diglycoaldehyde
Cisplatin	Suramin

DRUG-INDUCED AUTOIMMUNE HEMOLYTIC ANEMIA (DRUG INDEPENDENT)

Methylodopa	Procainamide
Mefenamic acid	Fludarabine
Levodopa	

IMMUNE COMPLEX OR NON-PENICILLIN–TYPE DRUG-DEPENDENT MECHANISM

Quinine	Methotrexate
Quinidine	Rifampicin
Phenacetin	Stibophen
Acetaminophen	Thiopental
Chlorpropamide	Cefotaxime
Melphalan	Ceftriaxone

available in the *Technical Manual*,[23] *Methods in Immunohematology*,[24] and Petz and Garratty.[4]

Immune Complex or Non-Penicillin–Type Drug-Dependent Mechanism

It has been proposed that the drug and its antibody form circulating immune complexes that may attach loosely to the red cell membrane, initiating complement activation. This complement activation may lead to intravascular or extravascular hemolysis. Red blood cells that are not hemolyzed have a positive DAT in which C3d is most often found, although IgG or IgM has also been reported in addition to

TABLE 18-4 Drugs Associated with Multiple Mechanisms and Red Cell Destruction

Drug	Mechanism
Streptomycin	AA + DA[37]
Nomifensine	AA + IC[38]
Tolmetin	AA + IC[39]
Cefataxime	DA + IC[40]
Ceftazidime	DA + IC[41]
Carboplatin	AA + DA + IC[42]
Cefotetan	AA + DA; DA + IC; AA + DA + IC[43-45]

AA, Autoantibody; DA, drug adsorption; IC, immune complex.

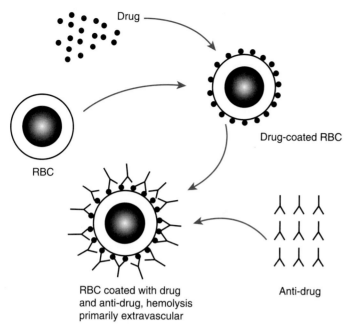

Fig. 18-2 The drug adsorption mechanism. *(From Petz LD, Branch DR: Drug-induced immune hemolytic anemia. In Chaplin H [ed]: Methods in Hematology: Immune Hemolytic Anemias. New York, Churchill-Livingstone, 1985.)*

C3d. As seen in Summary 18-1, many drugs have been reported to cause a positive DAT that may have included hemolysis via this mechanism. Many cases have demonstrated acute intravascular hemolysis, sometimes following small doses of the particular drug. Classic examples of drugs that have caused hemolysis by this mechanism are **quinine, quinidine, phenacetin,** and some second- and third-generation **cephalosporins.**[45,46] As stated earlier, the exact mechanism by which these drugs cause red cell destruction is unclear. Data suggest that these drug-dependent antibodies may also bind to specific receptors on the red cell membrane.[35,36,47]

Garratty[48] has proposed the unifying theory of drug-induced antibody reactions, presented in Fig. 18-3, to explain not only the immune complex mechanism, but also those situations where multiple types of drug-induced mechanisms appear simultaneously. In this theory, the drug antibody may bind loosely, or firmly, to cell membranes and antibodies may be made to (1) the drug, as in the drug-adsorption mechanism; (2) membrane components, resulting in autoantibody production; or (3) part-drug, part-membrane components to which the drug is loosely attached, negating the opportunity for antibody to bind to drug-sensitized cells but permitting antibody, in the presence of added drug, to bind readily to red cells, as noted in the immune complex mechanism.

Eluates are nonreactive, as are antibody screening tests, unless alloantibody is also present or antibody is directed toward membrane components. In vitro studies that demonstrate hemolysis and agglutination are possible when the patient's serum and reagent red cells are incubated in the presence of the drug.[4]

Since the first report of immune hemolysis associated with a third-generation cephalosporin, cefotaxime,[49] reports of drug-induced immune hemolytic anemias caused by second- and third-generation cephalosporins, including cefotetan, ceftriaxone, and ceftizoxime, have extensively appeared in the literature.[40,41,43,44,46,50] In fact, Petz and Garratty[4] report that cephalosporin-related cases now account for the most frequent type of drug-induced immune hemolytic anemia encountered in Garratty's laboratory. Many such cases with severe hemolysis have been well documented in the literature, and nearly 40% of such cases have resulted in fatal

Quinine and quinidine: Quinine is a malarial suppressant. Quinidine sulfate and quinidine gluconate are antimalarial schizonticides and antiarrhythmic drugs.

Phenacetin: An over-the-counter analgesic.

Cephalosporins: A family of broad-spectrum antibiotics divided into "generations." Included in the family are cephalothin, cephradine, cefuroxime axetil, ceftibuten, ceftriaxone, and cefepime.

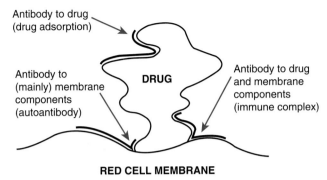

Fig. 18-3 Proposed unifying theory to account for the immune complex mechanism and other drug mechanisms. (*From Garratty G: Target antigens for red cell–bound antibodies. In Nance SJ [ed]: Clinical and Basic Science Aspects of Immunohematology. Arlington, VA, American Association of Blood Banks, 1991.*)

hemolytic anemia. Although some of these cases have been described as the immune complex type, it is of interest to note that many such cases clearly demonstrate multiple drug mechanisms that were responsible for the hemolysis, as shown in Table 18-4. Many have demonstrated immune complex and drug adsorption (both drug dependent), but in at least one third of the cases, autoantibodies (drug independent) were also noted.[4] For more extensive reviews of cephalosporin-induced immune hemolytic anemias, see Petz and Garratty[4] and Arndt and colleagues.[45]

Membrane Modification or Nonimmunologic Adsorption of Protein Mechanism

Cephalothin, cisplatin, diglycoaldehyde, and suramin can modify the red cell membrane, allowing the cells to adsorb protein nonimmunologically. This nonspecific adsorption of protein can result in a positive DAT that demonstrates IgG, IgM, IgA, C3, C4, and perhaps albumin and fibrinogen on the surface of the red cell. This mechanism is rarely associated with increased red cell destruction.

Eluates are nonreactive, as are antibody screening tests, unless alloantibody is also present. Studies with the patient's serum or eluate and the drug fail to demonstrate in vitro reactivity because there appears to be no drug antibody.

Drug-Induced Autoimmune Hemolytic Anemia or Drug-Independent Mechanism

A number of drugs have been shown to cause a positive DAT and immune hemolysis that is serologically indistinguishable from WAIHA. These include **methyldopa, levodopa, procainamide,** fludarabine, and **mefenamic acid.** For many years, methyldopa was the most commonly used of these drugs and therefore the most commonly encountered drug responsible for a positive DAT, with or without hemolysis. More recently, other antihypertensive drugs have replaced methyldopa, so this phenomenon is far less frequent than it once was. Historically, 15% of patients receiving methyldopa developed a positive DAT, and about 1% of these developed immune hemolysis.[4] It has been suggested that methyldopa interferes with suppressor T-cell function, leading to an elaboration of autoantibodies by B cells.[51] It has also been reported that absence of hemolysis in the majority of methyldopa patients is a result of impaired reticuloendothelial function.[52] No conclusive explanation as to why or how certain drugs induce autoimmunity has been put forward. The reader is encouraged to consult the excellent review of studies seeking to explain this phenomenon as detailed in Petz and Garratty.[4]

Cephalothin, cisplatin, diglycoaldehyde, and suramin: Cisplatin, diglycoaldehyde, and suramin are antineoplastic agents. In addition, suramin has been used to treat African trypanosomiasis. Cephalothin is a member of the cephalosporin family of antibiotics.

Methyldopa/levodopa (Aldomet): An antihypertensive drug.

Procainamide: A cardiac antiarrhythmic drug.

Mefenamic acid: A nonsteroidal agent with antiinflammatory, antipyretic, and analgesic activity.

Direct Antiglobulin Test

The DAT most often demonstrates only IgG, although cases of IgG and C3d sensitization have been reported.[4,5] The DAT becomes positive some 3 to 6 months after starting the drug and may persist for up to 2 years following cessation of the drug. An eluate prepared from the patient's red cells is reactive with normal red cells. Autoantibody specificities are as described previously for WAIHA. As a matter of routine practice, determining specificity of these autoantibodies has no value. As with patients with WAIHA, false-positive typing results that include primarily Rh are possible. Approaches for resolution are as described for WAIHA.

Serum Studies

The serum of these individuals should be evaluated for the presence of alloantibody, autoantibody, or a combination of alloantibody and autoantibody. Indeed, patients with hemolytic anemia nearly always demonstrate free serum autoantibody.[4] Autologous or allogeneic adsorption studies may be needed, based on the patient's transfusion history.

CHAPTER SUMMARY

1. Autoantibodies in warm autoimmune hemolytic anemia (WAIHA), cold agglutinin syndrome (CAS), mixed-type autoimmune hemolytic anemia (cold and warm autoantibodies), and paroxysmal cold hemoglobinuria (PCH) can cause decreased red cell survival and acquired immune hemolytic anemia. Drug-induced immune antibodies may also cause decreased red cell survival and acquired immune hemolytic anemia.

2. Most cases of acquired autoimmune hemolytic anemia are associated with IgG immunoglobulins that react optimally at 37° C and cause WAIHA. The DAT in WAIHA demonstrates IgG only, IgG and C3d, or C3d only. Rare cases of WAIHA demonstrate a negative DAT or demonstrate red cells sensitized with IgM or IgA immunoglobulins.

3. Approximately 57% of all patients with WAIHA demonstrate free serum autoantibody reacting at the antiglobulin phase of testing when antibody screening studies are performed.

4. In the presence of a reactive antibody screening test (antiglobulin phase), it is imperative that antibody identification studies be performed. If autoantibody is present, studies must also be undertaken to determine if clinically significant alloantibody is present. This generally requires adsorption studies, and these may be performed using autologous or allogeneic red cells.

5. Specificities of autoantibodies causing WAIHA include anti-D, anti-C, anti-c, anti-e, anti-A, anti-En[a], anti-Ge, anti-I[T], anti-Jk[a], anti-K1, anti-K4, anti-K5, anti-K13, anti-Lan, anti-LW[a], anti-N, anti-Sc1, anti-U, anti-Wr[b], anti-Di[b], anti-Vel, and anti-Xg[a].

6. Cold-reactive autoantibodies may cause CAS and account for approximately 16% of all cases of acquired immune hemolytic anemia.

7. Autoantibodies in CAS are usually IgM and react at up to 30° C. Specificities most often include anti-I, anti-i, and anti-IH. The DAT demonstrates C3d.

8. Antibody screening studies nearly always demonstrate autoantibody. Autologous or allogeneic red cells may be used for adsorption studies to evaluate the presence of clinically significant alloantibody.

9. PCH, or Donath-Landsteiner hemolytic anemia, is a rare type of acquired immune hemolytic anemia. This hemolytic anemia is caused by an IgG autoantibody that binds to red cells at low temperatures and then activates complement at 37° C, causing hemolysis. The DAT in PCH demonstrates C3d. Specificity is most commonly anti-P.

10. Mixed-typed autoimmune hemolytic anemia has serologic characteristics common to both WAIHA and CAS. Both IgG and C3d are found when DATs are performed.

11. Drug-induced immune antibodies may be responsible for a positive DAT, with or without hemolysis. Four mechanisms have been proposed to explain the formation of these antibodies: drug adsorption (penicillin-type drug-dependent mechanism), immune complex (non-penicillin–type drug-dependent mechanism), membrane modification (nonimmunologic protein adsorption), and drug-induced immune hemolytic anemia (drug-independent autoantibodies).

12. Some drugs, including the penicillins and cephalosporins, can bind to the red cell. These drugs or their metabolites then serve as receptors for drug antibodies, causing a positive DAT.

13. Cephalosporins are also purported to modify the red cell membrane, causing the nonspecific adsorption of proteins and a positive DAT.

14. It is postulated, but not proven, that certain drugs are responsible for increased red cell destruction due to circulating immune complexes that attach loosely to the red cell membrane, activate complement, and cause red cell destruction.

15. Certain drugs, including methyldopa, procainamide, fludarabine, and mefenamic acid, are capable of causing a positive DAT and immune hemolysis that is serologically indistinguishable from WAIHA.

REFERENCES

1. Kaplan HS, Garratty G: Predictive value of direct antiglobulin test results. Diagn Med 8:29-33, 1985.

2. Judd WJ, Barnes BA, Steiner EA, et al: The evaluation of a positive direct antiglobulin test (autocontrol) in pretransfusion testing revisited. Transfusion 26:220-224, 1986.

3. Laird-Fryer B: Application and interpretation of direct antiglobulin test results as applied to healthy persons and selected patients. In Wallace ME, Levitt JS (eds): Current Applications and Interpretations of the Direct Antiglobulin Test. Arlington, VA, American Association of Blood Banks, 1988.

4. Petz LD, Garratty G: Immune Hemolytic Anemias, 2nd ed. Philadelphia, Churchill-Livingstone, 2004.

5. Issitt PD, Anstee DJ: Applied Blood Group Serology, 4th ed. Durham, NC, Montgomery Scientific, 1998.

6. Sokol RJ, Booker DJ, Stamps R: The pathology of autoimmune haemolytic anemia. J Clin Pathol 45:1047-1052, 1992.

7. Sokol RJ, Hewitt S, Stamps BK: Autoimmune haemolysis: An 18 year study of 865 cases referred to a regional transfusion centre. BMJ 282:2023-2027, 1981.

8. Shulman IA, Branch DR, Nelson JM, et al: Autoimmune hemolytic anemia with both cold and warm autoantibodies. JAMA 253:1745-1748, 1985.

9. Gottsche B, Salama A, Mueller-Eckhardt C: Donath-Landsteiner autoimmune hemolytic anemia in children. Vox Sang 58:281-286, 1990.

10. Wilkinson SL: Serological approaches to transfusion of patients with allo- or autoantibodies. In Nance SJ (ed): Immune Destruction of Red Blood Cells. Arlington, VA, American Association of Blood Banks, 1989.

11. Edwards JM, Moulds JJ, Judd WJ: Chloroquine diphosphate dissociation of antigen-antibody complexes: A new technique for phenotyping red cells with a positive direct antiglobulin test. Transfusion 22:59-61, 1982.

12. Louie JE, Jiang AF, Zaroulis CG: Preparation of intact antibody-free red blood cells in autoimmune hemolytic anemia (abstract). Transfusion 26:550, 1986.

13. Wallhermfechtel MA, Pohl BA, Chaplin H: Alloimmunization in patients with warm autoantibodies: A retrospective study employing three donor alloabsorptions to aid in antibody detection. Transfusion 24:482-485, 1984.

14. Laine L, Beattie KM: Frequency of alloantibodies accompanying autoantibodies. Transfusion 25:545-546, 1985.

15. James P, Rowe GP, Tozzo GG: Elucidation of alloantibodies in autoimmune hemolytic anemia. Vox Sang 54:167-171, 1988.

16. Issitt PD, Combs MR, Bumgarner DJ, et al: Studies of antibodies in the sera of patients who have made red cell autoantibodies. Transfusion 36:481-486, 1996.

17. Leger RM, Garratty G: Evaluation of methods for detecting alloantibodies underlying warm autoantibodies. Transfusion 39:11-16, 1999.

18. Shirey RS, Boyd JS, Parwani AV, et al: Prophylactic antigen matched donor blood for patients with warm autoantibodies: An algorithm for transfusion management. Transfusion 42:1435-1441, 2002.

19. Morel PA, Bergren MO, Frank BA: A simple method for the detection of alloantibody in the presence of autoantibody (abstract). Transfusion 18:388, 1978.

20. Branch DR, Petz LD: A new reagent (ZZAP) having multiple applications in immunohematology. Am J Clin Pathol 78: 161-167, 982.

21. Burich MA, AuBuchon JP, Anderson HJ: Evaluation of a new rapid antibody dissociation technique (abstract). Transfusion 25:450, 1985.

22. Liew YW, Duncan N: Polyethylene glycol in autoadsorption of serum for detection of alloantibodies (letter). Transfusion 35:713, 1995.

23. Brecher M (ed): Technical Manual, 14th ed. Bethesda, MD, American Association of Blood Banks, 2002.

24. Judd WJ: Methods in Immunohematology, 2nd ed. Durham, NC, Montgomery Scientific, 1994.

25. Mollison PL, Engelfriet CP, Contreras M: Blood Transfusion in Clinical Medicine, 10th ed. Oxford, Blackwell Scientific, 1997.

26. Johnson ST, McFarland JG, Kelly KJ, et al: Transfusion support with RBCs from an M^k homozygote in a case of autoimmune hemolytic anemia following diphtheria-pertussis-tetanus vaccination. Transfusion 42:567-571, 2002.

27. Heddle NM, Kelton JG, Turchyn KL, Ali MA: Hypergammaglobulinemia can be associated with a positive direct antiglobulin test, a nonreactive eluate, and no evidence of hemolysis. Transfusion 28:29-33, 1988.

28. Toy PTCY, Chin CA, Reid ME, Burns MA: Factors associated with positive direct antiglobulin tests in pretransfusion patients: A case-control study. Vox Sang 49:215-220, 1985.

29. Moscow JA, Casper AJ, Kodis C, Fricke WA: Positive direct antiglobulin test results after intravenous immune globulin administration. Transfusion 27:248-249, 1987.

30. Wolach B, Heddle NM, Barr RD, et al: Transient Donath-Landsteiner hemolytic anemia. Br J Haematol 48:425-434, 1981.

31. Judd WJ: Investigation and management of immune hemolysis—autoantibodies and drugs. In Wallace ME, Levitt JS (eds): Current Applications and Interpretations of the Direct Antiglobulin Test. Arlington, VA, American Association of Blood Banks, 1988.

32. Reid ME: Autoagglutination dispersal utilizing sulphydryl-compounds. Transfusion 18:353-355, 1978.

33. Sokol RJ, Hewitt S, Stamps BK: Autoimmune haemolysis: Mixed warm and cold antibody type. Acta Haematol 69: 266-274,1983.

34. Kaji E, Miura Y, Ikemoto S: Characterization of autoantibodies in mixed-type autoimmune haemolytic anaemia. Vox Sang 60:45-52, 1991.

35. Mueller-Eckhardt C, Salama A: Drug-induced immune cytopenias: A unifying pathogenetic concept with special emphasis on the role of drug metabolites. Transfus Med Rev 4:69-77, 1990.

36. Petz LD, Mueller-Eckhardt C: Drug-induced immune hemolytic anemia. Transfusion 32:202-204, 1992.

37. Florendo NT, MacFarland D, Painter M, Muirhead EE: Streptomycin-specific antibody coincident with a developing warm autoantibody. Transfusion 20:662-668, 1980.

38. Salama A, Mueller-Eckhardt C: Two types of nomifensine-induced immune haemolytic anaemias: Drug-dependent sensitization and/or autoimmunization. Br J Haematol 64:613-620, 1986.

39. Squires JE, Mintz PD, Clark S: Tolmetin-induced hemolysis. Transfusion 25:410-413, 1985.

40. Shulman IA, Arndt PA, McGehee W, Garratty G: Cefotaxime-induced immune hemolytic anemia due to antibodies reacting in vitro by more than one mechanism. Transfusion 30:263-266, 1990.

41. Chambers LA, Donovan LM, Kruskall MS: Ceftazidime-induced hemolysis in a patient with drug-dependent antibodies reactive by immune complex and drug adsorption mechanisms. Am J Clin Pathol 95:393-396, 1991.

42. Marani TM, Trich MB, Armstrong KS, et al: Carboplatin-induced immune hemolytic anemia. Transfusion 36:1016-1018, 1996.

43. Garratty G, Nance S, Lloyd M, Domen R: Fatal immune hemolytic anemia due to cefotetan. Transfusion 32:269-271, 1992.

44. Gallagher NI, Schergen AK, Sokol-Anderson ML, et al: Severe immune-mediated hemolytic anemia secondary to treatment with cefotetan. Transfusion 32:266-268, 1992.

45. Arndt PA, Leger RM, Garratty G: Serology of antibodies to second- and third-generation cephalosporins associated with immune hemolytic anemia and/or positive direct antiglobulin tests. Transfusion 39:1239-1246, 1999.

46. Garratty G, Postoway N, Schwellenbach J, McMahill PC: A fatal case of ceftriaxone (Rocephin)-induced hemolytic anemia associated with intravascular hemolysis. Transfusion 31:176-179, 1991.

47. Salama A, Mueller-Eckhardt C: On the mechanisms of sensitization and attachment of antibodies to RBC in drug-induced immune hemolytic anemia. Blood 69:1006-1010, 1987.

48. Garratty G: Target antigens for red cell–bound autoantibodies. In Nance SJ (ed): Clinical and Basic Science Aspects of Immunohematology. Arlington, VA, American Association of Blood Banks, 1991.

49. Salama A, Gottsche B, Schleffer T, Mueller-Eckhardt C: "Immune complex" mediated intravascular hemolysis due to IgM cephalosporin dependent antibody. Transfusion 27: 460-463, 1987.

50. Calhoun BW, Junsanto T, Donoghue MD, et al: Ceftizoxime induced hemolysis secondary to combined drug adsorption and immune-complex mechanisms. Transfusion 41:893-897, 2001.

51. Kirtland HH, Mohler DH, Horwitz DA: Methyldopa inhibition of suppressor lymphocyte function: A proposed cause of autoimmune hemolytic anemia. N Engl J Med 302:825-832, 1980.

52. Kelton JG: Impaired reticuloendothelial function in patients treated with methyldopa. N Engl J Med 313:596-600, 1985.

FURTHER READINGS

Branch DR, Petz LD: Detecting alloantibodies in patients with autoantibodies (editorial). Transfusion 39:6-10, 1999.

Issitt PD, Anstee DJ: Applied Blood Group Serology, 4th ed. Durham, NC, Montgomery Scientific, 1998.

Garratty G: Target antigens for red cell–bound autoantibodies. In Nance SJ (ed): Clinical and Basic Science Aspects of Immunohematology. Arlington, VA, American Association of Blood Banks, 1991.

Garratty G, Petz LD: Approaches to selecting blood for transfusion to patients with autoimmune hemolytic anemia (editorial). Transfusion 42:1390-1392, 2000.

Mueller-Eckhardt C, Salama A: Drug-induced immune cytopenias: A unifying pathogenetic concept with special emphasis on the role of drug metabolites. Trans Med Rev 4:69-77, 1990.

Nance SJ (ed): Immune Destruction of Red Blood Cells. Arlington, VA, American Association of Blood Banks, 1989.

Petz LD, Garratty G: Immune Hemolytic Anemias, 2nd ed. Philadelphia, Churchill Livingstone, 2004.

Simon TL, Dzik WH, Snyder EL, et al: Rossi's Principles of Transfusion Medicine, 3rd ed. Philadelphia, Lippincott Williams & Wilkins, 2002.

Wallace ME, Levitt JS (eds): Current Applications and Interpretations of the Direct Antiglobulin Test. Arlington, VA, American Association of Blood Banks, 1988.

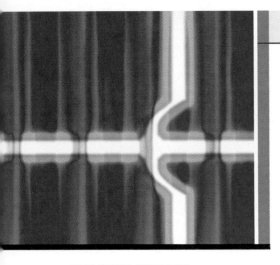

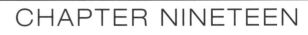

CHAPTER NINETEEN

Hematopoietic Stem Cells and Cellular Therapy

Maria Lukas

LEARNING OBJECTIVES

After reading and studying this chapter, the student should be able to:

1. List the sources of hematopoietic stem cells.
2. Discuss the rationale for hematopoietic transplantation.
3. Discuss the differences between various banking models.
4. Describe three procurement methods of stem cells.
5. Describe the donor selection process.
6. State the stem cell donor testing requirements.
7. Describe the quality control testing performed on stem cell products.
8. Describe three cryopreservation methods for stem cell preservation.
9. Define three types of stem cell transplantation.
10. Discuss transplant complications.
11. Discuss regulatory standards regarding HPC collection, storage, transportation, and transplantation.
12. Discuss future improvements and applications for cellular therapy.

OVERVIEW

Bone marrow transplantation (BMT) has been studied in animal models since the late 1940s as a treatment for lethal exposure to radiation.[1] Transplantation of hematopoietic stem cells (HSCs), a refinement of bone marrow transplant, is one of the great clinical medicine triumphs of the last 30 years. Early studies demonstrated that transfer of living cells mediated radiation protection and induced tolerance. Identification of the major histocompatibility complex (MHC) and identification of the role of the thymus in the development of the immune system were essential to developing strategies for marrow transplantation. Clinical allogeneic marrow transplantation from a human leukocyte antigen (HLA)–identical donor was performed in 1968 for the correction of severe combined immunodeficiency disease (SCID) and Wiskott-Aldrich syndrome.[2] It was also learned at this time that it was necessary to suppress the immune system to achieve engraftment and that additional radiation therapy and chemotherapy of the recipient were needed for treatment of the underlying malignant disease. By the 1970s, it was evident that HSC transplantation could lead to long-term survival and cure leukemia, SCID, and severe aplastic anemia.

The steady increase in the clinical application of HSC transplantation was paralleled by improvements in clinical benefits. National and international networks for donor registries (including the Laura Graves Foundation, which later became the National Marrow Donor Program [NMDP]) developed to meet the need for unrelated marrow transplantation, especially for patients with rare HLA phenotypes. By 1995 to 1996, 25% of all allogeneic transplants were from unrelated donors. This was due to several factors: the basis for clinical HSC was well developed; support for critically ill patients improved; and graft-versus-host disease (GVHD) prophylaxis and new antibiotics, including antiviral reagents, were more available.

HSC transplantation reconstitutes hematopoietic cell lineages with normal cells capable of self-renewal. Additionally, the engrafted HSCs can provide antitumor effects for patients with malignant disease. The major transplant-related complications are GVHD, graft rejection, graft failure, prolonged immunodeficiency, and toxicity from pretransplantation and posttransplantation radiation therapy and chemotherapy and GVHD prophylaxis[2] (Summary 19-1).

The first successful transplants were performed with stem cells derived from the marrow of identical twins (syngeneic transplantation). Application of transplantation therapy broadened with the use of stem cells obtained from either related or unrelated donors (allogeneic transplantation) suitably HLA matched, or the patient's own stem cells (autologous transplantation). Years of HSC transplant history have helped to define three basic transplant principles: (1) HSCs obtained from donor marrow or other sources can be infused into the venous blood system and engraft in the recipient's hematopoietic environment; (2) the recipient's immune system will tolerate engraftment of donor cells so that rejection does not occur; and (3) immune effector cells from the donor will tolerate host tissue so that fatal GVHD does not occur.[3]

STEM CELL TRANSPLANTATION OVERVIEW

Bone marrow transplant is the term historically applied to this stem cell transplantation; however, stem cells come from a number of sources in addition to bone marrow: peripheral blood, umbilical cord blood, and fetal liver. All blood cell lines

---

Summary 19-1

Major Transplant-Related Complications

Graft-versus-host disease (GVHD)
Graft rejection
Graft failure
Prolonged immunodeficiency
Toxicity from radiation therapy and chemotherapy
Adverse effects of GVHD prophylaxis

Stem cells: Precursor cells that have the capacity to both self-perpetuate and differentiate into a vast array of specialized tissue types.

Progenitor cells: Progenitor cells are committed to a blood cell lineage and do not have the ability to differentiate into all blood cell lineages.

Myeloablative: Therapy designed to eliminate marrow cells before HSC transplant.

Cytokines: Soluble polypeptides that are produced by both immune and nonimmune cells and that function in the regulation of the immune/inflammatory response.

CD34: A subset of cells that possess a transmembrane glycoprotein. Included in this cell cluster are those cells that are lineage committed, as well as pluripotent stem cells.

Graft rejection: An immune response against an engrafted organ or tissue resulting in failure of the graft to survive.

Graft-versus-host disease (GVHD): A disease that results when transplanted immunocompetent cells mount an immune response against the recipient. The disease can be either acute or chronic and most often affects the skin, gastrointestinal tract, and liver.

Hematopoiesis: The formation of blood cells.

Summary 19-2

Sources of Hematopoietic Stem Cells

Bone marrow
Fetal liver
Peripheral blood
Cord blood

are produced from primitive immature populations that consist of hematopoietic **stem cells** and **progenitor cells.** The major site of production of these rare immature cells is the bone marrow.[4] Hematopoietic stem cells from four different sources (Summary 19-2 and Figs. 19-1 and 19-2) have been used for reconstitution of the lymphohematopoietic function after **myeloablative,** near-myeloablative, or nonmyeloablative treatment. Bone marrow–derived stem cells were introduced by E.D. Thomas in 1963 and are considered the classical stem cell source. Fetal liver stem cell transplantation has been performed on a limited number of patients with aplastic anemia or acute leukemia, but only transient engraftment has been demonstrated. Peripheral blood as a source of stem cells was introduced in 1981. Cord blood was introduced as a source of stem cells in 1988.

Hematopoietic stem cells (HSCs) from the cord blood are in a slow or noncycling state but proliferate rapidly in response to stimulation by **cytokines** and can be expanded ex vivo in culture with a combination of cytokines. The primitive cells in cord blood express **CD34** antigens, and the cells expressing the highest density (Fig. 19-3) distribution of CD34 antigens on their surface can be enriched to yield the more immature subsets of stem and progenitor cells.[4] The percentage of CD34+ cells among the circulating total nucleated cells at steady state in a healthy donor is 0.06%. The percentage of CD34+ cells in the bone marrow is 1.1%.

HSCs are an effective treatment for a range of malignant, hematologic, immunologic, metabolic, and neoplastic diseases. Transplant of allogeneic stem cells requires careful HLA matching of the donor and recipient. Failure to match the donor and recipient can result in both **graft rejection** and **graft-versus-host disease (GVHD).** Rejection or GVHD occurs when the immunocompetent cells of the host or donor respond to alloantigen encoded by the MHC and peptides presented in association with these MHC antigens.[3] In an effort to provide a

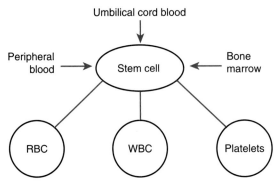

Fig. 19-1 Hematopoietic stem cells from one of three sources, bone marrow, peripheral blood, or umbilical cord blood, differentiate into a variety of cells and tissue types.

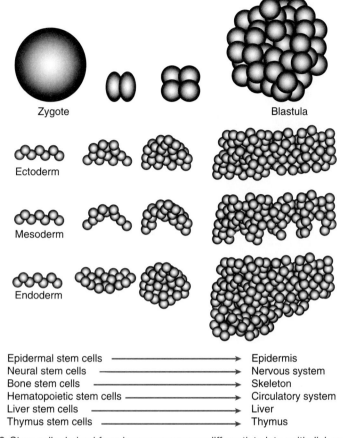

Epidermal stem cells ⟶ Epidermis
Neural stem cells ⟶ Nervous system
Bone stem cells ⟶ Skeleton
Hematopoietic stem cells ⟶ Circulatory system
Liver stem cells ⟶ Liver
Thymus stem cells ⟶ Thymus

Fig. 19-2 Stem cells derived from bone marrow can differentiate into epithelial, neural, bone, and liver cells.

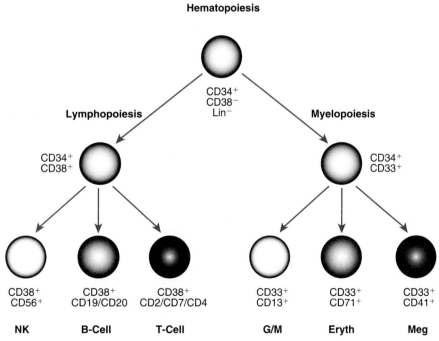

Fig. 19-3 CD34 is an indicator of the concentration of stem cells.

From stem cell....

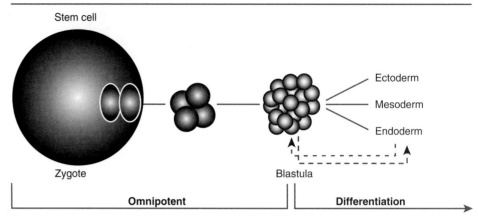

Fig. 19-4 Hematopoiesis: the development from stem cells to differentiated cells.

better HLA match, marrow transplantation has become a large-scale international cooperative endeavor.

STEM CELL PROCUREMENT
Cell Sources

The development of **hematopoiesis** occurs throughout the embryologic stages: mesodermal (yolk sac), hepatosplenic, and medullary (Fig. 19-4). After birth, human hematopoiesis comes solely from the bone marrow. Because of this, sources of HSCs in human adults are restricted to bone marrow and peripheral blood. Additional sources of stem cells include the fetal liver and umbilical cord blood (UCB). During the first and second trimester of fetal development, the liver is physiologically associated with the hematopoietic tissues. It is during this time that fetal liver cells could theoretically be used for transplantation. Because these cells can only be harvested from aborted fetuses, technical and ethical issues have yet to be resolved. At present there are no clinical applications for fetal liver–derived HSCs.

Collection Methods
Bone Marrow

Allogeneic bone marrow is obtained from donors who are matched to the HLA type of the recipient. The harvest is typically done under general anesthesia. Multiple small aspirates of bone marrow are drawn from the **posterior iliac crest** or **anterior iliac crest.** In children, bone marrow can be harvested from the head of the tibia if **epiphyseal closure** has not yet occurred (Fig. 19-5). The volume harvested is usually limited to 1500 mL. Once aspirated, the marrow is mixed with an anticoagulant such as adenine citrate dextrose (ACD) and/or heparin. After collection, the marrow may be manipulated and/or cryopreserved.

Apheresis (Peripheral Blood Stem Cell Collection)

Advantages such as rapid platelet and neutrophil engraftment, reduced early toxicity, and superior immune reconstitution without a significant increase in risk of acute GVHD make peripheral blood stem cell transplantation a preferable alternative to BMT. In **extramedullary** sources such as peripheral blood, HSCs exist in very low concentrations. To obtain sufficient numbers of HSCs, the donor is treated with a stem cell–mobilizing agent such as **granulocyte colony-stimulating factor (G-CSF)** over a multiday period. A final dose of G-CSF is given immediately before the stem cell apheresis procedure, to stimulate the release of HSCs from the bone marrow into the circulating blood. Most transplant centers use a 5-

Posterior iliac crest, anterior iliac crest: The superior portion of the hip bone.

Epiphyseal closure: Closure of the cartilaginous end of a long bone at the end of the growth period.

Extramedullary: Refers to outside of the bone marrow.

Granulocyte colony-stimulating factor (G-CSF): A growth factor used to mobilize granulocytes, thereby increasing the yield of stem cells in peripheral blood progenitor cell collection.

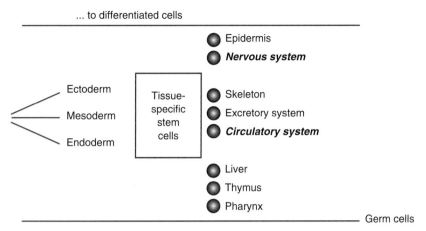

... to differentiated cells

Epidermis
Nervous system

Ectoderm
Mesoderm
Endoderm

Tissue-
specific
stem
cells

Skeleton
Excretory system
Circulatory system

Liver
Thymus
Pharynx

Germ cells

Fig. 19-4, cont'd for legend see opposite page.

day G–CSF regimen, starting peripheral stem cell collections on the fifth day. It has been reported that G–CSF causes a mean peripheral blood CD34+ cell concentration to increase from 3.8×10^9/L to 61.9×10^9/L, a 16.3-fold increase over baseline.[5]

Mononuclear cells are harvested by leukapheresis after treatment with G–CSF. Leukapheresis collection is less invasive than bone marrow collection. The leukapheresis procedure may be performed using peripheral venous access (usually the antecubital vein) or a double-lumen central venous catheter to support blood flows necessitated by the apheresis instrument. The cell compositions of unmanipulated peripheral blood stem cells (PBSCs) and bone marrow (BM) allografts differ

HSC Sources for Transplant

Comparison of different sources for unrelated hematopoietic (blood) stem cell transplants

FEATURE	CORD BLOOD	BONE MARROW	MOBILIZED PERIPHERAL BLOOD
Donor pain/discomfort during collection	Painless	Painful, requiring multiple bone needle punctures and general anesthesia	Growth factor shots/large needles or catheters/multiple, lengthy (3-6 hr) apheresis procedures
Donor risk	None	Risks of surgery and general anesthesia	Growth factor side effects and apheresis risks
Recipient tolerance of tissue type (HLA) mismatching	More tolerant	Less tolerant	Less tolerant
Ease of matching/ retrieval time	Short (less than 1 mo)	Long (2-6 mo)	Long (2-6 mo)
Risk of graft versus host disease (GVHD)	Lower	Higher	Highest
Risk of infectious disease in stem cells	Lower	Higher	Higher
Cost	Lower	Higher	Higher
Use in larger (adult) patients	Difficult to find large enough cord blood units	No significant problem	No significant problem
Time to engraftment	Longest (3-4 weeks)	Moderate (2-3 weeks)	Shortest (1-2 weeks)

Fig. 19-5 Comparison of features associated with bone marrow, peripheral blood, and cord blood transplants.

significantly. The total number of T cells, monocytes, and natural killer cells contained in a PBSC allograft are more than 10 times higher than in a BM allograft. Allografts of G-CSF–treated PBSCs contain two to four times more CD34+ cells than do those from untreated BM. When a BM donor is treated for 3 days with G-CSF, the number of CD34+ cells contained in the harvested BM averages 2.5 × 10^6/kg, which is similar to that obtained by steady state BM harvest.[5] Peripheral collections are the preferred source of HSCs over bone marrow in many centers.[5]

Cord Blood

Human umbilical cord blood (UCB) is a rich and readily accessible source of HSCs. The concentration of HSCs in UCB is greater than in peripheral blood but less than 10% of the cell dose administered in a typical BMT.[6] Additionally, immune competence is far less, allowing for diminished risk of GVHD in UCB transplants as compared with peripheral blood and bone marrow, thus allowing for the use of partially mismatched unrelated donors.[6] The relatively small number of nucleated cells in UCB limits the use of UCB transplantation in adults.

A dose equal to or greater than 1.7 × 10^5 CD34+ cells/kg of the recipient's weight is thought to be necessary to achieve hematopoietic reconstitution.

An advantage of the use of cord blood is the ease of collection.[6] UCB can be collected in a variety of ways. In an open collection method, needle aspirations of the placental vein are performed. Open systems have been replaced by closed systems with blood collection bags because, although the open collection is technically easier to perform, a closed collection system results in an optimum collection volume and reduces the risk of microbial and maternal cell contamination.[5]

The mode of birth may influence the white blood cell (WBC) content and collection volume. When a cesarean delivery is performed, cord blood collection is more efficacious if performed before delivery of the placenta.[7] Studies have shown that higher cord blood volume is collected following cesarean section than following vaginal delivery. However, UCB collected from vaginal delivery has a significantly higher WBC concentration than UCB collected from cesarean births.[8] Generally, UCB is collected by a simple venipuncture of the umbilical vein, followed by gravity drainage into a standard anticoagulant-filled blood collection bag.[9] UCB collection is performed using aseptic cord preparation and a closed system to minimize risk of bacterial or fungal contamination. The simple maneuver of placing the newborn on the maternal abdomen after delivery and before cord clamping may significantly increase the volume of UCB collected without harmful effects to the newborn.[7]

Embryonic

Fetal liver cells can be obtained from a fetus aborted in the first or second trimester. There is increasing interest in using these pluripotent embryonic stem cells to generate bone, muscle, brain, cartilage, and other tissues for the treatment of such diseases as diabetes, Alzheimer's, and Parkinson's. As previously mentioned, this is not a common source of HSCs because of the technical, ethical, and legal issues related to this source, which have to be resolved before the initiation of large-scale research endeavors.[5]

Adverse Events

Bone marrow harvesting is usually a one-time, single-day procedure that occurs under general anesthesia. It is associated with some limited procedural risks related to general or spinal anesthesia, as well as the potential for infection or injury at the site of marrow aspiration.[5,6] These risks significantly increase with the donor's age.[5]

Peripheral collections usually require multiple days, especially for autologous transplantations. Sophisticated flow cytometric analysis of the components is needed to ensure adequate HSC content. There is the risk that adequate CD34+

cells in the PBSC components cannot be collected from all patients and donors because of inadequate venous access. From 5% to 20% of donors may have inadequate peripheral venous access, and insertion of a central or femoral venous catheter may add to the risk and discomfort of the procedure. Last, there are risks associated with the administration of hematopoietic cytokines (such as toxicity) and to the apheresis procedure (such as fever, chills, and urticaria).[5] PBSC collection can be performed safely on donors ranging in age from 1 year to the eighties.[5]

Data on the long-term adverse effects of stem cell harvesting is scarce. One concern has been whether the short-term administration of G-CSF may trigger the development of malignancy. Studies, to date, have not detected any cases of leukemia or myelodysplasia in donors up to 40 months after donation.[5]

Concern has been raised that UCB collection will adversely affect the safety of the newborn. Early cord clamping leads to increased placental blood volume. Later clamping of the cord allows for greater transfer of placental blood to the fetus. In general, collection of approximately 100 mL of UCB during the third stage of labor or from the placenta ex utero within approximately 15 to 20 minutes of a healthy, full-term newborn delivery poses no significant risk to the mother or newborn. Early research raised the concern that early cord clamping on a premature infant may precipitate periventricular hemorrhage in premature infants. Later, randomized, controlled studies failed to confirm this finding.[10]

Donor Selection

Selection of the type of transplantation for a patient, autologous or allogeneic, depends on the type of malignant disease, age, availability of a suitable donor, ability to collect a tumor-free autograft, stage and status of disease, and chemosensitivity to conventional chemotherapy.

Autologous Transplants

An autologous transplant is technically not a transplant but rather a rescue of the patient with the patient's own HSCs. In autologous HSC transplants, the patient's hematopoietic stem cells are collected and cryopreserved to protect them from the lethal effects of therapeutic or ablative irradiation or chemotherapy. The autologous HSCs are reinfused in order to repopulate the patient's marrow. This most commonly occurs to support dose-intensive cytotoxic therapy for treatment of malignant diseases.

Autologous transplants have also been used for treatment of autoimmune diseases, as a vehicle for gene therapy, for correction of metabolic defects, and for immunotherapy. They cannot be used for genetic or acquired diseases because the salvaged HSCs would have the same genetic defect. Autologous transplantation is readily available, there is no need to identify a donor, and there is no risk of GVHD or need for immunosuppressive therapy. Immune reconstitution after autologous transplantation is faster and there is less risk of opportunistic infections. Graft failure rarely occurs. However, the autograft may be contaminated with clonigenic tumor cells that can contribute to relapse of the disease.[6]

Syngeneic Transplants

Syngeneic transplants involve hematopoietic cells from an identical twin donor. Such transplants are limited by the fact that most recipients do not have identical twin donors. In addition, malignant disease relapse is increased in syngeneic transplants.

Allogeneic Transplants

Allogeneic transplants are collected from related or unrelated donors. The HLA system is the MHC in humans, and the results of the allogeneic transplant depend on the histocompatibility between the donor and recipient.[6] Allogeneic transplants have the advantage that the graft is free of contaminating tumor cells. Additionally, the graft contains donor-immunocompetent cells that may produce an immune effect, immune-mediated graft-versus-malignancy (GVM), which may eradicate tumor cells surviving high-dose cytotoxic therapy. This generally leads to a lower risk of disease recurrence. Allotransplants may, however, be associated with certain potentially fatal complications such as graft rejection and GVHD. Immune reconstitution is slower and opportunistic infections are more frequent. The treatment-related mortality rate is significantly higher after allotransplants than autotransplants. Only 20% to 30% of patients have an HLA-identical related donor available. Treatment mortality rate is increased with mismatched or unrelated allotransplants. Allotransplants have been limited to younger patients in good general condition because of the risk of regimen-related toxicity and GVHD.

Allotransplant has been used predominantly to treat leukemia and malignant diseases. The outcome of HSC transplantation is based on the selection of patients and the timing of transplantation in the course of the malignant disease.

Xenogeneic Transplants

Xenogeneic transplantation involves HSCs collected from a nonhuman species. Currently, this source is not feasible because of insurmountable immunologic barriers and disease concerns.

Banked Umbilical Cord Blood

HSCs from banked umbilical cord blood are an alternative source of donor stem cells for use in allotransplantation. This therapy is currently used to treat patients with aggressive or recurrent malignancies, immunodeficiencies, certain genetic conditions, hemoglobinopathies, and congenital and acquired bone marrow failure syndromes. The most important advantage of cord blood stem cells is that they do not need to be fully HLA matched for a successful transplant. Additionally, cord blood is less likely to transmit infectious diseases transmissible by blood.

Cord blood donors are unique in that the birth mother is screened as the donor although the cord blood product is collected via the umbilical vein from the neonate. A maternal health history is obtained, and a sample from the birth mother is screened for transfusion-transmitted diseases (TTDs) before delivery. The birth mother (and, when possible, the biologic father) is required to complete a confidential health history questionnaire in order to identify behaviors that increase the risk of exposure to TTDs. This screening is done before collection, making the unit readily available for patients in need of a donor for stem cell transplant. The American Association of Blood Banks (AABB), the Foundation for the Accreditation of Cellular Therapy (FACT), and Netcord have developed worldwide standards for facilities involved in HSC services. Many state health departments have regulations regarding stem cell products, and the Food and Drug Administration (FDA) is in the process of finalizing national standards (good tissue practices [GTPs]) to regulate the practice of collecting, processing, testing, storing, shipping, and transplanting stem cell products.

Regardless of the type of model used to collect, process, and/or store the stem cell product for transplantation, bone marrow and apheresis donors are typically screened and tested before collection of the stem cell product. HSCs collected from the bone marrow or by apheresis are generally collected, processed, cryopreserved, and transplanted within a short period of time after collection. Stem cells recovered from cord blood can be collected, processed, and frozen for an extended period of time before transplantation. A variety of banking models have been developed for long-term storage of cord blood stem cells. These are discussed in the following section.

Banking Models
Public Banking

In the public banking model, established by Rubenstein and colleagues[11] in 1993, cord blood units are collected voluntarily from healthy, full-term placentas after obtaining maternal informed consent. These UCB units are processed, tested, and stored for allogeneic use in patients who do not have an identical HLA-matched relative. Through the development and efforts of organizations such as Netcord and NMDP, public cord blood banks have been established internationally and work together to identify HLA-matched donors. There are strict criteria for the storage of a UCB product by public banks regarding the volume, white blood cell count, and CD34 cell count, and absence of bacterial or fungal contamination. Products not meeting these criteria are discarded or used for research.

Private Banking (Family)

In the private or family banking model, the family pays for the collection and testing and maintains ownership of the UCB unit and directs the use of the product for their own family health needs. The family may also choose to use the UCB unit for treatment of an unrelated individual with an appropriate HLA match, to donate the product for research purposes, or to provide direct consent before the product is discarded. The family banking model grew out of the awareness of the potentially life-saving benefit by HPCs contained in the UCB, which, in the past, was discarded as medical waste. The ability to acquire cryopreserved UCB for immediate use has advantages over either BMT or PBSC. This is particularly advantageous for ethnic minority families and mixed ethnicity families who are generally underrepresented in the current unrelated public donor registries.[10,12]

Hybrid Model

This model provides both family and public banking in a single facility. This model affords the advantages of family banking to those who elect to use this service, while providing open registries for the provision of cord blood to the public.

DONOR SCREENING
Donor Testing
Autologous Donors

The major concern in autologous donor evaluation is the sensitivity of the malignancy to UCB testing. A second area of concern is the mobilization of sufficient cells from the patient to reconstitute the marrow after myeloablation. Before collection, the autologous marrow should be assessed for both residual malignancy and marrow cellularity.

Allogeneic Donors

Allogeneic donor selection is primarily based on HLA compatibility with the recipient. The high risk of morbidity and mortality associated with cytomegalovirus (CMV) infection makes the CMV status of the donor a deciding factor in the selection process. The use of parous females or sex-mismatched donors increases the risk of GVHD. Therefore the ideal allogeneic donor would be an HLA-identical match; CMV negative, if the recipient is CMV negative; the same gender as the recipient; and if female, nonparous and untransfused.

The allogeneic donor should be screened to minimize the risk of disease transmission to an already immunocompromised recipient. A blood sample from all cellular product donors is tested, and, in the case of cord blood, the maternal sample is tested within 30 days of donation/collection using an FDA-approved test for infectious disease markers (see Summary 19-1). This screening should occur within 30 days of collection. Confirmed human immunodeficiency virus (HIV)–positive donors should not be used as a source for the transplant. Other positive disease markers do not necessarily prohibit use of collections, but informed consent from the donor and recipient must be obtained before the transplant occurs. The cellular product donor is further tested for ABO/Rh and HLA-A, HLA-B, and HLA-DR antigens. A sample from the UCB is tested for abnormal hemoglobin if collected from ethnic groups at high risk for hemoglobinopathies.[13]

Cord Blood

In cord blood banking, maternal blood, fetal blood, or both are tested for infectious and genetic diseases transmitted through blood and stem cells. The maternal sample should be obtained from the mother within 48 hours of cord blood collection. The cord blood is tested for stem and progenitor cell content and for homozygous hemoglobinopathies. There is a review of the family's medical history and the medical records of both the infant and birth mother. Maternal donors are screened for hepatitis B and C viruses, human T-cell lymphotropic virus (HTLV), HIV, syphilis, and abnormal red cell antibodies. Maternal donors are also screened for exposure to TTDs by determining if they have traveled to or lived in countries where HIV, variant Creutzfeldt-Jakob disease (vCJD), or malaria is endemic; if they practice high-risk behaviors; or if they are known to have positive results of viral serologic or DNA tests for syphilis, hepatitis B or C, HTLV I or II, or HIV 1 or 2. The maternal sample is also tested for CMV. From 40% to 90% of mothers are seropositive for CMV immunoglobulin before pregnancy. Maternal IgG crosses the placenta and results in a positive serologic test in the cord blood. However, this is not indicative of the presence of active CMV viremia, disease, or infection but passive transfer of maternal IgG. Alternative means of viral detection in cord blood are being researched but are not available for clinical use.

Quality Control Testing

To determine the quality of the stem cell processing and cryopreservation methods, the stem cell units may be tested as follows: cells counts, differential counts to determine mononuclear cell and nucleated red cell dosing, cell viability, ABO and Rh typing, CD34 positivity, and bacterial and fungal growth.[14,15] HLA typing is performed on a pallet of red blood cells and granulocytes. DNA technology is generally used to determine HLA-A, HLA-B, and HLA-DRB1.[10] Monitoring and documenting days to engraftment for neutrophil and platelet lineage is required by regulatory agencies as a way to measure the quality of the transplanted product and the success of the transplant.[15,16]

STEM CELL PROCESSING AND STORAGE
Processing Methods

There are a number of current options for stem cell processing, all designed to increase the yield of CD34-positive cells in the product. Fluorescence-activated cell sorting (FACS) permits physical separation of CD34 cells based on the expression of molecules with predefined properties. This method is sensitive but not practical for large-scale purification of a graft. Immunomagnetic separation couples the CD34 antibody to a magnetic bead. After incubation, a magnet is used to separate the rosetting CD34 cells from the nonrosetting cells. Density gradient centrifugation uses silane-coated colloidal silica to separate HSCs based on their buoyancy during centrifugation. Counterflow centrifugal elutriation separates cells based on their size and density.

Stem Cell Storage

Long-term cryopreservation of human stem cells may be useful for those patients who achieve a complete remission after chemotherapy for whom immediate transplantation may not be indicated. HSCs can be cryopreserved for transplantation after relapse. Long-term storage of HSCs from cord blood improves the availability of allogeneic transplantation to unrelated recipients.[16] Cryopreservation permits transportation of cells to a clinical location, pooling of cells to reach a therapeutic dose, time for the completion of safety and quality control testing, and the development of national or regional cell processing centers.[17]

A controlled-rate freeze followed by storage in a mechanical freezer maintaining −80° C, or a freezer containing liquid nitrogen to ensure a steady temperature of −196° C, is typically used for storage of stem cell products after cryopreservation. Liquid nitrogen freezers may be filled with the gas (liquid phase) or may be maintained in a vapor phase to achieve a constant −196° C environment. The general freezing parameters include cryopreservation in **dimethyl sulfoxide (DMSO)** and a source of plasma protein with or without **hydroxyethyl starch (HES)**. The product is cooled at 1° to 3° C/min (controlled rate freeze) and stored at −80° C (mechanical) or colder (liquid nitrogen, −196° C).[18] A slow, controlled freezing rate can minimize the effects of thermal shock, phase transition time, and posttransition freezing rate. Mechanical or uncontrolled-rate freezing is a viable and cost-effective alternative to controlled-rate freezing. The mechanical freeze produces a freezing rate of 3° C/min. Widespread use of this method is limited by the availability of data on long-term storage and engraftment. Cryopreservation does result in the loss of an undefined but substantial portion of HPCs. There is also a considerable incidence of minor toxicity associated with the infusion of cryopreserved cells. Peripheral blood stem cell units are often much larger in quantity and therefore require the use of more cryopreservation material and the infusion of more cryopreservative.[15] The cryopreservative can be washed away after thawing, but there is increased risk of cell loss.

Since 1988, hundreds of thousands of cord blood collections have been frozen throughout the world, in anticipation of their potential use to treat a multitude of malignant and nonmalignant disorders in children and adults. The longest a cord blood collection is likely to be in frozen storage before clinical use is 3 to 5 years. Cord blood in the family model is likely to be stored longer. Therefore the effects of 5-year and 10-year storage on the retrieval of HSCs have been studied. The postfreeze HSC numbers have been compared directly with prefreeze numbers from the same cord blood samples. The numbers and proliferation of HSCs in vitro were studied. Further studies were performed on HSCs cryopreserved for 15 years. These samples were tested for HSC content and engrafting capability. The results demonstrated that cord blood could be cryopreserved for at least 15 years, and efficiently retrieved in a functionally competent form. There was no statistical difference in recovery after 10 and 15 years compared with prefreeze values of nucleated cells.[19] Engraftment failure or delay has not been attributed to variations in technique.[15] Umbilical cord blood stored as an unmanipulated whole blood requires large amounts of storage space in liquid nitrogen. Many studies have established techniques for volume reduction of UCB.[20]

HPC TRANSPLANTATION
Preparative or Conditioning Regimens

In most disease states, the intended recipient of an HSC transplant must receive some form of preparative or conditioning regimen to physiologically prepare for receipt of transplanted cells. This regimen eradicates or reduces abnormal or defective cells to a level below the limits of detection. A consequence of this preparative treatment is suppression of the patient's immune system in order to prevent rejection of donor cells and the elimination of marrow cells to make room for donor cell engraftment. The latter is particularly important in disease states such as thalassemia in which the marrow may be highly cellular. Methods of conditioning include irradiation, in the form of total body irradiation (TBI), total lymphoid irradiation (TLI), or thoracoabdominal irradiation, in addition to chemotherapy and

Dimethyl sulfoxide (DMSO): A cryoprotective agent.

Hydroxyethyl starch (HES): A sedimenting agent that causes red cell rouleaux formation. The red cells settle out, allowing for the separation of red cells from nucleated cells.

SECTION SIX **Clinical Considerations**

the administration of biologic reagents to suppress recipient immunity and reduce the potential for GVHD and host-versus-graft disease (HVGD).[21] Conditioning therapies are associated with significant toxicity and mortality rates.

Posttransplant clinical parameters that are typically measured are hematopoietic recovery, evidence of acute and chronic GVHD, treatment-related mortality, and disease relapse. The primary measure of hematopoietic recovery is the time after transplantation until a neutrophil count of at least 0.5×10^9/L is observed for 3 consecutive days. Additional measures of recovery are the times until a platelet count of at least 20×10^9/L (alternatively, a platelet count of at least 50×10^9/L) is achieved. The incidence of and time to develop grades II to IV acute GVHD and grades III to IV acute GVHD are measured in patients surviving 21 days after evidence of engraftment. Time to the occurrence of chronic GVHD is evaluated in patients surviving 90 days or longer after transplantation with engraftment.[21]

Complications

The diversity of the human population provides an ever-increasing challenge for histocompatibility testing. These problems have been resolved to a great extent by the conversion of HLA typing from serologic methods to DNA-based assays. The major transplant-related complications are GVHD, graft rejection, graft failure, prolonged immunodeficiency and toxicity from pretransplantation and posttransplantation radiation therapy and chemotherapy, and GVHD prophylaxis. Profound but transient immunodeficiency develops in all patients. Patients with an uncomplicated posttransplant course may achieve normal immunologic functions within 1 year of the transplant. Infectious complications and opportunistic infections are common. Epstein-Barr virus (EBV)–associated lymphoproliferative disease with EBV-positive B-cell lymphomas is observed in the posttransplant period. Improved outcome to UCB transplantation requires enhanced accessibility, improvements that would speed engraftment and lessen early morbidity, and prevention of GVHD.[22] Approximately 10% of patients develop chronic pulmonary disease after an allogeneic transplant.[23] The recipient may experience serious immunologic complications such as the following:

- An immediate, acute hemolytic reaction usually caused by donor-recipient ABO incompatibility
- Febrile, nonhemolytic reactions due to action of antibodies against white cells or the action of cytokines[13]
- Allergic reactions due to the presence of atopic substances or reactions to DMSO or HES[13]
- Anaphylactic reaction due to the presence of IgA antibodies, HES, or DMSO[13]
- Delayed hemolytic reactions caused by anamnestic production of antibody[13]
- Alloimmunization to antigens of red cells, white cells, platelets, or plasma proteins present in the donor product[13]
- GVHD, which occurs when T lymphocytes in the infused product engraft in the recipient and react against tissue antigens in the recipient[13]

Nonimmunologic complications that may result from cellular therapy include DMSO toxicity, septic reactions due to bacterial contamination of the cellular product, fat emboli that may block capillary perfusion, transmission of infectious diseases, bleeding due to excessive anticoagulation, circulatory overload, hypothermia, and nonimmunologic hemolysis.[13]

REGULATORY ISSUES

Cellular therapy involves the translation of scientific research from the laboratory bench to the recipient's bedside. As a result, cellular therapy is subject to good manufacturing practices (GMPs), good laboratory practices (GLPs), and current good tissue practices (cGTPs). Reagents, supplies, and devices involved in cellular therapy are regulated by the FDA in the United States and equivalent agencies in other countries.[24]

In 1977, the FDA proposed a comprehensive approach to the regulation of cellular and tissue-based products. This set of regulations requires that HPCs be handled according to standards that include proper handling, processing, labeling, record keeping, and maintenance of a quality program.

The American Association of Blood Banks (AABB) and the Foundation for the Accreditation of Cellular Therapy (FACT) have published separate but substantially similar standards for HPCs. AABB Standards address the collection, processing, storage, and distribution of HPCs.[16] FACT Standards address the issues covered by AABB, as well as clinical issues provided by HPC clinical transplant programs.[25,26] An institutional review board (IRB) is required when research on living human subjects is involved. The Health Information Portability and Accountability Act (HIPAA) protects the medical and health information of living and deceased patients involved in cellular therapy.[24] The development of industry standards has brought about the need for established standard operating procedures (SOPs), improvement in quality management programs, and comprehensive training and competency evaluation of personnel.[26]

NEW RESEARCH/FUTURE DIRECTIONS

We are currently observing an unprecedented expansion in the basic science and clinical applications of hematopoietic cytokines and stem cells. The future availability of a variety of highly purified progenitor populations and recombinant cytokines promises to revolutionize our understanding of how hematopoiesis is controlled and the best approaches to therapeutic intervention. Future bone marrow transplantation will involve peripheralized stem cells, stem cell expansion, and correction of genetic diseases by gene transfer technology.[27]

Improved Collection Methods

Improved collection methods, which will potentially lead to increased cell concentration and reduced bone marrow or peripheral blood donor discomfort and risk, are being researched.[28,29] The debate continues regarding which cord blood collection method yields the largest number of CD34 cells. Associated research continues to study the impact of such variables as the following:

- In utero versus ex utero collection
- The influence of early cord ligation and increased venous pressure
- Gravity drip versus syringe

New Developments in Clinical Transplantation
Stem Cell Plasticity

It was generally thought that only embryonic stem cells are pluripotent because plasticity in early development is critical. Recent data suggest that adult stem cells generate differentiated cells beyond their own tissue boundaries. This has been termed *developmental plasticity*.[30] It has been demonstrated that stem cells derived from bone marrow can differentiate into epithelial cells of the liver, lung, gastrointestinal tract, and skin.[31,32] Research suggests that cord blood may prove to be a new source of cells for cellular therapy for stromal, bone, and neural repair.[31] Additionally, umbilical cord blood contains a small population of nonhematopoietic progenitor (NHP) cells that are capable of differentiating into cells with bone, fat, and neural features in tissue culture.[33] The basic mechanisms of stem cell differentiation that lead to the formation of solid-organ tissue are still not completely understood. However, research and clinical studies are underway to develop additional potential treatment strategies.[30]

Prenatal Transplantation

Prenatal transplantation has tremendous potential to broaden the current indications for reconstitution therapy and to offer a safe, efficacious, and cost-effective alternative to conventional postnatal BMT for many congenital hematopoietic diseases.[34]

Stem Cell Expansion

In vitro expansion of progenitor cells has the potential to allow for the collection of a small number of stem cells that have the same effect as larger or more numerous collections. Expansion may also allow for purging of smaller volumes of cells in advance of expansion. Expansion may be directed at normal rather than malignant progenitors, allowing in vitro expansion to accomplish malignant cell removal. In vitro expansion may also allow for repeated clinical use of a single collection or limited numbers of collections of stem cells.[35]

Dendritic Cell Vaccine Therapy

The dendritic cell is a highly potent antigen-presenting cell that can present viral, bacterial, and tumor antigens. Dendritic cells can be isolated from mobilized peripheral blood but are more commonly cultured from mature mononuclear cells or CD34+ cells. When optimal protocols are developed for isolation and expansion of dendritic cells, these cells will be the preferred strategy for adoptive immunotherapy.[36]

Adoptive Cellular Therapy for Cancer

Adoptive cellular therapy is the process of transferring immune cells with antitumor activity into tumor-bearing patients to treat their cancer. To date, preclinical trials have been unsuccessful, but T-cell antitumor activity holds promise and has been successful in a limited number of patients.[36]

CHAPTER SUMMARY

1. Bone marrow transplantation opened the way for transplantation of hematopoietic stem cells.
2. Identification of the MHC, the role of the thymus, and the need to suppress the immune system led to the success of marrow transplantation.
3. HSC transplantation reconstitutes hematopoietic cell lineages with normal cells capable of self-renewal.
4. The major transplant-related complication is GVHD.
5. Stem cells are precursor cells that have the capacity to both self-perpetuate and differentiate into a vast array of specialized tissue types.
6. Bone marrow, fetal liver, peripheral blood, and cord blood are four identified sources of stem cells.
7. HSC therapy is an effective treatment for a range of malignant, hematologic, immunologic, metabolic, and neoplastic diseases.
8. Failure to HLA match the donor and recipient can result in graft rejection and GVHD.
9. Hematopoiesis occurs in the mesodermal, hepatosplenic, and medullary embryologic stages.
10. Stem cells from bone marrow are typically collected from multiple small aspirates drawn from the posterior or anterior iliac crests.
11. Peripheral blood stem cell transplantation is preferred to BMT because of rapid platelet and neutrophil engraftment, reduced early toxicity, and superior immune reconstitution without a significant increase in risk of acute GVHD.

12. G-CSF is used as a mobilizing agent to release HSCs from the bone marrow into the circulating blood.
13. The total number of T cells, monocytes, and natural killer cells contained in a PBSC allograft is more than 10 times higher than in a bone marrow allograft.
14. The concentration of HSCs in UCB is greater than that in peripheral blood but less than 10% of the cell dose administered in a typical BMT.
15. The risk of GVHD is diminished in partially mismatched, unrelated UCB transplants because immune competence is far less than in peripheral and bone marrow transplantation.
16. Collection methods may affect the volume of UCB collected and the cell concentration.
17. A closed collection system reduces the risk of microbial and maternal cell contamination in UCB collections.
18. Embryonic fetal liver cells are not a common source of HSCs because of the technical and ethical issues related to this source of stem cells.
19. Donor risk associated with bone marrow collection is related to the use of general anesthesia.
20. Risks to peripheral stem cell donors are associated with the administration of hematopoietic cytokines such as G-CSF.
21. There are no significant risks to the mother or newborn when umbilical cord blood is collected from a healthy, full-term newborn.

22. The type of transplant used to treat a patient depends on the type of malignancy, age, availability of a suitable donor, ability to collect a tumor-free autograft, stage and status of the disease, and chemosensitivity to conventional chemotherapy.
23. Autologous transplants have been used to treat autoimmune diseases, to support gene therapy, for correction of metabolic defects, and for immunotherapy. They cannot be used to treat genetic or acquired diseases.
24. The result of an allogeneic transplant depends on the histocompatibility between the donor and the recipient and the timing of the transplantation in the course of the malignant disease. Treatment-related mortality rate is significantly higher after allotransplants than after autotransplantation.
25. UCB transplantation is used to treat patients with aggressive or recurrent malignancies, immunodeficiencies, certain genetic conditions, hemoglobinopathies, and congenital and acquired bone marrow failure syndromes.
26. The advantages of UCB transplantation are that it does not have to be HLA matched and it is less likely to transmit infectious diseases.
27. There are three banking models for UCB: public, family or private, and hybrid banks.
28. Screening of cord blood before transplantation includes a family medical history, viral testing of the birth mother, and ABO/Rh and HLA testing.
29. Quality control testing performed on stem cell products includes enumeration of cell counts, differential counts to determine mononuclear cell

and nucleated red cell dosing, CD34 positivity, viability, and bacterial and fungal cultures.
30. Peripheral blood, bone marrow, and UCB can be frozen and stored following a controlled-rate freeze followed by storage in a mechanical freezer (–80° C) or a liquid nitrogen freezer (–196° C).
31. HPCs cryopreserved for 15 years have been retrieved in a functionally competent form.
32. Most disease states require preparative or conditioning regimens before the receipt of transplanted cells. The preparation suppresses the recipient's immune system to prevent rejection of donor cells. Conditioning therapies are associated with significant toxicity and mortality rates.
33. Transplant parameters typically measured are hematopoietic recovery, acute and chronic GVHD, treatment-related mortality, and disease relapse.
34. The major transplant-related complications are GVHD, graft rejection, graft failure, prolonged immunodeficiency and toxicity from pretransplantation and posttransplantation radiation therapy and chemotherapy, and GVHD prophylaxis.
35. Infectious complications and opportunistic infections are common in the recipient after transplant.
36. Donor screening, stem cell collection and quality control testing, donor infectious disease, processing, storage, transportation, and transplantation are regulated by such agencies as AABB, FACT, FDA, and state health departments.
37. Stem cell plasticity, prenatal transplantation, and stem cell expansion are several of the predicted future advances in stem cell therapy.

REFERENCES

1. Avichai S, Champlin R: Bone marrow and peripheral blood stem cell transplantation. In Hillyer CD, Silberstein LE, Ness PM, Anserson KC (eds): Blood Banking and Transfusion Medicine: Basic Principals and Practice. Philadelphia, Churchill Livingstone, 2003.
2. Dupont B: Immunology of hematopoietic stem cell transplantation: A brief review of its history. Immunol Rev 157:5-12, 1997.
3. McGlave P: Overview of stem cell transplantation. In Hoffman R, Edward J, Banz J, et al (eds): Hematology: Basic Principles and Practice, 3rd ed. Philadelphia, Churchill Livingstone, 2000.
4. Broxmeyer HE: Cord blood stem and progenitor cell therapy for immunodeficiency and other disorders. Immunol Allergy Clin 16(2):439-450, 1996.
5. Körbling M, Anderlini P: Peripheral blood stem cell versus bone marrow allotransplantation: Does the source of hematopoietic stem cells matter? Blood 68:2900-2906, 2001.
6. Avichai S, Champlin R: Bone marrow and peripheral blood stem cell transplantation. In Hillyer CD, Silberstein LE, Ness PM, Anderson KC (eds): Blood Banking and Transfusion Medicine: Basic Principles and Practice. Philadelphia, Churchill Livingstone, 2003.

7. Grisaru D, Deutsch V, Pick M, et al: Placing the newborn on the maternal abdomen after delivery increases the volume and CD34+ cell content in the umbilical cord blood collected: An old maneuver with new applications. Am J Obstet Gynecol 180(5):1240-1243, 1990.
8. Sparrow RL, Cauchi JA, Ramadi LT, et al: Influence of mode of birth and collection on WBC yields of umbilical cord blood units. Transfusion 42:210-214, 2002.
9. Bertolini F, Lazzari L, Lauri E, et al: Comparative study of different procedures for the collection and banking of umbilical cord blood. J Hematother 4:29-36, 1995.
10. Surbek DV, Visca E, Steinmann C, et al: Umbilical cord blood collection before placental delivery during cesarean delivery increase cord blood volume and nucleated cell number available for transplantation. Am J Obstet Gynecol 183(1):218-221, 2000.
11. Rubinstein, P, Dobrila L, Rosenfield RE, et al: Processing and cryopreservation of placental/umbilical cord blood for unrelated bone marrow reconstitution. Proc Natl Acad Sci 92:10119-10122, 1995.
12. Ballen KK, Hicks J, Dharan B, et al: Racial ethnic composition of volunteer cord blood donors: Comparison with volunteer unrelated marrow donors. Transfusion 42:1279-1284, 2002.

13. Circular of Information for the Use of Cellular Therapy Products. Bethesda, American Association of Blood Banks, Oct 2003.

14. Brecher M (ed): Technical Manual, 14th ed. Bethesda, American Association of Blood Banks, 2002.

15. Rowley SD, Bensinger WI, Gooley TA, et al: Effect of cell concentration on bone marrow and peripheral blood stem cell cryopreservation. Blood 83(9):2731-2736, 1994.

16. Attarian H, Feng Z, Buckner CD, et al: Long-term cryopreservation of bone marrow for autologous transplantation. Bone Marrow Transpl 17:425-430, 1996.

17. Hubel A: Parameters of cell freezing: Implications for the cryopreservation of stem cells. Transfus Rev 11(3):224-233, 1997.

18. Scott RD: Practical aspects of stem cell collection. In Hoffman R, Edward J, Banz J, et al (eds): Hematology: Basic Principles and Practice, 3rd ed. Philadelphia, Churchill Livingstone, 2000.

19. Broxmeyer HE, Srour EF, Hangoc G, et al: High-efficiency recovery of functional hematopoietic progenitor and stem cells from human cord blood cryopreserved for 15 years. PNAS 100(2):645-650, 2003.

20. Zingsem J, Strasser E, Weisbach V, et al: Cord blood processing with an automated and functionally closed system. Transfusion 43:806-813, 2003.

21. Champlin RE, Schmitz N, Horowitz MM, et al: Blood stem cells compared with bone marrow as a source of hematopoietic cells for allogeneic transplantation. Blood 95(12):3702-3709, 2000.

22. Rubinstein P, Carrier C, Scaradavou A, et al: Outcomes among 562 recipients of placental blood transplants from unrelated donors. N Engl J Med 339(22):1565-1577, 1998.

23. Copelan EA, Penza S: Preparative regimens for stem cell transplantation. In Hoffman R, Edward J, Banz J, et al (eds): Hematology: Basic Principles and Practice, 3rd ed. Philadelphia, Churchill Livingstone, 2000.

24. Sharp JG: Regulatory issues in cellular therapies. Cytotherapy 5(4):277-278, 2003.

25. Warkentin PI: Voluntary accreditation of cellular therapies: Foundation for the Accreditation of Cellular Therapy (FACT). Cytotherapy 5(4):299-305, 2003.

26. Kelly LL: The role and activities of the ISCT Regulatory Affairs Committee. Cytotherapy 5(4):279-283, 2003.

27. Spangrude GJ: Biological and clinical aspects of hematopoietic stem cells. Annu Rev Med 45:93-104, 1994.

28. Surbek DV, Visca E, Steinmann C, et al: Umbilical cord blood before placental delivery during cesarean delivery increase cord blood volume and nucleated cell number available for transplantation. Am J Obstet Gynecol 183(1):218-221, 2000.

29. Grisaru D, Deutsch V, Pick M, et al: Placing the newborn on the maternal abdomen after delivery increases the volume and CD34+ cell content in the umbilical cord blood collected: An old maneuver with new applications. Am J Obstet Gynecol 180(5):1240-1243, 1999.

30. Körbling M, Estrov Z: Adult stem cells for tissue repair—a new therapeutic concept? N Engl J Med 349(6):570-582, 2003.

31. Krause DS, Theise ND, Collector MC, et al: Multi-organ, multi-lineage engraftment by a single bone marrow–derived stem cell. Cell 105:369-377, 2001.

32. Blau HM, Brazelton, Weimann JM: The evolving concept of a stem cell: Entity or function? Cell 105:829-841, 2001.

33. Goodwin HS, Bricknese AR, Chien SN, et al: Multilineage differentiation activity by cells isolated from umbilical cord blood: Expression of bone, fat, and neural markers. Biol Blood Marrow Tr 7:581-588, 2001.

34. Flake AW, Zanjani ED: Cellular therapy. Obstet Gynecol Clin North Am 24(1):159-177, 1997.

35. Rudmann SV: Transfusion issues in selected patient populations. In Rudmann SV (ed): Textbook of Blood Banking and Transfusion Medicine. Philadelphia, WB Saunders, 1995.

36. Reys SD: Embryonic stem cells. In Szczepiorkowski ZM, Snyder E (eds): Current Perspectives in Cellular Therapy 2002. Bethesda, MD, American Association of Blood Banks; 2001.

Expert Opinion

COLLECTION AND EXPANSION OF BLOOD-FORMING (HEMATOPOIETIC) CELLS FROM CORD BLOOD

Larry C. Lasky, MD

Copious published data have shown that the number of cells available for and transfused during a cord blood transplant is a prime determinant of outcome. Two approaches to increase the number of cells available are (1) collecting and storing more cells and (2) expanding cells in vitro before infusion.

COLLECTING AND STORING MORE CELLS

Collecting maximum numbers of cells is highly technique dependent. Whether the collection is done before or after the placenta is delivered may help determine the quantity of cells collected and their quality. When the two methods were compared, the volume and total nucleated cell count of collected cord blood before processing, as well as after processing CFU-GM and CD34+ cells, showed no advantage of either method.[1] In utero collections resulted in more rejections of collected units (due to labeling problems, bacterial contamination, clotting, and delay between collection and processing) than ex utero collections. There were fewer medical exclusions of units collected in utero, presumably because a more thorough medical history was available and evaluated for rejection criteria before the collection. Storing the cord cells collected is also important for maximizing the number eventually infused. The most straightforward method is to freeze all of the cord blood white cells collected. This method is somewhat wasteful of expensive freezer space, and it can lead to large volumes and lysed red cells at the time of infusion. The method used in some other banks entails centrifugation of the cord blood unit, removal of white cell–rich plasma from the heavier red cell layer, and a subsequent spin to separate the desired white cells from the plasma.[2] Many white cells (including a portion of the blood-forming cells) are lost in this process. One method to decrease this loss is to perform a gravity sedimentation in the presence of hydroxyethyl starch to separate the red cells from the white cells.[3] This increases the number of cells eventually frozen, but still falls short of freezing all of the white cells.

EXPANDING CELL NUMBERS

Because the number of cells in the frozen unit is limited by the number collected, there is no way to collect additional cord blood cells from a given donor, should it be needed. The donor may be a very rare and desirable HLA type, but a low dose of cord blood cells may be collected.

One straightforward but still very experimental approach to overcome this limitation is to use more than one unit of cord blood to perform a transplant in large recipients. This seems to lead to faster recovery of blood cell production and prolonged engraftment of at least one of the cord blood types infused. Most often, in the reported cases, a single unit is responsible for long-term posttransplant blood cell production. The degree of matching between the units and the recipient patient, and among the units themselves, may be important; results on this point are still forthcoming.

In another approach, researchers are developing ways to expand the number of blood-forming cells in vitro before transplant. These methods generally involve incubation of cord cells with cloned growth factors or other proteins. This begs the question of which cells should be expanded. If the goal of infusing these blood-forming cells is to cause rapid recovery of blood cell production, then cells already committed to differentiation, that is, more differentiated cells, seem to be indicated. On the other hand, to ensure long-term engraftment early cells capable of self-renewal should be infused.

Although many methods have been proposed or reported in the literature, no one has yet reported a documented increase in the speed of recovery with in vitro (ex vivo) cord blood expansion. However, several potentially effective methods have been described. Important parameters that characterize

these methods include length of ex vivo treatment; the nature of the media, growth factors, and other supporting proteins used; whether and what "feeder" layer of nonhematopoietic cells is used; the type of culture vessel or bioreactor; and the geometry and other details of the cell-matrix construct, if any.

The most reported and easiest to implement is short-term incubation of the cells in suspension in plastic bags with growth factors. The bags can be gas-permeable transfer packs as used for platelet storage. A group in Colorado has reported use of this method to increase the number of committed blood-forming cells in cord blood. They feel that this allows them to transplant larger recipients with a single expanded unit.

The growth factors that have been most used are those utilized in vivo to promote blood cell production. Additional growth factors that are not yet routinely used in vivo have also been used. This allows the use of these factors for their specific effect, but avoids at least some of their in vivo toxicity. Recently, intracellular and transmembrane signaling proteins have been used in vitro for experimental blood cell progenitor expansion.[4]

More complex bioreactors that allow external control of culture conditions based on such culture parameters as pH and dissolved oxygen level have been described. Some methods use a flat surface to grow the cells, and some provide a three-dimensional scaffold on which the cells (either the blood-forming cell precursors or the supporting "feeder" cells) can grow.[5] This three-dimensional structure mimics the in vivo growth environment of these cells in vivo.

REFERENCES

1. Lasky LC, Lane TA, Miller JP, et al: In utero or ex utero cord blood collection: Which is better? Transfusion 42:1261-1267, 2002.
2. Rubinstein P, Dobrila L, Rosenfield RE, et al: Processing and cryopreservation of placental/umbilical cord blood for unrelated bone marrow reconstitution. Proc Natl Acad Sci USA 92:10119-10122, 1995.
3. Alonso JM III, Regan DM, Johnson CE, et al: A simple and reliable procedure for cord blood banking, processing, and freezing: St. Louis and Ohio Cord Blood Bank experience. Cytotherapy 3:429-433, 2001.
4. Amsellem S, Pflumio F, Bardinet D, et al: Ex vivo expansion of human hematopoietic stem cells by direct delivery of the HOXB4 homeoprotein. Nat Med 9:1423-1427, 2003.
5. Li Y, Ma T, Kniss D, et al: Human cord blood cell hematopoiesis and expansion in three-dimensional non-woven fibrous matrices: In vitro simulation of bone marrow microenvironment. J Hemat Stem Cell Res 10:355-368, 2001.

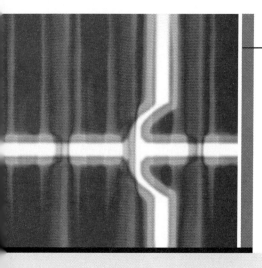

Safety, Quality Assurance, and Data Management

The goal of transfusion medicine is the delivery of the safest and most efficacious product to the patient. Inherent in this goal is the provision of a safe work environment for the blood bank staff. To provide optimal transfusion outcomes for the patient, the blood bank must develop a system of quality assurance and quality improvement. Appropriate methods of data collection, retrieval, and analysis are essential to the process of monitoring quality. Assurance of a quality product includes issues of safety, reagent quality control, equipment repair and maintenance, employee competency and proficiency, continuing education and training, peer review of transfusion practice, and development of and compliance with standards of practice.

A safe laboratory environment requires attention to issues of universal precautions, personnel protection devices, waste management, hazardous chemical handling, accident management, and fire safety. Product quality management assumes that all steps are taken to provide the most positive patient outcome. Issues of cost, convenience, safety, efficacy, and patient satisfaction are essential to this outcome. Quality begins with the donor and ends with the patient and cannot be confined to the walls of the blood bank. Adequate record keeping is essential to

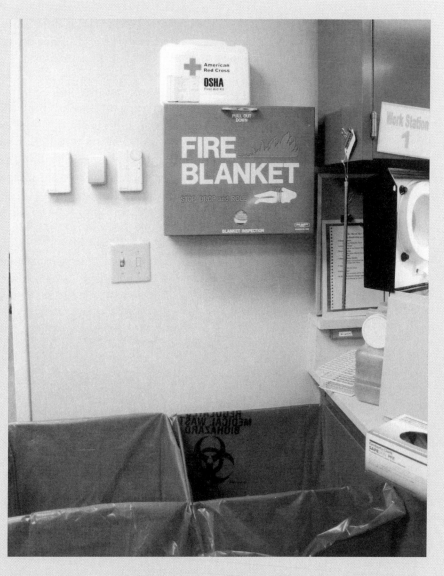

the process of quality and safety assurance. Records—whether paper or computer—must be legible, accurate, thorough, retrievable, and complete. All regulations regarding record retention, confidentiality, and release must be understood and complied with.

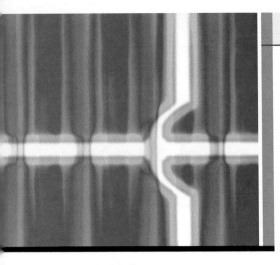

Safety

Suzanne H. Butch

LEARNING OBJECTIVES

After reading and studying this chapter, the student should be able to:

1. Identify employee and employer responsibilities for safety.
2. List regulatory and accrediting agencies with safety standards.
3. Apply general safety practices to daily laboratory work.
4. Use safety labels to determine appropriate safety precautions.
5. Define *standard precautions.*
6. Select the safety equipment appropriate for the prevention of infectious disease transmission.
7. Define the elements of an infection control plan.
8. Identify tasks at higher risk for exposure to blood-borne pathogens.
9. Properly dispose of laboratory waste.
10. Package a specimen for transport.
11. List the elements of a chemical hygiene plan.
12. Use a material safety data sheet to obtain chemical information.
13. Select appropriate safety equipment for prevention of injury from chemicals.
14. Define *exposure limits.*
15. Interpret labels on chemical bottles.
16. Outline actions in the case of a chemical spill or fire.
17. List the safety precautions necessary when using equipment, compressed gases, radioactive substances, and cryogenic liquids.
18. Identify the goals of accident reporting.

SAFETY REGULATIONS

In 1970, the **Occupational Safety and Health Administration (OSHA)** was created by passage of the Occupational Safety and Health Act. This act established the employer's responsibility to "assure safe and healthful working conditions for working men and women."[1] The legislation defined "separate but dependent responsibilities and rights"[1] for employees and employers in maintaining a safe work environment.

Employer's Responsibilities

It is the employer's responsibility to
- Maintain a plan for minimizing risks and accidents
- Train staff and conduct refresher courses periodically
- Provide protective equipment
- Survey for potential risks
- Maintain records of training and injuries
- Monitor unsafe working activities
- Take prompt corrective action when unsafe work activities or hazardous conditions occur

Employee's Responsibilities

Each employee has the responsibility to

- Read the OSHA information provided by the employer
- Follow work safety rules
- Report real or potential hazards
- Control accidents

Employees have the right to request an OSHA inspection whenever they believe there is a violation of an OSHA regulation that threatens their health and safety. The reporting employee's name is held confidential if the employee desires.

Voluntary and Professional Association Guidelines

Other federal agencies, as well as several state agencies (Summary 20-1), also issue regulations, standards, and guidelines that affect safety in the workplace. The federal regulations and standards are printed in the Code of Federal Regulations.[2-8] In addition, professional organizations (Summary 20-2) and voluntary accrediting agencies such as the Clinical and Laboratory Standards Institute (formerly known as NCCLS) and the College of American Pathologists (CAP) have issued voluntary guidelines. These organizations provide educational materials, checklists, and other materials to assist employers and employees in meeting regulatory requirements.[9-16]

Occupational Safety and Health Administration (OSHA): Agency of the federal government that develops standards and regulations for safety and health in the workplace.

Summary 20-1

Federal Agencies with Safety Regulations or Guidelines

Occupational Safety and Health Administration (OSHA): www.osha.gov
Centers for Disease Control and Prevention (CDC): www.cdc.gov
Food and Drug Administration (FDA): www.fda.gov
Department of Transportation (DOT): www.dot.gov
Environmental Protection Agency (EPA): www.epa.gov
Nuclear Regulatory Commission (NRC): www.nrc.gov

Summary 20-2

Agencies with Voluntary Guidelines

Clinical and Laboratory Standards Institute (CLSI): www.nccls.org
College of American Pathologists (CAP): www.cap.org
Joint Commission on Accreditation of Healthcare Organizations (JCAHO): www.jcaho.org
National Fire Protection Association (NFPA): www.nfpa.org

Laboratory safety program: A systematic laboratory plan that sets safety and health goals for the laboratory work environment. This plan must be described in a laboratory safety manual that provides program goals, policies, and procedures for all aspects of laboratory safety. The laboratory safety committee is generally the formal body responsible for the development, maintenance, and review of the safety program.

Personal protective equipment: Clothing and equipment designed to protect the laboratory worker from risk of infection or injury. Examples of personal protective equipment include chemical-resistant gloves, fluid-impervious garments, face shields, explosion-proof cabinets, hoods, and masks.

The Safety Plan

The basis for a safe working environment is the **laboratory safety program.** Each laboratory is required to have a safety manual that covers all of the potential employee risks and methods to reduce those risks. The components of a safety plan are listed in Summary 20-3.

Employees may fail to follow safety guidelines because they wish to save time and effort or increase comfort or because they lack proper training. It is the employer's responsibility to ensure that safety rules are followed. However, all employees have an obligation to follow the safety rules as they perform their daily work. Summary 20-4 lists general safe work practices.

Personal protective equipment (PPE) must be used when working with substances defined as hazardous in the safety plan.[4,5] While performing tasks that carry risks of exposing the employee to blood-borne pathogens, protective equipment such as gloves, laboratory coats, and eye/face protection must be used. When exposure to toxic, carcinogenic, or corrosive chemicals is a risk, chemical-resistant gloves and aprons should be used. Face protection must be used when splashes are possible. Fume hoods must be used when inhalation of the chemical poses a risk (Fig. 20-1).

Summary 20-3

Components of a Safety Plan

General facility maintenance
Chemical safety
Infection control
Handling sharp objects
Use of equipment
Compressed gases
Cyrogenic liquids
Radiation
Accident reporting
Use of safety and emergency equipment
Drills
Shipping of hazardous materials
Waste disposal

Summary 20-4

General Rules for Safety

Do
1. Follow safety instructions.
2. Perform only authorized procedures.
3. Wear gloves, protective clothing, and eyewear as necessary.
4. Clean up spills immediately.
5. Wash hands frequently.
6. Use household gloves for general-purpose cleaning such as instrument cleaning and decontamination.
7. Report all accidents.

Don't
1. Eat, drink, or smoke in the laboratory.
2. Use defective equipment.
3. Clutter hallways and aisles with boxes and equipment.
4. Touch electrical equipment with wet hands.
5. Lick labels, chew pencils, or pipette by mouth.
6. Wash gloves.

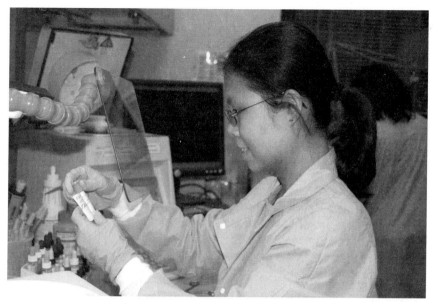

Fig. 20-1 Personal protective equipment: splash guard, gloves, and lab coat.

The cleanup of spills requires special attention. They must be cleaned up immediately after the occurrence using appropriate protective equipment. Chemical-resistant gloves and protective clothing must be used when cleaning up chemical spills. Household gloves should be used when performing general cleaning and disinfection procedures.

Accidents, exposures, and injuries must be reported to ensure that employees receive appropriate medical attention. The occurrence must be investigated and measures taken to prevent future incidents.

STANDARD PRECAUTIONS AND INFECTION CONTROL
Standard Precautions

Preventing the spread of infectious diseases to health care workers and patients is a critical part of a safety program. The federal regulation, "Occupational Exposure to Bloodborne Pathogens,"[2] requires the employer to maintain an infection control plan, including the use of **standard precautions.** Employees are responsible for following general safe work practices (Summary 20-5), as well as the institution's policies for the prevention of occupational exposures to infectious diseases.

Standard precautions (formerly known as "universal precautions") is the name for the concept that all body fluids are to be handled as if they were potentially

Standard precautions: Procedures and methods that reduce the risk of exposure to blood-borne infection. Standard precautions are based on the assumption that all body fluids are potentially infectious. Standard precautions in the donor phlebotomy setting are discussed in Chapter 8.

Summary 20-5

Safe Work Habits: Standard Precautions

Use safety needles.
Do not recap, bend, or reuse needles.
Wash your hands after removing gloves or other personal protective equipment or after contact with body fluids.
Remove overtly contaminated personal protective equipment as soon as possible.
Use techniques to minimize splashing, spraying, and aerosolization.
Use gloves, gowns or laboratory coats, head and foot coverings, face shields or masks, eye protection, mouthpieces, resuscitation bags, or ventilation devices.
Do not store food with potentially infectious material.
Report accidental exposure immediately.

infectious, and laboratory procedures and patient care should be performed by methods that minimize the risk of accidental exposure.

Training

Laboratory workers must receive information and training to minimize their risk of exposure. Areas with increased risk of exposure should be restricted to only those individuals who must be present. All workers, including volunteers, who perform duties in restricted areas must be trained to prevent accidental exposures to infectious diseases. More frequent training may be necessary for those who perform the work infrequently. The training program should be designed specifically for the group and given in language that is understandable, given the education and ethnic background of the individuals being trained. In patient care areas or donor collection areas, children must be closely supervised. Training must include the modes and rates of transmission; tasks that are at increased risk; the types, use, and limitations of protective clothing and equipment; actions to be taken if an accident occurs; reporting procedures; and recommended health monitoring.

Medical Treatment

Hepatitis B vaccination must be offered to all employees who have a potential for occupational exposure to hepatitis B on an average of one or more times per month.[2] The laboratory must provide for follow-up when exposure to an infectious disease has occurred. Policies must be in place for immediate reporting of an accident to ensure that proper counseling, testing, and treatment are made available to the injured person. There are additional requirements for training and use of protective equipment and health monitoring when performing work with a live virus.[2]

Risk of Exposure

The employer implements standard precautions by providing workers with personal protective equipment and designing the work to reduce the potential for accidental exposure to blood-borne diseases. OSHA has classified risk levels into three **infectious risk categories** (Summary 20-6).[4]

1. Common category I tasks include removing stoppers from specimen tubes, compatibility testing, centrifugation, and operation of cell-separation devices.
2. Category II excludes routinely performing tasks at increased risk but allows for the unplanned performance of category I tasks. For example, transporting blood specimens may create an increased risk if the specimen container becomes broken.
3. Category III tasks include clerical work that involves no risk of exposure.

Hand Washing

Probably the most effective infection control measure is hand washing. Hands should be washed with a liquid soap before donning gloves, after removing gloves, before leaving the laboratory, and before eating. An alcohol-based hand cleaner may be used when hands are not visibly contaminated.

Hepatitis B vaccine: A formalin-inactivated vaccine derived from the surface antigen of the hepatitis B virus. The vaccination is indicated for immunization against all subgroups of hepatitis B but does not protect against hepatitis A, C, or non-A, non-B, non-C. The immunization is required for all laboratory professionals. The vaccine is administered intramuscularly in three doses: initial, 1 month, and 6 months.

Infectious risk categories: Classifications based on probable risk of exposure to blood-borne pathogens from I (routine exposure) to III (no risk of exposure).

Summary 20-6

OSHA Categories of Exposure

Category I: Tasks that involve exposure to blood, body fluids, or tissues
Category II: Tasks that involve no exposure to blood, body fluids, or tissues, but employment may require performance of unplanned category I tasks
Category III: Tasks that involve no exposure to blood, body fluids, or tissues

Work Design and Exposure Prevention

The methods used to perform tasks should minimize the risk of exposure. For example, stoppers should be removed from specimen tubes behind a shield or with an absorbent material covering the top of the tube to prevent aerosols or splashes. Aerosols that may be created during centrifugation can be minimized by capping tubes before centrifugation, inspecting all tubes for chips and cracks, balancing the centrifuge, and keeping the centrifuge cover closed until the rotor has come to a complete stop.

Using Personal Protective Equipment

The employer is responsible for providing personal protective clothing and equipment such as gloves, laboratory coats, goggles, and masks to be used for tasks designated to cause increased risk. Open skin lesions must be covered with a bandage. Long-sleeve, fluid-resistant laboratory coats and gloves must be worn whenever handling open containers of blood and body fluids.

Gloves

The use of gloves is required when performing finger and/or heel punctures and phlebotomies. The only exception is that during the collection of units of blood from volunteer donors, the use of gloves is optional. If gloves become torn, punctured, or visibly contaminated, they must be changed. Gloves must also be worn when cleaning up spills or handling waste materials. Cotton glove liners and specially treated gloves are available for personnel who have an allergic reaction to vinyl or latex gloves.

Gloves are potentially contaminated and should not be worn outside the laboratory or when using equipment such as computer terminals or telephones if the equipment is designated safe for use without gloves. In some laboratories, equipment is designated "clean" or "dirty." The "dirty" equipment may be used only when wearing gloves.

Protective Clothing

Protective clothing such as a fully buttoned, fluid-resistant laboratory coat should be worn over street clothes in areas where splashes and spills are possible. If the coat becomes visibly contaminated, it should be changed. Coats must be removed before leaving the laboratory. Coats worn as a protective barrier must not be worn while eating, drinking, or applying makeup. Lip balm should not be carried in laboratory coat pockets.

Face Protection

Plastic face masks or goggles and masks covering nose and mouth must be worn when there is an increased risk of splashes such as when removing tubing from an automated blood cell processor.

Housekeeping
General Cleaning

In addition to daily general housekeeping, equipment and surfaces must be cleaned when they appear contaminated with blood or body fluids (Summary 20-7). A solution of 10% sodium hypochlorite (household bleach) prepared the day of use is the most commonly used disinfectant. Metals and plastics should not be soaked in bleach solutions for extended periods, because this may cause pitting of metals and deterioration of the plastic. Other cleaning agents such as phenol or glutaraldehyde disinfectants may be used at the dilution recommended by the manufacturer. The instructions on the label must be followed to ensure that the correct dilution is made and the correct contact time is used.

Summary 20-7

Cleaning Up a Biohazardous Spill

Wear heavy-weight gloves.

Absorb the spill: Soak up liquid with paper towel, dispose in container marked "BIOHAZARD."

Clean up any glass or sharp objects with a dust pan or cardboard. Do NOT use your fingers.

Remove visible spill with toweling soaked in bleach solution or with detergent.

Soak cleaned area with 10% bleach solution and allow solution to remain on the surface for 10 to 20 minutes.

Wipe up disinfectant.

Dispose of materials in biohazard container.

Cleaning Instruments

Scissors, rotors, and other tools must be cleaned routinely. Any visible contamination must be removed, and then the instruments must be soaked in a disinfectant solution. Alternatively, the instruments may be autoclaved.

Labeling Biohazardous Containers and Waste

To minimize the risk of accidental exposure of personnel to biohazards, refrigerators and freezers, contaminated laundry, and waste containers must be labeled as containing biohazardous materials. The biohazard symbol, a fluorescent orange or orange-red with white or black lettering, is used to label containers (Figs. 20-2 and 20-3). Alternatively, red bags may be used for laundry and waste so that housekeeping and laundry personnel can easily identify potentially hazardous materials.

Transporting Biohazardous Materials
Within the Institution

Specimens should be transported to the laboratory in a secondary container such as a plastic bag. The bag should be large and sturdy enough to contain the contents if the specimen spills or the primary container breaks. To avoid contamination of

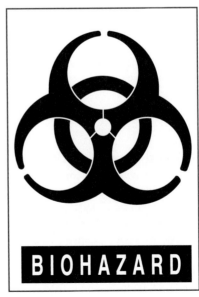

Fig. 20-2 Biohazard label.

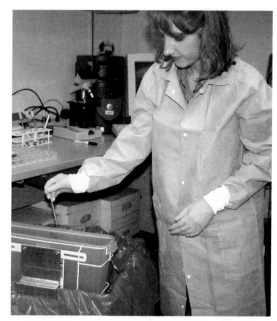

Fig. 20-3 Disposal of hazardous waste and sharps.

the paperwork, it should not be placed in the same compartment as the specimen. The paperwork should be attached to the outside of the bag or placed in a special section of the bag.

Shipping Outside of the Institution

When specimens must be shipped by common carrier such as the U.S. Postal Service or an overnight delivery service, special packaging must be used to prevent the accidental exposure of workers who handle the package during transport.[6] In general, specimens must be securely capped and placed in a waterproof container. This container should be placed in a second watertight container with enough absorbent material to absorb the entire contents if all of the containers are broken. This second container should be securely sealed and placed into a shipping container. Accompanying paperwork should be sealed in waterproof pouches to prevent contamination. The outer container must be labeled with the special "Etiologic Agents/Biomedical Material" label.

Tested blood components that do not contain any infectious substances are exempt from biohazard labeling regulations. When specimens are transported via commercial airlines, a shipper's declaration for dangerous goods may also be required. Special hazard labeling also is required when dry ice is used as the coolant. It is always best to check with the carrier for correct packaging and labeling requirements.

HAZARDOUS CHEMICALS

The blood bank or transfusion service has fewer chemicals than the average chemistry or research laboratory. However, some of the routinely used chemicals are significant hazards. Summary 20-8 defines the classes of hazardous chemicals. In 1987, OSHA published regulations known as the **Hazard Communication Standard**.[3] These regulations are commonly referred to as the "right to know" law.

The Hazard Communication Standard

The standard requires employers to maintain a hazard communication program that includes the following:

Hazard Communication Standard: OSHA regulation that requires employers to identify workplace hazards and have written policies for documentation of employee hazard training.

Summary 20-8

General Classes of Hazardous Chemicals

Carcinogen: A chemical known to cause or have the potential to cause cancer

Mutagen: A chemical that may cause heritable changes in genetic material

Toxin: A substance that, when inhaled, consumed, or in contact with skin, causes a serious biologic effect

Irritant: A substance that causes a reversible inflammatory effect on living tissue by chemical action at the site of contact

Sensitizer: A chemical that causes a substantial portion of exposed persons to develop an allergic reaction in normal tissue after repeated exposure

Corrosive: An aqueous liquid that has a pH of less than 2.1 or greater than 12.5, or a liquid waste that can corrode SEE 1020 steel more than 0.250 inch per year at 50° C; also used to describe a substance that can cause visible destruction or irreversible alteration in human tissues at the site of contact

Ignitable: A liquid that has a low flash point and/or boils at normal atmospheric pressure; combustible liquids have a flash point of greater than 37.8° C

Asphyxiant: A chemical that can prohibit metabolic use of available oxygen or have an adverse effect by displacing atmospheric oxygen

Explosive: A chemical (reactant) that may violently decompose at normal temperatures and pressures

Material Safety Data Sheets (MSDSs): Information regarding hazardous chemicals designed to reduce risk. MSDSs are required by OSHA as a part of the Hazard Communication Standard.

- Hazard determination
- Development of a written hazard communication program listing the hazardous chemical present
- Labeling of the contents in English
- Maintenance of **Material Safety Data Sheets (MSDSs)**
- Development, implementation, and documentation of employee hazard communication training

Chemical Hygiene Plan

In 1990 OSHA published rules for occupational exposure to hazardous chemicals in laboratories.[4] This regulation requires the development and implementation of practices to minimize laboratory employee exposures to hazardous chemicals. The keystone of this rule is development of the chemical hygiene plan (Summary 20-9). The chemical hygiene plan defines the duties of the chemical hygiene officer or committee to define the hazards in the laboratory, provide protective equipment and training to reduce exposure, and provide medical consultation when exposure limits have been exceeded.

Information about Chemicals

Each employee must be able to locate the laboratory list of chemicals on hand (Summary 20-10) and the MSDS for those chemicals (Fig. 20-4). The employee should read the MSDS before using a chemical for the first time. The MSDS is designed to provide the user of the chemical with information concerning the following:

- The route of entry into the body
- Permissible exposure limits
- Whether the chemical is listed as a carcinogen
- Precautions for safe handling
- Protective measures for repair and maintenance of equipment
- Cleanup of spills and leaks
- Control practices such as use of safety hoods or protective equipment
- Emergency and first-aid procedures

Summary 20-9

Chemical Hygiene Plan Requirements

Standard operating procedures contain safety and health considerations when hazardous chemicals are used.

Criteria the employer uses to determine and implement measures to reduce employee exposure to hazardous chemicals.

Permissible exposure limits and threshold exposure values for chemicals must not be exceeded.

Protective equipment such as fume hoods must be maintained and operations and performance monitored.

Program for employee training and information.

The employer must define procedures that require prior approval.

Medical consultation and examination.

Chemical hygiene officer and optional committee.

Special precautions for work with particularly hazardous substances.

Personal Protective Equipment

Personal protective equipment such as chemical safety goggles and chemical-resistant gloves and aprons or coats must be worn when indicated. When recommended by the chemical label or MSDS, fume hoods or respiratory protection should be used. The protective gloves and aprons described here are chemical resistant and are made of different materials than those used for biohazard protection. Each employee must know where to find emergency equipment such as showers, eyewashes, and chemical spill kits, as well as how to use them (Fig. 20-5).

Exposure Limits

Some chemicals have **permissible exposure limits** that define the exposure limits below which no adverse effect has been noted. When these limits are exceeded, additional health monitoring is required. References for determining

Permissible exposure limits: Levels of chemical exposure below which there have been no substantiated reports of adverse reaction.

Summary 20-10

Blood Bank and Transfusion Service: Chemical Inventory

Revised: 03-20-04
Storage Location: Open Shelves Reference Laboratory

Shipping Name	Class	Hazard Quantity	Manufacturer	MSDS
p-Aminobenzoic acid	Irritant	10 g	Eastman	Yes
Ammonium sulfate, purified	Irritant	120 g	Baker	Yes
p-Chloromercuribenzoic acid	Poison	5 g	Benton-Dickinson	Yes
Citric acid Corrosive	Irritant	450 g	Drake Brothers	Yes
Chloroquine diphosphate	Irritant	250 g	Sigma	Yes
Calcium chloride, anhydrous Irritant	Corrosive	1 lb	Allied Chemical	Yes
Dipotassium ethylenediamine tetra-acetate (EDTA)	Poison	50 g	Cambridge Chemicals	Yes
Digitonin	Irritant	5 g	Baker	Yes
N-Ethyl malenmides	Poison	2 g	Benton-Dickinson	Yes
Ethyl *p*-hydroxybenzoate 99%	Irritant	100 g	Aldrich	Yes
Glycine	Irritant	500 g	EM Science	Yes
Glycine	Irritant	250 g	Matheson Coleman Bell	Yes

MSDS, Material Safety Data Sheet.

MATERIAL SAFETY DATA SHEET

This form may be used to comply with OSHA's Hazard Communication Standard, 29 CFR 1910.1200. To be valid, all information required by § 1910.1200 (g) of the Standard must appear on this form. Consult the Standard for specific requirements. Note: Blank spaces are not permitted. If any item is not applicable, or no information is available, the space must be marked to indicate that.

IDENTITY *(As Used on Label and List)*

Section I

Manufacturer's name Chemical Corporation	Emergency telephone number 1-800-555-5555
Address *(Number, Street, City, State, and ZIP Code)* 1234 Main Street	Telephone number for information 1-800-555-5555
Anytown, Anystate 10000	Date prepared January 1, 1987
	Signature of preparer (optional)

Section II – Hazardous Ingredients/Identity Information

Hazardous components (specific chemical identity/common name (s)	OSHA PEL	ACGIH TLV	Other limits recommended	% *(optional)*
Methanol (methyl alcohol; carbinol)	200 ppm	200 ppm		100

Section III – Physical/Chemical Characteristics

Boiling point 760 mm Hg	148 F	Specific gravity (H_2O= 1) @ 68 F	0.7925
Vapor pressure (mm Hg.)	96.0	Melting point	−144 F
Vapor density (AIR =1)	1.11	Evaporation rate (butyl acetate= 1) 5.91	

Solubility in water
Soluble

Appearance and odor
Clear, colorless liquid with a characteristic alcohol odor.

Section IV – Fire and Explosion Hazard Data

Flash point *(method used)* 54 F	Flamable limits	LEL 6.0	UEL 36.0

Extinguishing media
Alcohol-foam, water, carbon dioxide

Special fire-fighting procedures
Addition of water will reduce flame intensity.

Unusual fire and explosion hazards
Methanol burns with a faint blue flame which may not be visible.

Based on Draft of OSHA, 174, September 1985
Replaces obsolete OSHA Form 20 MSDS.

Fig. 20-4 Material Safety Data Sheet (MSDS).

Section V – Reactivity Data

Stability	Unstable	X	Conditions to avoid
			Sparks, heat, fire.
	Stable		

Incompatibility *(materials to avoid)*
Strong oxidizers

Hazardous decomposition or byproducts
Carbon monoxide

Hazardous Polymerization	May Occur		Conditions to avoid
	Will Not Occur	X	

Section IV – Health Hazard Data

Route(s) of entry:	Inhalation?	Skin?	Ingestion?
	Yes	Yes	Yes

Health hazards *(acute and chronic)*

Acute exposure: May cause irritation.

Chronic exposure: Proloned or repeated exposure may cause eczema, blurred

vision, and/or visual impairment.

Carcinogenicity:	NPT?	IARC monographs?	OSHA regulated?
None	N/A		

Signs and symptoms of exposure
Inhalation or swallowing may cause inebriation, headache, nausea, and vomiting leading to severe illness, blindness,

and perhaps death.

Medical conditions
generally aggravated by exposure   N/A

Emergency and first aid procedures
Flush skin and eyes with water. Get medical attention for eye contact. If swallowed, induce vomiting

and then administer two tablespoons of baking soda in a glass of water. Call a physician at once.

Section VII – Precautions for Safe Handling and Use

Steps to be taken in case material is released or spilled
Eliminate all ignition sources. Absorb spills with absorbent materials and place in a sealed container.

Waste disposal method
Use an approved waste processing facility.

Precautions to be taken in handling and storing
Methanol may be fatal or cause blindness. Avoid breathing vapors.

Keep away from heat, sparks, and fire.

Other precautions
Avoid contact with skin.

Section VIII – Control Measures

Respiratory protection *(specify type)*
Organic cartridge, half-mask

Ventilation	Local exhaust		Special
	Preferred		
	Mechanical *(general)*		Other
	Acceptable		

Protective gloves		Eye protection

Other protective clothing or equipment
Boots made of neoprene, butyl rubber and aprons where splashing may occur. An eye wash/safety shower should be available

Work/hygienic/maintenance practices

Fig. 20-4, cont'd. Material Safety Data Sheet (MSDS).

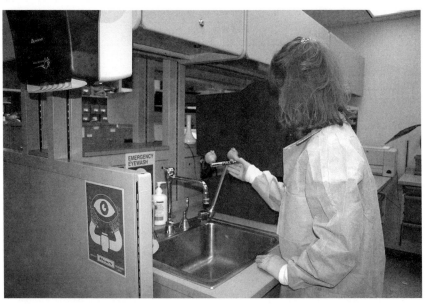

Fig. 20-5 Emergency eyewash station.

the current exposure limits for chemicals include MSDSs and the NIOSH Pocket Guide to Chemical Hazards (NPG) (www.cdc.gov/niosh/npg/npg.html),[16] updates of which are published by the National Institute of Occupational Safety and Health (www.cdc.gov/niosh). Chemicals found in the laboratory that have defined exposure limits include formaldehyde and ether, as well as other air contaminants.

Chemical Labeling

Chemical containers that have a large enough label area contain warnings or symbols indicating physical and health hazards, as well as the laboratory protective equipment required. The **National Fire Protection Association (NFPA)** has developed a system of labeling that was designed to identify hazards to firefighters.[15] Some chemical manufacturers have modified the labeling to include additional safety information. The NFPA label is diamond shaped and is divided into four additional color-coded diamonds. The color code is blue for health hazard, red for flammability, yellow for reactivity, and white for special precautions. The diamonds contain hazard ratings from a "0" minimal rating to "4," an extreme hazard.

Chemical Spills

If a chemical spill occurs, the first step is to remove any injured person from the area and initiate first aid. Then the following steps should be taken:
- Wear chemical protective clothing.
- Stop the spill, if possible.
- Alert other personnel.
- Use an appropriate spill cleanup kit.

When the spill is serious and cannot be handled by routine cleanup methods, employees should know how to activate the emergency chemical spill plan, and, if necessary, evacuate the area.

FIRE SAFETY
Fire Response Plan

Each employee must be familiar with the laboratory fire response plan that details his or her responsibilities in case of fire (Summary 20-11). A map with the exit

National Fire Protection Association (NFPA): An organization that provides information regarding the risks associated with chemical exposure.

Summary 20-11

Fire Response Plan

YOUR RESPONSIBILITY IN CASE OF FIRE IN THE BLOOD BANK

1. Person discovering fire should do the following:
   Remove person from immediate danger area.
   Close door to room on fire.
   Report the fire (code F): Dial 911 or use a pull station; state the following: "This is a code F (or code F drill) for level 2, blood bank room 225" and give your name.
2. Obtain fire extinguisher and bring to the scene (exercise fire-fighting skills and containment techniques only if safe to do so).
3. Protect the blood supply and equipment (if possible).
4. Alert other areas, check lounges and bathrooms for patients and staff, and direct them to an exit.
5. Assign personnel to listen for messages on the corridor intercom and relay messages to staff until the all clear (or evacuation).
6. Prevent the use of passenger and service elevators in affected areas.
7. Stand by to assist with evacuation if directed by fire marshals, hospital administrator, supervisor, or hospital fire safety team. If evacuation is required, use wheelchairs and stretchers from hall or reception area. Collect blankets and other linen from storage area or main laboratory.
8. If evacuation is required and time permits, prepare to remove patient charts and medications using pillowcase or linen bag.
9. Move patients beyond a smoke barrier door or near an exit.
   Fire emergency phone numbers: fire, 911; radiation safety, 4-4420
   Revised 9/04.

routes and fire protection devices must be posted in the laboratory (Fig. 20-6). The evacuation plan may be used in other emergencies such as a chemical spill. Each employee should

- Become familiar with the layout of the laboratory
- Review all possible exit routes
- Locate the designated evacuation meeting spot
- Locate each fire extinguisher and fire blanket (Fig. 20-7)
- Learn to use the fire-fighting equipment (Summary 20-12)
- Participate in fire drills and evacuations

Storage and Use of Flammables

Summary 20-13 lists general fire prevention practices. Storage should be limited to the smallest practical quantities. Flammables should be stored in safety cans and explosion-proof refrigerators or cabinets (Fig. 20-8). Chemicals should be used in well-ventilated areas, and a fume hood should be used when indicated. Flammables should not be used near a flame.

EQUIPMENT SAFETY

Many accidents and injuries are caused by misuse of equipment. The manufacturer's recommendations for routine maintenance and servicing of equipment should be followed. Parts must be replaced as needed even though the cost may be considerable. For example, an ultracentrifuge rotor costs several thousand dollars but must be replaced periodically owing to metal fatigue. Failure to replace the rotor may cause serious injuries if it disintegrates during operation. Although other equipment failures may be less dramatic, each poses a potential hazard to the employee. Simple commonsense rules apply (Summary 20-14).

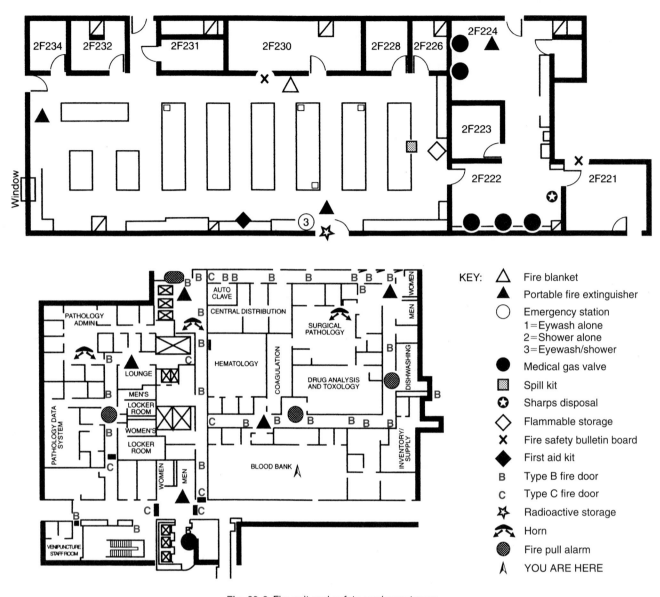

Fig. 20-6 Fire exit and safety equipment map.

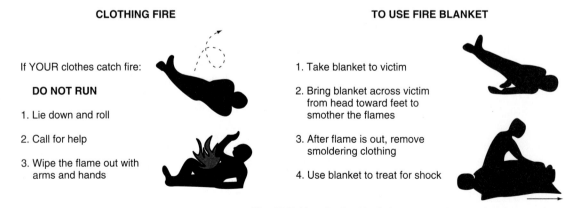

CLOTHING FIRE

If YOUR clothes catch fire:

DO NOT RUN

1. Lie down and roll

2. Call for help

3. Wipe the flame out with arms and hands

TO USE FIRE BLANKET

1. Take blanket to victim

2. Bring blanket across victim from head toward feet to smother the flames

3. After flame is out, remove smoldering clothing

4. Use blanket to treat for shock

Fig. 20-7 Use of a fire blanket.

Summary 20-12

Use of Fire Extinguishers

Class of Fire	Types of Extinguishers	Directions for Use
A. Ordinary combustibles: paper, cloth, wood	Water extinguisher or ABC	1. Swing horn up and squeeze handle. 2. Sweep under flames.
	Fire hose	DO NOT USE. Used only by professional fireman.
	Fire blanket	SMALL FIRES ONLY: 1. Pull loop with right hand. 2. Revolve body to left. 3. Throw blanket on fire.
B. Flammable liquids: gas, ether, oil, grease, paint	CO_2 extinguisher or ABC	1. Remove locking pin. 2. Pull trigger up and keep erect. 3. Point horn to base of fire. 4. Squeeze handle. 5. To lock open, pull trigger in and push latch, then release trigger to shut off. 6. Sweep under flames.
C. Electrical	Fire blanket or ABC extinguisher	SMALL FIRES ONLY.

Summary 20-13

Fire Prevention

Store the smallest quantity possible.
Use explosion-proof refrigerators and cabinets.
Use chemicals in a well-ventilated area.
Use a fume hood with a flow of 100 ft/min.
Use safety cans for storage and transfer.
Do not use chemicals near a source of ignition.

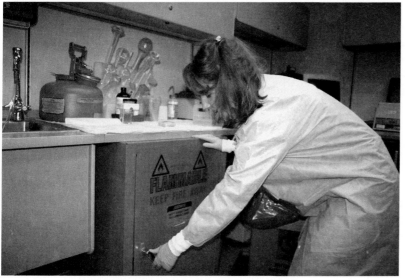

Fig. 20-8 Flammable storage cabinet.

Summary 20-14

Equipment Safety

1. Use equipment as described in the operator's manual.
2. Perform periodic maintenance and function checks.
3. Do not continue to operate defective equipment.
4. Check for electrical voltage leaks annually.
5. Unplug equipment before beginning a repair.
6. Do not touch equipment with wet hands.
7. Do not use equipment with frayed electrical cords.
8. Avoid the use of extension cords.
9. Do not obstruct switches and circuit breaker boards.

RADIATION SAFETY

Laboratory tests that use low-level radionuclides are becoming less common. However, the use of lasers, ultraviolet (UV) light, and gamma irradiators for the irradiation of blood components has become more frequent. As with other laboratory hazards, the employee must be trained to use the material or device, use protective equipment, and report any accidents. In addition, exposure monitoring may be required.

Liquid Radioisotopes

The Nuclear Regulatory Commission (NRC) regulates radioactive materials and their use. When liquid radioisotopes are used, additional precautions are required. Bench tops should be covered with an absorbent material with waterproof backing to protect them from contamination. Testing using radioactive materials should be confined to a specific area that is posted with radiation warning signs (Fig. 20-9). Laboratory work area radiation levels should be monitored monthly to detect contamination. All equipment and supplies must be discarded in containers designed for disposal of radioactive waste. In addition, personnel must be monitored for radiation exposure using film badges.

Blood Irradiators

Blood irradiators vary in design and the amount of radiation leakage and scatter. Thus not all personnel using these irradiators are required to wear monitors. However, even if operators are not monitored individually, area monitors are used. For solid-source irradiators, periodic wipe tests are used to detect leakage of radiation. The best protection is to move away from the radiation source. With most irradiators in use today, the radiation emission drops to background level within a few feet of the irradiator. Regulatory agency requirements restrict the use of irradiators to trained individuals, and records of training and exposure are required. State agencies regulate the use of irradiators when the source of irradiation is x rays.

Lasers

Lasers can produce burns and eye damage. Personnel should wear protective goggles appropriate for the wavelength being used when the potential exists for exposure to direct or indirect laser light greater than 0.005 watt. Areas where lasers are used should be posted.

Ultraviolet Irradiation

Overexposure to UV radiation causes reddening of the skin, sunburn, and skin cancer. To avoid eye injury, personnel should wear protective goggles when using wavelengths shorter than 250 nm.

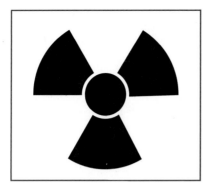

Fig. 20-9 Radiation warning symbol.

Summary 20-15

Safe Handling of Gas Cylinders
Use the smallest container appropriate for the purpose. Do not store empty cylinders. Transport cylinders on wheeled carts. Store cylinders upright and secured to a support.

COMPRESSED GASES AND CRYOGENIC LIQUIDS

The improper handling of compressed gas cylinders may cause significant injury. The release of gas from a cylinder could propel the cylinder through a wall. Summary 20-15 describes the safe handling of compressed gases. **Cryogenic liquids** may condense enough moisture to block pressure relief valves, may displace air when they vaporize resulting in difficulty breathing, and may cause injury to skin and eyes. One should use cryoprotective gloves whenever working with cryogenic liquids and use face protection when splashes are possible.

Cryogenic liquids: Liquids under pressure that generate low temperatures on vaporization.

WASTE MANAGEMENT

Local regulations and recycling options vary and influence the waste disposal methods used in your area. Abide by the waste disposal and recycling "rules" of your institution.

Waste Reduction

The first principle of waste management is to reduce the amount of waste created. New techniques use a smaller specimen, and less potentially infective body fluids may need to be collected from the patient. Exercise care when deciding to reuse and recycle laboratory supplies and paper. Used laboratory supplies are generally contaminated, and most are designed to be discarded after a single use. Uncontaminated paper may be recycled unless confidentiality of the information printed on the paper is a concern. Alternatively, the paper can be shredded before recycling or incineration.

Separation of waste is essential in proper waste management. To avoid injury to co-workers, patients, and housekeeping staff, dispose of glass and other sharp objects in puncture-resistant containers. Separate radioactive waste and dispose of it separately in labeled containers. Biohazardous materials may be incinerated or decontaminated via autoclaving and then disposed of in a landfill. Proper labeling of materials that will be transported is essential.

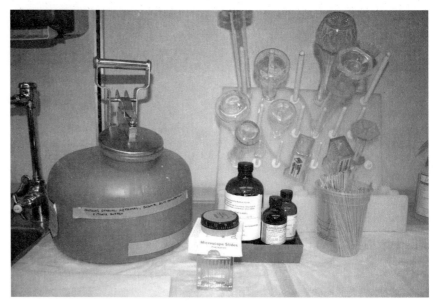

Fig. 20-10 Chemical disposal container.

Disposal of Body Fluids

Regulations vary by location, but in most facilities, blood and body fluids may be discarded in a sanitary sewer.[10] However, it is recommended that units of blood found to be positive for infectious diseases be autoclaved or incinerated.

Disposal of Waste Chemicals

Waste chemicals must be appropriately labeled and stored for pickup by hazardous materials specialists (Fig. 20-10). Small amounts of diethyl ether may be disposed of by evaporation, and small amounts of other chemicals may be disposed of in a sink followed by flushing with large amounts of water. Review local regulations for chemical disposal.

EMERGENCY MANAGEMENT

It is essential that all employees know how to report emergencies and obtain assistance, as well as know the location of emergency equipment and how to use it. In the event of an injury, employees may administer first aid if they are trained. The initial first aid must be followed by medical evaluation.

Accident Reporting

Once the emergency has been resolved, the events must be documented. Accident reporting is an essential part of maintaining a safe working environment. The goals of accident reporting are to ensure that the employee obtains appropriate medical assessment and/or treatment and to prevent future accidents. Investigation of an accident involves determining the factors that contributed to the event. Slippery floors, lack of training, haste, and defective equipment all contribute to accidents. Prevention of future accidents may involve job redesign, use of protective equipment, or employee training.

Safety Committee

A safety committee is useful in coordination of safety training and monitoring in a large facility. A safety audit should be conducted periodically to identify areas of noncompliance. Institutional rules and safety equipment alone cannot ensure a safe working environment; it takes the continuous effort of all employees to follow the rules and identify and remove hazards.

CHAPTER SUMMARY

1. Both employers and employees are responsible for maintaining a safe working environment.
2. A laboratory safety plan outlines the safety guidelines and procedures to be followed in the event of an accident.
3. Every employee must be trained in how to work safely with chemicals and patient specimens and to respond to accidents and emergencies.
4. Employers are responsible for providing personal protective equipment such as gloves, fluid-resistant laboratory coats, chemical-protective gloves, face shields, and masks. Employees are responsible for using them when indicated in the standard operating procedures of the laboratory.
5. Using "standard precautions" means treating every specimen as if it were infectious.
6. Hand washing is the most effective infection control method. Frequent general cleaning and immediate cleanup of accidents are essential to a safe environment.
7. The "right to know" regulations require that employees be trained concerning the potential hazards of using the chemicals available in the laboratory. A laboratory chemical hygiene plan defines laboratory chemical hazards, protective equipment and clothing required, and the appropriate medical consultation if an employee is injured or exceeds exposure limits.
8. Each employee must be familiar with the institution's fire response plan.
9. Equipment must be used according to the manufacturer's safety guidelines. Periodic maintenance must be performed, and malfunctioning equipment must not be used.
10. Guidelines for the use of radioactive materials and personnel monitoring must be followed.
11. Laboratory waste must be disposed of using methods that prevent injuries and accidental exposure to hazards. Local waste disposal and recycling requirements vary.
12. Accidents must be reported to aid in the prevention of future occurrences.

REFERENCES

1. Occupational Safety and Health Act of 1970. Public Law 91-596.
2. Occupational Exposure to Bloodborne Pathogens, 29 Code of Federal Regulations Part 1910.1030.
3. Hazard Communication, 29 Code of Federal Regulations Parts 1910, 1915, 1917, 1918, 1926, and 1928.
4. Occupational Exposure to Hazardous Chemicals in Laboratories, 29 Code of Federal Regulations Part 1910.1450.
5. Air Contaminants—Permissible Exposure Limits, 29 Code of Federal Regulations Part 1910.1000.
6. Department of Transportation, 49 Code of Federal Regulations Parts 100-177 Transportation of Dangerous Goods.
7. Public Health Service, Department of Health and Human Services, 42 Code of Federal Regulations Part 72.
8. Nuclear Regulatory Commission, 10 Code of Federal Regulations Parts 9 and 10.
9. Clinical Laboratory Standards Institute: Protection of Laboratory Workers from Occupationally Acquired Infections—Approved Guidelines, 2nd ed. M29-A2. Wayne, PA, Sept 2001.
10. Clinical Laboratory Standards Institute: Clinical Laboratory Waste Management, Approved Guideline GP5-A2, 2nd ed. Wayne, PA, NCCLS, 2002.
11. Commission on Laboratory Accreditation: 2002 Inspection Checklist, Laboratory General, Section I. Northfield, IL, College of American Pathologists, 2002.
12. Clinical Laboratory Standards Institute: Clinical Laboratory Safety, Approved Guidelines GP17-A. Wayne, PA, NCCLS, 1996.
13. Joint Commission on Accreditation of Healthcare Organizations: 2004 Hospital Accreditation Manual, Management of the Laboratory Environment. Oakbrook Terrace, IL, Joint Commission on Accreditation of Healthcare Organizations, 2003.
14. National Fire Protection Association: Fire Protection Guide to Hazardous Materials 2001. Quincy, MA, National Fire Protection Association, 2001.
15. National Fire Protection Association: NFPA 99 Standard for Health Care Facilities, 2002 edition. Quincy, MA, National Fire Protection Association, 2002.
16. National Institute of Occupational Safety and Health/Occupational Safety and Health Administration: NIOSH Pocket Guide to Chemical Hazards (NPG), NIOSH Publication No 97-140. Washington, DC, US Government Printing Office, 2004.

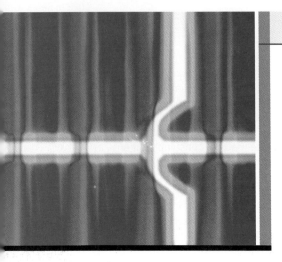

CHAPTER TWENTY-ONE

Quality Control, Quality Assurance, Quality Improvement, and Peer Review

Suzanne H. Butch

LEARNING OBJECTIVES

After reading and studying this chapter, the student should be able to:

1. Define the following terms:
   Quality systems   Continuous quality improvement
   Quality control   Utilization review
   Quality assurance
2. Define the AABB "quality essentials."
3. Describe the organizational structure of a quality function.
4. List the elements of a technical procedure according to the Clinical and Laboratory Standards Institute (formerly NCCLS) guidelines.
5. List the components of a position description.
6. Use a training checklist to document training.
7. Identify the requirements for calibrating and testing laboratory instruments.
8. Describe a situation that requires an agreement with a supplier.
9. List three ways processes are controlled.
10. Define *proficiency testing*.
11. List the requirements for testing laboratory reagents.
12. Describe the requirements for tracing the disposition of unsatisfactory components and reagents.
13. Describe a method to document the lot number of reagents used.
14. List the minimum standards for quality control of blood components.
15. Describe a process for documenting nonconformances.
16. Describe the purpose of the FMEA process.
17. Develop an indicator for quality monitoring of blood transfusion service activities.
18. Describe the use of an audit.

OVERVIEW

The patient care goals of the transfusion service or blood bank should be to efficiently provide blood and blood components that are safe, pure, potent, and effective. In addition, any component administered should be needed. To this end, the laboratory and the medical care facility must have policies and procedures in place which ensure that these goals are met. Each institution is required to have a documented quality system. Quality control, quality assurance, utilization review, and continuous quality improvement are complementary, yet distinctly different, concepts that are part of a quality system.

DEFINITION OF TERMS

Quality System

The quality system consists of the policies, processes, and procedures that define the various quality activities in an institution. The American Association of Blood Banks (AABB) has designated 10 "quality essentials" making up the quality system for blood banks and transfusion services (Summary 21-1).[1] A number of accrediting and regulatory agencies require a quality monitoring function (Summary 21-2).

Quality Control

Quality control (QC) is management of the testing process itself. It includes assessment of the accuracy and reproducibility of a test. Thus equipment or instruments used to perform a test must be installed, verified as appropriate for use, and monitored to determine if they are functioning properly. Reagents must be tested on or before initial use and each day of use thereafter to determine if they have maintained their specificity and sensitivity.

Quality Assurance

Quality assurance (QA) includes the entire process of providing patient care, from the time the physician selects a test to be performed to development of a treatment

---

Summary 21-1

Quality System Essentials for Transfusion Services

Organization
Resources
Equipment
Supplier and customer issues
Process control
Documents and records
Deviations, nonconformances, and complications
Assessment: internal and external
Process improvement through corrective and preventive action
Facilities and safety

Summary 21-2

Accrediting and Regulatory Agencies with Quality Assessment Requirements

American Association of Blood Banks (AABB):* www.aabb.org
Joint Commission on Accreditation of Healthcare Organizations (JCAHO):† www.jcaho.org
College of American Pathologists (CAP):‡ www.cap.org
Food and Drug Administration (FDA):§ www.fda.gov
Center for Medicare and Medicaid Services (CMS):¶ www.cms.gov

*Menitove JE (ed): Standards for Blood Banks and Transfusion Services, 21st ed. Bethesda, MD, American Association of Blood Banks, 2002.
†Joint Commission on Accreditation of Healthcare Organizations: Comprehensive Accreditation Manual for Hospitals: The Official Handbook. Oakbrook, IL, Joint Commission on Accreditation of Healthcare Organizations, 2004.
‡College of American Pathologists, Commission of Laboratory Accreditation: Inspection Checklist (Section I, Laboratory General). Northfield, IL, College of American Pathologists, 2003.
§Current Good Manufacturing Practice for Blood and Blood Components (Part 606); Additional Standards for Human Blood and Blood Products (Part 640), 21 Code of Federal Regulations.
¶Center for Medicare and Medicaid Services. Laboratory Requirements Relating to Quality Systems and Certain Personnel Qualifications; Final Rule. CMS-2226-F. January 2003.

plan based on the results of testing. The process includes preanalytic, analytic, and postanalytic segments. In other words, did the physician order pretransfusion hematology or coagulation tests appropriately, assess patient needs, and order the correct blood component? Was the component prepared and transfused properly, and did the patient obtain the anticipated benefit of the transfusion without sustaining an adverse reaction?

Utilization Review

Utilization review (UR) is the process of monitoring the appropriateness of the transfusion of blood components. It is frequently termed *peer review* because physicians participate in reviewing the transfusion practices of other physicians.

Continuous Quality Improvement

Continuous quality improvement (CQI) involves reviewing the process of providing patient care with the goal of reducing rework, waste, and inappropriate care.

In all of these quality processes, observations are made and conclusions are drawn. The focus of the processes is determining whether appropriate patient care was provided. Corrective actions must be taken when expectations are not being met. In the following sections of this chapter, specific examples of quality control and quality assurance are given that lead to continuous quality improvement.

Regulatory and accrediting agencies have outlined minimum quality monitoring standards, which the institution may choose to exceed. The requirements of each organization for quality control and quality assurance are essentially the same, although some variations exist. The written plan and documentation of testing and review must be available to inspectors/assessors. If no document records that an activity was planned or performed, no evidence proves that it was done. Each facility designs forms for recording quality control and quality assessment activities to provide an audit trail of plans, values obtained, conclusions made, and corrective actions taken.

ORGANIZATION

The reporting relationships and responsibilities for the management and quality functions of an organization must be defined. An organizational chart defines the reporting arrangements. A quality system must be defined, implemented, and maintained.[1] The person designated the responsible head (according to FDA regulations[4]) or the laboratory director (according to Clinical Laboratory Improvement Act [CLIA] regulations[5]) of a blood bank or transfusion service must ensure that quality monitoring activities are performed. The actual performance of quality monitoring is usually delegated to a compliance officer or technical director, who reports directly to the responsible head. Ideally, the individuals responsible for the quality review functions are not responsible for reviewing their own work and do not report to supervisory staff responsible for the operation of the laboratory.

PROCEDURE MANUALS

Standard operating procedures are required for all laboratory, quality, and administrative procedures,[1] including quality assessment activities.[2-4] The procedures manual defines the methods used to control processes and activities. It should be organized to match the workflow in the laboratory and separate preanalytical, analytical, and postanalytical processes and procedures. The Clinical Laboratory and Standards Institute (former known as NCCLS) has written guidelines for the preparation of technical procedures.[6] Policies and nontechnical procedures may have another format. Summary 21-3 lists the components of a procedure for analytical procedures. The common elements in all procedures are as follows:

Title
Principle or purpose
Procedure instructions
References
Author
Approval signatures
Version and effective date

Summary 21-3

Recommended Elements of a Procedure Manual

*Title
*Purpose
*Policy—if applicable
Reagents
*Equipment
*Supplies
Specimen
*Safety precautions
Quality control
*Procedure
Interpretation/Results
Calculations (quantitative procedures)
Expected values (quantitative procedures)
Method limitations
*Procedure notes
*References
*Related documents
*Appendixes (forms, labels, tags, tables)
Analytical procedures

*Sections for preanalytical and postanalytical procedures as required.
Source: Clinical Laboratory Standards Institute: Clinical Laboratory Technical Procedure Manuals, 4th ed. GPO2-A4. Wayne, PA, NCCLS, 2002.

Other sections are needed based on the purpose of the procedure. Preanalytical procedures for test ordering, specimen collection, special transport, and processing may include the following:[6]

Patient preparation
Specimen collection
Equipment
Forms
Safety
Specimen handling
Specimen storage
Problems or pitfalls
Computer activities

Postanalytical procedures may include the following:

How results are prioritized
Entry of results
Guidelines for notification of individuals of critical test results
Archiving results and report documents
Specimen retention

Technical procedures for chemical assays, such as those for testing donor blood for infectious diseases, should also contain instructions for instrument calibration, calculations, and limitations of the procedure. The CLSI guidelines are consistent with the requirements for procedure manuals in the Clinical Laboratory Improvement Act of 1988 regulations.[5]

Administrative policies and technical procedures may be maintained in separate manuals. Procedures should be written in a consistent style. Page numbers are essential. The manual must be reviewed annually to ensure that the written procedure conforms to actual practice. Superseded pages, as well as documents used as references, should be maintained for at least 5 years.[1]

Technical procedures must be consistent with the recommendations of the manufacturers of any reagents, equipment, or instruments used in the procedure. These recommendations may be found in the reagent or test kit product circulars and instrument operator's manuals.

PERSONNEL RESOURCES

Personnel who perform tests and prepare components must have adequate education and training.[1-5] The first step is to define the tasks performed and levels of competence needed and then develop a position description, which might consist of the following sections:

Title
Brief description of general function and responsibility
Description of specific duties
Supervision
Qualifications
Special factors

A sample position description for a medical technologist (clinical laboratory scientist) is shown in Summary 21-4. The percentage of time spent performing specific duties may be included, as shown in the example. Special factors might include shift hours, special physical requirements such as lifting, or special hazards of the job.

Once the job has been defined, the education and training requirements can be developed. When employees are interviewed for a position, their education and previous experience must be evaluated in light of the duties required for the position.

On-the-job training is essential for all employees. A written training plan and an assessment of employee competency must be documented. Employee understanding of policies and procedures may be assessed by testing and/or observation

Summary 21-4

Job Description

POSITION: MEDICAL TECHNOLOGIST (CLINICAL LABORATORY SCIENTIST)—BLOOD BANK TRANSFUSION SERVICE

Basic Function

Perform and interpret pretransfusion tests on donor blood and patient samples, select and prepare blood components for transfusion, resolve antibody problems, and instruct students.

Duties and Responsibilities

20%: Assess sample suitability, perform and interpret routine and stat typing and screening, determine the need for additional pretransfusion testing.

20%: Perform and interpret routine and stat crossmatches, including selection of donor units.

20%: Prepare, inspect, and issue components for transfusion.

5%: Perform and interpret testing for transfusion reaction investigations.

14%: Perform quality control activities.

10%: Perform and interpret routine antibody identification studies.

1%: Assess blood supply and procure additional components from supplier; assess requests to ship to other institutions.

5%: Teach routine blood bank testing to students.

1% to 4%: Attend mandatory continuing education programs.

Communicate effectively with co-workers, health care professionals, and institution guests.

Supervision Exercised

Student training

Supervision Received

Blood bank supervisor

Qualifications

Bachelor of science majoring in clinical laboratory science or equivalent combination of education and experience.

Certification as a clinical laboratory scientist or equivalent by a certifying organization of clinical laboratory science.

Special Factors

Participate in rotating weekend, holiday, and on-call schedule.

---

of the trainees performing their work. A checklist is frequently used to document that competency has been attained. Fig. 21-1 is an example of a partial checklist that might be used as part of a training program.

Because procedures and policies are frequently modified, training is an ongoing process. Periodic documentation of employee competence is also required. An evaluation of competency may include observing the employee performing assigned tasks and reviewing the documentation of work performed, including quality control records and proficiency testing. The employee's performance should be judged using predetermined performance standards. Summary 21-5 lists several sample performance standards. Providing an employee with samples to test and comparing the employee's result with the expected result is known as proficiency testing. Proficiency testing challenges could include assessment of reading and recording results, detection of mixed-field agglutination, or detection and

Municipal Blood Bank
New Employee Training Checklist

Name _____   Date of hire _____

Position _____

	Employee	Supervisor	Date
1. Unpack and inspection blood and blood components unassisted.			
a. Red Blood Cells	_____	_____	_____
b. Frozen Red Blood Cells	_____	_____	_____
c. Apheresis Red Blood Cells	_____	_____	_____
d. Apheresis Platelets	_____	_____	_____
e. Plasma and Cryoprecipitated AHG	_____	_____	_____
#f. Granulocytes	_____	_____	_____
g. Component transported with patient	_____	_____	_____
2. Enter units received into the computer system.			
a. Red Blood Cells	_____	_____	_____
b. Autologous Red Blood Cells	_____	_____	_____
c. Directed Red Blood Cells	_____	_____	_____
d. Apheresis Red Blood Cells	_____	_____	_____
e. Frozen Red Blood Cells	_____	_____	_____
f. Random Platelets	_____	_____	_____
g. Apheresis Platelets	_____	_____	_____
h. HLA Apheresis Platelets	_____	_____	_____
i. Plasma	_____	_____	_____
#j. Granulocytes	_____	_____	_____
k. Cryoprecipitated AHG	_____	_____	_____
3. Perform typing, enter results and verify	_____	_____	_____
4. Distribute units			
a. Acceptable units into available storage	_____	_____	_____
b. Unacceptable units into quarantine	_____	_____	_____

# Indicates infrequently performed task. Procedure may be discussed and procedure manual reviewed.

Employee initials indicate that the employee feels that he or she is proficient. Supervisor's initials indicate that the supervisor has observed the employee performing the task and that the employee is proficient.

Form 76545   Rev mm/dd/yy

Fig. 21-1 Training checklist.

Summary 21-5

Sample Performance Standards for a Medical Technologist (Clinical Laboratory Scientist)
35%: Perform routine pretransfusion testing of patient specimens and donor units. Complete typing and screening of six patient specimens within 45 minutes of initiating testing.
Stat type and crossmatch for two units of red blood cells completed within 30 minutes of receipt of specimen.
All procedures performed according to procedure manual instructions.
No more than one valid occurrence report filed per year concerning communication with patient care personnel.

identification of antibodies. A paper-and-pencil test of donor eligibility requirements or safety regulations could also be used as an assessment tool. Online programs are particularly useful as a means of providing (24 × 7) opportunities for access to education, training, and assessments on all shifts.

EQUIPMENT

It should be possible to trace the acceptance testing and calibration, routine maintenance, repairs, and testing performed on an instrument from the time of receipt until the instrument is permanently removed from service. This assists in detecting frequently failing equipment, as well as in documenting appropriate monitoring and calibration. Equipment must be calibrated and tested before initial use and periodically thereafter for proper performance while in use. In general, recalibration of most of the equipment routinely used in a transfusion service must be performed only after repair or a change in procedures. The manufacturer's recommendations should be followed in determining the frequency of routine maintenance. Recalibration of instruments used in chemical assays must be performed in accordance with the manufacturer's instructions.[4] Summary 21-6 lists the minimum requirements for blood bank equipment testing, as specified in *Current Good Manufacturing Practice for Blood and Blood Components.*[4] Summary 21-7 suggests monitoring schedules of additional equipment. Fig. 21-2 is a sample serologic centrifuge quality control record. This form may be used to record preventive maintenance, repairs, and the results of testing.

Temperature monitoring is a critical element in quality control (Fig. 21-3). The temperature of refrigerators, freezers, incubators, and water baths must be recorded each day of use. Recording charts or temperature logs must be reviewed to ensure that the storage of blood components has not been compromised. Alarms on blood component refrigerators and freezers and incubators for platelets must be tested periodically to ensure that the alarm sounds before the components have reached an unsatisfactory temperature.

SUPPLIER AND CUSTOMER ISSUES

Policies, processes, and procedures are needed to evaluate supplier performance and customer needs.[1] Materials and supplies critical to the operation of the facility must be identified and suppliers for these supplies must be approved. Agreements are required between blood centers and transfusion services that outline expectations.

Incoming blood, components, tissue, and derivatives, as well as critical reagents and supplies, must be inspected and tested on receipt. Records for receipt of reagents and supplier should contain the date of receipt, the manufacturer, the lot

Summary 21-6

FDA Equipment Performance Monitoring Requirements

EACH TIME OF USE

Autoclave: Observe temperature

EACH DAY OF USE

Temperature recorder: Compare against thermometer
Refrigerated centrifuge: Observe speed and temperature
Hematocrit centrifuge: Calibrate initially, after repair, annually; timer every 3 months
Automated blood typing instrument: Observe for correct results
Hemoglobinometer: Standardize against cyanmethemoglobin standard
Refractometer: Standardize against distilled water
Blood container scale: Standardize against known weight
Vacuum blood agitator: Observe with first container filled each day
Water bath/dry heat block: Observe temperature
Rh view box: Observe temperature
Serologic rotators: Observe control for correct results

MONITOR MONTHLY

Electronic thermometers: Calibrate

MONITOR EVERY 6 MONTHS

General laboratory centrifuge: Tachometer

Summary 21-7

Other Equipment Monitoring

Platelet incubator/storage area: Observe temperature; any rotation alarms
pH meter: Before use
Blood irradiator: Annually assess dose, exposure time; rotation per manufacturer
Refrigerators and freezers: Quarterly alarm activation check
Liquid nitrogen freezer: Nitrogen level—daily, weekly; alarm check quarterly
Blood warmer: Quarterly alarm and temperature check
Infusion devices: Manufacturer's recommendation
Platelet rotator/agitator: Initially, after repair
Automated Pipettes: Quarterly

number, the outdate, and if they met specified requirements. With each shipment, the manufacturer's circular must be reviewed for changes. Before the reagent or supply is placed into routine use, it should be inspected for damage and, in the case of reagents, tested for specificity and sensitivity. Fig. 21-4 shows an example of an inventory record for antisera.

PROCESS CONTROL
Change Control

To provide a consistent product, the processes and procedures used must be defined and validated to ensure that the end product meets quality standards. When changes are made in the process, the new requirements must be defined and validated before the new process is implemented. Equipment changes require appropriate documentation of installation qualification, operational qualification, and performance qualification. Summary 21-8 lists the elements of a change control document.

Municipal Blood Bank
Serofuge Quality Assurance Record

Blood Bank designation _____

Manufacturer's serial number _____

Criteria: Timer 1 min = 65 to 64 sec, ± 3 sec from last check
15 sec = 14 to 16 sec, ± 1 sec from last check

Speed = 3100 to 3500, ± 70 rpm

Date	Procedure and Results	OK	Tech

From 12345   Rev mm/dd/yy

Fig. 21-2 Serologic centrifuge quality control record.

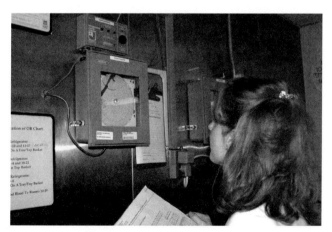

Fig. 21-3 Temperature monitoring.

Proficiency Testing

Proficiency testing is used by accrediting and regulatory agencies to assess the competency of the laboratory.[1-4] Competency and proficiency differ, yet these terms are sometimes used interchangeably. Competency is the measure of the individual's ability to perform a job. Competency is based on the job description/task

Municipal Blood Bank

Routine antisera order/inventory record _____

(Product)

Date ordered				
Quantity				
Manufacturer				
Received				
Quantity				
Date				
Lot #				
Expiration				
Revision				
Comments				
Tech				
Date tested				
1. cells				
source				
result				
2. cells				
source				
result				
3. cells				
source				
result				
Comments				
Tech				

Form 23456   Rev mm/dd/yy

Fig. 21-4 Antisera inventory receipt record.

analysis. Proficiency, on the other hand, is the measure of the laboratory's performance in testing given analytes. Proficiency is broader than competency and measures the procedure, equipment, and other variables, as well as the competency of the staff performing the task.

Samples are sent to the laboratory two to four times a year. These samples must be tested as routinely as possible. The results are then submitted for review and comparison to other laboratories. A passing score is determined. The results

Summary 21-8

Change Control Plan Documentation

Reason for the change
Process modifications required
Risk assessment and critical steps
Equipment installation, operational, and performance qualification
Procedure changes required
Training plans and competency assessment
Postimplementation evaluation process
QA and management review of plans and readiness before implementation
Follow-up evaluation after implementation

are also reported to the Center for Medicare and Medicaid Services (CMS). Current CLIA proficiency testing regulations require 100% accuracy for ABO, Rh, and antibody screening and crossmatching.[5] In antibody identification and other laboratory test events such as hematology and biochemical tests, 80% is the minimum passing score. In addition to indicating potential quality problems, two successive failures or two out of three successive failures to meet or exceed the passing score has serious consequences for the laboratory. Reimbursement for testing performed for patients with Medicare and Medicaid health insurance may be lost.[5]

Quality Control

Quality control encompasses monitoring the use of equipment, reagents, materials, and processes to ensure that they function as expected.

Assessment of Supplies and Reagents

Summary 21-9 lists the Food and Drug Administration (FDA) requirements for reagent testing. Reagents may be made on site or purchased from a manufacturer. When a reagent is made on site, the quality control that is required of the manufacturer must be performed by the facility making the reagent. Thus, if group A reagent red cells are prepared from a tube of blood collected from a donor or patient, the sample must be tested to determine that the reagent red cells react at the appropriate strength with anti-A and do not cause agglutination when mixed with anti-B. Consideration must be given to the potential infectivity of the reagent, and testing for transmission of blood-borne diseases may be necessary. Because of the additional quality assessment requirements, most routine blood bank reagents are purchased from a manufacturer who has performed the initial testing.

   Each day of use, reagents must be tested to determine if they have been contaminated or have lost their potency. A sample recording form for daily cell and serum testing is shown in Fig. 21-5. Note that the expected reactivity is shown on the form to facilitate interpretation of the appropriateness of the reaction. The form also contains blanks for the lot numbers and expiration dates of the reagents being tested because it is essential to know the lot number of reagents used to perform a test and that the reagents were within the dating period specified by the manufacturer. Most large institutions test the routine reagents at the beginning of the day; however, it is necessary to rotate performance of quality control testing among all those who perform testing.[6] Reagents need be tested only if used, and special antigen-typing sera such as anti-Jk[a] are tested when used. Reagents used for testing for blood-borne diseases require additional monitoring. With each test

Summary 21-9

FDA Requirements for Reagent Testing

REAGENTS TO BE TESTED EACH DAY OF USE

Antihuman serum
Blood grouping serum
Lectins
Antibody screening cells
Reverse grouping cells
Enzymes

REAGENTS TO BE TESTED EACH RUN

Hepatitis testing reagents
Human immunodeficiency virus (HIV) testing reagents
Human T-cell lymphotropic virus types I and II (HTLV-I/II) reagents
Alanine aminotransferase (ALT) testing reagents
Syphilis serology reagents

performance, positive and negative controls must be performed and the sensitivity of the test must be monitored with dilutions of antibody or antigen. A sample from each lot number of items such as radiation indicators must be tested in parallel with a sample from the old lot before use.

Supplies and reagents that are received damaged or found to be unsatisfactory must not be used, and their final disposition must be documented.[4] For example, if in-date vials of reagents are returned to the manufacturer for investigation of a possible manufacturing problem, laboratory records should indicate the lot number and quantity returned. Figure 21-6 displays a sample of a reagent/equipment quality assurance report describing the disposition of antisera found to be unsatisfactory. The form has blanks for a description of the instrument or reagent used by serial or lot number and a description of the problem. The bottom half of the form has blanks to record initial response to the problem, further investigation, final resolution, and supervisory review.

Identification and Traceability

It should be possible to trace each critical material used, procedures performed, and the date, time, and person performing each step from the time the donor is received in the donor room to the time a unit is transfused. This includes documentation of processing, component preparation, handling, storage, inspection, distribution, and transportation of blood components.

Component Preparation

The preparation of blood components is considered manufacturing,[4] and each step in the process must be documented. The equipment used to prepare the components and test the donor sample must be functionally assessed. Because it is not always possible to test every individual component itself for potency, efficacy, and purity, samples of the components prepared are tested. Summary 21-10 lists the quality monitoring required for components. Fig. 21-7 is a sample quality control recording form for a leukocyte-reduced apheresis platelet component quality control. Note that the form contains the evaluation criteria to assist the reviewer in identifying possible manufacturing problems. If the minimum standards are not met, corrective action must be taken. This may include monitoring performance of component preparation, modification of the method, or recalibration of equipment.

Municipal Blood Bank
Daily Testing of Reagent Red Cells and Antisera

Date _____   Tech _____   Reagent rack tested _____

Water bath temperature _____   (37 $\pm$ 1° C)

	Source/ Lot number		Source/ Lot number	Results
Tube #				
1. Anti-D	_____	SCl	_____	_____ 2+
2. Anti-D	_____	A$_1$ cells	_____	_____ 0
3. Anti-D	_____	SCll	_____	_____ 2+
4. Rh control	_____	B cells	_____	_____ 0
5. Anti-A	_____	A$_1$ cells	_____	_____ 4+
6. Anti-B	_____	B cells	_____	_____ 4+
7. Anti-A,B	_____	A$_1$ cells	_____	_____ 4+
8. Anti-A,B	_____	B cells	_____	_____ 4+

Antiglobulin
Reagent Lot # _____   LISS Lot # _____

Indirect antiglobulin test with diluted antisera, screening cells suspended in LISS with incubation for 10 minutes at 37 °C.

		Results
9. Anti-C (dil) & SCl	_____	_____ 2+
10. Anti-C (dil) & SCll	_____	_____ 0
11. Anti-E (dil) & SCl	_____	_____ 0
12. Anti-E (dil) & SCll	_____	_____ 2+
13. Tube #10 after addition of IgG collated cells	_____	_____ MF

Reagents performed satisfactorily except as noted below:

Reviewed by _____   Date _____

Form 34556   Rev mm/dd/yy

Fig. 21-5 Antisera quality control testing record.

In some circumstances periodic testing of components is not required once proficiency in preparation is established. Washed and frozen deglycerolized components may not require testing if the procedure used to prepare the component is a "method known to" result in a satisfactory component.[1] However, equipment, reagents, and actual performance of component preparation must be monitored to ensure that the component is adequate.

Control of Donor Units and Patient Testing

Policies and procedures control the processes used in testing donor and patient specimens. Quality control of reagents, equipment, and supplies helps ensure that

Municipal Blood Bank
Reagent/Equipment Quality Assurance Report

Date _____8/23/04_____   Tech _____SHB_____

Equipment description/manufacturer _____

Serial number _____

Reagent name/lot number _____Anti-D   Lot 677_____

Description of problem (please be specific):

Cloudy with particulate matter.

Immediate action taken:

___√___ Removed from service   ___√___ Quarantine

_____ Work order number

Additional action taken (test results, letters sent, phone inquiries):

Quarantined all 3 bottles left of the lot.
Notified manufacturer. SHB 8/23/04

Returned to manufacturer on 8/31/04. SHB

Resolution:

QA review by _____   Date _____

Form 55555   Rev mm/dd/yy

Fig. 21-6 Reagent/equipment quality assurance.

Summary 21–10

Component Quality Control Requirements of Selected Components

Red Blood Cells (RBCs) Pheresis	≥50 g hemoglobin or ≥150 mL packed cell volume	95% of units tested
Red Blood Cells Leukocytes Reduced	85% red cell recovery	75% of units tested
	$<5 \times 10^8$ residual leukocytes	
Red Blood Cells Deglycerolyzed	Prepared by a method known to ensure 80% recovery of post–leukocyte reduction RBCs	
	Minimum free hemoglobin	
	Adequate removal of cryoprotective agents	
Platelets	Platelet count 5.5×10^{10}	90% of units tested
	pH 6.2 at end of storage	
	No clumping	
Pheresis Platelets	Platelet count 3×10^{11}	90% of units tested
	pH 6.2 at end of storage	
Platelets Pheresis, prestorage Leukocyte Reduced	$<8.3 \times 10^5$ residual leukocytes	75% of units tested
	Platelet count $\geq3 \times 10^{11}$	90% of units tested
	pH 6.2 at end of storage	
Cryoprecipitated Antihemophilic factor	≥80 IU Factor VIII/unit	All units tested
	≥150 mg fibrinogen	
Granulocytes	$>1.0 \times 10^{10}$	75% of units tested

*The reader is advised to check current standards for any changes.

Municipal Blood Bank
Automated Plateletpheresis Donor and Product QC Data

Date				
Donor				
Unit #				
Product volume				
Instrument #				
Drawn by				
Donor pre-aphersis				
Spun Hct				
Hct				
Plt × 10³				
Donor post-aphersis				
Spun Hct				
Plt × 10³				
Product counts				
Hct				
Plt × 10³				
WBC × 10³				
Platelet yield				
WBC yield				
Interpretation				
QC calculations by				
Comments				

Platelet yield = $10^6 \times \{$(Product platelet count expressed in thousands/mm³) × (Product volume)$\}$
Example: $\{(2000) \times (250)\} \times 10^6 = 5.0 \times 10^{11}$

WBC yield = $10^6 \times \{$(Product WBC count expressed in thousands/mm³) × (Product volume)$\}$
Example: $\{(1.0) \times (250)\} \times 10^6 = 2.5 \times 10^8$

Interpretation "OK" indicates that results are within the acceptable ranges as defined unless otherwise indicated in comments.

Acceptable results: Donor pre- and postplatelet count ≥150,000
                  Product platelet yield ≥ 3.0×10^{11}
                  Product WBC yield ≥ 1.0×10^{10}
                  Product hematocrit < 1.5%

Form 66777   Rev mm/dd/yy

Fig. 21-7 Automated plateletpheresis donor and product quality control.

the testing is accurate. Policies and procedures for the administration of blood components control patient care at the time of transfusion.

RECORD KEEPING

Documentation is the keystone of quality monitoring, and a written plan is essential. The plan must be based on the individual institution's activities, levels of service, and patient mix. See Chapter 22 for more information on record keeping.

DEVIATIONS, NONCONFORMANCES, AND COMPLICATIONS

A process for documenting errors, accidents, and intentional deviations from standard operating procedures is needed. Appropriate documentation and follow-up

Process Step	Potential Failure Mode	Effects of Failure	Severity	Potential Causes	Occurrence	Current Controls	Detection	RPN*	Recommended Action
ABO/Rh	Mislabeled specimen	Hemolytic transfusion reaction	10	Prestamped labels at nursing station	9	SOP	10	900	Barcoding of patient Wristbands/labels produced at bedside Or require two specimens from each patient
		Hemolytic transfusion reaction	10	Carelessness	4	Training	10	400	
	Wrong specimen tested	Hemolytic transfusion reaction	10	Similar names	5	Two ABO/Rh on file or type specimen twice	6	300	Use barcoded specimen label to test units
		Hemolytic transfusion reaction	10	Lack of organization	3	SOP	6	180	
Antibody screen	Missed positive	Transfusion reaction	8	Improper reagent	4	SOP	10	320	
Electronic crossmatch	Positive screen overlooked	Regulatory BPDR	9	Human error	6	Computer check	2	108	
	Antibody history	Regulatory BPDR	9	Human error	4	Computer check	2	64	
	Missed ABO/Rh disagreement	Regulatory BPDR	9	Human error	6	Computer warning	2	108	
	No ABO/Rh confirmation on unit	Regulatory BPDR	9	Human error	3	Physical separation of units not confirmed; tested units labeled	7	189	Ask for computer warning

*RPN, Risk priority number = Severity × Occurrence × Detection

Fig. 21-8 Sample FMEA analysis.

of all incidents, whether they caused patient harm or not, is essential to preventing future problems. See Chapter 22 for a sample form. When the preparation of blood components is not done according to standard operating procedures or the quality, storage, or testing of a unit does not meet specifications, the unit is considered "nonconforming." When events occur that could potentially harm the safety, potency, and purity of a blood component, it must be quarantined. If nonconforming units are issued, a Biological Product Deviation Report (BPDR) must be submitted to the FDA within 45 days.[7] The report requires an analysis of the incident, including a root cause analysis, contributing factors, and a plan to prevent or reduce the likelihood of recurrence. Transfusion reactions must be documented and reported to the transfusion service. Deaths must be reported within 24 hours.[4]

ASSESSMENTS: INTERNAL AND EXTERNAL

Each facility should schedule internal reviews or audits of its practices and outcomes. System audits review a specific area of the quality essentials. Focused audits

FMEA Rating Scales

Rating		Severity	Occurrence	Probability	Detection
10 (Bad)		Injure a customer or employee	More than once per day	>30%	Not detectable
9		Illegal/regulatory requirement	Every 3-4 days	<30%	Occasional units checked for defects
8		Render product or service unfit for use	Once per week	<5%	Units are systematically sampled and inspected
7		Cause extreme customer dissatisfaction	Once per month	<1%	All units are manually inspected
6		Result in partial malfunction	Once in 3 months	<0.03%	Manual inspection with mistake-proofing modifications
5		Cause a loss of performance likely to result in a complaint	Once in 6 months	1/10,000	Process is monitored through statistical process control (SPC) and manually inspected
4		Cause minor performance loss	Once per year	6/100,000	SPC used with an immediate reaction to out-of-control conditions
3		Cause a minor nuisance, no loss	Once every 1-3 years	6/1,000,000	SPC as above with 100% inspection surrounding out-of-control conditions
2		Be unnoticed, minor effect on performance	Once every 3-6 years	<3/100,000,000	All units are automatically inspected
1 (Good)		Be unnoticed and no performance effect	Once every 6-100 years	<2/1,000,000,000	Defect is obvious and can be kept from affecting customer

Fig. 21-8, cont'd. Sample FMEA analysis.

address areas of high risk or of concern to the facility. Audits must be scheduled and reviewed by management, and action must be taken to resolve problems identified. Blood banks and transfusion services are assessed by regulatory and accrediting agencies at regular intervals. Reports of these assessments must be reviewed by the heads of each department, and action must be taken to correct any deficiencies uncovered.

PROCESS IMPROVEMENT THROUGH CORRECTIVE AND PREVENTIVE ACTION

Process improvement is a broad term that includes the review of patient care outcomes with the goal of overall quality, that is, optimal patient care, efficiency, and cost-effectiveness. Within this context are such quality activities as quality control, quality assurance, and peer review. It is essential to document all aspects of quality improvement in the laboratory and to maintain these documents as required by law. "If it is not in writing, it has not been done."

Risk Assessment

Rather than waiting for a critical incident to occur, the facility can use a process known as failure modes and effects analysis (FMEA). This process evaluates the risks associated with each step in the process and assigns a weight to the frequency and serious consequence of a process failure. Using this process a facility can identify the possible preventive actions to be taken and implement those with a higher likelihood of success. Fig. 21-8 is sample FMEA chart for the electronic crossmatch.

Quality Assessment

The **quality assessment plan** for the institution defines the personnel responsible for coordinating quality assessment activities. In addition, the written plan describes the activities and reporting mechanisms used in the facility. Definition of the facility's important aspects of care allows appropriate quality assessment **indicators (monitors)** to be selected. An indicator is a definable, reliable measure of service quality. Summary 21-11 lists some possible indicators. The monitors selected should be related to identified problems or should monitor high-volume or high-risk activities. The monitors may include omission of appropriate care, as well as performing unnecessary activities. Only a few monitors should be selected. If they prove to be nonproductive, they should be replaced with other monitors. The JCAHO requires assessment of physician ordering practices and use of blood components.[2] In addition, other indicators of transfusion service activities should be considered. Graphic displays of ongoing monitors are recommended.

Fig. 21-9 is a sample quality indicator report assessing whether the patient's medical record contains the reason for transfusion. In the example, the important aspect of care was "transfusion." The class was listed as "high volume," indicating that transfusion was a very frequent occurrence at the facility. The "indicator" was documentation of the reason for transfusion. The criterion for making the assessment was that the indications for transfusion would be recorded in the patient's medical record for each "transfusion episode." Note that by using the term *transfusion episode* the reviewers would not expect the justification for each unit transfused to be documented separately.

A threshold is set at a point above (or below) which there is reason to believe that a problem in patient care exists. In the example monitor, the threshold of 50% (clearly a low target) was based on an estimate of adequate performance. If the facility had a written policy requiring documentation of the indications of transfusion, the threshold might be 95%, and the basis for the threshold would be "institutional policy."

The data collection should be described. In the sample monitor, the sample size was defined as 100 charts (individual medical records). The data source was defined as medical records randomly selected from a list of all transfused patients. The frequency of analysis column indicates that one report was expected. The lead/contact column names the person responsible for submitting the report.

The data collected indicate that the documentation of the reason for transfusion was less than expected and corrective action was required. After consideration of possible causes for the lack of documentation, the transfusion committee decided that the medical staff lacked knowledge of the importance of documenting the indications for transfusion. Possible corrective actions or interventions include systems analysis, in-service education programs, letters, and increased one-on-one communication. The corrective actions selected were writing to the clinical department chairmen and presentations to the residents at grand rounds. The effectiveness of the corrective actions will be assessed by repeating the audit.

Transfusion Committee

In a hospital service the medical staff of the institution has the responsibility of assessing the adequacy of transfusion services, as well as the performance of the medical staff in using blood components appropriately.[2] This is usually done through a committee of the medical staff usually known as the transfusion committee (or tissue and transfusion review committee). The blood usage review process must include all categories of blood components issued by the transfusion service. Usage must be reviewed against screening criteria to identify cases or patterns of use requiring more intensive investigation. The committee must

Summary 21-11

Quality Assurance Monitors

DONOR COLLECTION MONITORS

Donor arm preparation technique
Donor history and physical examination
Number of short drawn/inadequate venipunctures
Donor reactions
Number/indications for therapeutic procedures

COMPONENT PROCESSING

Mislabeled units released
Inappropriate release of components

SHIPPING

Temperature maintained
Incorrect components shipped

TRANSFUSION SERVICE LABORATORY MONITORS

Number of mislabeled specimens
Volume of samples inadequate
Number of corrected reports
Number of service complaints
Turnaround time
Blood delivery time

Municipal Blood Bank
Quality Assurance Monitor Report

Report date: _____   Submitted by _____

Monitor: Documentation of the reason for transfusion

Criteria: Indications for transfusion will be recorded in the patient's medical record for each transfusion episode.

Data source: 100 medical records selected from emergency, surgical, medical, and pediatric patients.

Threshold: 80%

Benchmark data: Compare to previous results

Data collection period: Jan-March, 200x

Numerator: Number of charts meeting criteria   65

Denominator: Number of charts reviewed   100

Indicator results: 65%

Actions taken:

1. Letters sent to clinical chairpersons with response date of May 5
2. Presentation at Medical, Surgical and Pediatric Grand Rounds for June
3. Continue monitor

Reviewed by_____   Date _____

Fig. 21-9 Sample quality assurance monitor report form.

evaluate all confirmed transfusion reactions; develop policies and procedures relating to the distribution, handling, and administration of blood components; review the adequacy of the transfusion service to meet patient care needs; and review the ordering practices for blood and blood components. The transfusion committee may have the assistance of medical record professionals in coordinating data collection.

Utilization Review

A utilization review program is required by the various agencies.[1,2] A program must be in place to assess the blood ordering and transfusion practices of the medical staff. A sample of utilization review monitors is listed in Summary 21-12. Fig. 21-10 is a sample summary report for blood usage statistics such as total number of components ordered, transfused, and wasted. The crossmatch:transfusion ratio (C:T ratio) is the number of units crossmatched divided by the number of units transfused. This statistic is often used as an indicator that too much blood is being requested to be "on hold." A high outdate rate could indicate overordering by physicians. A high waste rate could indicate inadequate management of the blood supply. Other monitors of transfusion practices include the number of autologous transfusions and the number of units issued without complete pretransfusion testing (emergency release). In addition to institution utilization rates, facilities may calculate statistics by physician or by clinical service such as oncology, obstetrics, and general surgery, or compare utilization rates with published data. Peer review and the role of the transfusion committee are further discussed in Chapter 11.

Physician ordering practices also may be assessed by comparing the documented reasons for administering a transfusion with predefined audit criteria. The audit cri-

---

Summary 21-12

Utilization Review Monitors

Number of cases of infectious disease transmission
Number of transfusion reactions reported
Number of hemolytic transfusion reactions
Use of white cell removal filters
Crossmatch:transfusion ratio
Wasted units
Outdated units
Use of uncrossmatched blood
Percentage of red blood cells used
Number/percentage of autologous units collected and transfused
Number/percentage of autologous units transfused
Indications for transfusion documented in the patient's medical record
Patient response to transfusion documented in the patient's medical record
Blood transfusion where
    Hct/Hgb >24 Hct/8 g/dL
    Platelet count >20,000/mL
Fresh frozen plasma (FFP) where activated partial thromboplastin time (aPTT) <60 and
    prothrombin time (PT) <16
Transfusion of granulocytes
Blood use in cardiac surgery; transplant surgery
Use of factor concentrates/serum albumin
Blood use per patient/admission

May-03

Product	# XM	#TX'd	#U OD	%U OD	#NTNO	%NTNO	WASTE	TOTAL%	Comments
Total Allo RBC	684	328	2	0.09%	22	0.94%	24	1.02%	
Red Blood Cells	6	3	0	0.00%	0	0.00%	0	0.00%	
LR RBC	3207	1865	2	0.11%	16	0.85%	18	0.96%	"A2, C12, E2"
LR RBCI Irradiated	471	457	0	0.00%	6	1.30%	6	1.30%	"C2, P4"
Resusp.LP WB	0	2	0	0.00%	0	0.00%	0	0.00%	
Washed RBC	0	1	0	0.00%	0	0.00%	0	0.00%	
Total DD and Autos	51	27	11	27.50%	2	5.00%	13	32.50%	
Directed RBC	15	4	1	14.29%	2	28.57%	3	42.86%	C2
Auto RBC/WB	36	23	10	30.30%	0	0.00%	10	30.30%	
Partial/Aliquot Units	56	222	0	0.00%	6	2.63%	6	2.63%	
LP Half Units	2	1	0	0.00%	0	0.00%	0	0.00%	
LP Half Units IRR	2	3	0	0.00%	0	0.00%	0	0.00%	
LRRP Partial Units	28	55	0	0.00%	1	1.79%	1	1.79%	C1
LRRP Part IRR	20	19	0	0.00%	0	0.00%	0	0.00%	
Aliquots	4	144	0	0.00%	5	3.36%	5	3.36%	"A1, E4"
Total Random Platelets		3884	15	0.37%	137	3.39%	152	3.77%	
LR Random Plts		3884	15	0.37%	137	3.39%	152	3.77%	"A14, C16, E97, I5, P5"
Total Apheresis Plts		12	0	0.00%	0	0.00%	0	0.00%	
LP Apheresis Plts		5	0	0.00%	0	0.00%	0	0.00%	
XM LR Apheresis Plts		7	0	0.00%	0	0.00%	0	0.00%	
Total Plasma Units		873	0	0.00%	14	1.58%	14	1.58%	
SDPL		116	0	0.00%	0	0.00%	0	0.00%	
FFPL		757	0	0.00%	14	1.82%	14	1.82%	"A1, C12, I1"
Plasma Aliquots		16	0	0.00%	1	5.88%	1	5.88%	E1
Plasma Half Units		4	0	0.00%	2	33.33%	2	33.33%	C2
Total Cryo Units		470	0	0.00%	83	15.01%	83	15.01%	
CRYO		27	0	0.00%	8	22.86%	8	22.86%	"A4, EA"
CRYO pooled		63	0	0.00%	15	19.23%	15	19.23%	"C5, E10"
CRYO prepooled		380	0	0.00%	60	13.64%	60	13.64%	"A10, E50"
RHIG		63	0	0.00%	0	0.00%	0	0.00%	
VZIG		2	0	0.00%	0	0.00%	0	0.00%	
WRHO		72	0	0.00%	0	0.00%	0	0.00%	
SKIN		0	0		0		0		

Indicators:

	Threshold	Actual
C/T Ratio	1.8	1.6
Wasted RBC	1.0%	1.02%
Wasted Plt	4.0%	3.77%
Wasted Plasma	4.0%	1 0.58%
Wasted Cryo	7.00%	22.86%

Legend:
XM = Crossmatched
TX = Transfused
OD = Outdated
NTNO = "Not transfused, not outdated (wasted)"
A = Broken Bag
C = Improper storage
E = Entered, not transfused
P= Pneumatic tube problem
I= Misc

Broken bags returned for credit
Cryo
Pcryo   4
Plasma   10
         FFP   23

Fig. 21-10 Blood utilization statistics.

teria (or threshold for additional investigation) may be based on published references such as the AABB *Technical Manual*[8] or may be locally defined. These audit criteria are used to screen medical records to determine if the transfusions administered were "justified." If the reasons for transfusion are not included in the audit criteria, the patient's medical record is set aside for additional review. If, following a second review, the transfusion cannot be justified on the basis of information included in the patient's medical record, the transfusion is classified as unjustified. The rate or number of unjustified transfusions may be reported by physician or by clinical service. For example, a facility may define the audit criteria for the transfusion of red blood cells as documentation in the medical record of one or more the following:

Hematocrit of less than 24%

Hemoglobin of less than 8 g/dL

Symptoms due to anemia

Recent estimated blood loss of greater than 10% of blood volume

If the medical record being reviewed indicates that the patient's pretransfusion hematocrit was documented as 27%, the medical record is marked for a second level review. If, in the opinion of the reviewers, no other circumstances in the medical record justified the transfusion, the transfusion is classified as unjustified. The physician ordering the transfusion is notified and given an opportunity to respond.

The records of the audit plan, criteria, results obtained, and any communications with physicians must be retained for review by accrediting agency personnel. As with all medical records, quality assessment documents are considered confidential, and the data collected must be protected from accidental disclosure to unauthorized individuals.

Facilities and Safety

A safe and adequate environment for donors, patients, volunteers, and staff is expected. Policies and procedures that safeguard personnel, reagents, and equipment are needed. See Chapter 20 for a discussion of safety issues.

CHAPTER SUMMARY

1. The process of providing a blood component to a patient is quite complex, and system problems may occur at various points.

2. The facility must be organized to facilitate quality monitoring and management review.

3. The quality system essentials define the systems that need to be in place to ensure efficient, safe, and effective services.

4. A procedures manual must be available that describes the details of performing all tests or procedures, including quality assurance procedures, in order to control processes.

5. Personnel must be trained and their performance assessed.

6. Reagents, supplies, equipment, and temperature-sensing devices must be monitored when used. Unsatisfactory reagents and supplies and malfunctioning equipment and instruments must not be used.

7. Periodic monitoring of the preparation of blood components must be documented.

8. The goal of quality monitoring should be to continuously improve service to patients. Monitoring for the sake of regulatory compliance is not a fruitful task. The goal of quality monitoring should be to continuously improve service to patients.

9. Medical staff blood ordering and transfusion practices must be evaluated.

10. Monitors or quality care indicators must be defined, and corrective action must be taken when thresholds are exceeded.

11. A quality audit plan must be written, criteria for assessing performance defined, and the results of studies and corrective actions "documented.

12. The entire process is reviewed to ensure that the patient obtains the appropriate care.

REFERENCES

1. Menitove JE (ed): Standards for Blood Banks and Transfusion Services, 21st ed. Bethesda, MD, American Association of Blood Banks, 2002.
2. Joint Commission on Accreditation of Healthcare Organizations: Comprehensive Accreditation Manual for Hospitals: The Official Handbook. Oakbrook, IL, Joint Commission on Accreditation of Healthcare Organizations, 2004.
3. College of American Pathologists, Commission of Laboratory Accreditation: Inspection Checklist (Section I, Laboratory General). Northfield, IL, College of American Pathologists, 2003.
4. Current Good Manufacturing Practice for Blood and Blood Components (Part 606); Additional Standards for Human Blood and Blood Products (Part 640), 21 Code of Federal Regulations.
5. Center for Medicare and Medicaid Services. Laboratory Requirements Relating to Quality Systems and Certain Personnel Qualifications; Final Rule. CMS-2226-F. January 2003.
6. Clinical and Laboratory Standards Institute: Clinical Laboratory Technical Procedure Manuals, 4th ed. GPO2-A4. Wayne, PA, NCCLS, 2002.
7. Food and Drug Administration, CBER: Reporting of Biological Product Deviations in Manufacturing Blood and Blood Components; Final Rule, November 7, 2000.
8. Brecher M. (ed): Technical Manual, 14th ed. Bethesda, MD, American Association of Blood Banks, 2002.

FURTHER READING

Clinical and Laboratory Standards Institute: A Quality System Model for Healthcare; Approved Guideline, HS1-A, 2002.

Expert Opinion

THE TECHNOLOGY OF PATIENT IDENTIFICATION

Gerald A. Hoeltge, MD

Transfusion safety depends on accuracy. Two thirds of all transfusion errors follow misidentification of the patient at the bedside.[1] Whether at the time of collection of the pretransfusion blood sample or before administration of the blood component, failure to identify the patient with absolute certainty risks serious consequence. The incidence of misidentification errors reported voluntarily is more than 1 in 17,000 units transfused, although the actual rate may be much greater.[1,2] In other words, between 500 and 1000 units of Red Blood Cells are transfused each year to the wrong patients in the United States.

Misidentification of the patient is 100% preventable. The standard of care in hospital medicine is for patients to wear identification bracelets. Wristbands applied at the time of hospital admission provide positive patient identification even for unresponsive or confused patients. Unfortunately, wristbands are too often ignored. In a hospital survey of 1.7 million phlebotomies, 3% of the time the bracelet was either missing, illegible, or erroneous.[3] If pretransfusion samples were collected only from patients who had proper wristbands and if every transfusion was preceded by a careful review of the wristband information, the risk of mistransfusion would be less. Too often, however, missing wristbands are ignored because the caregiver "knows" the patient or gives the wrist a cursory glance.

The technology to prevent misidentification errors exists. Secure, accurate identification systems are used every day for package shipments, retail inventories, and credit card sales. That these systems work is not because of computers. Computers make them fast. They are effective because they block human error.

A simple technology is to assign a unique identifier to each pretransfusion blood specimen. This identifying number is copied to the patient's wrist, to the pretransfusion blood sample, and to the crossmatched unit intended for transfusion. The identification routine at the patient's bedside at the time of blood administration includes a comparison of the identifier on the bag with the identifier on the patient's wrist. Such a system supplements the usual "two forms of identification" (usually the patient's name and hospital number). A variation on this is a special fastener that secures the plastic bag used to transport the blood component from the laboratory to the patient care area. To open the plastic bag containing the blood component, the bedside nurse must use a dial on the fastener to enter the special identifying number.

All identifiers can be bar-coded. A bar code is simply a font that is easy for a computer to read. Several formats are in common use, including two-dimensional bar codes that can embed much data in a very small space. Faster than manual systems, they can incorporate check digits for internal verification of the read signal.

A fully electronic system will capture digitized identifiers at each point along the path of workflow:

1. At the time of pretransfusion sample collection, the phlebotomist scans the patient's wristband and her own identification badge using a handheld device downloaded with data from the laboratory information system (LIS). The device compares the patient's identification with the phlebotomist's work list and enables the next step only if all information matches the data in memory. The device then prints a machine-readable specimen label.

2. In the laboratory the specimen label is scanned as the sample is typed. The LIS automatically retrieves all previous serologic information for comparison. If the blood type of the sample does not match the historical type, the LIS blocks further data entry until the problem is resolved.

3. The compatibility label applied to each unit prepared for transfusion includes bar-coded identifiers. At the patient's bedside and before blood administration, the transfusionist scans the patient's wristband, his or her identification badge (and the badge of the second nurse if required by hospital policy), and the compatibility label using a handheld device that contains relevant data from the LIS. Only if all information matches will the display on the device signal that it is safe for the nurse to proceed with the transfusion.

Such a system is only as good as the readability of the data. Scanners should be fully portable and untethered by a cable. Bar codes curved around wrists or tubes are difficult for scanners to read. Dirt, debris, and smudged ink interfere with smooth data transmission. The portable computer used as an input device must be returned to its dock promptly after each use so that its information is current (and to enable the next user to find it!).

Wireless technology simplifies the task. Information from the LIS can be downloaded to the handheld device in real time, precluding the need to return the dock before each use. Of course each additional function made portable increases the weight and size of the device carried by the nurse or phlebotomist.

In the future, we may see wireless transponders tagged to patients' wrists or to unit labels. Small, wireless transponders are used today to identify automobiles, pets, and golf balls. Computers in patient care areas could sense transfusion errors before they occur by comparing data from a transponder on the patient's wrist with another on the unit even without visual comparison or the need for a scanner.

We may also find that digitized identifiers such as bar codes will be replaced by biometry. Finger, palm, face, retina, and iris scans provide unique identifiers that can never be left at home, removed, or placed on the wrong wrist. They would work as well for outpatient transfusion as for inpatients. Finger scanning is already used in some methadone clinics for patient identification.[4]

REFERENCES

1. Linden JV, Wagner K, Voytovich AE, Sheehan J: Transfusion errors in New York state: An analysis of 10 years' experience. Transfusion 40:1207-1213, 2000.
2. Serious Hazards of Transfusion Steering Group: Annual report 2000-2001. Manchester, SHOT, 2002.
3. Howanitz PJ, Renner SW, Walsh MK: Continuous wristband monitoring over 2 years decreases identification errors: A College of American Pathologists Q-Tracks study. Arch Pathol Lab Med 126:809-815, 2002.
4. Moser L: Positive identification: Fingerprint images identify patients under any circumstances. Health Manag Technol 21:22, 2000.

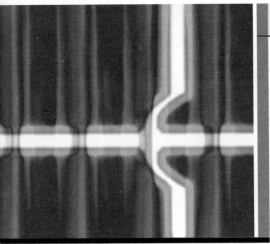

Record Keeping and Computers

Suzanne H. Butch

LEARNING OBJECTIVES

After reading and studying this chapter, the student should be able to:

1. Identify circumstances in which confidential patient information may be discussed or reported to a third party.
2. Define the four levels of documentation in an organization.
3. List two records that must be maintained indefinitely.
4. List three records that should be maintained for at least 5 years.
5. Identify the resource for interpreting locally defined abbreviations.
6. Contrast and compare the terms *results* and *conclusions*.
7. List the items required to document the infusion of a blood component.
8. Identify the agency to be notified in the event of a transfusion-related death.
9. Describe the method for correcting an original entry on a laboratory report.
10. List the documentation required when a computer system is used in a blood bank or transfusion service.
11. Define the following terms and give an example of each:
    Critical control function
    Validation
12. List two methods of preventing unauthorized access to a computer system.
13. Describe the testing necessary if a change is made to the computer system.
14. Complete a validation testing report.
15. Describe the purpose of a disaster recovery plan.

RECORD-KEEPING SYSTEMS

Each blood bank and transfusion service must have a record-keeping system—either manual, computerized, or a combination of manual and computerized systems—that is documented (described in procedure manuals) and allows the retrieval of information in a timely manner.[1,2] The records must document all significant steps in the collection, storage, testing, processing, and distribution of the blood or blood component. The records must be preserved and protected from accidental and unauthorized modification or destruction. In addition, the system must ensure the confidentiality of donor and patient information.[3]

Confidentiality of Information

Medical records and information concerning a donor or patient are considered confidential. Thus information may not be discussed or shared with others unless they need to know the information in order to provide patient care or perform their duties. Regulations promulgated from the **Health Insurance Portability and Accountability Act (HIPAA)** influence the release of information. Many states have specific provision for disclosure of the results of human immunodeficiency virus (HIV) test results.

At patient or donor request, test results may be sent to physicians and insurance carriers. Requests for patient information are usually handled by the medical information section of the institution to ensure compliance with institutional and state regulations. However, some blood banks and transfusion services provide information concerning blood group antibodies and transfusion history when the information is necessary for the immediate treatment of the patient. It is essential that the transfer of this information be done in keeping with the institution's patient confidentiality policies.

Health Insurance Portability and Accountability Act (HIPAA): Legislation passed in 1996 intended to ensure confidentiality of medical information and to prevent discrimination based on health status. HIPAA training of employees is required in all health care institutions.

Reporting Positive Infectious Disease Testing Results

Although state public health laws differ, the health department must be notified of the results of persons testing positive for certain diseases. These often include HIV, human T-cell lymphotropic virus (HTLV), West Nile virus, syphilis, and hepatitis. Blood donors must be advised that positive results will be reported, and a statement concerning result reporting must be included in the consent for donation.

RECORD-KEEPING REQUIREMENTS

Federal, state, and local laws and regulations influence the records maintained. The regulatory and voluntary agencies that require record keeping are listed in Summary 22-1. The most recent editions of their requirements must be reviewed periodically to determine if any changes in the requirements require a modification of the current record-keeping system.[1,2]

A complete, indelible, legible record must be made concurrently with performance of a test or activity. From the record it should be possible to determine who, what, when, where, why, and how for each significant step in the process. Regulatory agencies do not define a standard form or format for keeping information. Each

---

Summary 22-1

Regulatory and Voluntary Agencies with Requirements for Blood Bank Record Keeping

Food and Drug Administration (FDA): www.fda.gov
American Association of Blood Banks (AABB): www.aabb.org
Joint Commission on the Accreditation of Healthcare Organizations (JCAHO): www.jcaho.org
College of American Pathologists (CAP): www.cap.org

Summary 22-2

Levels of Documents[2]
Level I Policies: What to do **Level II** Processes: How it happens **Level III** Procedures: How to do it **Level IV** Documents: Forms, templates, data, records, labels

---

facility is free to design a system tailored to its individual needs. Summary 22-2 lists four levels of documentation needed in a facility.[4] Level I provides the policies, or "what is done." Level II defines the processes, or "how it happens." Level III describes the "specific instructions of how to do it." The reports, labels, records, data, and forms make up level IV. From these documents it should be possible for a blood bank to be able to trace a unit of blood from collection to final disposition, including all of the steps in processing, tracing transmission of infectious diseases, identification of possible manufacturing defects, and comparison with previous results.

Record Retention

Local and state regulations may result in the retention of blood bank and transfusion service records indefinitely. Summaries 22-3 and 22-4 are based on the American Association of Blood Banks (AABB) requirements for record retention.[2] The tables separate records into those that may be discarded after 5 years and those that should be kept at least 10 years.[2] Records may be stored on paper, on microfilm or microfiche, or on computer disks and magnetic tape. The AABB requires that ABO and Rh typing results be available for review for at least 5 years.[2] Records of typing and antibody problems should be maintained for at least 10 years. Before discarding records, the requirements of all accrediting and regulatory agencies, as well as any state laws, should be reviewed.

Summary 22-3

Information that MUST Be Maintained 10 Years or More

INDEFINITE
Difficulty in blood typing, clinically significant antibodies, significant unexpected adverse reactions to transfusion, and special transfusion requirements
Notification of donor significant abnormal findings; donors placed on indefinite deferral list
 	
10-YEAR RETENTION
Donor records
Informed consent of donors
Notification of nonconforming products
    Donor information
    Predonation history
    Physical examination results
    Donor ABO and Rh type
    Interpretation of infectious disease markers
    Confirmatory testing results

Summary 22-3, cont'd

10-YEAR RETENTION—cont'd

Notification to donors who are permanently deferred

Quarantine of units from prior collections

Lookback (tracing the recipients of previously donated blood components from a donor who is subsequently found to be positive for an infectious disease transmissible by blood, such as HIV or hepatitis C)

Final review of records relating to testing and acceptability criteria

BLOOD COMPONENTS RECEIVED FROM OUTSIDE SOURCES

Collection facility name and address

Component

Date received

Outdate

Unit identification (number or alphanumeric)

Identity of any facility preparing the component

Function performed by the preparing facility

PATIENT INFORMATION

Transfusion information

Component name

Donor unit or pool identification number

Date and time of transfusion

Vital signs and identification of transfusionist

Amount transfused

Consent for transfusion

Adverse reaction to transfusion, including investigation and follow-up

Notification of potential exposure to infectious diseases

OTHER RECORDS

Component preparation

Blood component irradiation logs

Final check of records at unit issue

Quarantine and release records

Final disposition, including method of destruction if not transfused

Reissue

Emergency issue, including physician request

Recall of issued components

Errors and accidents, including follow-up

Identification of personnel who have authority to sign forms and procedures

  Name

  Signature

  Initials

  Computer identification codes

  Dates of employment

HLA testing

Bone marrow collection, processing, and infusion

Therapeutic apheresis procedures

Forms

Forms or templates facilitate record keeping because they contain blanks for required information. The information routinely needed on a form is listed in Summary 22-5,[4] and a sample form for recording compatibility testing and plasma component reservations is shown in Fig. 22-1. For example, the compatibility testing record form identifies the facility and the kind of testing being recorded. The form has blanks for

Summary 22-4

Information with a Minimum 5-Year Retention Period

DONOR RECORDS

ABO and Rh typing results
Severe reaction to donation
Hemapheresis procedure clinical records
Inspection of blood components before issue
Shipping records
   Date and time
   Identity of units shipped
   Name of person performing task
   Receiving facility name and address

PATIENT RECORDS

ABO and Rh typing results
Antibody screening results
Verification of patient identification before transfusion
Evaluation of immediate and delayed transfusion reactions
Compatibility testing records
Therapeutic phlebotomy
Request for emergency release of blood components
Outpatient transfusion

COMPUTER RECORDS

Validation of system software, hardware, databases, and user-defined tables
Fulfillment of applicable life-cycle requirements
Numerical designations of system versions with inclusive dates of use
Monitoring of data integrity for critical data elements

QUALITY CONTROL RECORDS

Superseded procedures (manuals and references)
Initialed temperature recording charts
Inspection of incoming blood, components, and tissue
Inspection of weld integrity and identification of disposables
Verification of irradiation dose delivery
Distribution of units before completion of testing
Quality control testing of
   Reagents
   Components
   Proficiency
Maintenance of equipment and physical plant
Calibration and standardization of equipment
Sterilization records
Reagents and supplies
   Date of receipt
   Lot number
   Supplier
   Expiration date
Sterility testing
Disposition of rejected supplies
Shipping container—temperature maintenance
Staff training, evaluations, and continuing education records

Summary 22-5

Information Needed on a Form

Title descriptive of the use of the form
Facility identification
Identity of the patient, unit number, lot number, and/or specimen
Identity of the person performing each significant step
Results or readings
Interpretations
Date (and time, if relevant) the activity was performed

Municipal Blood Bank

Compatibility testing and component reservation Form 105 Rev 11/03

Patient name _____ Test, Patient _____   Blood type __A POS__
Medical record number ____ 1234567 ____   Antibody history:
Date/time specimen _____ 4/15/03 _____   Irradiated Components
Accession number _____   Anti-Kell

Anti-A	Anti-B	Anti-D	A Cells	B Cells	Anti-D	Rh Cont	ABO/RhInterp
4+	0	4+	0	4+	NP	NP	A POS

1W	2W	1G	2G	1C	2C	ABSC Interp	Date	Tech
0	0	1+	0	NP	mf	NEG	4/15/03	SHB

Date	Unit #	Antigen Neg	IS	Liss 37	IAT	CCC	Conc.	Tech	Label
4/3/04	85GG12345	K−	NP	0	0	MF	Neg	SHB	

Unit numbers

85GG22222	FFP	

Abbreviations

0	Negative, No reactivity
±, 1+, 2+, 3+, 4+	Degrees of reactivity
mf	Mixed field
Neg	Negative
Pos	Positive
H	Hemolysis

Fig. 22-1 Compatibility testing and component reservation form.

recording the identification of the patient by name and identification number. The specimen is identified by the accession number. There are labeled columns to record the date, the unit number tested, the results of all phases of the tests, the conclusion, and the identification of the person performing the testing.

Symbols and Abbreviations

Note that the entries on the form in Fig. 22-1 include symbols and abbreviations. The approved symbols and abbreviations should be a part of the procedures manual. It is often helpful to print the abbreviations on the form, but owing to space constraints this cannot always be done. The meaning of approved symbols must be documented because they do not have the same meaning in all facilities. The symbols should be unambiguous. In Fig. 22-1, the "−" symbol means "not performed" and the conclusion "antigen typing negative" is indicated by the "K−" notation. In some facilities, the "−" symbol means "tested and found to be negative." As shown in Fig. 22-1, the negative test result is also indicated by the symbol "0." The symbols "0" or NEG are preferred over "−" in computerized records because the "−" may be easily overlooked.

Results and Conclusions

When multiple test results or readings of a device are used to draw a conclusion, both the individual results and the conclusion (or interpretation) should be recorded. For example, the conclusion that a patient is A-positive is made from the interpretation of the seven reactions of the patient's red blood cells and serum with antisera and reagent red cells (see Fig. 22-1). The conclusion that a thermometer is suitable for use is based on a comparison of the readings of the thermometer being tested and the readings on a calibrated thermometer. It is necessary to record the results of the reference thermometer and the test thermometer, as well as the conclusion "satisfactory" or "unsatisfactory."

Records of Transfusion

Records of the actual transfusion must include documentation that the transfusionist matched the container label information with the patient's identification wristband in the presence of the recipient and before administration of the transfusion.[2] Nursing and facility policies and forms differ significantly. Fig. 22-2 includes documentation of a patient's vital signs and instructions on reporting a suspected transfusion reaction. The patient's vital signs may be recorded in other places on the patient's medical record, and the instructions for responding to a transfusion reaction could be published in a nursing manual.

PROCEDURE MANUALS

The procedure manual serves as documentation of how a task or procedure is to be performed. A more complete discussion of procedure manuals based on the Clinical Laboratory Standards Institute Guidelines[5] is found in Chapter 21.

In the example of testing a thermometer, the method used to test the thermometer and the conclusion that the thermometer is defective or suitable for use must be based on the criteria defined in the procedure manual. The performance criteria must be based on the manufacturer's specifications and documented in the procedure manual.

When the method used deviates from the standard method, the record must indicate the nature of the deviations. For example, if the standard method of performing an ABO forward grouping calls for the use of unwashed patient cells, but it was necessary to use four-times–washed cells to eliminate rouleaux, the record should indicate that four-times–washed cells were used.

1187512

	Patient

Registration number	Crossmatch

Bedside Verification

Date	Time	Donor Unit Number

Give blood product immediately after verification. Do not separate blood product from the patient after the double-checking process has occured. If the blood is removed from the patient room, repeat the bedside verification.

ABO/Rh	Tech

We have verified that:
1. The recipient's name and hospital registration number on the recipient's wristband matches the corresponding information on the blood bag and this form.
2. The donor unit number and blood product name on the bag label match the corresponding information on this form.
3. The donor and recipient blood groups are compatible, and
4. This blood product is not outdated.

Recipient Component/Volume	Donor

Transfusion started by:

Double checked by: Date and time begun   /   /

Vital Signs

Vital signs recorded on another record: (check one)
☐ ED Flowsheet   ☐ 24 Hr Flow Sheet
☐ Dialysis Record   ☐ Anesthesia Record
☐ OR Record   ☐ TAW
☐ Recovery Note   ☐ Other: _____

		Time	Temp.	Blood Pressure	Pulse	Resp.
Pre-transfusion						
During Transfusion	15 min					
	30 min					
	1½ hrs					
	2½ hrs					
	3½ hrs					
After Transfusion	1 hr					

Reaction suspected (complete reaction report form) ☐   No reaction ☐

Date and time completed: / /   Amount administered ☐ All ☐ Part _____ mL estimate

Physician/Nurse Responsibilities When Reporting A Suspected Transfusion Reaction

Note: A temperature rise of 1.0 C (1.5 F) is a febrile response.

1. Stop the transfusion.

2. Immediately verify identification of unit and patient.

3. Notify patient's physician.

4. Consult with Blood Bank regarding samples required for serological investigation.

5. Consult with Blood Bank House Officer.

6. Submit both copies of the Transfusion Reaction and Consultation Request and Report Form to the Blood Bank **immediately.**

7. Refer to the Blood Transfusion Policies and Standard Practices Booklet for further guidance.

Fig. 22-2 Blood transfusion record form.

RECORDS OF ERRORS AND ACCIDENTS

Records of accidents, errors, and adverse reactions must be maintained.[1] The records must include all the pertinent details of the occurrence—its discovery, investigation, and steps taken to avoid recurrence. Fig. 22-3 is a sample report form for documenting errors and accidents. Errors such as issuing the wrong blood component to a patient or mislabeled units must be reported to the FDA.[6]

TRANSFUSION REACTIONS

Adverse reactions to transfusion include the transmission of infectious diseases, as well as serologic incompatibility, febrile reactions, urticaria, transfusion-related acute lung injury (TRALI), and shock due to a bacterially contaminated unit.

Municipal Blood Bank
OCCURRENCE REPORT FORM

Laboratory _____Transfusion Service_____ Date of report ___4/10/03___

Report completed by _____LLG_____ Date/time of occurrence ___4/09/03__

Brief description of error/occurrence: _____

_____ Market withdrawal of red blood cells _____

Blood bank unit number(s) _____85P12345_____

(Information on tube/label)   (Correct patient information if known)

Patient name _____   Patient name _____

Reg. No. _____   Reg. No. _____

1st specimen _____ Accn# _____   Test code(s) _____

2nd specimen_____ Accn# _____   Test code(s) _____

Where did error occur _____   Patient location _____

Person involved _____   Service/

                                              position _____

- -

Correction in computer? _____ Yes _____ NA   Tech ID _____

Person Notified:

Dr. _____ Date _____Time _____

Other _____ Date _____Time _____

Signature of person making correction _____Date _____

Name (printed) of person making correction _____Date _____

Laboratory personnel

involved _____

- -

Further description and action taken in laboratory:

**Call received from blood supplier 4/10/03 at 16:45 to quarantine unit. Removed unit from
shelf and placed into quarantine status in computer and moved unit to quarantine shelf.
Shb 4/10/03**

Unit returned to supplier on 4/11/03. Packed at 10:15. Documented on return form 22222. Placed
unit in final status: returned to supplier in computer. Hhs 4/11/03

Supervisor's review _____QA Tech_____ Review Date ___4/12/03___

QA review by/date _____Q Control_____

Copy to risk management ____NO____   04/14/91 Quality Assurance Document

                                       Confidential MCLA 33.21515,.20175

Fig. 22-3 Occurrence report form.

Fig. 22-4 is a transfusion reaction report, and Fig. 22-5 is a form for recording the results of serologic testing. When a complication of blood collection or transfusion is confirmed to be fatal, the Director of the Center for Biologics Evaluation and Research must be notified as soon as possible by the transfusing facility.[1]

RECORD CORRECTIONS

Any corrections to an original entry must be clearly identifiable.[1,4] The original entry must be legible and not be obliterated by ink, error correction tape, or opaque fluids. A single line should be drawn through the original entry and/or conclusion. The revised entry must be dated and must identify the person performing the correction (Fig. 22-6). Corrections to computer records must identify the previous result, the new result, the date and time, and the person changing the results.

TRANSFUSION REACTION REPORT AND CONSULTATION REQUEST FORM	**Results Reporting Location Code:**	Birth date_____ Name _____ CPI number _____ Sex: M F Visit no. _____

If a transfusion reaction is suspected:
1. Stop the transfusion.
2. Immediately verify the patient and blood component identification
3. Notify the patient's physician.
4. Consult with the Blood Bank regarding samples required for serological investigation.

5. Consult with the Blood Bank House Officer and/or refer to booklet Blood Transfusion Policies and Standard Practices for further guidance.
6. Submit the top copy of the completed form to the Blood Bank immediately.

Answer the following questions:
Date of report: _____ Clinical house
Report submitted by: _____ Dr. No. _____ Officer notified _____ Dr. No. _____
Attending physician _____ Dr. No. _____

1. Patient and product identification were checked and agree   □ Yes □ No
2. Date and time of reaction _____
3. Blood component _____ Unit ID Number   _____
4. Volume transfused _____ mL
5. Other transfusions in the last 3 hours? _____
6. Was a blood warmer used □ Yes □ No
7. IV solution used _____
8. Was medication added to the unit or IV tubing? □ Yes _____ □ No
9. Premedication □ None □ Tylenol □ Benadryl □ Other _____
10. Signs and symptoms

Sign/symptom	Pretransfusion	At time of reaction
Pulse		
Temperature		
Blood pressure		
Respirations		

□ Chills □ Back Pain □ Dyspnea □ Hives □ Chest Pain □ Hemoglobinuria □ Rigors
□ Other _____

11. Why was patient transfused? _____
12. Medical history (main diagnoses) _____
13. Has the patient been routinely spiking temperatures throughout the day?   □ Yes □ No
14. What is the maximum temperature in the past 24 hours? _____
15. Input/output   Last 8 hours _____ Last 24 hours _____
16. Is the patient on ACE inhibitor? □ Yes □ No
17. Is the patient on pressors? □ Yes □ No

Rev.3/1/04	Ply 1 Blood Bank Copy Ply 2 Medical Record	BLOOD BANK LABORATORY Transfusion Reaction Consult Form

Fig. 22-4 Blood bank transfusion reaction consultation request and report.

USING COMPUTERS IN THE BLOOD BANK OR TRANSFUSION SERVICE

A computer system is made up of the equipment (hardware), programs (software), institutional database, and operating policies and procedures for using them. Hardware includes the central processing unit (CPU), display monitors, keyboards, bar-code readers, tape, disk or optical drives, terminal servers, and printers (Fig. 22-7). The software includes the operating programs and interfaces, as well as utility programs to manage the data. The database consists of locally defined infor-

Transfusion Reaction Studies

Name _____ Medical record number _____

Date/time of reaction _____ Accn number_____

Patient location _____ Pathology house officer _____

Donor unit numbers _____

Product codes_____

Clerical Check and First Tier

Record check and label check _____ IgG DAT Pre _____

Visual serum hemolysis check   Pre _____   Post _____

Post _____   Unit(s)_____

ABO/Rh Recheck

	Anti-A	Anti-B	Anti-D	A cells	B cells	MTD	Cont	Interp
Pre								
Post								

Tech _____ Date/time _____ Computer entry _____ Date/time _____

Second Tier

	Anti-A	Anti-B	Anti-D	A cells	B cells	MTD	Cont	Interp
Units								

Antibody screen _____ Screen cell lot number _____

Patient's Pre				Patient's Post			
	LISS 37 C	IAT	CCC	Conc.	LISS 37 C	IAT	CCC	Conc.
I								
II								

Major crossmatches

	Patient's Pre				Patient's Post			
Units	LISS 37 C	IAT	CCC	Conc.	LISS 37 C	IAT	CCC	Conc.

Additional testing ordered (Circle)

Bilirubin   Culture
Haptoglobin   Other_____

Tech _____ Date/time _____

Abbreviations 0 = no reactivity, blank = not tested, 4+, 3+, 2+, 1+ = degrees of reactivity, MF = Mixed field.

Form 11222   Rev mm/dd/yy

Fig. 22-5 Form for recording testing for a transfusion reaction investigation.

mation and the data records. Examples of information that is locally defined include such items as length of a patient identification number, abbreviations used to define a blood component, test codes and names, and number of days data are retained in active records.

Although two computer systems may have the same hardware and software, they are not exactly the same because of institutional variation in the locally defined information, software options chosen, and operating policies and procedures of the institution. Thus, before use a computer system must be tested as set up by the facility to determine that it performs as expected.[1,2]

Interpretation	Tech	Date
O Neg shb 4/25/03		
A ~~Pos~~	shb	4/24/03

Fig. 22-6 Correcting an entry.

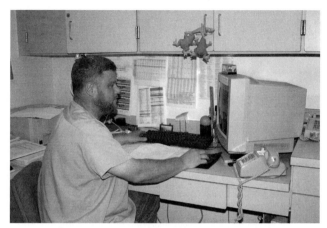

Fig. 22-7 Using computers for record keeping.

Computer Records

Computer-stored records and printed computer reports must meet the same requirements as a manual paper records system.[2] Confidentiality must be maintained,[3] and the procedure manuals must describe the computerized record-keeping system. When computer records are modified, the record must indicate that the record was changed and the original record must be retrievable. When a computer system is used to maintain records and assist in decision making, there must be documentation of the following:[2]

Program development, if done internally

Installation of the system

Validation of functionality and data integrity

Training of personnel

Policies and procedures for system maintenance and operations

Defining the System and Control Functions

Some computer systems primarily perform reporting and billing functions and maintain a log of blood component final dispositions. Most systems capture actual test results and perform a number of **control functions.** System interpretation of results, prohibition of action, and provision of information that a scientist uses to make decisions are control points. For example, if the computer interprets the ABO and Rh test results to conclude group A Rh positive, the computer is performing a control function.

For the system to be used effectively, the users must understand how it operates and the limitations of the system.[7,8] Diagrams of the hardware configuration and documentation manuals that outline the interactions of the system are required. A narrative description of how the computer operations replace the manual system and definition of the computer critical control functions assist users in understanding how their system works. The institutionally defined options (parameters),

Control functions: Computer functions in which the computer provides interpretations or suggests actions, that is, serves in a consultative role. Examples of a control function are the interpretation of serologic data and suggestions for further testing, limitations on outdates of components, and prevention of the release of ABO- and Rh-incompatible blood.

such as test code names, abbreviations, and operating options, are based on how the system is intended to operate. Then standard operating procedures can be written (the procedure manual) to perform specific tasks. This is termed "integration" of the computer into ongoing operations.

System Security

Methods for ensuring the security of data and programs must be set.[8] Systems vary in how security is accomplished. The ability to view data, record information, modify or delete records, and modify the operating parameters requires different levels of system access. Passwords, program restrictions, and terminal lockouts may be used to prevent unauthorized access. Passwords should be changed frequently to prevent unauthorized use. Passwords must not be given to others. In most facilities, sharing passwords is cause for disciplinary action up to and including discharge.

VALIDATION AND TESTING

Once all of the operating parameters are set, users must be trained and the system must be tested to determine if it is functioning as expected. The extent of control over laboratory operations influences the extent of testing required before a computer system may be used in the laboratory.[2,7-9] If the computer system is used to prevent the issue of outdated or incompatible components, the function must be tested or "validated." The **validation** of the computer system is analogous to the testing required of other laboratory instruments. It must be tested initially and after modification.[2,7,8] The entire system must be included in the test to make sure that each application program has the screen displays, prompts, messages, and blocks that are needed. Each method of data entry (keyboard, computer transfer, bar-code reader) and method of sorting and retrieving data (computer screens or printed report), as well as purging and restoring data from tape or disk, are tested. The system security must be tested to ensure that unauthorized individuals cannot access or alter data records.[7] Although parallel testing (simultaneous use of both manual and computer record keeping) is frequently used to test a system, additional test challenges that include unusual scenarios and deliberate tests to evaluate the control mechanisms must be included. For example, if the computer system is expected to prevent incompatible blood from being released, the system must be tested to determine if it allows appropriate units to be issued and blocks incompatible units. The system should be tested to determine if it detects invalid entries such as the letter "O" instead of zeros in a number field.

The evaluation must be documented.[7-9] Required documentation is listed in Summary 22-6. Fig. 22-8 is a test plan for verifying that the computer can detect that an ABO-incompatible unit is being assigned to a patient. Testing documents must contain both the testing input and the output. The input, such as the patient identification, blood component identification, and results entered, must produce the expected output, such as the acceptance or rejection of an attempted issue of a blood unit. If errors are detected, the source of the problem must be found, the problem fixed, and the system retested before implementation.

While the system is in use, it should be monitored for proper function.[2,7,8] Errors or problems must be documented. Fig. 22-9 is a form for recording computer problems. Although the cause of problems is most often user error, software programming errors (bugs) may be found in commercially available software. Problem tracking identifies training or procedure deficiencies, as well as the need for software changes.

Control of Computer Changes

When it is necessary to make changes in the system, the system must be retested to determine that the operations have not been compromised by the change.[7-9]

Validation: Testing whether the computer system does what it purports to do. Documentation of computer validation is required.

Summary 22-6

Evaluation Documentation Requirements

Intentions/expectations
Evaluation plan
Who is responsible?
What was done?
When was it done?
What were the results?
What were the conclusions?
Review and approval
Implementation date

Municipal Blood Bank
Computer Change and Validation Report

Program/module environment	Product modification vendor change notice #66543 Certification environment
Description	To verify that the system warns the user when a new product's expire date is greater than the maximum allowed. The following scenarios tested: • When the expire date is greater than the original product • When the expire date is greater than the original product and the modification conversation is backdated • When an invalid expire date is entered for the new product
Expectations/ critical points	The message "Days entered is greater than maximum allowed" if: • The days entered for a new product is greater than the expire date of the original product • The days entered for a new product is greater than the expire date of the original product when the modification conversation is backdated • An invalid expire date is entered for the new product
Validation plan	1. Print table 1150 2. Follow client certification guidelines for Scenario 1-4 - see attachment 3. Use downtime forms to record data input 4. Attach hard copies of output to downtime form
Impact/repetitions	One
Criteria for acceptance	"Days entered is greater than maximum allowed" as described in in expectations/critical points.

Plan approved by: _____GGF_____ **Date:** _____7/15/04_____

Testing performed by: _____ **Date:** _____

Testing results   Criteria for acceptance is met.

Decision   **Acceptable:** _____ **Not acceptable:** _____

Corrective action:

Retested by: _____ **Date:** _____

Conclusion: **Acceptable:** _____ **Not acceptable:** _____

Final review by: _____ **Date:** _____

Fig. 22-8 Change validation plan and report.

Municipal Blood Bank
Laboratory Information System Computer Problem Report

Date/time: _____ Reported by: _____ Lab: _____ Phone: _____

Patient name _____

Med record no. (__) _____ Specimen accession no. ___ - ___ - ___

Unit no. _____ Component: _____

Error message displayed

Problem description

Is the problem reproducible?   N   Y
Hard copy examples provided: N   Y
- LIS STAFF USE BELOW THE LINE - - - - - - - - - - -

Report received by_____ Date/time_____

LIS immediate action/response

- -
Reported to vendor _____ on ___/___/___ By_____ Service request # _____
Resolution:

- -
Person who reported the problem notified?   N   Y   Other users notified?   N   Y
Final resolution on (date)___ / ___ / ____   Completed by: _____

Bill or credit patient

Date_____ Clerical ID _____

Form# C12345   Rev MM/DD/YYYY

Fig. 22-9 Computer problem report form.

A change may be something as simple as adding a new test code or comment, or it may be the installation of revised software (upgrades). The change and the testing must be documented. A log of changes helps to identify the source of problems that may not have been detected during the validation procedure (Fig. 22-10).

Down Time and Manual Backup Procedures

Most computer systems have down time associated with maintenance and version changes. In addition, any system may have unexpected computer malfunctions. During these periods, a manual record-keeping system is necessary in order to continue operations.[2] The form displayed in Fig. 22-1 could be used to collect type and screen and serologic crossmatch information when a computer is not available.

Municipal Blood Bank
Change Planning and Validation

Description of new/revised policy or procedure and process validation:

Use EDTA tubes for routine pretransfusion and prenatal ABO, Rh, antibody screen, antibody identification, and titers.

The purpose of the change is to facilitate automation. The change will reduce and eventually eliminate the use of 3, 5, 7, and 15 mL red-topped tubes.

The plan needs to be coordinated with and communicated to Materials Services, Plebotomy, Nursing Services, Outpatient Clinics, and Outreach clients.

References:

Westhoff CM, Sipherd BL, Toalson LD. Advantages of EDTA Plasma in Transfusion Service Testing. Lab Med 25:573, 1994.

Menitove J. Standards for Blood Banks and Transfusion Services, Bethesda, MD, American Association of Blood Banks, 2003.

Training/Inservice needed? (if yes, describe plan) __√__Yes _____No

1. Change information in the Pathology and MLabs handbooks at the next revision
2. Modify SOPs for main laboratory
3. Issue notice in the Spectrum
4. Notice in communication notes
5. Distribute fliers
6. Complete direct observation and paper/pencil test competency assessment
7. Develop audit of compliance

Evaluation of effectiveness:

Initial evaluation after 1 month and final evaluation after 3 months.
Criteria for success: 90% of specimens submitted in EDTA tubes. No problems arising from change.

Reviewed by: _____   Date: _____

Final review of effectiveness:

Comments:

Reviewed by: _____
Date: _____
QA 96   Rev 9/04

Fig. 22-10 Computer change log form.

Once functionality has been restored, a plan for verifying computer function and data integrity, as well as entry of manually collected information, is required. In addition, a disaster recovery plan for extended down periods and recovery of lost data is necessary.[7]

Bar Codes and Uniform Blood Labeling

A significant advantage of a computer system is the reduction of clerical errors such as transcription and labeling errors. This advantage can be enhanced by the use of bar codes and the uniform blood labeling system. *ISBT 128,* an international system of identifying a unit of blood by country, donor site, and individual

Collection Date   N 29433

EXPIRES
6-5-2004 15:42

FORM #S-1052PK

FORM #3135CM

PLATELETS POOLED
LEUKOCYTES REDUCED

Approx. 200 mL from
CP2D Anticoagulant
Store at 20°–24° C

12061

See Circular of Information for
indications, contraindications,
cautions, and methods of infusion.

VOLUNTEER DONOR

This product may transmit infectious agents.

℞ ONLY

Properly Identify Intended Recipient

AB
Rh NEGATIVE

Accurate Blood Center
Home town, VA

Registration # 1111111

W1234 96 **123456** ⧺ | S |

Accurate Blood Center
Anywhere, Worldwide

FDA Registration Number _____
US License Number _____

Properly Identify Intended Recipient

See Circular of Information for indications, contraindications, cautions, and
methods of infustion. This product may transmit infectious agents.

℞ only
VOLUNTEER DONOR

8400

AB
Rh POSITIVE

9972322359

RED BLOOD CELLS
ADENINE-SALINE (AS-1) ADDED

From 450 mL CPD Whole Blood
Store at 1° to 6° C

9972322359

Expiration
Date

20 AUG 2005

Special Testing label goes here

1BA04R1424

0M96B28044

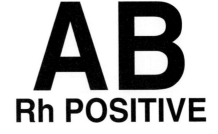

Fig. 22-11 Bar-coded blood bag labels.

donor, is being implemented.[10] The list of bar codes for specific products is being expanded to include more components. Systems are being expanded to include bedside verification of blood component compatibility. Fig. 22-11 pictures blood labels using Codabar and *ISBT 128* bar codes.

Although it may appear that the record keeping and testing associated with the use of computer systems are onerous, the additional speed and accuracy are well worth the effort. The use of computers and bar codes will undoubtedly increase in an effort to reduce errors.

CHAPTER SUMMARY

1. A record-keeping system must be in place to trace the significant steps in the processing of donor blood and patient samples and must include the final disposition of units.
2. The record-keeping system may be manual, computerized, or a combination of both methods.
3. The system must be documented.
4. Symbols and abbreviations used must be defined.
5. Both results and conclusions must be recorded.
6. Records must be retrievable in a reasonable period of time.
7. The system must ensure confidentiality and security of the information.
8. Records must include reports of testing, transfusion reactions, errors, and accidents.
9. Records must be legible and corrections must be identifiable.
10. If a computer system is used, it must be tested to ensure that it operates as expected (validated). Critical control functions are to be tested using both usual and unusual occurrences, as well as invalid entries.

REFERENCES

1. 21 Code of Federal Regulations, Parts 200-299, 606.160, 606.170.
2. Blood Bank/Transfusion Service Standards Program Unit: Standards for Blood Banks and Transfusion Services, 22nd ed. Bethesda, MD, American Association of Blood Banks, 2003.
3. 45 Code of Federal Regulations, Parts 160 and 164, Standards for Privacy of Individually Identifiable Health Information.
4. Quality systems. In Brecher ME (ed): Technical Manual. Bethesda, MD, American Association of Blood Banks, 2002.
5. Clinical and Laboratory Standards Institute: Clinical Laboratory Technical Procedures Manuals, 4th ed. GP2-A4. Wayne, PA, National Committee for Clinical Laboratory Standards, 2002.
6. Food and Drug Administration: Reporting Biological Deviations in Manufacturing, Final Rule. November 7, 2000.
7. Food and Drug Administration: Draft Guidelines for Validation of Blood Establishment Computer Systems. Rockville, MD, Food and Drug Administration, 1994.
8. Center for Devices and Radiological Health, Food and Drug Administration: General Principles of Software Validation; Final Guidance for Industry and FDA Staff. January 11, 2002.
9. College of American Pathologists: Commission of Laboratory Accreditation. Inspection checklist (Section I, Laboratory General—Computer Services). Northfield, IL, College of American Pathologists, 2002.
10. United States Industry Consensus Standard for the Uniform Labeling of Blood and Blood Components Using ISBT-128. November 19, 1999.

FURTHER READING

21 Code of Federal Regulations, Part 11, Electronic Records and Signatures.
21 Code of Federal Regulations 606.10, Automatic, Mechanical, and Electronic Equipment, 211.68: Standard Operating Procedures.

Butch SH, Simpson MD: Information Technology in Transfusion Medicine. Bethesda, MD, American Association of Blood Banks, 2002.

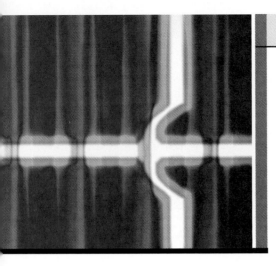

Study Questions and Answers

Chapter 1

1. Mendel made a series of crosses between true-breeding strains of plants that differed by only one characteristic: short versus tall plants. The first filial generation was all tall plants. Which of the following statements describes the relationship between the tall and short traits?
   A. Tall is a dominant trait.
   B. Tall is an incomplete dominant trait.
   C. Short is a dominant trait.
   D. Tall and short are codominant traits.

2. From monohybrid crosses Mendel determined that yellow pea seeds (Y) are dominant and green seeds (y) are recessive. When heterozygous yellow-seeded plants are crossed with green-seeded plants, what is the expected ratio of yellow to green seeds in the offspring?
   A. 3 yellow to 1 green
   B. 2 yellow to 2 green
   C. 1 yellow to 3 green
   D. All yellow

3. The product of meiosis is:
   A. Gametes with twice the genetic complement of the mother cell.
   B. Gametes with one half the genetic complement of the mother cell.
   C. Gametes with the same genetic complement as the mother cell.
   D. Cells identical to the mother cell.

4. When studying a pedigree it was noted that the trait was transmitted by affected fathers to all of their daughters and none of their sons. The pattern of inheritance of this trait is:
   A. X-linked recessive.
   B. X-linked dominant.
   C. Autosomal recessive.
   D. Autosomal dominant.

5. The simultaneous transmission of nonallelic genes through successive generations violates Mendel's Law of Independent Assortment. This phenomenon is termed:
   A. Incomplete dominance.
   B. Crossing over.
   C. Linkage.
   D. Polymorphism.

6. Mr. Smith was admitted to your institution for surgery. The physician has ordered four units of blood. Mr. Smith's presurgical testing showed that he has an anti-C and anti-D. Approximately how many units of ABO-compatible blood would you have to screen to find four that are negative for both C and D antigens?
   Antigen Frequencies
   D positive: 85%
   C positive: 70%
   A. 10
   B. 45
   C. 60
   D. 89

Two hypothetical blood group antigens, T and R, are coded for by two codominant alleles, T and R. In the population, 25% of the individuals are T positive and R negative, whereas 9.5% are positive for both the T and R antigens. Using these data, answer questions 7 and 8:

7. What is the frequency of the *T* gene in the population?
   A. 3%
   B. 5%
   C. 9%
   D. 25%

8. A patient has an anti-R and the blood bank wishes to find blood that is negative for the R antigen for transfusion. Which of the following mathematical equations would be used to calculate the percentage of population that would meet these transfusion criteria?

Key:

p = frequency of the *T* gene
q = frequency of the *R* gene
A. p^2
B. q^2
C. $2pq$
D. $p^2 + 2pq$

9. In the pedigree at top right, identify the inheritance pattern of the trait indicated.
A. Autosomal dominant
B. X-linked dominant
C. Autosomal recessive
D. X-linked recessive

10. The pattern of inheritance **MOST** frequently expressed by blood group genes is:
A. Autosomal dominant.
B. Autosomal recessive.
C. Autosomal codominant.
D. Sex-linked codominant.

11. In a family study, the mother's red cell genotype is SS and the father's is ss. What are the possibilities for the genotypes of the children?
A. 25% SS; 50% Ss; 25% ss
B. 50% SS; 50% ss
C. 75% Ss; 25% ss
D. 100% Ss

12. Molecular antigen typing techniques could potentially yield more reliable information than traditional hemagglutination techniques in each of the following situations **EXCEPT:**
A. Testing samples from patients who have recently been transfused.
B. Testing samples from patients whose red cells are coated with immunoglobulin.
C. Testing sera for the presence of ABO system antibodies.
D. Forensic testing of blood from a crime scene.

13. The following enzyme allows for the analysis of viral RNA in donor blood by PCR:
A. Reverse transcriptase.
B. T4 ligase.
C. RFLP.
D. Eco RI.

14. The technique in which DNA sequences are identified by hybridization with labeled probes is:
A. Northern blotting.
B. Western blotting.
C. Fluorescence in situ hybridization (FISH).
D. Southern blotting.

15. In humans, the physiologic function of the *RHD* gene, which codes for the normal $Rh_o(D)$ antigen, would **BEST** be explored by examining red cells from individuals of the following phenotype:
A. $Rh_o(D)$ positive.
B. Rh null.
C. $Rh_o(D)$ negative.
D. AB.

Chapter 2

1. Processes of the adaptive immune system include:
A. Production of antibody on exposure to foreign antigens.
B. Inflammation.
C. Increased capillary permeability.
D. Phagocytosis of viral particles.

2. The change in production of IgM to IgG is an example of:
A. Epitope switching.
B. Isotype switching.
C. Immune surveillance.
D. Antibody specificity.

3. Which of the following is an example of innate immunity?
A. Antigen processing by APCs
B. Antibody production
C. Phagocytosis
D. Graft rejection

4. The tuberculin skin test reaction is an example of what type of immune response?
A. Production of humoral antibody
B. Antibody-independent cell-mediated cytotoxicity
C. Delayed hypersensitivity
D. Antibody-dependent cell-mediated cytotoxicity

5. In humans B cells mature in:
A. The bursa.
B. The liver.
C. The bone marrow.
D. The thymus.

6. Tissue macrophages can be found in:
   A. The spleen.
   B. The liver.
   C. Lymph nodes.
   D. All of the above.

7. Human B cells carry which cell surface markers?
   A. Immunoglobulin
   B. Fc receptors
   C. CD4 antigen
   D. B antigen

8. Analysis of T-cell subsets has shown that approximately what percentage of T cells are helper T cells?
   A. 35%
   B. 50%
   C. 65%
   D. 80%

9. In general, antibody produced to T-independent antigens is:
   A. IgA.
   B. IgD.
   C. IgG.
   D. IgM.

10. For an immune process to take place, the antigen-processing cells and helper T cells must have compatible:
   A. Fc receptors.
   B. Major histocompatibility antigens.
   C. Monokines.
   D. CD4 antigens.

11. Which is true of the primary immune response?
   A. Antibody may be detected within hours of antigen stimulation.
   B. Antibody is of relatively low titer.
   C. Antibody is of relatively high titer.
   D. Antibody is predominantly of the IgG class.

12. Which of the following is true of immunoglobulins (Ig) of the IgM class?
   A. They are the most abundant in human serum.
   B. They exist only as monomers.
   C. They are the only Ig class that crosses the placenta.
   D. Each molecule has a J chain.

13. The major factor affecting the electrostatic repulsion between red cells is the:
   A. Dielectric constant.
   B. pH of the medium.
   C. Zeta potential.
   D. Immunoglobulin class.

14. An agglutination reaction in which there are many small agglutinates in a turbid background would be graded as:
   A. 1+.
   B. 2+.
   C. 3+.
   D. 4+.

15. The direct antiglobulin test is useful for which of the following?
   A. The detection of hemolytic disease of the newborn
   B. The identification of unknown serum alloantibodies
   C. The identification of antigens on the surface of red cells
   D. The determination of compatibility between donor and recipient red cells

16. A patient has been transfused with two units of blood. The recipient was previously sensitized to the antigens present on the transfused red cells and has an anamnestic response. Which of the following would **MOST** probably be true of this case?
   A. The transfused red cells will survive normally.
   B. The patient will have no physical signs.
   C. The patient will shift from IgM to IgG production.
   D. Antibody production will not take place for at least 2 weeks.

17. Interleukin-3 is a substance that stimulates T-cell proliferation and is an example of:
   A. A red cell alloantibody.
   B. A skin-reactive factor.
   C. A red cell membrane glycophorin.
   D. A lymphokine.

18. The "attack sequence" of the classic complement pathway includes:
   A. C1q, C1r, and C1s.
   B. C2, C3, and C4.
   C. C1 through C9.
   D. C6 through C9.

19. The following statement best describes which of the antiglobulin reagents? "Contains anti-IgG and anti-C3d; may contain other anticomplement and other anti-Ig activities."
   A. Polyspecific antihuman globulin
   B. Anti-IgG
   C. Anti-IgG (heavy chain)
   D. Anti-C3d (murine monoclonal)

20. NK cells arise from which precursor cell?
    A. Hematopoietic stem cell
    B. Granulocyte/monocyte precursor
    C. B-cell progenitor
    D. Lymphopoietic stem cell

21. Class I MHC recognition molecules:
    A. Present processed antigen derived from intracellular sources.
    B. Present processed antigen derived from extracellular sources.
    C. Bind the recognition unit, C1q-C1r-C1s, of the complement system.
    D. Appear only on antigen-presenting cells.

22. Class II MHC recognition molecules:
    A. Present processed antigen derived from intracellular sources.
    B. Present processed antigen derived from extracellular sources.
    C. Act as co-receptors to stimulate effector functions in cytotoxic T cells.
    D. Are expressed by most cell types.

23. Cells targeted by cytotoxins:
    A. Up-regulate macrophages to increase phagocytosis.
    B. Down-regulate antibody production.
    C. Die through apoptosis.
    D. Fuse to form hybridomas.

24. A decrease in functional T_H2 cells could result in:
    A. Decrease in cytotoxin production.
    B. Down-regulation of macrophage clearance of extracellular pathogens.
    C. Increase in opsonization.
    D. Down-regulation of antibody production.

25. Cytokines are effector molecules with:
    A. Cytotoxic functions.
    B. Regulatory functions.
    C. MHC-independent functions.
    D. T-cell–independent functions.

26. Isotype switching is directed by:
    A. Macrophages.
    B. Dendritic cells.
    C. T_H2 cells.
    D. T_H1 cells.

27. All of the following are characteristics of NK cells **EXCEPT:**
    A. They produce cytotoxins.
    B. They possess MHC class I receptors.
    C. Affinity maturation does not occur in their effector responses.
    D. They are guided by immunologic memory.

28. Based on sequence homology, immunoglobulins and T-cell receptors are:
    A. In the immunoglobulin superfamily.
    B. Components of MHC class I and II molecules.
    C. Macrophage recognition molecules.
    D. Both on dendritic cells.

29. The diversity of the B- and T-cell response to immune challenge is the result of:
    A. Clonal selection.
    B. Clonal expansion.
    C. Germ line gene rearrangement.
    D. Linkage disequilibrium.

30. All of the following are examples of type II hypersensitivity reactions **EXCEPT:**
    A. Hemolytic transfusion reaction.
    B. Hemolytic disease of the newborn.
    C. Autoimmune hemolytic anemia.
    D. Hyperacute organ rejection.

Chapter 3

1. Which of the following statements is **NOT** true of the H antigen?
   A. Inheritance of the H antigen is necessary for the normal expression of the ABO antigens.
   B. The amount of H antigen varies for different ABO types.
   C. The antibody directed toward the H antigen (anti-H) is naturally occurring in the serum of most adults.
   D. H antigen may be present in the secretions.

2. Which of the following is true of type 2 precursor chains?
   A. They have a β1-3 linkage between the terminal sugars.
   B. They are found only as glycolipids on the red cell membrane.
   C. They are found only as glycoproteins in body secretions.
   D. They are found both as glycoproteins in body secretions and as glycolipids on the red cell surface.

3. An individual has the following ABH genotype: *AO, hh*. Which of the following antigens would be present on the red cells of this individual?
   A. A only
   B. A and H
   C. A and O
   D. None of the above

4. A group A man marries a group AB woman. The father of the group A man was group O. What possible ABO groups would be expected from this mating?
   A. A, B, AB, and O
   B. A and B
   C. A, B, and AB
   D. A and AB

5. Given the data in question 4, what percentage of the offspring could be expected to be group A?
   A. 5%
   B. 25%
   C. 50%
   D. 75%

6. Which of the following is true regarding the ABO serology of newborns?
   A. ABH antigens are complex branched structures.
   B. ABH antigens are strongly expressed at 5 to 6 weeks of gestation.
   C. ABO antibodies are produced at birth.
   D. None of the above.

7. Which of the following is true of anti-A,B but not true of anti-A and anti-B?
   A. Anti-A,B efficiently binds complement.
   B. Anti-A,B is present in the serum of group O individuals.
   C. Anti-A,B is clinically significant.
   D. Anti-A,B is predominantly IgM.

8. A patient has the following serologic results:

Anti-A	Anti-B	Anti-A,B	A_1 Cells	B Cells
4+	0	4+	2+	4+

Which of the following causes would be the **BEST** explanation for these results?
   A. An elderly patient
   B. A subgroup of A
   C. Hypogammaglobulinemia
   D. Deterioration of reagents

9. A patient has the following ABO typing results:

Anti-A	Anti-B	Anti-A,B	A_1 Cells	B Cells
4+	4+	4+	0	0

This patient's ABO blood type is:
   A. O
   B. A
   C. AB
   D. Not able to be determined with the information given

10. Given the typing results in question 9, indicate what ABO type red cells (plasma removed) could be safely selected for transfusion to this patient.
    A. AB
    B. AB or O
    C. AB, O, A, or B
    D. O

11. The products of genes inherited at the *ABO* locus are:
    A. Carbohydrates.
    B. Glycolipids.
    C. Transferases.
    D. Kinases.

12. The immunodominant sugar that confers B blood group specificity is:
    A. l-fucose.
    B. d-galactose.
    C. *N*-acetylgalactosamine.
    D. l-glucose.

13. The *O* gene has no detectable product and is therefore termed:
    A. Recessive.
    B. Dominant.
    C. Codominant.
    D. Amorphic.

14. A transfusion error in which group A blood is transfused to a group O recipient could result in:
    A. Rapid destruction of transfused red cells.
    B. Renal failure.
    C. Disseminated intravascular coagulation.
    D. All of the above.

Chapter 4

1. All of the following statements are true regarding the Lewis blood group system **EXCEPT:**
   A. Lewis antigens are soluble antigens found in body fluids.
   B. Lewis phenotypes in the secretions result from the interaction of the *Se* and *Le* genes.
   C. All Lewis antigens are type 1 structures.
   D. Lewis phenotypes in the secretions depend on the interaction of *ABO* genes and *Le* genes.

2. Which of the following statements is true of the secretor system?
   A. The gene *Se(FUT2)* is necessary for the secretion of soluble Le^a substance.
   B. Approximately 20% of the population is secretors.
   C. Homozygous *sese* individuals secrete ABH antigens.
   D. Secretion of the Le^b antigen substance depends on the interaction of the *Le* and *Se* genes.

3. The *Se(FUT2)* gene codes for the production of which of the following enzymes?
   A. Glucosyltransferase
   B. Galactosyltransferase
   C. *N*-acetylgalactosyltransferase
   D. Fucosyltransferase

4. Type 1 H antigen in secretions is a product of which of the following genes?
   A. Le
   B. H
   C. Se
   D. le

5. Most newborns type as which of the following Lewis phenotypes?
   A. Le(a–b–)
   B. Le(a+b–)
   C. Le(a–b+)
   D. Le(a+b+)

Use the following answer key for questions 6 through 14:
   A. 1 and 2 are correct.
   B. 1, 2, and 3 are correct.
   C. Only 2 is correct.
   D. All of the responses are correct.

6. A patient has the following genotype: *AO, sese, Lele, Hh*. Which of the following soluble antigens is (are) present in the saliva?
   1. A
   2. Le^a
   3. H
   4. Le^b

7. Using the information in question 6, which of the following antigens is/are present on the red blood cells of this patient?
   1. A
   2. Le^a
   3. H
   4. Le^b

8. A patient has the following genotype: *OO, SeSe, lele, Hh*. Which of the following antigens would be present in the saliva?
   1. Type 1 H
   2. Type 2 H
   3. Le^a
   4. Le^b

9. A patient has group A Le(a–b+) red cells. Which of the following statements is (are) true regarding this patient?
   1. The patient is a secretor.
   2. The patient has group A substance in his or her saliva.
   3. The patient has some Le^a antigen in his or her saliva.
   4. The patient has inherited at least one *H* gene.

10. Which of the following statements is (are) true of anti-Le^a?
    1. It is made by Le(a–b–) secretors.
    2. It is usually clinically insignificant.
    3. It sometimes activates complement.
    4. It causes severe hemolytic disease of the newborn.

11. Which of the following cells would be expected to react strongly with anti-Le^{bH}?
    1. A$_1$, Le(a–b+)
    2. O, Le(a–b+)
    3. O, Le(a–b–)
    4. A$_1$, Le(a+b–)

12. Which of the following statements describe anti-I?
    1. It is a fairly common autoantibody.
    2. It reacts optimally at 4° C.
    3. It is associated with cold agglutinin syndrome.
    4. It may be associated with *Mycoplasma pneumoniae* infection.

13. Which of the following antigens is (are) present on the red cells of an individual of the P$_1$ phenotype?
    1. P$_1$
    2. P
    3. P^k
    4. P$_2$

14. Which of the following statements is (are) true regarding anti-P$_1$?
    1. It is usually clinically insignificant.
    2. It is produced by P$_2$ individuals.
    3. It shows variable reactivity with a panel of random P$_1$-positive red cells.
    4. It is inhibited by hydatid cyst fluid.

Chapter 5

1. The specificity of the antibody described by Landsteiner and Wiener that was produced in rabbits injected with rhesus monkey red cells was later found to be:
   A. Anti-D.
   B. Anti-C.
   C. Anti-LW.
   D. Anti-Rh29.

2. Anti-D is a clinically significant antibody because:
   A. It is capable of activating complement.
   B. It is naturally occurring in all D-negative healthy adults.
   C. It can cause hemolytic transfusion reactions.
   D. It does not cross the placenta.

3. A patient has the following Rh antigen typing (phenotyping) results: D+, C+, E−, c−, e+. The patient could have which of the following Rh haplotypes?
   A. R_1R_1
   B. R_2r'
   C. rr
   D. r'r

4. The frequency of the R_0 haplotype in the white population is:
   A. 0.42.
   B. 0.37.
   C. 0.14.
   D. 0.04.

5. The frequency of the r haplotype in the black population is 0.26. Given a sample of 50 persons from this population, how many would you predict to be rr?
   A. 3
   B. 6
   C. 9
   D. 12

6. A patient types as D-negative with high-protein anti-D at immediate spin and 37° C incubation. The test is positive at the antihuman globulin phase of testing. The Rh control is negative throughout. This patient should receive:
   A. D-positive blood only.
   B. D-negative blood only.
   C. D-negative blood usually.
   D. No blood until further testing is performed to determine the D type of the patient.

7. The **MOST** common cause of false-positive anti-D testing is:
   A. The deterioration of reagents.
   B. Failure to follow manufacturer's directions.
   C. Spontaneous agglutination of red cells due to a positive DAT.
   D. Rouleaux formation.

8. Which of the following Rh phenotypes would be positive for the compound antigen ce(f)?
   A. CDe/cDE
   B. cDE/Cde
   C. cde/cde
   D. All of the above

9. Which of the following is (are) true of amorph type Rh_{null} patients?
   A. They are LW(a−b−).
   B. They have abnormal red cell survival.
   C. They demonstrate stomatocytes in peripheral blood smears.
   D. All of the above.

10. Patient number 1 has the following phenotype: Cde/CDe, LW^aLW^a. Patient number 2 has the following phenotype: Cde/cde, LW^aLW^a. Which of the following statements **BEST** describes the relative expression of LW antigens by these patients?
    A. Patient number 1 will produce more LW^a than patient number 2.
    B. Patient number 1 will produce less LW^a than patient number 2.
    C. Both patients will produce the same amount of LW^a.
    D. Neither patient will produce LW^a.

Chapter 6

1. The mode of inheritance of the Kell antigens K(KEL 1) and k(KEL 2) is:
   A. X-linked dominant.
   B. X-linked recessive.
   C. Autosomal recessive.
   D. Autosomal codominant.

2. In vitro preparation of K_0 cells can be accomplished by the treatment of red cells with which of the following?
   A. Ficin
   B. ZZAP (dithiothreitol plus cystein-activated papain)
   C. 2-aminoethylisothiouronium bromide (AET)
   D. Both B and C are correct

3. Which of the following is true of the antibody anti-Kx?
    A. It does not react with red cells from patients with the McLeod phenotype.
    B. It reacts strongly with K_0 red cells.
    C. Both A and B are correct.
    D. Neither A nor B is correct.

4. Which of the following is associated with the McLeod syndrome?
    A. Reticulocytosis and decreased haptoglobin levels
    B. Increased levels of creatinine phosphokinase (MM band)
    C. Both A and B
    D. Neither A nor B

5. Genes at the *MN* locus are responsible for the production of which of the following?
    A. MN sialoglycoprotein
    B. Glycophorin A
    C. A transmembrane, glycosylated protein
    D. All of the above

6. The En(a–) phenotype results in:
    A. The absence of glycophorin A on the red cells.
    B. Increased expression of MN antigens on the red cell.
    C. The absence of the Ss sialoglycoprotein on the red cells.
    D. The diminished expression of the U antigen on the red cells.

7. An individual who is M+N+U– lacks which of the following antigens?
    A. S
    B. M
    C. 'N'
    D. En^a

8. Which of the following techniques/reagents may be useful in increasing the reactivity of anti-M?
    A. Papain pretreated cells
    B. Anticomplement antihuman globulin reagents
    C. Acidified serum techniques
    D. Heterozygous MN cells

9. Of the following MNSs system antibodies, which is almost always cold-reacting, IgM, and clinically insignificant?
    A. Anti-S
    B. Anti-U
    C. Anti-s
    D. Anti-N

10. Anti-Fy3 reacts with cells from individuals with which of the following genotypes?
    A. FyFy
    B. Fy4Fy4
    C. Both A and B
    D. Neither A nor B

11. Which of the following techniques/reagents is useful in the detection of anti-Fy^a?
    A. Heat-treatment of red cells at 56° C
    B. Ficin pretreatment of red cells
    C. Indirect antiglobulin technique
    D. Incubation at room temperature and below

12. Anti-Fy^a and anti-Fy^b are implicated in which of the following?
    A. Hemolytic transfusion reactions
    B. Hemolytic disease of the newborn
    C. Both A and B
    D. Neither A nor B

13. Which of the following antigens is a weakened form of the Fy^b antigen?
    A. Fy
    B. Fy^x
    C. Fy3
    D. Fy4

14. Which of the following red cell phenotypes would be the **LEAST** susceptible to infection with *Plasmodium vivax*?
    A. Fy(a–b–)
    B. Fy(a+b+)
    C. Fy(a–b+)
    D. Fy(a+b–)

15. Which of the following techniques/reagents would be the **LEAST** useful in the detection of anti-Jk^a?
    A. Low ionic strength saline (LISS)
    B. Proteolytic enzymes
    C. Polyethylene glycol (PEG)
    D. Saline room temperature

16. All of the following statements are true of anti-Jk^a **EXCEPT:**
    A. It is often implicated in delayed hemolytic transfusion reactions.
    B. The strength of in vitro reactions correlates well with the degree of in vivo red cell destruction.
    C. It often reacts only with homozygous Jk^a-positive red cells.
    D. It decreases in strength during storage.

17. The Lutheran null phenotype may be inherited by which of the following mechanisms?
    A. Inheritance of a dominant suppressor gene
    B. Inheritance of two recessive null genes at the *LU* locus
    C. Inheritance of a gene on the X chromosome
    D. All of the above

18. Which of the following is true of the Lutheran blood group system?
    A. Anti-Lu^a is often naturally occurring.
    B. Anti-Lu^a is associated with severe hemolytic transfusion reactions.
    C. Anti-Lu^a and anti-Lu^b are frequently implicated in hemolytic disease of the newborn.
    D. The Lu^a antigen is a high-incidence antigen.

19. Which of the following antigens is destroyed by proteolytic enzymes?
    A. K
    B. Jk^a
    C. Xg^a
    D. Lu^a

20. Which of the following is a low-incidence antigen?
    A. Yt^a (Cartwright)
    B. Co^a (Colton)
    C. k (KEL2 or Cellano)
    D. Di^a (Diego)

21. All of the following statements are true regarding Chido and Rogers **EXCEPT:**
    A. They are antigenic determinants of human complement C4.
    B. Antibodies react strongly with enzyme-premodified red cells.
    C. The antibodies are clinically insignificant.
    D. Antibodies can be neutralized by fresh human serum.

Chapter 7

1. MHC class II molecules are found on the surfaces of which one of the following groups of cells in the body?
   A. All nucleated cells
   B. Macrophages, dendritic cells, and B lymphocytes
   C. All bone marrow–derived cells
   D. Dendritic cells, eosinophils, and basophils

2. Class II MHC proteins are:
   A. Recognized by the CD4 T cells.
   B. Used to mark a cell for killing by CD8 cytotoxic T cells.
   C. Used to participate in CDC.
   D. Encoded by HLA-A, HLA-B, and HLA-C loci.

3. The biologic function of major histocompatibility complex proteins is to:
   A. Degrade CD4 and CD8 polypeptides.
   B. Prevent organ allografts.
   C. Bind complement for cell lysis.
   D. Bind antigen fragments for presentation to T cells.

4. C2, C4, and properdin B are associated with:
   A. Class I HLA loci or gene products.
   B. Class II HLA loci or gene products.
   C. Class III HLA loci or gene products.
   D. Hyperacute allograft rejection.

5. If both the recipient and a sibling inherit the same paternal and maternal sixth chromosomes, they are said to be:
   A. Haploidentical (half matched).
   B. HLA identical.
   C. Clones.
   D. Twins.

6. The HLA antigens from all HLA loci that are inherited on a chromosome are called:
   A. An antigen profile.
   B. A genotype.
   C. Haploidentical.
   D. A haplotype.

7. A high PRA means that the patient:
   A. Has antibody against many HLA antigens.
   B. Has a high level of immunosuppression.
   C. May have a strong cellular rejection response.
   D. Is likely to have a negative crossmatch.

8. What is the **BEST** reason for not routinely performing HLA-C typing on apheresis platelet donors?
   A. Platelets do not have DNA, and therefore it is not possible to type donors for HLA-Cw.
   B. Anti-Cw antibodies are irrelevant in all transplant situations.
   C. Platelets do not express Cw.
   D. Cw is a form of HLA class II, and platelets do not express HLA class II antigens.

9. Which of the following HLA antigens corresponds to Bgb?
   A. HLA-B7
   B. HLA-B17
   C. HLA-B27
   D. HLA-A28

10. A strong linkage disequilibrium exists between:
    A. HLA-A1 and HLA-B8.
    B. HLA-A1 and HLA-B27.
    C. HLA-A30 and HLA-B27.
    D. HLA-A1 and HLA-B45.

11. Which assay is commonly used to identify serologically defined antigens?
    A. MLC
    B. PCR
    C. RFLP
    D. CDC

12. A purified suspension of B lymphocytes is required for:
    A. Class I antigen typing.
    B. HLA-DR and HLA-DQ antigen typing by CDC.
    C. C2, C4, and Factor B typing.
    D. All HLA testing procedures.

13. For solid organ transplants, recipients and donors are often tested for:
    A. HLA-A, HLA-B, and HLA-DR antigens.
    B. HLA-A and HLA-B antigens.
    C. HLA-DR antigens only.
    D. HTLA antigens.

14. A patient with an anti–HLA-A2 antibody would be most likely to have a positive T-cell crossmatch with which of the following donors?
    A. A1, A3, B8, B35, DR4, DR17
    B. A1, A25, B7, B8, DR1, DR17
    C. A24, A68, B7, B64, DR1, DR7
    D. A11, A29, B38, B62, DR4, DR7

15. A PRA specificity of B40, B44, B45, and B49 is **MOST** likely due to:
    A. B7 CREG antibody.
    B. B8 CREG antibody.
    C. B12 CREG antibody.
    D. Multiple specific antibodies.

16. Which of the following diseases is associated with an HLA class I allele?
    A. Ankylosing spondylitis
    B. Type 1 insulin-dependent diabetes mellitus
    C. Narcolepsy
    D. Rheumatoid arthritis

17. Which of the following is true about HLA nomenclature?
    A. The HLA number assigned to an allele represents its location, in centimorgans, from the centromere.
    B. The first two digits of a DNA allele usually correspond to the serologic antigen.
    C. The first two digits of a split represent the parent antigen.
    D. The "w" prefix was dropped from the C locus because of the confusion with the complement factors.

18. A flow cytometric crossmatch was performed for a patient against an unrelated potential donor. Results of the crossmatch were T-cell negative and B-cell positive. The patient's serum **MOST** likely contains:
    A. Anti-HLA class I antibodies.
    B. Anti-HLA class II antibodies.
    C. Anti-HLA class I and anti-HLA class II antibodies.
    D. A high PRA.

19. Antibodies in the serum of a transplant recipient that react with HLA class I (HLA-A, HLA-B, HLA-C) antigens on the donor are particularly dangerous in that they can induce:
    A. Type IV hypersensitivity reactions.
    B. Cytotoxic T cells.
    C. Chronic rejection.
    D. Hyperacute rejection.

20. If the six (6) HLA-A, HLA-B, and HLA-DR genes are compared between a parent and a child, how many would you typically expect to be matched?
    A. 1
    B. 3
    C. 6
    D. Impossible to predict without DNA testing

Chapter 8

1. Which of the following agencies or organizations provides mandatory regulations for transfusion medicine practice?
    A. American Association of Blood Banks (AABB)
    B. College of American Pathology (CAP)
    C. Food and Drug Administration (FDA)
    D. Joint Commission on Accreditation of Healthcare Organizations (JCAHO)

2. The National Committee for Clinical Laboratory Standards provides which of the following services?
    A. Voluntary accreditation
    B. Guidelines for procedure manual formats
    C. Regulations regarding interstate commerce
    D. Good manufacturing practices for blood and blood products

3. Blood donors in the United States make up approximately what percent of the population?
    A. 1%
    B. 4%
    C. 15%
    D. 25%

4. Which of the following is **NOT** an outcome of the donor screening process?
   A. Reduction of the risk of adverse donor reactions
   B. Reduction in the risk of harm to the recipient
   C. Useful health information for the donor
   D. A blood product that will not transmit disease

5. A donor reports that he suffered a nerve injury from a needle-stick injury 3 months ago, but has recovered. All other screening is acceptable. This donor should be:
   A. Allowed to donate.
   B. Deferred for 12 months from the incident.
   C. Deferred for 12 months from the day of screening.
   D. Permanently deferred.

6. A donor with an unacceptable hemoglobin level due to nutritional iron deficiency is deferred for what period?
   A. 6 months
   B. 12 months
   C. Permanently
   D. Until the hemoglobin reaches the acceptable limit

7. Hypertensive donors who are taking medication and who have controlled their blood pressure are:
   A. Acceptable to donate.
   B. Deferred for 6 months.
   C. Deferred for a year.
   D. Permanently deferred.

8. A donor weighing 80 pounds can donate what volume of whole blood?
   A. 450 mL
   B. 405 mL
   C. 385 mL
   D. 325 mL

9. Which of the following is **NOT** true regarding confidential unit exclusion?
   A. The donor form will be held in strict confidence.
   B. The donor blood will not be tested if the donor indicates that his or her blood may not be safe.
   C. The donor will be notified of positive test results.
   D. The excluded unit will not be used for transfusion regardless of the test results.

10. Which of the following is **NOT** characteristic of hyperventilation reactions?
    A. They may be associated with an increased respiratory rate.
    B. They may be associated with an increased depth of respiration.
    C. They result in O_2 depletion.
    D. They result in CO_2 depletion.

11. Which of the following donor records must be maintained indefinitely?
    A. Temporary deferral
    B. Donor typing (ABO and Rh)
    C. Quality control records for typing antisera
    D. Signed consent forms

12. Which of the following blood components may carry a risk of CMV infection?
    A. Fresh Frozen Plasma
    B. Cryoprecipitated AHF
    C. Platelets
    D. All of the above

13. Which of the following is an absolute contraindication to autologous donation?
    A. Weight less than 110 pounds
    B. Bacteremia
    C. Systolic blood pressure of 200 mm Hg
    D. Pulse of 42 beats per minute

14. Which of the following is **NOT** true regarding plateletpheresis donation?
    A. Posttransfusion platelet counts remain close to pretransfusion levels.
    B. Aspirin ingestion is a cause for temporary deferral.
    C. The plateletpheresis product is equivalent to six units of platelet concentrates.
    D. Predonation platelet counts must be $150 \times 10^9/L$ or greater.

15. Why is "NAT" testing used in testing donor blood for WNV, HIV, and HCV?
    A. NAT is a neutralization antibody test that is used to confirm a previously positive result by removing reactive antibodies resulting in a negative test.
    B. NAT is nucleic amplification testing to enhance low quantities of antigen material that can indicate infectious disease before antibodies can be detected.
    C. NAT is a native antibody amplification test to increase the antibody detection levels in blood samples.
    D. None of the above.

16. Bacterial detection testing for platelet concentrate products can be accomplished using which of the following methods?
    A. Swirling a pooled product just before issue for transfusion
    B. A Gram stain of each individual concentrate
    C. A dipstick test of each individual concentrate for pH and glucose levels
    D. Either B or C

17. Bacterial detection testing for platelet products is now mandated because:
    A. Current apheresis platelet storage requirements are favorable for bacterial growth.
    B. The most common transfusion-associated infectious disease risk in the United States is from bacteria in platelets.
    C. It is impossible to collect blood products aseptically no matter what cleansing agents or protocols are used.
    D. All of the above.

Chapter 9

1. Which of the following is **NOT** an advantage of blood component therapy?
    A. It allows for the optimum storage of each component.
    B. It provides products that can better meet patients' individual needs.
    C. It decreases the risk of transfusion-transmitted disease.
    D. It maximizes the use of donated whole blood.

2. Which of the following is **NOT** true of satellite bags?
    A. They serve as the main collection bag for whole blood.
    B. They are sterile and pyrogen free.
    C. They are attached to the collection bag via a sterile tubing system.
    D. They can be used to make smaller aliquots from whole blood collections.

3. In general, which of the following principles apply to the outdate of a component that has been exposed to a nonsterile environment (open system)?
    A. For a product stored at 20° to 24° C, the outdate is changed to 24 hours.
    B. For a product stored at 1° to 6° C, the outdate is changed to 4 hours.
    C. Neither B nor C.
    D. Both B and C.

4. Most components are separated using differential centrifugation, which separates components based on their relative:
    A. Surface charge
    B. Zeta potential
    C. Size
    D. Specific gravity

5. When using a standard 450 mL collection bag, what is the acceptable range for the volume of whole blood collected?
    A. 350 to 550 mL
    B. 400 to 500 mL
    C. 405 to 495 mL
    D. 425 to 475 mL

6. Which of the following is not a licensed anticoagulant/preservative for the collection of whole blood?
    A. Heparin
    B. Acid-citrate-dextrose
    C. Citrate-phosphate-dextrose
    D. Citrate-phosphate-dextrose-adenine

7. The licensure of anticoagulant/preservatives is done by:
    A. American Association of Blood Banks.
    B. Food and Drug Administration.
    C. College of American Pathologists.
    D. American Medical Association.

8. Which of the following is a desirable characteristic for a centrifuge that will be used to separate blood components?
    A. A fixed temperature of 4° C
    B. A fixed temperature of 22° C
    C. Highest yield with the longest spin time
    D. Highest yield with the shortest spin time

9. Of the following criteria, which is used to determine the shelf life of Red Blood Cells?
    A. 65% cell viability in vitro at the end of the storage period
    B. 75% cell viability in vitro at the end of the storage period
    C. 65% of transfused red cells in the recipient's circulation 24 hours after transfusion
    D. 75% of transfused red cells in the recipient's circulation 24 hours after transfusion

10. Whole Blood is generally limited to patients who are:
    A. Normovolemic and hypoxic.
    B. Hypervolemic and hypoxic.
    C. Hypovolemic and hypoxic.
    D. All of the above.

11. When compared with Whole Blood at the end of its shelf life, fresh blood (less than 5 days old) has:
    A. A lower concentration of potassium.
    B. A lower concentration of 2,3-DPG.
    C. A lower concentration of ATP.
    D. All of the above.

12. Which of the following categories of patients may be considered suitable candidates for fresh blood (less than 5 to 7 days)?
    A. Low birth weight infants
    B. Massively transfused patients
    C. Recipients of exchange transfusions
    D. All of the above

13. The separation of plasma from red cells must be done:
    A. Within 4 hours of collection.
    B. Within 8 hours of collection.
    C. Within 24 hours of collection.
    D. Anytime before outdate.

14. Which of the following is true of additive solutions (AS)?
    A. They extend the red cell outdate to 42 days from collection.
    B. They can be prepared up to 3 days after outdate of the original unit.
    C. They have higher hematocrit than red blood cells.
    D. All of the above.

15. A patient who has developed anti-IgA and who has experienced a previous anaphylactic reaction during the transfusion of a Red Blood Cell product should receive which of the following red cell–containing components?
    A. Whole Blood
    B. Red Blood Cells Irradiated
    C. Red Blood Cells Leukocyte Reduced
    D. Red Blood Cells Washed

16. Which of the following is true of the high-glycerol method of freezing Red Blood Cells?
    A. The final concentration of glycerol is 20%.
    B. Glycerol added during preparation is removed before freezing.
    C. The glycerolization process is performed at 25° to 32° C.
    D. Frozen red cells are stored at –20° C.

17. Red Blood Cells in CPDA-1 without additive solution must be frozen:
    A. Within 8 hours of collection.
    B. Within 24 hours of collection.
    C. Within 6 days of collection.
    D. Anytime before the expiration date.

18. Once deglycerolized, Red Blood Cells Frozen are stored at what temperature?
    A. –65° C
    B. –20° C
    C. 1° to 6° C
    D. 20° to 24° C

19. Red Blood Cells Leukocytes Reduced must contain fewer than how many leukocytes?
    A. 5×10^6
    B. 5×10^8
    C. 5×10^{10}
    D. 5×10^{12}

20. The leukocyte-reduction procedure that is most effective in reducing the incidence of cytokine-related reactions in the recipient is:
    A. Centrifugation.
    B. Bedside filtration.
    C. Prestorage laboratory filtration.
    D. Post-storage laboratory filtration.

21. A rare unit of autologous blood was outdated yesterday. The recipient's surgery has been postponed for a month. What procedure would be suitable to preserve this unit?
    A. Addition of AS-1 and continued storage at 1° to 6° C
    B. Addition of AS-1 and preparation for frozen storage using a standard procedure
    C. Addition of a rejuvenation fluid and continued storage at 1° to 6° C
    D. Addition of a rejuvenation fluid and preparation for frozen storage using a standard procedure

22. Administration of a single unit of Platelets should raise the recipient's platelet count by:
    A. 1 to 3×10^9/L.
    B. 3 to 5×10^9/L.
    C. 5 to 10×10^9/L.
    D. 10 to 15×10^9/L.

23. Platelet concentrate quality control data must indicate that at least 75% of the units counted have a minimum platelet count of:
    A. 5.5×10^8.
    B. 5.5×10^{10}.
    C. 1.0×10^8.
    D. 1.0×10^{10}.

24. Preparation of random-donor Platelets from Whole Blood involves the following sequence of steps:
    A. A light spin, separation of platelet-rich plasma, followed by a light spin.
    B. A hard spin, separation of the buffy coat, followed by another hard spin.
    C. A light spin, separation of platelet-rich plasma, followed by hard spin.
    D. A hard spin, separation of platelet-rich plasma, followed by light spin.

25. The minimum acceptable pH of stored platelets is:
    A. 6.0.
    B. 6.2.
    C. 6.4.
    D. 6.6.

26. Which of the following is true of platelets collected by apheresis?
    A. They are suspended in 50 to 75 mL of plasma.
    B. They are equivalent to 2 to 4 random donor units.
    C. They are stored at 1° to 6° C.
    D. They contain a minimum of 3×10^{11} platelets in 90% of units tested.

27. A patient who exhibits less than the expected response to Platelets transfusion is termed:
    A. Immunocompromised.
    B. Refractory.
    C. Insensitive.
    D. Sensitized.

28. Which of the following is true of Fresh Frozen Plasma?
    A. Contains all coagulation factors except for Factor V and Factor VIII
    B. Can be stored for up to 10 years after preparation
    C. Is thawed at 30° to 37° C
    D. Is indicated as a volume expander

29. According to the AABB, cryoprecipitated antihemophilic factor (Cryoprecipitated AHF) must contain a minimum of:
    A. 80 IU of Factor VIII.
    B. 150 mg of fibrinogen.
    C. Both A and B.
    D. Neither A nor B.

30. If being used as a source of Factor VIII, thawed Cryoprecipitated AHF may be stored at:
    A. 1° to 6° C for 4 hours.
    B. 20° to 24° C for 4 hours.
    C. 1° to 6° C for 24 hours.
    D. 20° to 24° C for 24 hours.

31. Which of the following is true of Granulocytes?
    A. The product does not contain red cells.
    B. The product is prepared from a Whole Blood unit by centrifugation.
    C. The product, if not irradiated, has a high risk of GVHD.
    D. The product is recommended as a prophylactic measure for prevention of infection.

32. When components are irradiated, the minimum dose of radiation at the container midplane is:
    A. 1000 cGy
    B. 1500 cGy
    C. 2000 cGy
    D. 2500 cGy

33. If a unit of blood that outdates in 14 days is irradiated, what is the outdate after irradiation?
    A. 24 hours after irradiation
    B. 4 days from the date of irradiation
    C. Same as the original unit
    D. 28 days after irradiation

Chapter 10

1. Storage of Platelets concentrate requires:
    A. Continuous agitation at 1° to 6° C.
    B. Occasional agitation at 37° C.
    C. Continuous agitation at room temperature.
    D. Occasional agitation at room temperature.

2. Stored RBCs' ability to deliver O_2 to the tissues is most directly affected by the:
    A. Plasma hemoglobin level.
    B. 2,3-BPG level.
    C. ATP concentration.
    D. pH.

3. Which of the following concentrations increases during storage of a unit of blood?
   A. pH
   B. NH_3
   C. 2,3-BPG
   D. ATP

4. Rejuvenation solutions can be administered up to:
   A. 8 hours after the blood is collected from the donor
   B. 5 days after the blood outdates
   C. 24 hours after the blood is collected from the donor
   D. 3 days after the blood outdates

5. Which of the following blood components should be shipped with dry ice?
   A. FFP
   B. Platelets
   C. Thawed Cryoprecipitated AHF
   D. Washed RBCs

6. Blood collected in CPDA-1 has an expiration date of:
   A. 21 days.
   B. 42 days.
   C. 35 days.
   D. 5 days.

7. Which of the following chemicals is the calcium chelator used in the anticoagulant/preservatives to store blood?
   A. Adenine
   B. Citrate
   C. Phosphate
   D. Dextrose

8. Who is considered to be the "father of blood transfusion"?
   A. James Blundell
   B. Philip Syng Physick
   C. William Harvey
   D. Oswald Robertson

9. Who established the first recognizable blood bank during World War I?
   A. John Elliott
   B. Bernard Fantus
   C. Oswald Robertson
   D. Karl Landsteiner

10. Which of the following statements is true regarding the structure of the RBC?
    A. Actin and spectrin are integral RBC membrane proteins.
    B. The RBC membrane is a semipermeable lipid bileaflet layer interspersed with proteins.
    C. The cytoskeleton of the RBC is composed of glycophorin A and B.
    D. Interaction between the membrane integral proteins and lipids gives the RBC its properties of flexibility.

11. Which of the following statements is true about hemoglobin's structure?
    A. It is made of two polypeptide chains.
    B. It contains one heme group, which binds four O_2 molecules.
    C. It is made of two α and two β chains.
    D. It contains two tetrapyrrole rings with Fe^{2+} in the center.

12. How does hemoglobin buffer the blood?
    A. It generates the bicarbonate ion, increasing the blood pH.
    B. It generates H^+ when it binds O_2, increasing the blood pH.
    C. It binds CO_2 in the oxyhemoglobin state, decreasing the blood pH.
    D. It binds H^+ in the deoxyhemoglobin state. decreasing blood pH.

13. What is the role of 2,3-BPG?
    A. It binds with oxyhemoglobin in the central cavity, causing O_2 release to the tissues.
    B. It binds with deoxyhemoglobin in the central cavity, causing O_2 release to the tissues.
    C. It binds with the terminal amino group of hemoglobin, causing it to bind O_2.
    D. It binds with the bicarbonate ion and causes hemoglobin to release O_2.

14. Which of the following conditions causes the O_2 dissociation curve to shift to the left?
    A. Anemia
    B. Fever
    C. Massive transfusion
    D. Hypoxia

15. In preparing a unit of RBCs with additive solution, when is this solution added to the RBCs?
    A. After the plasma is separated from the RBCs
    B. Immediately after the collection of the whole blood
    C. 5 days after the blood is collected
    D. Before centrifugation of the whole blood

16. Which of the following statements is true regarding regulations for RBC refrigeration?
    A. The units must be continuously agitated.
    B. There must be at least one visual thermometer to record temperatures.
    C. At a minimum, refrigeration temperatures should be recorded every 4 hours.
    D. Alarm systems must be able to alert personnel when the temperature goes below $0°$ C.

17. Which of the following levels affects stored platelet viability?
    A. pH
    B. NH_3
    C. ATP
    D. 2,3-DPG

18. Storage lesions that occur in stored Platelets include:
    A. Loss of nuclei.
    B. Change from sphere to disc shape.
    C. Loss of both α and dense granules.
    D. Increased response to single aggregating agents.

19. Which of the following would result in the quarantine of a blood component?
    A. Greenish color in the plasma
    B. RBCs with a brown supernatant fluid
    C. Platelets with a greenish color
    D. Cryoprecipitated AHF with a whitish-yellow color

20. AABB regulations for shipping blood components require that:
    A. RBCs be kept at $1°$ to $6°$ C during transport.
    B. Thawed Cryoprecipitated AHF be shipped at $1°$ to $6°$ C.
    C. Platelets be shipped at $20°$ to $24°$ C.
    D. Granulocytes be occasionally agitated during transport.

Chapter 11

1. Which of the following would **NOT** be considered a part of routine pretransfusion testing?
   A. ABO and Rh of the donor
   B. Review of the patient's past records
   C. Screening the recipient's serum for unexpected antibodies
   D. A minor crossmatch

2. A potential recipient has a record of a previous anti-K antibody. The antibody is no longer demonstrable in his serum even when enhancement techniques are used. Blood for transfusion to this patient should be:
   A. K-negative and crossmatch compatible.
   B. K-positive and crossmatch compatible.
   C. K-negative; crossmatch not performed.
   D. Crossmatch compatible; K antigen typing not performed.

3. The AABB requires that the blood/component request form contain the following minimum information:
   A. Two unique identifiers and the date of collection.
   B. All information in A plus the patient's age.
   C. All information in A plus the patient's diagnosis.
   D. All information in A plus the patient's Social Security number.

4. Which of the following would make a specimen unacceptable for routine compatibility testing?
   A. An anticoagulated tube was drawn
   B. The specimen was stored at $4°$ C for 24 hours
   C. The specimen was hemolyzed
   D. All of the above

5. AABB requires that blood specimens be stored at $1°$ to $6°$ C in the transfusion service for which of the following time periods?
   A. 72 hours after transfusion
   B. 7 days after collection
   C. 7 days after transfusion
   D. 10 days after collection

6. Which of the following is **NOT** required when repeating donor typing in the transfusion service?
   A. Retesting of blood drawn at the same facility
   B. ABO typing
   C. Rh typing on units labeled Rh-negative
   D. Rh typing on units labeled Rh-positive

7. A 23-year-old woman is admitted to your institution with an acute gastrointestinal bleed. The attending physician has requested two units of blood and has indicated that this is a life-threatening emergency. The patient's records indicate that she was previously typed B positive. She has no history of transfusion. The typing results on the current specimen confirmed the B typing, but the Rh control tube was positive, making the Rh type uninterpretable. Of the following units of blood, which one would be the **MOST** suitable for emergency release to this patient?
   A. B-positive blood
   B. A-negative blood
   C. O-negative blood
   D. O-positive blood

8. AABB Standards require that antibody detection testing include the use of:
   A. Pooled screen cells.
   B. Room-temperature incubation.
   C. Antihuman globulin testing.
   D. Low ionic strength testing.

9. In a group B patient, which of the following antibodies would be considered unexpected and clinically significant?
   A. Anti-A
   B. Autoanti-I
   C. Anti-Le^a
   D. Anti-C

10. An enhancement technique that destroys red cell antigens Fya, M, and N is:
    A. Albumin.
    B. Enzymes.
    C. Low ionic strength saline.
    D. Low ionic polycations.

11. A false-negative antibody screen could be due to:
    A. An antibody to a low-incidence antigen.
    B. A weak antibody reacting with selected homozygous cells only.
    C. Pooled screen cells.
    D. All of the above.

12. A pretransfusion test that uses red cells from the donor unit and the plasma from the patient is known as:
    A. A major crossmatch.
    B. A minor crossmatch.
    C. An antibody screen.
    D. An autocontrol.

13. If a potential recipient has no clinically significant antibodies and no record of previous antibodies, which of the following applies?
    A. No further compatibility testing is required.
    B. The crossmatch can be abbreviated to immediate spin to demonstrate ABO compatibility.
    C. The crossmatch must include 37° C incubation and the anti–human globulin phase of testing.
    D. The crossmatch must be done using enhancement techniques such as LISS or enzymes.

14. A neonatal patient has the following serologic results:
    Neonate: A-negative
    Antibody screen: anti-A,B
    DAT: positive
    Mother: O-positive
    Antibody screen: negative
    Which of the following units of blood would be the **MOST** suitable for transfusion to this infant?
    A. A-negative red cells.
    B. A-positive red cells.
    C. O-negative red cells.
    D. O-positive red cells.

15. A patient has the following pretransfusion profile:
    Antibody screen: negative
    Autocontrol: negative
    Major crossmatch: positive (incompatible)
    Which of the following conditions could **BEST** explain this profile?
    A. The patient has a potent cold autoanti-I.
    B. The patient has an alloantibody directed against a high-incidence antigen.
    C. The donor has an alloantibody directed against an antigen on the recipient's cells.
    D. The unit has a positive direct antiglobulin test.

16. Which of the following crossmatch:transfusion ratios would be considered a target for acceptability?
    A. >7.5:1
    B. 7.5:1 to 5.0:1
    C. 4.9:1 to 2.0:1
    D. ≤2.0:1

17. The maximum surgical blood schedule should result in which of the following outcomes?
    A. An increase in the total number of units crossmatched.
    B. An increase in the number of type and screen procedures.
    C. An increase in the number of units transfused.
    D. A decrease in the rate of transfusion reactions.

Use the following key to answer questions 18 to 21:
    A. Standard blood filter
    B. Microaggregate filter
    C. Leukocyte-reduction filter
    D. No filter required

18. Which filter would be **MOST** suitable for the prevention of adult respiratory distress syndrome following the massive transfusion of stored blood?

19. Which filter would be **MOST** appropriate for the administration of fresh frozen plasma?

20. Which filter would be **BEST** suited for the infusion of red cells to a recipient with a history of multiple severe febrile transfusion reactions?

21. Which filter would be required for the administration of 5% albumin?

Chapter 12

1. Which of the following situations would indicate the possible presence of a blood group alloantibody?
    A. A negative antibody screen but an incompatible crossmatch
    B. A recently transfused patient who fails to maintain the expected hematocrit but has no evidence of bleeding
    C. An obstetric patient whose newborn has a positive direct antiglobulin test
    D. All of the above

2. If a patient's RBC phenotype is D+C+E–c–e+S– s+K–Fy(a–b+) Jk(a–b+), which alloantibodies is the patient capable of forming?
    A. Alloanti-E, –s, –K, –Fy^a, –Jk^a
    B. Alloanti-E, –c, –K, –Fy^a, –Jk^b
    C. Alloanti-E, –c, –S, –K, –Fy^a, –Jk^a
    D. Alloanti-E, –c, –S, –Fy^b, –Jk^a

3. An agglutination reaction described as "many medium-sized clumps, clear supernatant" would be graded as:
    A. 1+.
    B. 2+.
    C. 3+.
    D. 4+.

4. If hemolysis were noted in grading a reaction, it could be attributed to which of the following serologic explanations?
    A. An IgG antibody
    B. An IgM antibody
    C. A complement-activating antibody

5. Which of the following are reasons to use a blood sample less than 3 days old when performing antibody identification?
    A. The patient may be pregnant
    B. The patient may have been recently transfused
    C. A reliable transfusion history is not available.
    D. For the sake of having a consistent policy
    E. All of the above

6. Which of the following are purposes of using IgG-coated "check" cells in indirect antiglobulin testing?
    A. To ensure that the crossmatch is compatible
    B. To ensure that serum proteins were effectively washed off the test RBCs
    C. To ensure that anti-IgG was added to the test tubes
    D. Both B and C

7. When beginning the antibody exclusion process after testing a panel of RBCs, the technologist should first:
    A. Start ruling-out with the first panel cell.
    B. Start ruling-out with the first reactive panel cell.
    C. Start ruling-out with the first nonreactive panel cell.
    D. Try to match the pattern of reactivity with each column on the worksheet to see if any patterns match exactly.

8. In which of the following situations might mixed-field reactions be expected to be seen?
    A. In the serum reactions with a single alloantibody
    B. In the serum reactions with a warm autoantibody
    C. In the RBC phenotyping of a blood donor
    D. In the RBC phenotyping of a recently transfused patient

9. Ficin treatment of red blood cells will destroy which of the following antigens?
   A. B
   B. Le^a
   C. Fy^a
   D. D

10. DTT treatment will denature which of the following antigens?
    A. E
    B. K
    C. S
    D. Jk^b

11. Which of the following methods or enhancement media are acceptable to detect most clinically significant alloantibodies?
    A. Room temperature incubation of the patient's serum with test RBCs
    B. 37° C incubation of serum and test RBCs, followed by the indirect antiglobulin test
    C. Testing ficin-treated panel RBCs with the patient's serum
    D. Testing an eluate of the patient's RBCs

12. If an antibody identification panel is tested and the auto control is negative but all panel RBCs react 2+ with the patient's serum, which of the following scenarios is **MOST** likely?
    A. A warm autoantibody
    B. Multiple alloantibodies
    C. An antibody to an antigen of high incidence
    D. An antibody to an antigen of low incidence

13. If anti-c has been tentatively identified in the patient's serum, but anti-E, anti-K, and anti-S have not been excluded, RBCs of which of the following phenotypes would need to be included in a selected cell panel?
    A. E–c+S–K–
    B. E+c+s–K–
    C. E+c–S+K+
    D. E–c–S–K–

14. If a patient has a positive direct antiglobulin test and there is a need to phenotype the patient's RBCs, which of the following cell treatments could be used to remove IgG from the patient's RBCs?
    A. Chloroquine diphosphate (CDP)
    B. Dithiothreitol (DTT)
    C. LISS
    D. Ficin

15. If a patient's serum contains alloanti-E, alloanti-K, and alloanti-Fy^a and the blood bank record indicates the patient has a history of anti-c, which is not currently detectable, which of the following antigens must be lacking from a unit of Red Blood Cells to be transfused?
    A. E
    B. K
    C. Fy^a
    D. c
    E. All of the above

Chapter 13

1. Which of the following patterns is consistent with polyagglutination?
   A. Antibody screening test with PEG is nonreactive.
   B. Patient's serum is incompatible with all donor cells.
   C. Testing of the patient's cells with cord serum demonstrates no reactivity.
   D. All of the above.

2. A patient sample demonstrates the following reactivity in LISS 37° C:

Screening cell	I	II	III	Auto
AHG	3+	3+	3+	3+

Which of the following would be consistent with this serologic finding?
   A. Reactivity with the enhancement medium
   B. A warm autoantibody
   C. Rouleaux
   D. All of the above

3. The following are nonserologic causes of serologic discrepancies:
   A. Fibrin clots in the serum sample.
   B. There is a sample tube mix-up.
   C. Glass fragments in the tube.
   D. All of the above.

4. Patient JGB has an ABO/Rh typing discrepancy and requires immediate transfusion, due to unexpected surgical bleeding. What type blood should be released on an emergency basis?
   A. AB-negative red cells and O plasma
   B. O-negative red cells and AB plasma
   C. O-positive red cells and O plasma
   D. All of the above are suitable
   E. None of the above

5. The following antibodies are present in the serum of a Bombay individual:
   A. Anti-H.
   B. Anti-Le^a.
   C. Anti-P$_1$.
   D. All of the above.

6. Given the following results, determine the **MOST** likely cause(s) of the following ABO discrepancy:

Anti-A	Anti-B	Anti-A,B	A$_1$ cells	A$_2$ cells	B cells
0	4+	4+	0	0	0

   A. Newborn sample
   B. Acquired B
   C. Transfusion chimera
   D. All of the above

7. Which of the following is (are) consistent with the following ABO discrepancy?

Anti-A	Anti-B	Anti-A,B	Anti-A$_1$	A$_1$ cells	A$_2$ cells	B cells
4+	+ weak	4+	4+	0	0	4+

   A. Excess blood group substance from a tumor
   B. Room temperature reactive autoantibody
   C. Acquired B antigen
   D. All of the above

8. Which of the following is (are) true statement(s) about the following discrepancy?

Anti-A	Anti-B	Anti-A,B	Anti-A$_1$	A$_1$ cells	A$_2$ cells	B cells
4+	+weak	4+	4+	0	0	4+

   A. Saline replacement will most likely resolve the discrepancy.
   B. This sample is most likely an A positive.
   C. Rare donor registries will most likely provide the only source of compatible blood.
   D. All of the above.

9. Which of the following is (are) consistent with the following serologic findings?

Anti-B	Anti-B	Anti-A,B	A$_1$ cells	A$_2$ cells	B cells
+^{mf}	0	+^{mf}	3+	0	4+

   A. An acquired chimera
   B. Contamination with Wharton's jelly
   C. Polyagglutination
   D. All of the above

10. Which of the following is (are) consistent with the following serologic findings?

Anti-A	Anti-B	Anti-A,B	A$_1$ cells	A$_2$ cells	B cells	O cells
0	3+	3+	2+	3+	4+	3+

   A. A room temperature reactive alloantibody
   B. A subgroup of A with anti-A$_1$
   C. Excessive blood group substances
   D. All of the above

11. Which of the following is a logical step in the resolution of the following discrepancy?

Anti-A	Anti-B	Anti-A,B	Anti-D	A$_1$ cells	A$_2$ cells	B cells
+^{weak}	+ weak	+ weak	3+	4+	4+	4+

   A. Wash patient cells and repeat testing
   B. Perform antibody identification with a panel of cells with known low-incidence antigens
   C. Repeat forward grouping at 18° and 4° C
   D. All of the above

12. Which of the following is (are) consistent with the following serologic discrepancy?

Anti-A	Anti-B	Anti-A,B	A$_1$ cells	A$_2$ cells	B cells
4+	4+	4+	2+	2+	2+

   A. A cold autoantibody
   B. A Bombay phenotype
   C. An immunocompromised patient
   D. All of the above

13. Which of the following is (are) consistent with the following serologic discrepancy?

Anti-A	Anti-B	Anti-A,B	Anti-A$_1$	A$_1$ cells	A$_2$ cells	B cells
4+	0	4+	0	2+	0	4+

   A. An A$_2$ with anti-A$_1$
   B. An acquired B
   C. Polyagglutination
   D. All of the above

14. Which of the following is/are consistent with the following serologic discrepancy?

Anti-A	Anti-B	Anti-A,B	Anti-D	Rh control	A₁ cells	A₂ cells	B cells
0	0	+ weak	3+	0	0	0	4+

    A. Polyagglutination
    B. Cells will type positive with *Ulex europaeus*
    C. Rouleaux
    D. All of the above

15. Which of the following may be used when a patient exhibits a coagulopathy resulting in the formation of fibrin clots in vitro?
    A. Perform testing with plasma
    B. Use saline replacement techniques
    C. Remove fibrin clots and continue testing to compensate for the coagulopathy
    D. All of the above

16. Hemolysis is noted in testing of reverse grouping cells. Which of the following solutions should be considered?
    A. The reverse grouping cells are contaminated.
    B. The reverse grouping cells are outdated.
    C. The patient demonstrates a high-titered, complement-binding antibody.
    D. All of the above.

17. Rouleaux:
    A. Appear microscopically as distinctive coinlike stacks of RBCs.
    B. May be observed following transfusion of dextran.
    C. Are not generally observed in the antiglobulin phase of testing.
    D. All of the above.

18. A chimera:
    A. May be observed after transfusion.
    B. May be observed after a bone marrow transplant.
    C. Is derived from twin-to-twin transfusion in utero.
    D. All of the above.

19. What does the following indicate?
    $O > A_2 > A_2B > B > A_1 > A_1B$
    A. Frequency of ABO typing from greatest to least
    B. Amount of H antigen on red cells from greatest to least
    C. Frequency of ABO types from least to greatest
    D. Amount of Leᵃ antigen on red cells from least to greatest

20. Which of the following D typing requires a negative control?
    A. Saline anti-D
    B. Monoclonal-polyclonal blend
    C. Monoclonal-monoclonal blend
    D. High protein

21. A patient has the following serologic data:

Anti-A	Anti-B	Anti-A,B	A₁ Cells	A₂ Cells	B Cells
3+	3+	3+	1+	0	0

Auto	DAT	Antibody screen
0	0	Negative

Of the following, which is the **MOST** probable explanation for these results?
    A. A warm-reacting autoantibody
    B. Excessive blood group substances
    C. A subgroup of A with anti-A₁
    D. Polyagglutination

22. A multiply transfused trauma patient has the following serologic data:

Anti-A	Anti-B	Anti-A,B	A₁ Cells	A₂ Cells	B Cells
1 +mf	0	1 +mf	0	0	4+

Auto	DAT	Antibody screen
0	0	Negative

Of the following, which is the **MOST** probable explanation for these results?
    A. Reduced immunoglobulin levels
    B. A cold-reacting alloantibody
    C. A group B patient transfused with O plasma
    D. A group A patient transfused with O blood

23. A leukemia patient is admitted to your institution with a history of multiple Red Blood Cell and Plateletpheresis transfusions. The admission serologic data are:

Anti-A	Anti-B	Anti-A,B	A₁ Cells	A₂ Cells	B Cells
4+	0	4+	1+	1+	4+

Auto	DAT	Antibody screen
1+	1+	Negative

Of the following, which is the most probable explanation for these results?
A. Administration of group O platelets
B. A warm autoantibody
C. A cold autoantibody
D. Rouleaux

24. A patient has the following admission serologic data:

Anti-A	Anti-B	Anti-A,B	A₁ Cells	A₂ Cells	B Cells
4+	2+	4+	2+	2+	4+

Auto	DAT	Antibody screen
2+	0	All cells react 2+

The **BEST** next step in the resolution of this discrepancy would be:
A. Perform an eluate panel.
B. Wash patient cells for ABO forward grouping.
C. Incubate all tests at 4° C.
D. Perform an enzyme panel.

25. Resolution of ABO discrepancies due to polyagglutinable cells can be accomplished by using which of the following?
A. DTT-treated patient cells
B. Monoclonal or antisera
C. Anti-A₁ lectin
D. Enzyme-treated patient cells

26. The acquired B antigen is **MOST** often associated with which of the following blood groups?
A. A
B. AB
C. O
D. All of the above

27. A 96-year old woman has the following serologic data:

Anti-A	Anti-B	Anti-A,B	A₁ Cells	A₂ Cells	B Cells
0	0	0	0	0	0

Auto	DAT	Antibody screen
0	0	0

Of the following, which is the **MOST** probable explanation of these results?
A. Decreased immunoglobulin levels
B. A weak subgroup of B
C. An A₂ subgroup
D. Contaminated reagents

28. A potential blood donor has the following initial serologic reactions:

Anti-A	Anti-B	Anti-A,B	A₁ Cells	A₂ Cells	B Cells
0	0	1+	1+	0	4+

Auto	DAT	Antibody screen
0	0	0

Which of the following subgroups of A would **MOST** likely be associated with this reaction pattern?
A. A₂
B. A₃
C. Aₓ
D. Aₘ

29. Mixed field reactions can be associated with which of the following?
A. Weak subgroups of A and B
B. Genetic chimeras
C. Transfusion
D. All of the above

30. A patient has the following serologic data:

Anti-A	Anti-B	Anti-A,B	A₁ Cells	A₂ Cells	B Cells
0	0	0	4+	4+	4+

Auto	DAT	Antibody screen
0	0	All cells 4+

Of the following, which is the **MOST** probable explanation for these results?
A. A warm autoantibody
B. Rouleaux
C. A transfusion reaction
D. The Bombay phenotype

31. Which of the following tests would be the **MOST** useful in resolving the problem in question 10?
A. Typing with *Dolichos biflorus* lectin
B. Typing with *Ulex europaeus* lectin
C. An eluate from patient's cells
D. Prewarmed techniques

Chapter 14

1. The most important consideration in the selection and administration of blood and blood components is (are) the:
A. Clinical condition of the patient.
B. Results of laboratory testing.
C. Cost of the treatment.
D. Component inventory.

2. Blood component therapy may be indicated in all of the following instances **EXCEPT:**
   A. Restore functional leukocytes in a septic patient.
   B. Treat congenital hemostatic disorders.
   C. Treat hypoxia secondary to acute blood loss.
   D. Treat hypovolemia without associated loss of oxygen-carrying capacity.

3. The component best suited for the treatment of a patient with chronic anemia complaining of fatigue and shortness of breath is:
   A. Whole Blood.
   B. Red Blood Cells.
   C. Red Blood Cells Leukocytes Reduced.
   D. Red Blood Cells Washed.
   E. Factor VIII concentrate.

4. The component best suited for an acute trauma victim in hemorrhagic shock is:
   A. Whole Blood.
   B. Red Blood Cells.
   C. Red Blood Cells Leukocytes Reduced.
   D. Red Blood Cells Washed.
   E. Factor VIII concentrate.

5. Which of the following components is best suited for a patient who shows clinical signs of hypoxia due to chronic gastrointestinal blood loss and who has a history of two previous severe febrile transfusion reactions after the administration of Red Blood Cells?
   A. Whole Blood.
   B. Red Blood Cells.
   C. Red Blood Cells Leukocytes Reduced.
   D. Red Blood Cells Washed.
   E. Factor VIII concentrate.

6. The component best suited for a patient deficient in IgA who has had a previous anaphylactic reaction to transfusion is:
   A. Whole Blood.
   B. Red Blood Cells.
   C. Red Blood Cells Leukocytes Reduced.
   D. Red Blood Cells Washed.
   E. Factor VIII concentrate.

7. The component **BEST** suited for a normovolemic, nonbleeding hemophiliac with a 5% Factor VIII level is:
   A. Whole Blood.
   B. Red Blood Cells.
   C. Red Blood Cells Leukocytes Reduced.
   D. Red Blood Cells Washed.
   E. Factor VIII concentrate.

8. A physician has ordered two units of red cells for an outpatient with iron deficiency anemia. The patient has a 9 g hemoglobin and shows no signs of hypoxia. In the patient history there was a reported mild febrile response to a previous postsurgical transfusion. You would:
   A. Recommend to the physician that a leukocyte-reduced product is warranted to minimize the risk of febrile reactions.
   B. Suggest the transfusion of Whole Blood to prevent dilutional thrombocytopenia.
   C. Process the request because it is the component of choice for this patient.
   D. Suggest to the physician that the patient does not need transfusion at this time because the risk of transfusion in this case exceeds the benefit.

9. A recipient is typed B-positive with a negative antibody screen. Based on the AABB Standards for the selection of blood and components for transfusion, which of these components would be suitable for transfusion to this recipient?
   A. Group A Granulocytes Pheresis
   B. Group AB Platelets
   C. Group O, Whole Blood
   D. Group O, Fresh Frozen Plasma

10. Which of the following crossmatch/transfusion ratios would be considered a target for acceptability?
    A. >7.5:1
    B. 7.5:1 to 5.0:1
    C. 4.9:1 to 2.5:1
    D. <2.5:1

11. The maximum surgical blood order schedule should result in an increase in the:
    A. Total number of units crossmatched.
    B. Number of type and screen procedures.
    C. Total number of units transfused.
    D. Hemoglobin and hematocrit.

12. A single unit of platelet concentrate should have a minimum of:
    A. 3.0×10^{10} platelets.
    B. 3.0×10^{11} platelets.
    C. 5.5×10^{10} platelets.
    D. 5.5×10^{11} platelets.

13. The component of choice for a fibrinogen deficiency is:
    A. Fresh Frozen Plasma.
    B. Cryoprecipitated AHF.
    C. Activated Factor IX.
    D. DDAVP.

14. Platelet transfusions are most suitable for which of the following conditions?
    A. Dilutional thrombocytopenia
    B. Autoimmune thrombocytopenic purpura
    C. Untreated disseminated intravascular coagulation
    D. Thrombotic thrombocytopenic purpura

15. Which of the following components is **MOST** suitable for a recipient who has become refractory to platelet transfusion owing to the development of HLA antibodies?
    A. Leukocyte-reduced platelet concentrates
    B. Irradiated platelets
    C. HLA-matched platelets pheresis from unrelated donors
    D. HLA-matched platelets pheresis from family members

16. All of the following are true concerning granulocyte concentrates **EXCEPT** they:
    A. May be indicated in patients with documented septicemia.
    B. Must be crossmatched if they contain more than 5 mL of red cells.
    C. Are used prophylactically to prevent infection.
    D. Should be irradiated before transfusion to bone marrow transplant recipients.

17. Fresh Frozen Plasma is the component of choice for the management of:
    A. Multiple factor deficiencies.
    B. Factor VIII deficiency.
    C. Factor IX deficiency.
    D. Hypovolemia.

18. Cryoprecipitate AHF is indicated:
    A. For the management of FactorVII deficiencies.
    B. As a source of viable granulocytes.
    C. For patients with Factor VIII inhibitors.
    D. To treat Factor XIII deficiencies.

19. Which of the following is an immune cause of unresponsiveness to platelet transfusion that would be associated with the failure of HLA-matched platelets to yield satisfactory posttransfusion increments?
    A. Septicemia
    B. Disseminated intravascular coagulation
    C. Antibodies to platelet-specific antigens
    D. Graft-versus-host disease

20. Which of the following components should be irradiated to prevent graft-versus-host disease in the recipient?
    A. Fresh Frozen Plasma to be transfused to a bone marrow transplant recipient
    B. Red cells to be transfused to an immunocompetent adult
    C. Granulocytes donated by a husband for his spouse
    D. Platelets donated by a son for his father

21. Which of the following may be a complication associated with the rapid administration of plasma protein fraction?
    A. Hypertension
    B. Hypotension
    C. Intestinal dehydration
    D. Graft-versus-host disease

22. Which of the following products increases intravascular fluid volume by increasing osmotic pressure and subsequently drawing water into the vascular compartment from the extravascular spaces?
    A. 5% albumin
    B. 25% albumin
    C. Ringer's lactate
    D. Plasma protein fraction

23. Which of the following components/products is the **MOST** suitable for the treatment of hemophilia B?
    A. Cryoprecipitated AHF
    B. Fresh Frozen Plasma
    C. Anti-inhibitor coagulation complex
    D. Factor IX concentrate

24. A 50-kg girl has a hematocrit of 40% (0.40). Her initial Factor VIII level is 5%. The physician has requested that her presurgical Factor VIII activity be raised to 45%. How many International units of Factor VIII would be necessary to achieve this desired outcome?
    A. 840
    B. 630
    C. 560
    D. 480

25. Which of the following components/products is indicated in conjunction with the administration of vitamin K for patients actively bleeding as a result of Coumadin overadministration?
    A. Cryoprecipitated AHF
    B. Fresh Frozen Plasma
    C. Factor VIII concentrate
    D. Factor IX concentrate

Chapter 15

1. The **MOST** commonly reported acute transfusion reaction is:
   A. Hemolytic.
   B. Febrile nonhemolytic.
   C. Transfusion-related acute lung injury (TRALI).
   D. Physical/chemical hemolysis.

2. The **MOST** common cause of morbidity and mortality linked to hemolytic transfusion reaction is:
   A. Hypoxia.
   B. Respiratory failure.
   C. Acute renal failure.
   D. Cardiac failure.

3. Acute intravascular hemolysis is **MOST** commonly associated with antibodies of which blood group system?
   A. ABO
   B. Rh
   C. Kidd
   D. Duffy

4. The **MOST** common initial clinical manifestation of a hemolytic transfusion reaction is:
   A. Shock.
   B. Shortness of breath.
   C. Fever.
   D. Bleeding.

5. Which antibody is commonly associated with delayed hemolytic transfusion reactions?
   A. Anti-A,B
   B. Anti-D
   C. Anti-Jk^a
   D. Anti-Lu^b

6. A patient requiring transfusion of six units of platelet concentrates has a history of multiple severe febrile reactions during red cell administration. Which of the following strategies would be **MOST** effective in minimizing the risk of subsequent febrile reactions during platelet administration?
   A. Pretransfusion administration of antipyretics
   B. Reduce the plasma volume of the platelet concentrates
   C. Infuse the platelets slowly
   D. Administer the leukocyte-reduced platelets

7. According to the AABB Standards, a transfusion is **NOT** required to be discontinued if the patient:
   A. Has an extreme elevation in body temperature.
   B. In flushed and short of breath.
   C. Exhibits hives on his or her extremities.
   D. Has nausea, vomiting, and intestinal cramps.

8. Noncardiogenic pulmonary edema is **MOST** frequently associated with:
   A. The transfusion of preformed leukocyte antibodies from a sensitized donor.
   B. The transfusion of donor leukocytes into a previously sensitized recipient.
   C. A deficiency of IgA in the donor.
   D. A deficiency of IgA in the recipient.

9. Which of the following components is **MOST** frequently associated with transfusion reactions due to bacterial contamination?
   A. Fresh Frozen Plasma
   B. Red Blood Cells
   C. Granulocytes pheresis
   D. Platelet concentrates

10. A patient has laboratory evidence of hemolysis (hemoglobinemia, decreased haptoglobin) 2 hours after the transfusion of two units of red cells. The serologic results are as follows:
    A positive
    Antibody screen negative
    DAT negative
    The patient has no physical symptoms and other laboratory findings are within normal ranges. Which of the following would **MOST** probably be associated with this clinical picture?
    A. Acute immune hemolysis
    B. Delayed immune hemolysis
    C. Nonimmune hemolysis
    D. Bacterial contamination

11. Posttransfusion purpura is **MOST** commonly associated with:
    A. Transfusion of preformed leukoagglutinins in donor plasma.
    B. Transfusion of HLA-incompatible white cells from the donor.
    C. Bacterial contamination of platelet concentrates.
    D. Transfusion of Pl^{A1}-positive platelets to a recipient with anti-Pl^{A1}.

12. Cytomegalovirus can be transmitted in which of the following products?
    A. Red cells
    B. Fresh Frozen Plasma
    C. Albumin
    D. Intravenous immune globulin

13. The first step the patient care staff should take when a hemolytic reaction is suspected is to:
    A. Stop the transfusion.
    B. Call the laboratory.
    C. Call the patient's physician.
    D. Administer intravenous fluids.

14. Which of the following steps should be included in the preliminary laboratory investigation of a suspected transfusion reaction?
    A. Perform a DAT on the pretransfusion specimen.
    B. Perform an antibody screen on the posttransfusion specimen.
    C. Repeat the crossmatches.
    D. Visually check the posttransfusion serum/plasma for hemolysis.

15. A patient is readmitted to your institution with a hemoglobin of 7 g/dL (70 g/L) 2 weeks after the transfusion of three units of Red Blood Cells. The initial serologic results are as follows:
    A positive
    Antibody screen negative
    DAT 2+
    During the time interval since the last transfusion, the patient complained of no symptoms except fatigue and shortness of breath on exertion. The physical findings are unremarkable. The patient's physician has contacted the blood bank requesting an investigation of this posttransfusion episode. Which of the following tests should be run next in order to better explain this adverse posttransfusion reaction?
    A. Antibody identification panel on the patient's serum
    B. Culture on the donor blood bag
    C. Antibody identification panel on the patient's eluate
    D. Repeat ABO type on the units transfused

Chapter 16

1. A group A-positive, Kell-negative woman is carrying a group O fetus. The father is group O, Kell-negative. Which of the following statements is true regarding the potential for this infant to be affected by HDN?
   A. It is at risk for anti-Kell HDN, but not ABO-HDN.
   B. It is at risk for ABO-HDN, but not anti-Kell HDN.
   C. It is at risk for both anti-Kell and ABO-HDN.
   D. It is not at risk for either anti-Kell or ABO-HDN.

2. The most common antibody specificity associated with HDN is:
   A. ABO.
   B. Anti-D.
   C. Anti-Kell (K1).
   D. Anti-C.

3. Which of the following conditions can be associated with thrombocytopenia and bleeding in the newborn?
   A. Maternal warm autoimmune hemolytic anemia
   B. A newborn infected with rubella
   C. Maternal autoimmune thrombocytopenia
   D. All of the above

4. Of the following signs and symptoms, which is associated with severe fetal (before delivery) HDN?
   A. Hydrops fetalis
   B. Icterus gravis neonatorum
   C. Kernicterus
   D. All of the above

5. Rh immune globulin is effective in the prevention of HDN due to which of the following antibodies?
   A. Anti-D
   B. Anti-CD
   C. Anti-E
   D. All of the above

6. The **MOST** common cause of fetal-maternal bleeding is:
   A. Amniocentesis.
   B. Trauma.
   C. Placental separation at delivery.
   D. Placental malformation.

7. In HDN bilirubin levels are generally normal at birth but begin to elevate during the first few hours after delivery. Which of the following statements **BEST** explains the reason for this clinical feature?
   A. The newborn experiences rapid red cell destruction.
   B. Newborn antibody titers continue to rise.
   C. Newborns are deficient in glucuronyl transferase.
   D. Newborns are deficient in serum albumin.

8. Which of the following tests is the **MOST** useful in predicting ABO-HDN?
   A. Maternal ABO type
   B. Paternal ABO type
   C. Maternal antibody screen
   D. None of the above

9. Which of the following antibodies is **NOT** associated with HDN?
   A. Anti-Le^a
   B. Anti-A,B
   C. Anti-Fy^a
   D. Anti-Kell (K1)

10. Which of the following techniques is **MOST** useful when titering the serum of a mother who has a mixture of IgM and IgG antibodies in her serum?
    A. Enzyme techniques
    B. Dithiothreitol (DTT)
    C. Low ionic strength saline
    D. Polybrene

11. Which of the following would be the **LEAST** effective in the control of variables affecting the results of titration procedures?
    A. Use of commercial screen cells
    B. Procedural control of incubation time/temperature
    C. Repeating previous serum sample when the subsequent sample is tested
    D. Using standard media and techniques

12. If no data regarding critical titer are available, which of the following titer values is frequently used as a cutoff?
    A. 8
    B. 16
    C. 32
    D. 64

13. Amniotic fluid analysis showed a marked increase into zone III of the Liley graph. Lecithin/sphingomyelin ratios indicated that the fetal lungs were not mature. Which of the following is the **MOST** appropriate decision regarding medical intervention?
    A. No immediate need for intervention; repeat amniocentesis to establish a trend
    B. Delivery by cesarean section
    C. An intrauterine transfusion
    D. A cordocentesis

14. A turbid amniotic fluid was centrifuged at high speed to remove turbidity. Which of the following is true regarding this specimen?
    A. It can be used for both bilirubin and L/S measurements.
    B. It can be used for L/S but not for bilirubin.
    C. It can be used for bilirubin but not for L/S.
    D. It cannot be used for either test.

15. A mother's titer has risen above the critical level and the father is unavailable for testing. The **MOST** useful procedure to determine the antigen type of the fetus is:
    A. Family studies involving grandparents and siblings.
    B. Typing a cord specimen at the time of delivery.
    C. Cordocentesis.
    D. Amniocentesis.

16. Assuming ABO and Rh compatibility, which of the following conditions makes a unit of blood unsuitable for intrauterine transfusion to an infant suffering from anti-Fy^a HDN?
    A. CMV-negative red cells
    B. Washed red cells donated by the father
    C. Washed red cells donated by the mother
    D. Washed red cells from a random donor with an 80% hematocrit

17. After delivery, which of the following test combinations is the **MOST** useful in predicting the severity of HDN?
    A. Bilirubin and cord hematocrit
    B. Bilirubin and heel-stick hematocrit
    C. Maternal antibody titer and bilirubin
    D. Maternal antibody titer and cord hematocrit

18. Which of the following tests is required only if other than group O blood is selected for exchange transfusion?
    A. Maternal antibody identification
    B. Hemoglobin S screen on donor unit
    C. Testing infant's serum for anti-A and anti-B using the antiglobulin test
    D. ABO and Rh type of the infant

19. An A-positive mother with anti-Kell (K1) gives birth to a B-negative, Kell (K1)–positive infant with HDN. The physician requests blood for exchange transfusion. Which of the following units is **MOST** suitable?
    A. A-negative, Kell-negative blood
    B. O-negative, Kell-positive blood
    C. B-negative, Kell-negative blood
    D. O-negative, Kell-negative blood

20. An infant has the following history and serologic findings: first born, weakly positive direct antiglobulin test, slight rise in bilirubin at 48 hours. These findings are **MOST** consistent with hemolytic disease due to:
    A. Anti-D.
    B. Anti-Le^a.
    C. Anti-A,B.
    D. Anti-Kell (K1).

21. A technologist reported seeing no fetal cells on the Kleihauer-Betke slide on a mother with a positive rosette test. How many vials of RhIG should be administered to this patient?
    A. 0
    B. 1
    C. 2
    D. 3

22. The pathophysiology of HDN is associated with both anemia and bilirubinemia. From a treatment standpoint, which of the following statements is true regarding the clinical concerns in these two periods?
    A. Bilirubinemia is of primary concern in the antenatal period, whereas anemia is of primary concern in the postpartum period.
    B. Anemia is of primary concern in the antenatal period, whereas bilirubinemia is of primary concern in the postpartum period.
    C. Anemia is the primary concern in both periods.
    D. Bilirubinemia is the primary concern in both periods.

Chapter 17

1. Which of the following is considered to be a massive transfusion in a 70 kg adult?
   A. The transfusion of 4 units of Whole Blood in 24 hours
   B. The transfusion of 6 units of Red Blood Cells in 24 hours
   C. The transfusion of 8 units of Red Blood Cells in 24 hours
   D. The transfusion of 10 units of Red Blood Cells in 24 hours

2. Approximately 12 hours after a massive bleed, a patient's hemoglobin may underestimate the amount of blood lost owing to:
   A. Fluid shifts from the extravascular spaces into the vasculature.
   B. The accumulation of ascitic fluid.
   C. A loss of protein from the vascular compartment.
   D. Increased capillary permeability.

3. Infusion of large amounts of citrate in AS-3 red cells can result directly in which of the following?
   A. A shift to the left in the oxygen-dissociation curve
   B. Hyperkalemia
   C. Hypocalcemia
   D. Platelet dysfunction

4. Whole blood is generally reserved for those patients losing at **LEAST** what percent of their blood volume?
   A. 10%
   B. 15%
   C. 20%
   D. 25%

5. Hypothermia can be associated with which of the following clinical features?
   A. Decreased citrate metabolism
   B. Acidosis
   C. Impaired hemostatic function
   D. All of the above

6. According to AABB Standards, blood warmers must:
   A. Warm blood to 40° C.
   B. Have a visible alarm.
   C. Maintain blood in a closed system.
   D. All of the above.

7. Which of the following is **NOT** true regarding the emergency release of blood?
   A. Rh-positive blood is safe for a nonimmunized Rh-negative recipient if Rh-negative blood is not available.
   B. It is sufficient to use previous blood bank records to determine the ABO type of a trauma recipient.
   C. An emergency release must be signed by the physician if pretransfusion testing protocols are not followed.
   D. If other than type-specific blood is given, the donor red cells must be ABO compatible with the recipient's serum.

8. With regard to the transmission of viral disease, which of the following blood components is considered the safest?
   A. Whole Blood
   B. Red Blood Cells Irradiated
   C. Red Blood Cells Leukocytes Reduced
   D. Autologous Red Blood Cells

9. Which of the following is **NOT** true regarding physiologic characteristics of neonates?
   A. Hematologic values differ from those of adults.
   B. Blood volume per kilogram of body weight is constant for the first 6 months.
   C. Blood group alloantibodies are maternal in origin.
   D. Fetal hemoglobin has a high oxygen affinity.

10. In infants, what dose of red cells raises the hemoglobin by approximately 1 g/dL?
    A. 1 mL Red Blood Cells/kg
    B. 3 mL Red Blood Cells/kg
    C. 5 mL Red Blood Cells/kg
    D. 7 mL Red Blood Cells/kg

11. A number of techniques are used to obtain small aliquots of blood for infant transfusion. Which of the following techniques carries the **HIGHEST** risk of contamination?
    A. Multiple pack system
    B. A single unit sampled through a coupler into a syringe
    C. Preparation of frozen aliquots
    D. Reduced volume donations

12. In which of the following cases should additive solutions (AS) be removed before transfusion?
    A. Routine adult transfusion
    B. Routine infant transfusion to replace blood lost in laboratory sampling
    C. Exchange transfusion in neonates
    D. All of the above

13. A neonate is admitted to your nursery. Admission serologic results are as follows:

	Anti-A	Anti-B	Anti-A,B	A_1 Cells	B Cells	Antibody Screen	DAT
Infant	4+	0	4+	NT	NT	NT	0
Mother	0	0	0	4+	4+	Neg	NT

NT, Not tested.
The physician has requested a transfusion of ABO type-specific blood for this infant. What additional testing (if any) is necessary to determine suitable blood for transfusion?
    A. A test for anti-A at the anti–human globulin phase of testing
    B. An antibody screen on the infant
    C. A reverse grouping on the infant
    D. A DAT on the mother

14. Irradiated blood is recommended for exchange transfusion in order to:
    A. Decrease the incidence of graft-versus-host disease.
    B. Shift the oxygen dissociation curve to the right.
    C. Decrease the risk of CMV transmission.
    D. Decrease the risk of febrile transfusion reactions.

15. An exchange transfusion has been ordered to treat hyperbilirubinemia and anemia in an infant affected by hemolytic disease of the newborn. The serologic results on the mother and the infant are as follows:

	Anti-A	Anti-B	Anti-A,B	A_1 Cells	B Cells	Anti-D	Antibody ID	DAT
Infant	4+	0	4+	NT	NT	3+	NT	3+
Mother	0	4+	4+	4+	0	0	Kell	NT

Which of the following units of Red Blood Cells is **MOST** suitable for exchange transfusion? (Note: All units are less than 5 days old, CMV negative, hemoglobin S negative, and irradiated.)
    A. B-positive, Kell-negative
    B. A-positive, Kell-negative
    C. O-positive, Kell-negative
    D. B-negative, Kell-negative

16. Plasma exchange has been found effective in removing which of the following substances from the plasma?
    A. Abnormal paraproteins
    B. Excessive numbers of red blood cells
    C. Dysfunctional white cells
    D. All of the above

17. Which of the following plasma exchange techniques is the **MOST** specific?
    A. Simple exchange
    B. Exchange with filtration
    C. Exchange with cryofiltration
    D. Exchange with immunoadsorption

18. In plasma exchange procedures, which of the following statements is true with regard to the relative effectiveness of Ig removal?
    A. IgM and IgG can be removed with equal efficacy.
    B. IgM can be removed more effectively than IgG.
    C. IgG can be removed more effectively than IgM.
    D. Neither IgG nor IgM can be removed by this procedure.

19. Plasma exchange has been found effective in the treatment of:
    A. DIC.
    B. Sickle cell anemia.
    C. Myasthenia gravis.
    D. Hemolytic disease of the newborn.

20. In which of the following disorders has plasma exchange been successful because of the resultant reduction in blood viscosity?
    A. Dysproteinemia
    B. Sickle cell anemia
    C. Hypercholesterolemia
    D. Glomerulonephritis

21. Cytapheresis procedures can be used to reduce:
    A. Erythrocytes.
    B. Leukocytes.
    C. Platelets.
    D. All of the above.

22. Which of the following is the **MOST** common cause of morbidity and mortality in burn patients?
    A. Loss of water from the skin
    B. Ascites
    C. Red cell destruction
    D. Loss of the skin barrier to infection

23. Hypoperfusion, shock, and increased blood viscosity during the first 24 hours in severely burned patients are due to:
    A. Loss of protein-containing fluid from capillaries.
    B. Direct heat destruction of red cells.
    C. Infection.
    D. Decreased erythropoiesis.

24. The loss of normal serum opsonic activity associated with burns can be **BEST** treated by which following blood component/derivative?
    A. Red Blood Cells
    B. Lactated Ringer's solution
    C. Cryoprecipitated AHF
    D. 25% albumin

25. Which of the following is associated with end-stage liver disease?
    A. Abnormal bleeding
    B. Decreased blood ammonia levels
    C. Increased serum albumin levels
    D. Portal hypertension

26. Massively transfused liver disease patients are at risk for hypocalcemia due to:
    A. The inability to conjugate steroids.
    B. The inability to excrete potassium.
    C. The inability to synthesize albumin.
    D. The inability to metabolize citrate.

27. End-stage liver disease may be associated with a hemolytic anemia due to:
    A. Gastrointestinal blood loss.
    B. Accumulation of lipids on red cell surface.
    C. Nutritional deficiencies.
    D. Alcohol-induced marrow suppression.

28. Which of the following components is **BEST** suited for the replacement of multiple factor deficiencies in liver disease patients?
    A. Fresh Frozen Plasma
    B. Prothrombin complex
    C. Cryoprecipitated AHF
    D. Plasma protein fraction

29. In which of the following periods is the liver transplant patient **MOST** at risk for hemorrhage?
    A. Before surgery
    B. During the ahepatic stage
    C. 1 hour after the donor liver revascularization
    D. In the immediate postsurgery period

30. Which of the following is **NOT** true regarding the production of donor-derived antibodies in liver transplant patients?
    A. It occurs most frequently when patients receive ABO-incompatible transplants.
    B. Antibodies usually appear within 24 hours.
    C. A positive direct antiglobulin test may result.
    D. It can be associated with overt hemolysis.

Chapter 18

1. A history of previous transfusion is important in the investigation of autoimmune hemolysis because it helps:
   A. Differentiate between primary and secondary disease.
   B. Determine the type of adsorption studies to be run.
   C. Predict the category of autoimmune hemolysis.
   D. Determine the urgency of the serologic evaluation.

2. A nonreactive eluate is frequently associated with which type of autoimmune hemolysis?
   A. Autoimmune hemolytic anemia
   B. Methyldopa-induced immune hemolysis
   C. Mixed-type autoimmune hemolysis
   D. Cold agglutinin syndrome (CAS)

3. Warm autoimmune hemolytic anemia is characterized most frequently by which of the following serologic patterns?
   A. A DAT positive for both IgG and C3 with a reactive eluate
   B. A DAT positive for IgG only with a nonreactive eluate
   C. A DAT positive for C3 only with a reactive eluate
   D. A DAT positive for both IgG and C3 with a nonreactive eluate

4. Which of the following statements describes both harmless and pathologic cold autoantibodies?
   A. They usually react at 30° to 37° C.
   B. They usually have titers greater than 1000 at 4° C.
   C. They are usually polyclonal.
   D. They are usually IgM.

5. Which of the following drugs is associated with the drug adsorption (drug-dependent) mechanism in drug-induced immune hemolysis?
   A. Penicillin
   B. Methyldopa
   C. Quinine
   D. Acetaminophen

6. A patient has bluing of the hands and feet after cold exposure. The patient's hematologic and serologic findings are as follows: hemoglobin of 10 g/dL (100 g/L), polychromasia, hemoglobinemia, hemoglobinuria, an elevated reticulocyte count, and a positive DAT: C3 only. The **MOST** probable explanation for these findings is:
   A. Warm autoimmune hemolysis (primary).
   B. Penicillin-induced immune hemolysis.
   C. Mixed-type autoimmune hemolytic anemia.
   D. Cold agglutinin syndrome.

7. In warm autoimmune hemolytic anemia, serum can contain:
   A. Autoantibody alone.
   B. Alloantibody alone.
   C. Both autoantibody and alloantibody.
   D. All of the above.

8. Identification of alloantibody(ies) in the serum of a patient with autoantibody is essential for the selection of blood for transfusion. Which of the following specimens is **MOST** appropriate to identify an alloantibody in the serum of an untransfused patient who has a strong autoantibody that reacts with all panel cells at the anti–human globulin phase of testing?
   A. Serum adsorbed with autologous cells
   B. Serum adsorbed with allogeneic cells
   C. An elute from the patient's red cells
   D. Untreated serum using a prewarmed technique

9. If autologous cells are pretreated with ZZAP before adsorption, which of the following autoantibodies is **NOT** adsorbed out?
   A. Anti-e
   B. Anti-Jk^a
   C. Anti-K
   D. Anti-C

10. Which of the following techniques is inappropriate for preparing eluates of autoantibody in WAIHA?
    A. Digitonin-acid
    B. Glycine-HCl
    C. Organic solvents (e.g., methylene chloride)
    D. Freeze-thaw

11. Which of the following is true of paroxysmal cold hemoglobinuria (PCH)?
    A. The autoantibody is usually IgM.
    B. The antibody is biphasic.
    C. The antibody usually has broad Rh specificity.
    D. The disease is often secondary to infections such as infectious mononucleosis.

12. Which of the following statements is true of mixed-type autoimmune hemolytic anemia?
    A. Only C3 is present on the red cells.
    B. The eluate is generally nonreactive.
    C. Patients generally do not have severe hemolysis.
    D. It has serologic features of both CAS and WAIHA.

Chapter 19

1. The first successful stem cell transplant was which of the following types?
   A. Syngeneic
   B. Autologous
   C. Allogeneic
   D. Xenogeneic

2. Which of the following is **NOT** true regarding hematopoietic stem cell transplantation?
   A. Engrafted stem cells can provide antitumor effects.
   B. GVHD is a major transplant-related complication.
   C. Fetal liver stem cells have resulted in long-term engraftment.
   D. Progenitor cells from cord blood can be expanded ex vivo with cytokines.

3. In the case of an allogeneic transplant, failure to HLA match donor and recipient can result in:
   A. Graft rejection.
   B. Graft-versus-host disease.
   C. Both A and B.
   D. Neither A nor B.

4. After birth, hematopoiesis takes place in:
   A. Spleen.
   B. Bone marrow.
   C. Liver.
   D. Both B and C.

5. When compared with bone marrow transplantation, untreated peripheral blood stem cells:
   A. Are associated with more rapid platelet and neutrophil engraftment.
   B. Are more difficult to collect.
   C. Are associated with increased risk for GVHD.
   D. Have higher concentrations of stem cells.

6. Which of the following is true regarding umbilical cord blood as a source of stem cells for transplantation?
   A. Umbilical cord blood has a lower concentration of stem cells than either bone marrow or peripheral blood.
   B. Umbilical cord blood has a decreased risk of GVHD.
   C. Umbilical cord blood is difficult to collect.
   D. All of the above.

7. Possible risks and/or adverse effects of peripheral blood stem cell collection by apheresis include all of the following **EXCEPT:**
   A. Risk associated with general anesthesia.
   B. Toxicity associated with administration of cytokines.
   C. Inadequate venous access.
   D. Discomfort associated with the insertion of a venous catheter.

8. The decision to select autologous or allogeneic stem cells for transplantation will depend on which of the following factors?
   A. Age of the patient
   B. Type of malignant disease
   C. Ability to collect a tumor-free allograft
   D. All of the above

9. Unlike allogeneic stem cell transplants, autografts:
   A. Provide more graft-versus-tumor effect.
   B. Do not require HLA matching.
   C. Lack contaminating tumor cells.
   D. Are associated with higher posttreatment mortality rates.

10. Preparative regimens for stem cell transplant recipients result in:
    A. An increased risk of host-versus-graft disease (HVGD).
    B. Reduction or eradication of abnormal marrow cells.
    C. Proliferation of stem cells in the marrow.
    D. All of the above.

11. The primary measure of posttransplant hematopoietic recovery is:
    A. Evidence of GVHD.
    B. Evidence of disease relapse.
    C. A neutrophil count of $\geq 0.5 \times 10^9$/L.
    D. A platelet count of $\geq 100 \times 10^9$/L.

12. Immediate posttransplant hemolytic reactions are **MOST** frequently due to:
    A. Donor-recipient ABO incompatibility.
    B. HLA mismatches.
    C. Allergic reactions to DMSO.
    D. GVHD.

13. Standards and regulations regarding the collection, processing, storage, and transplant of stem cells are developed by the:
    A. Food and Drug Administration (FDA).
    B. American Association of Blood Banks (AABB).
    C. Foundation for the Accreditation of Cellular Therapy (FACT).
    D. All of the above.

14. The term used to describe the ability of stem cells to differentiate outside of their own tissue boundaries is:
    A. Plasticity.
    B. Elasticity.
    C. Durability.
    D. Vulnerability.

Chapter 20

1. A laboratory task that is considered a category III risk level (no risk of exposure) is:
   A. Clerical work.
   B. Centrifugation.
   C. Compatibility testing.
   D. Removing stoppers from tubes.

2. The **MOST** effective measure to prevent the spread of infection is:
   A. Wearing a face mask.
   B. Washing hands frequently.
   C. Using bulbed pipettes.
   D. Wearing a laboratory coat.

3. Gloves should be worn for all of the following tasks **EXCEPT:**
   A. Pipetting.
   B. Handling papers.
   C. Uncapping specimens.
   D. Cleaning biologic spills.

4. A protective laboratory coat that has been worn in the laboratory to perform testing should be:
   A. Changed every hour.
   B. Worn unbuttoned to reduce heat.
   C. Taken home to launder when soiled.
   D. Removed before leaving the laboratory.

5. The **MOST** commonly used disinfectant in the laboratory is:
   A. Phenol.
   B. Glutaraldehyde.
   C. 10% sodium hydroxide.
   D. 10% sodium hypochlorite.

6. A label indicating that the materials inside are biohazardous is required for all of the following **EXCEPT:**
   A. Specimen storage refrigerators.
   B. All blood specimens shipped on a common carrier.
   C. Laboratory waste such as test tubes and pipettes.
   D. Tested blood that does not contain infectious substances.

7. Information about a chemical's permissible exposure limits and protective equipment required for use is found in the:
   A. Merck Index.
   B. Safety plan.
   C. Material safety data sheet.
   D. Laboratory procedure manual.

8. A list of the chemical hazards found in a particular laboratory is found in the:
   A. College of American Pathologist's Safety Manual.
   B. Laboratory's chemical hygiene plan.
   C. Test kit package inserts.
   D. Infection control plan.

9. Latex laboratory gloves are used to:
   A. Protect against chemical spills.
   B. Protect against biohazardous materials.
   C. Clean laboratory benches with disinfectant.
   D. Protect against burns from liquid nitrogen.

10. A diamond-shaped label with four triangles is used to identify:
    A. Biohazard levels.
    B. Chemical properties.
    C. Fire extinguishers.
    D. Radioisotopes.

11. A "wipe test" is used to monitor:
    A. Radiation levels.
    B. Chemical levels.
    C. Biohazard levels.
    D. Liquid nitrogen levels.

12. The recommended disposal method for a unit of blood that is positive for infectious diseases markers is:
    A. Incineration.
    B. Burial in a landfill.
    C. Draining the bag in a laboratory sink.
    D. Mixing with 10% hypochlorite solution.

13. The term for the concept that every specimen should be treated as if it were infectious is:
    A. Biohazard safety plan.
    B. Standard precautions.
    C. Exposure limitation.
    D. Class III safety steps.

14. One purpose of requiring accident reporting is:
    A. Disciplinary action against the employee.
    B. Disciplinary action against the employer.
    C. To ensure that appropriate protective equipment was used.
    D. To ensure that the employee obtains appropriate treatment.

Chapter 21

1. The management of the testing process that documents accuracy and reproducibility of a test is called:
   A. Quality control.
   B. Quality assessment.
   C. Quality assurance.
   D. Quality improvement.

2. Assessment of the entire process of providing patient care, from selecting a test to be performed to the treatment being administered, is called:
   A. Quality control.
   B. Quality assessment.
   C. Quality assurance.
   D. Quality improvement.

3. The practice of physicians monitoring the appropriateness of other physicians' transfusion practices is called:
   A. Quality control.
   B. Asset management.
   C. Utilization review.
   D. Quality improvement.

4. An essential component of quality monitoring is:
   A. Documentation.
   B. Exceeding regulatory requirements.
   C. Defining physician services.
   D. Monitoring a list of specific patient care activities.

5. The agency that has published a guideline for the preparation of the technical procedure manuals is the:
   A. Clinical and Laboratory Standards Institute (formerly NCCLS).
   B. College of American Pathologists.
   C. Joint Commission on Accreditation of Healthcare Organizations.
   D. American Society for Clinical Laboratory Science.

6. Each laboratory procedure must be consistent with:
   A. The instructions (product insert) of the manufacturer of the reagents used in the procedure.
   B. The instructions for use of the reagent as outlined in the material safety data sheets.
   C. The procedures used in other institutions performing the same test.
   D. The procedures used in other institutions in the area.

7. Before routine use of a new lot number of reagent, all of the following must be done **EXCEPT:**
   A. Document the date of receipt, manufacturer, lot number, and outdate.
   B. Perform parallel testing of the new and old reagent with 50 specimens.
   C. Review the product circular (insert) for changes.
   D. Testing for sensitivity and specificity.

8. Reagents found unsatisfactory during use should be:
   A. Sent to the FDA for further testing.
   B. Tested in duplicate with other reagents.
   C. Removed from use and the final disposition documented.
   D. Tested to determine if altering the amount of reagent used will provide satisfactory results.

9. The minimum frequency of documenting the accuracy of the timer on a serologic centrifuge is:
   A. Daily.
   B. Weekly.
   C. Monthly.
   D. Quarterly.

10. The minimum frequency of documenting the temperature of refrigerators, freezers, and water baths is:
    A. Each day of use.
    B. Weekly.
    C. Monthly.
    D. Quarterly.

11. The Failure Modes and Effects Analysis is a quality tool primarily used to:
    A. Prevent injury to employees.
    B. Assess process risks and select preventative actions.
    C. Report responses to employee accidents to federal regulatory agencies.
    D. Collate error reports and make quarterly reports to the Food and Drug Administration.

12. A compliance officer is responsible for:
    A. Routine laboratory testing.
    B. Ensuring that quality monitoring is performed.
    C. Performing quality control procedures.
    D. Hiring and firing laboratory personnel.

13. The transfusion committee is responsible for monitoring all of the following **EXCEPT:**
    A. Use of blood components.
    B. Transfusion policies.
    C. Transfusion reactions.
    D. Daily quality control data.

14. In quality monitoring, the set point above which corrective action should be initiated is called the:
    A. Threshold.
    B. Action point.
    C. Cutoff.
    D. Break point.

15. A hospital has a waste rate for red blood cells of 6.4%; the national average is below 1.0%. This indicates a need for further investigation of:
    A. Waste of blood components.
    B. Supplier blood delivery schedule.
    C. Emergency release procedures.
    D. Physician requests for crossmatching blood.

Chapter 22

1. Information concerning a patient is considered confidential and should be discussed only with those persons with a need to know. Which of the following is an appropriate discussion of patient data?
   A. Answering a telephone inquiry from an attorney
   B. Answering a question about the patient's diagnosis from a worker in another section of the laboratory who is a close friend of the patient
   C. Answering a question about the patient's diagnosis from a worker in another section of the laboratory who is investigating the cause of abnormal results before issuing a final report of the results
   D. Discussing an interesting case while at lunch in the cafeteria

2. Reporting the identity of persons with positive tests for infectious diseases to public health agencies is:
   A. Voluntary.
   B. Required in many states.
   C. Forbidden by hospital confidentiality policies.
   D. Allowed only if written consent of the patient has been obtained.

3. Records of test results should be complete and recorded in the computer or on record forms:
   A. Concurrent with performance.
   B. After completing the entire test run.
   C. On a piece of scratch paper and transcribed at the end of the shift.
   D. Without errors; therefore the records should be erased and record forms rewritten if errors were made.

4. The standard method used to perform a procedure in a specific laboratory is documented by:
   A. The laboratory procedures manual.
   B. Detailed steps attached to each record form.
   C. Circling the procedure used on the product insert that came with the reagents used.
   D. Making a notation on the recording form referring to the reference document used for the method.

5. A record that should be kept indefinitely is a record of:
   A. Compatibility testing.
   B. Refrigerator temperature.
   C. Blood inspection before issue.
   D. Donor medical history and physical examination.

6. Definition of symbols and abbreviations used in a laboratory must be defined in the:
   A. American Association of Blood Banks *Technical Manual.*
   B. Laboratory procedures manual.
   C. Standard medical dictionary.
   D. Hospital formulary.

7. Federal regulations require that the transfusion service report a transfusion-related death to the:
   A. State health department.
   B. Supplier of the unit of blood.
   C. American Association of Blood Banks.
   D. Director, Center for Biologics Evaluation and Research.

8. A correction to a record should be made by:
   A. Correction tape covering the original record.
   B. Opaque fluid cover of the original record and overwriting the correct entry.
   C. A single line through the record with date and identification of the person making the correction.
   D. Obliterating the original entry with an ink pen and making the correct entry above the original entry.

9. An example of computer software is a:
   A. Disk drive.
   B. Bar-code reader.
   C. Database.
   D. Utility program.

10. Before a computer system is used, all of the following must be performed **EXCEPT:**
    A. Training of personnel to use the system.
    B. Validation that the system works as intended.
    C. Development of system operations and maintenance procedures.
    D. Duplicate entry of records into the new system and the old system for 2 months.

11. All of the following are examples of computer critical control functions **EXCEPT:**
    A. Connection of a printer to a CPU.
    B. Interpretation of ABO and Rh testing results.
    C. Warning that a unit of blood is outdated at the time of issue.
    D. Disallowing an ABO-incompatible unit from being used.

12. All of the following are used to prevent unauthorized personnel from accessing information **EXCEPT:**
    A. Individual passwords.
    B. Terminal lockout.
    C. Program restrictions.
    D. Minimal training of users.

13. Testing of the computer system to determine if it is working as expected is called:
    A. Validation.
    B. Quality assurance.
    C. Operations review.
    D. Control point assessment.

14. Retesting a computer system is required:
    A. Each day of use.
    B. Monthly.
    C. Annually.
    D. When making changes to the system.

15. Most often, problems encountered with the use of a computer are associated with:
    A. User error.
    B. Software "bugs."
    C. Hardware malfunction.
    D. Unreadable bar codes.

ANSWER KEY

Chapter 1
1. A
2. A
3. B
4. B
5. C
6. D
7. B
8. A
9. A
10. C
11. A
12. C
13. A
14. D
15. B

Chapter 2
1. A
2. B
3. C
4. C
5. C
6. D
7. A
8. C
9. D
10. B
11. B
12. D
13. C
14. A
15. A
16. C
17. D
18. D
19. A
20. D
21. A
22. B
23. C
24. D
25. B
26. C
27. D
28. A
29. C
30. D

Chapter 3
1. C
2. D
3. D
4. C
5. C
6. D
7. B
8. B
9. C
10. C
11. C
12. B
13. D
14. D

Chapter 4
1. D
2. D
3. D
4. C
5. A
6. C
7. B
8. A
9. D
10. B
11. C
12. D
13. A
14. D

Chapter 5
1. C
2. C
3. A
4. D
5. A
6. C
7. C
8. C
9. D
10. C

Chapter 6
1. D
2. D
3. C
4. C
5. D
6. A
7. A
8. C
9. D
10. D
11. C
12. C
13. B
14. A
15. D
16. B
17. D
18. A
19. C
20. D
21. B

Chapter 7
1. B
2. A
3. D
4. C
5. B
6. D
7. A
8. C
9. B
10. A
11. D
12. B
13. A
14. C
15. C
16. A
17. B
18. B
19. D
20. A

Chapter 8
1. C
2. B
3. B
4. D
5. A
6. D
7. A
8. D
9. B
10. C
11. A
12. C
13. B
14. A
15. B
16. D
17. D

Chapter 9
1. C
2. A
3. C
4. D
5. C
6. A
7. B
8. D
9. D
10. C
11. A
12. D
13. D
14. A
15. D
16. C
17. C
18. C
19. A
20. C
21. D
22. C
23. A
24. C
25. B
26. D
27. B
28. C
29. C
30. B
31. C
32. D
33. C

Chapter 10
1. C
2. B
3. B
4. D
5. A
6. C
7. B
8. A
9. C
10. B
11. C
12. D
13. A
14. C
15. A
16. C
17. A
18. C
19. B
20. C

Chapter 11
1. D
2. A
3. A
4. C
5. C
6. D
7. C
8. C
9. D
10. B
11. D
12. A
13. B
14. C
15. D
16. D
17. B
18. C
19. A
20. C
21. D

Chapter 12
1. D
2. C
3. B
4. C
5. E
6. D
7. C
8. D
9. C
10. B
11. B
12. C
13. C
14. A
15. E

Chapter 13
1. C
2. D
3. D
4. B
5. A
6. A
7. C
8. B
9. A
10. A
11. A
12. A
13. A
14. B
15. A
16. D
17. D
18. D
19. B
20. D

21.	C	**Chapter 15**		21.	B	3.	A	11.	A

21. C
22. D
23. A
24. B
25. B
26. A
27. A
28. C
29. D
30. D
31. B

Chapter 14
1. A
2. D
3. B
4. A
5. C
6. D
7. E
8. D
9. B
10. D
11. B
12. C
13. B
14. A
15. C
16. C
17. A
18. D
19. C
20. D
21. B
22. B
23. D
24. A
25. D

Chapter 15
1. B
2. C
3. A
4. C
5. C
6. D
7. C
8. A
9. D
10. C
11. D
12. A
13. A
14. D
15. C

Chapter 16
1. D
2. A
3. C
4. A
5. A
6. C
7. C
8. D
9. A
10. B
11. A
12. C
13. C
14. C
15. C
16. B
17. A
18. C
19. D
20. C

21. B
22. B

Chapter 17
1. D
2. A
3. C
4. D
5. D
6. C
7. B
8. D
9. B
10. B
11. B
12. C
13. A
14. A
15. C
16. A
17. D
18. B
19. C
20. A
21. D
22. D
23. A
24. C
25. A
26. D
27. B
28. A
29. B
30. B

Chapter 18
1. B
2. D

3. A
4. D
5. A
6. D
7. D
8. A
9. C
10. D
11. B
12. D

Chapter 19
1. A
2. C
3. C
4. B
5. A
6. B
7. A
8. D
9. B
10. B
11. C
12. A
13. D
14. A

Chapter 20
1. A
2. B
3. B
4. D
5. D
6. D
7. C
8. B
9. B
10. B

11. A
12. A
13. B
14. D

Chapter 21
1. A
2. C
3. C
4. A
5. A
6. A
7. B
8. C
9. D
10. A
11. D
12. B
13. D
14. A
15. A

Chapter 22
1. C
2. B
3. A
4. A.
5. D
6. B.
7. D.
8. C
9. D
10. D
11. A
12. D
13. A
14. D
15. A

Glossary

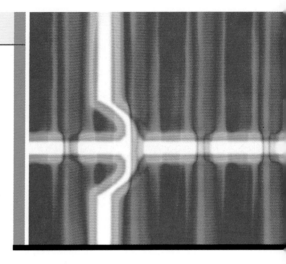

2-aminoethylisothiouronium bromide (AET): A chemical that removes the activity of antigens of the Kell system (with the exception of Kx) from red cells.

2-α-fucosyltransferase: The product of the H gene that transfers fucose to type 2 chains on the red cells to produce H antigen.

2,3-BPG: Produced in a side pathway of RBC glycolysis, the Luebering-Rapaport shunt, it binds to hemoglobin and facilitates O_2 delivery to the tissues. 2,3-BPG was previously known as 2,3-DPG. The term 2,3-DPG still appears in much of the literature on the topic.

2,3-DPG: Refer to 2,3-BPG above.

3-α-galactosyltransferase: Transfers the sugar galactose to the H antigen, conferring B blood group specificity.

3-α-N-acetylgalactosaminyltransferase: Transfers the sugar N-acetylgalactosamine (GalNAc) to the H antigen, conferring group A specificity.

AABB: The professional organization for practitioners in the field of transfusion medicine and cellular therapies. The AABB provides international standards of excellence for transfusion medicine practice and cellular therapies and has a voluntary inspection and accreditation program.

abbreviated crossmatch: An immediate-spin, saline major crossmatch used to determine ABO compatibility in patients with no demonstrable clinically significant antibodies and a negative history of antibody formation. Under some conditions, this determination of ABO compatibility can also be accomplished by an electronic (computer) crossmatch.

acanthocytosis: An abnormal red cell morphology characterized by cytoplasmic projections resembling thorns.

acid-citrate-dextrose: An anticoagulant/preservative containing citric acid, sodium citrate, and dextrose. Blood stored in acid-citrate-dextrose (ACD) has a shelf life of 21 days. ACD is no longer used for the collection of donor blood because solutions are available that allow for extended shelf life. Owing to the acid pH, 2,3-BPG levels are not well maintained in this solution.

acidosis: An increase in the hydrogen ion concentration (decreased pH), which can result from the accumulation of acid substances or the loss of buffering capability.

acute normovolemic hemodilution: A procedure whereby blood is removed before surgery and reinfused during or after surgery.

adaptive immune response: Immune system mechanisms that recognize antigens as non-self, specifically respond to the antigens, and respond faster and more vigorously on subsequent exposure to the antigen. Prototypic examples are antibody-mediated and T-cell–mediated immune reactions.

adaptive immunity: The ability of the immune system to specifically respond to antigenic challenge, that is, the ability to discriminate between self and non-self. Adaptive immunity can be divided into cellular and humoral immunity.

additive solutions (AS): Solutions that contain saline, adenine, glucose, and mannitol that when added to RBCs increase the shelf life of stored blood to 42 days. The adenine and glucose increase RBC ATP levels, and the mannitol decreases RBC lysis during storage.

adenine: Added to preservative solutions to maintain the adenine nucleotide pool and thus enhance red cell viability.

adsorption: The attachment of antibody to the red cell surface via binding with specific antigen. For example, A cells adsorb anti-A from solution. Adsorption is a blood bank technique in which red cells and plasma are mixed, and antibody is adsorbed onto the red cell surface. Adsorptions can be autologous or allogeneic and can remove autoantibody, alloantibody, or both.

affinity: The degree of fit between an antigen and antibody.

agglutination: The clumping together of antigen-bearing cells (such as red blood cells) in the presence of specific antibody.

albumin: A protein potentiating agent that enhances the reactions of some clinically significant alloantibodies. Albumin reagents such as 22%, 30%, and polymerized bovine albumin are available commercially. Although it is of historical significance, albumin is rarely used in today's blood bank testing because newer reagents allow for similar enhancements accomplished with shorter incubation times.

allele: Any alternate form of a gene that can occupy a given chromosomal location (locus). Each individual inherits one allele from the mother and one from the father, making up a homologous pair for each trait.

alloantibodies: Antibodies against foreign red cells (non-self).

allogeneic/homologous: Referring to antigens that are from the same species but are antigenically distinct. Blood group antibodies can be formed when an individual receives red cells from another individual that carry allogeneic antigens. Antibodies made to these alloantigens are known as alloantibodies.

amniocentesis: The withdrawal of fluid from the sac surrounding the fetus (amniotic sac).

amphotericin B: An antifungal agent used for patients with progressing, potentially fatal fungal infections.

amyloidosis: A group of conditions associated with the deposition of insoluble proteins (amyloids) in organs and tissues resulting in organ dysfunction.

anamnestic (secondary) immune response: The characteristics of the immune response to a second or subsequent exposure to a specific antigen. This response differs in a number of ways from the typical first (primary) response.

anaphylactic reaction (anaphylaxis): A severe immunologic response to transfusion that is both rapid and life-threatening. Systemic anaphylaxis produces changes in circulation and bronchioles consistent with shock and is characterized by a number of symptoms including dyspnea, cyanosis, fever, redness of the skin, and urticaria. Anaphylactic reactions cannot be predicted by routine pretransfusion testing.

anaphylatoxin: A substance that stimulates the release of mediators such as histamine from mast cells and basophils resulting in the symptoms of immediate sensitivity independent of IgE.

anisocytosis: An abnormal red cell morphology characterized by marked variation in red cell size.

ankylosing spondylitis: An inflammatory disorder of unknown etiology that primarily affects the axial skeleton, resulting in the loss of spine flexibility.

antepartum: Before delivery.

antibody repertoire: The total variety of antibodies made by an individual.

antibody: An immunoglobulin molecule produced in response to stimulation by a specific antigen and capable of reacting with the antigen that elicited its production.

anticoagulant/preservative: A solution designed to preserve the viability and function of the collected blood (preservative) and prevent clotting (anticoagulant). Such solutions provide buffering capability and nutrients for cellular metabolism during storage.

antigen: A substance capable of eliciting an immune response and reacting specifically with the product of that response.

antigenic determinant/epitope: That portion of the antigen molecule with which antibody can combine.

antigen-presenting cells (APCs): Cells that process antigen into peptides and display complexes of MHC molecules and peptides on their surfaces.

antiglobulin phase: The phase of in vitro testing that uses antihuman globulin reagent to detect in vivo or in vitro binding of IgG or complement to red cells.

antihistamine: An agent that opposes the action of histamine and thus reduces the symptoms associated with histamine release, including increased gastric secretion, flushing of the skin, headache, hypotension, and constriction of bronchial smooth muscle.

antipyretics: Agents that reduce fever.

anti-Rh29: An antibody produced by Rh_{null} patients that is frequently termed "anti–total Rh."

antithetical genes: Genes that can reside at the same genetic locus.

apheresis/hemapheresis: The process of removing whole blood from a donor or patient, processing the blood to separate selected elements, and returning the unharvested portion to the donor or patient. Apheresis can be cytapheresis, in which cellular components are harvested, or plasmapheresis, in which plasma is harvested.

apoptosis: A mechanism of controlled cell death in which cells are induced to degrade themselves from within.

Apt test: A test that differentiates adult hemoglobin and fetal hemoglobin, based on the principle that adult hemoglobin is less resistant to alkali denaturation than is fetal hemoglobin and is converted to alkaline globin hematin.

ascites: An accumulation of fluid in the peritoneal cavity, often associated with obstruction of the portal vein.

autocontrol: A control test with patient's own serum and cells run in parallel with antibody detection and compatibility testing. Positive autocontrols require further investigation.

autologous donation: The donation of blood for the donor's own use.

autosomal codominant: A pattern of inheritance in which alleles are located on autosomes and are expressed whenever present. Since *A* and *B* are autosomal codominant, if both are inherited both A and B antigens will be expressed (group AB).

autosomal inheritance: Alleles that are carried on any autosome (except the X or Y sex chromosome).

avidity: The strength of the bond between an antigen and its respective antibody.

azathioprine: An immunosuppressive antimetabolite drug used to reduce disease symptoms in autoimmune disorders and to extend allograft survival in transplantation.

azurophilic: The ability to stain with blue aniline dyes.

Bg antigens: HLA antigens present on red cells that may cause weak and variable reactions with sera containing the corresponding antibody. These antibodies may interfere with the interpretation of pretransfusion antibody detection and identification and may be present as contaminating antibodies in commercial antisera.

bilirubin (unconjugated): A breakdown product of hemoglobin. The unconjugated form is the lipid-soluble form that circulates, bound to serum proteins, en route to the liver, where it is conjugated.

biologic product deviation: A blood product that does not meet the good manufacturing standards of the FDA.

blood center (blood bank): A facility that is generally responsible for all activities leading to the preparation of suitable blood products for transfusion, including such areas as donor recruitment, phlebotomy, processing, storage, and shipment. Some blood centers have expanded roles, including pretransfusion testing, antigen screening, and reference services.

blood group antigens: Membrane chemical structures capable of inducing the production of antibody in foreign hosts. Red cell antigens differ among members of the species (alloantigens); therefore individuals can produce antibodies directed against antigens on transfused red cells. This is the basis for much of the science of immunohematology.

blood sample label: A label completed and attached to the sample before leaving the patient's bedside. This label must contain the following minimum information: two unique identifiers (usually the patient's name and identification number) and the date of collection. There must also be a mechanism to determine who drew the specimen.

blood transfusion form: A form completed for each unit of crossmatched blood that contains the following minimum information: two unique identifiers (usually the patient's name and identification number), ABO and Rh type of the recipient and the donor, donor unit number, pool number (if applicable), interpretation of compatibility testing, and identification of the person performing the tests.

blood volume: Approximately 75 mL/kg (about 10 units in a 70 kg adult).

blood warmers: Devices that warm blood to 37° C in-line during infusion.

B lymphocytes (B cells): Bursa-dependent lymphocytes that are the precursors of antibody-producing plasma cells and are primarily involved in humoral immunity. B-cell maturation takes place predominantly in the bone marrow, and the cells are characterized by the presence of surface immunoglobulin.

Bombay phenotype: The rare inheritance of two *h* genes at the *Hh* locus and the subsequent lack of the H antigen. Such individuals are unable to express other ABO antigens. True Bombay individuals also have mutant alleles at the *Se* locus.

bradykinin: A polypeptide substance capable of inducing hypotension, increasing the permeability of capillaries, and eliciting pain.

cardiomyopathy: Disease of the heart muscle.

CD34: A subset of cells that possess a transmembrane glycoprotein. Included in this cell cluster are those cells that are lineage committed, as well as pluripotent stem cells.

cellular (cell-mediated) immunity: Immune responses mediated by T lymphocytes either as a result of direct cytotoxicity or through the liberation of lymphokines.

cephalosporins: A family of broad-spectrum antibiotics divided into "generations." Included in the family are cephalothin, cephradine, cefuroxime axetil, ceftibuten, ceftriaxone, and cefepime.

cephalothin, cisplatin, diglycoaldehyde, and suramin: Cisplatin, diglycoaldehyde, and suramin are antineoplastic agents. In addition, suramin has been used to treat African trypanosomiasis. Cephalothin is a member of the cephalosporin family of antibiotics.

Chagas' disease: An insect-transmitted parasitic *(Trypanasoma cruzi)* disease that can be transmitted by transfusion.

chimera: An individual who has more than one cell population from different sources. In the blood bank, chimerism may result in multiple red cell populations with differing antigens thus resulting in discrepant cell typing.

chlorambucil and cyclophosphamide: Alkylating agents with antineoplastic activity.

chloroquine diphosphate and glycine acid EDTA: Reagents that dissociate IgG from the red cell membrane while retaining membrane integrity. This technique is useful for removing bound antibody so that cells can be antigen typed using antisera that require the indirect antiglobulin phase of testing.

choreiform movements: Involuntary movement of the limbs and facial muscles.

chorionic villi: A branching, vascular process of the embryonic membrane forming part of the placenta.

chronic granulomatous disease (CGD): An inherited disorder in which polymorphonuclear leukocytes are able to phagocytize but not kill certain microorganisms. The disease is characterized by chronic severe bacterial infections.

Circular of Information: The *Circular of Information for the Use of Human Blood and Blood Components* is a publication that provides a review of blood and blood components including composition, indications, contraindications and precautions, instructions for administration, and adverse reactions. The *Code of Federal Regulations,* Title 21, requires that the *Circular of Information* be available to medical personnel involved in transfusion processes.

cirrhosis: Liver disease characterized by loss of normal cellular structure and fibrosis.

citrate: A calcium-chelating agent that prevents coagulation by interfering with calcium-dependent steps in the coagulation cascade. Anticoagulation is only one of the many functions of anticoagulant/preservative solutions.

citrate-phosphate-dextrose (CPD): An anticoagulant/preservative solution with phosphate that is associated with higher levels of RBC 2,3-BPG when compared with RBCs stored in ACD. Blood stored in CPD has a shelf life of 21 days. Adding adenine to CPD (CPDA-1) extends the shelf life to 35 days. CPDA-1 storage results in higher levels of RBC ATP.

citrate toxicity: An adverse effect of citrate administration due to the chelation of calcium and subsequent hypocalcemia.

class I genes: Alleles at the HLA-A, HLA-B, and HLA-C loci that are defined (serologically) by complement-dependent cytotoxic reactions using known antisera from immunized humans and monoclonal sources.

class II genes: Alleles at the HLA-D locus. The gene products are defined by the mixed lymphocyte culture technique.

class III genes: Alleles of the MHC that produce a number of functionally diverse molecules.

clinically significant antibodies: Red cell alloantibodies that react at 37° C and are capable of causing decreased survival of transfused red cells.

clonal selection: Adaptive immune responses derive from a single antigen-specific lymphocyte that proliferates in response to antigen.

CMV negative: Negative for the antibody to the cytomegalovirus (CMV). CMV-negative blood is preferred for immunocompromised recipients to decrease the risk of CMV infection.

CMV-safe (CMV risk–reduced) blood: Blood that carries minimal risk of CMV infection, including blood from CMV-seronegative donors or blood that has been leukocyte reduced (less than 5×10^6 leukocytes).

Code of Federal Regulations **(CFR):** A publication of the FDA that includes regulations pertaining to the manufacture of blood, blood components, and blood products.

codominance: Inherited traits that are expressed whether the allele is present in the homozygous or heterozygous form.

cold agglutinin syndrome: A condition resulting from the agglutination of red blood cells by a cold-reacting autoantibody. A disease associated with hemolytic anemia and/or obstruction of the microcirculation.

collateral circulation: Secondary side branching of the circulatory system that carries blood from areas otherwise occluded.

College of American Pathologists (CAP): A professional organization for clinical pathologists and clinical laboratory scientists. CAP develops standards of practice for clinical laboratories and has a voluntary inspection and accreditation program.

colloid solution: A solution with particles too large to pass through animal membranes. Colloids therefore remain in the vasculature and exert an oncotic effect, drawing water into the vascular space. Colloids are indicated for volume expansion.

compatibility label: A firmly attached unit label that contains the following minimum information: two unique identifiers (usually the recipient's name and identification number), donor number, interpretation of compatibility testing, and identification of person who performed the tests.

compatibility testing: All serologic testing and clerical checks involved in determining compatibility between a potential recipient and donor. Compatibility testing policies are based on prevailing standards of practice and ensure a high probability of a successful transfusion outcome but cannot guarantee safety.

complement: A system of at least 20 functionally related serum proteins that cause immune cytolysis and other biologic activities.

complement-dependent cytotoxicity (CDC) test: Laboratory procedures that use complement fixation and resultant cell lysis as an end point.

component: A product made from the source product, Whole Blood. Components are broken into two general classes: cellular products and plasma products.

compound antigen: A distinct antigen, formed when two additional antigens are produced by the same gene.

congenital adrenal hyperplasia: Defects associated with the blockage of one or more enzymes necessary for the production of cortisol and resulting in decreased plasma cortisol, increased ACTH, and hyperplasia of the adrenal cortex.

constant and variable domains or regions: Portions of the immunoglobulin and T-cell receptor molecules that have constant amino acid sequences are known as constant regions and those with variable amino acid sequences are known as variable regions. Portions of the variable regions have extreme variability. These hypervariable regions give the antibody molecule its specificity for a particular antigen.

control functions: Computer functions in which the computer provides interpretations or suggests for actions, that is, serves in a consultative role. Examples of a control function are the interpretation of serologic data and suggestions for further testing, limitations on outdates of components, and prevention of the release of ABO- and Rh-incompatible blood.

cooperativity: Refers to the fact that every time an O_2 molecule binds to one heme in hemoglobin, it becomes easier for other O_2 molecules to bind to the other heme subunits. This is because there is a change in the conformation or shape of hemoglobin toward a more compact tetramer, facilitating O_2 binding.

cordocentesis: The technique of obtaining blood from the umbilical cord vein.

CPD, CP2D, and CPDA-1: Licensed anticoagulant-preservative solutions that can be used for the collection of blood and components for transfusion.

creatine kinase, MM band: An isomer of creatine kinase (CK) also known as CK-3. This enzyme is present predominantly in skeletal muscle and myocardium.

critical titer: That titer at or below which no severely affected infants or stillbirths have been reported. This value is determined by data from the institution. If no data are available, a titer of 32 is often used as a benchmark.

crossed over: The process of placing unused predeposit autologous units into the homologous blood supply.

cross-reactive groups (CREGs): Groups of antigens based on their common reactivity with antibodies to public epitopes.

cross-reactivity: The quality of broad specificity and the ability to react with more than one antigenic determinant or epitope.

cryogenic liquids: Liquids under pressure that generate low temperatures on vaporization.

Cryoprecipitated Antihemophilic Factor (AHF): The cold-insoluble portion of plasma. The component is rich in factor VIII:C, Factor VIII:vWF, Factor XIII, fibrinogen, and fibronectin.

cryoprotective agent: A chemical agent, such as glycerol, capable of protecting cells from freeze injury.

cryptantigen: An antigen hidden from detection on normal red cells.

crystalloid solution: A solution that can be diffused through animal membranes. Crystalloids such as normal saline can be used to restore blood volume up to approximately 20% blood loss.

confidential unit exclusion (CUE): The opportunity for a blood donor to indicate in confidence that the donated unit should not be used for transfusion. In such cases, all donor testing is completed and the donor is notified of any abnormal results and offered any necessary consultation.

$CuSO_4$ method: Donor hemoglobin screening can be accomplished by using $CuSO_4$ solutions. The test is based on the relative specific gravity of the solution and the blood. Blood will either float on the surface or sink to the bottom of the $CuSO_4$ solution depending on the hemoglobin concentration.

cyanosis: Bluish discoloration of the skin due to decreased oxygen saturation of the blood.

cytokines: Soluble polypeptides that function in the regulation of the immune/inflammatory response.

cytomegalovirus (CMV): One of a group of herpes viruses transmitted by the viable leukocytes in blood components, which is of special concern when transfusing immunocompromised recipients. Leukocyte depletion of components and the transfusion of CMV-negative blood are methods of reducing risk.

D-deletion phenotypes: Phenotypes that lack many Rh antigens and may result when some of the Rh genetic material is rearranged.

defense: Immunologically mediated resistance to infection.

deglycerolize: Removal of glycerol (cryoprotective agent) from red cells during the thawing process.

delayed hemolytic transfusion reaction: Destruction of transfused red cells that happens days to weeks after transfusion. These reactions are difficult to identify and resolve. Anti-Jka is frequently associated with delayed hemolytic events.

delayed serologic transfusion reaction (DSTR): Delayed reaction associated with the production of RBC alloantibodies after transfusion in which there is no clinical evidence of hemolysis.

desferoxamine: An investigative drug (ICL670) that functions as a chelator of iron. It has been shown to be effective in the treatment of iron overload in multiply transfused patients.

desmopressin (DDAVP): A synthetic form of vasopressin useful in the treatment of hemostatic disorders due to its ability to release stores of high-molecular–weight von Willebrand factor (vWF) with a subsequent increase in Factor VIII. Because of the function of vWF in platelet adhesion and formation of the platelet plug, DDAVP has also been used in a variety of platelet disorders.

dextrose: Provided as a nutrient for red cells to support the generation of ATP by glycolysis, thus enhancing red cell viability and extending shelf life.

diastolic pressure: That period of lowest pressure in the arterial system, which corresponds to the time in the heart cycle when fibers lengthen and the heart dilates and fills (diastole).

differential centrifugation: The separation of components of differing densities by centrifugation. This technique is used for most blood component preparation.

dilutional coagulopathy: Dysfunction of hemostasis due to the dilution of coagulation factors and platelets during the massive administration of blood, components, and derivatives.

dimethylsulfoxide (DMSO): A cryoprotective agent.

diploid: The condition of having two sets of chromosomes (maternal and paternal). The somatic cells of higher organisms are diploid.

direct antiglobulin test (DAT): A one-step test used to identify red blood cells that have been sensitized with antibody or complement in vivo.

directed donations: The process by which donors designate specific recipients for their donated blood or blood components.

disseminated intravascular coagulation: A condition associated with the activation of the coagulation cascade within the vasculature. DIC causes fibrin deposition in the microcirculation and consumption of platelets and fibrinogen. The major complication of DIC is clinical bleeding.

dithiothreitol (DTT): A potent reducing agent that cleaves the intersubunit disulfide bonds of IgM molecules, thereby abolishing both agglutinating and complement-binding properties of the molecule. 2-Mercaptoethanol can also be used for this purpose. DTT inactivates antigens in the Kell system.

diuretic: A substance that increases urine output either by increasing the rate of glomerular filtration or by decreasing tubular reabsorption.

Dolichos biflorus: A lectin with anti-A_1 specificity.

dominance: Expression of inherited trait when the allele is present in either the homozygous or heterozygous form.

Duchenne muscular dystrophy: A disease inherited as an X-linked trait associated with progressive degeneration of muscle fibers starting with the pelvic girdle and progressing to the shoulder girdle.

dyspnea: Shortness of breath.

edema: A general term for the accumulation of fluid in the tissues.

electromechanical infusion devices: Devices that control the flow of intravenous fluids.

elution: The process by which adsorbed antibody (on the red cell surface) is removed and returned to solution. Elutions can be performed by a number of physical and chemical procedures.

enhancement: Strengthening antigen-antibody reactions through a variety of chemical and nonchemical techniques. In some cases, the most convenient and least expensive of these techniques involve no special reagents or equipment, such as increasing the serum-cell ratio.

enteric administration, parenteral administration, or hyperalimentation: The administration of nourishment through a variety of routes (enteric: small intestine; parenteral: subcutaneous/intramuscular) or in greater than optimum (hyper) amounts.

enzyme techniques: Enhancement and differential detection techniques using proteolytic enzymes.

enzymes: The use of proteolytic enzymes in in vitro test systems to facilitate antibody identification. Blood group antigen-antibody reactions are differentially affected by enzyme treatment.

epinephrine: A hormone produced by the adrenal medulla that can be used as a vasoconstrictor and bronchiole dilator.

epiphyseal closure: Closure of the cartilaginous end of a long bone at the end of the growth period.

equivalence: Optimal antigen-antibody concentrations that facilitate the development of visible agglutinates.

erythema: Redness of the skin caused by capillary dilation.

erythroblastosis fetalis: A synonym for hemolytic disease of the newborn. The hemolytic disease is associated with anemia, jaundice, splenomegaly, edema, and the presence of immature red cells in the circulation (erythroblasts).

erythropoiesis: The production of red cells.

erythropoietin: A hormone produced predominantly by the kidneys in response to hypoxia.

esophageal varices: Enlarged veins or arteries in the esophagus that tend to rupture and bleed.

exchange transfusions: The simultaneous withdrawal of blood and infusion of compatible donor blood to infants with hemolytic disease of the newborn. The procedure removes antigen-positive cells, provides cells that are compatible with maternal antibodies, decreases bilirubin levels, and corrects anemia.

exogenous/endogenous: Exogenous means "outside" and endogenous means "within." An endogenous disease, for example, arises from circumstances within the organism.

exon: Transcribed region of a gene that is present in mature messenger RNA.

expiration date: The last date on which stored blood can be used for transfusion. Storage periods are based on in vivo viability standards.

extramedullary: Refers to outside of the bone marrow.

extramedullary erythropoiesis: Production of red cells outside of the bone marrow.

extravascular hemolysis: The premature removal of incompatible transfused red cells from the circulation by the phagocytic cells of the reticuloendothelial system (liver and spleen).

Factor IX complex (prothrombin complex): A commercial lyophilized product containing Factors II, VII, IX, and X. Factor IX makes up about 5% of this product.

Factor IX concentrate: A commercial product similar to Factor IX complex except that it is more highly purified and the final concentration of Factor IX is 30%. Both products are indicated for the management of Factor IX deficiency.

Factor VIII concentrate: A lyophilized commercial product prepared from the fractionation of plasma that contains Factor VIII:C. The product is treated to reduce the risk of viral transmission and is indicated for the management of hemophilia A.

Factor XII/Hageman factor: A serine protease (molecular weight 80,000) in the intrinsic coagulation pathway. Factor XII activation during the process of immune hemolysis contributes to both intravascular coagulation and activation of the kinin system.

febrile nonhemolytic transfusion reactions: Fever responses due to a reaction between HLA and/or leukocyte antigens on donor white cells and antibodies in transfusion recipients. These reactions can be associated with the transfusion of any component containing residual donor white cells and can be reduced by transfusing leukocyte-reduced components.

fetal lung maturity: A measure of the ability to inflate alveolar spaces and allow oxygen transport to red blood cells, which is related to the production of pulmonary surfactant (lipids). Lung maturity is often monitored using the lecithin/sphingomyelin (L/S) ratio. Other tests for fetal lung maturity include phosphatidylglycerol.

fetal-maternal hemorrhage: The passage of red cells from the maternal to the fetal circulation due to placental trauma or at delivery.

fibrin glue: The combination of thrombin and cryoprecipitate used topically to arrest surgical bleeding.

Food and Drug Administration (FDA): Federal agency that promulgates regulations and guidance documents for blood product manufacture and transfusion.

forward testing (typing): ABO testing that uses reagent antisera (anti-A and anti-B) to identify antigens on the red cells.

fresh blood: Whole blood or red cells selected for transfusion early (generally less than 5 to 7 days) within the storage period to minimize the infusion of cellular breakdown products and metabolic waste and to optimize levels of red cell 2,3-DPG and ATP.

Fresh Frozen Plasma: Plasma separated from whole blood within 8 hours of donation and frozen at −18° C or below. This process preserves levels of stable and labile coagulation factors for the storage period of 1 year.

gene: Composed of deoxyribonucleic acid (DNA); the basic unit of inheritance.

genomics: The field of genetics concerned with the structural and functional studies of the genome.

genotype: The genetic makeup of an individual.

ghost cells: Cells that appear pale and unstained.

glucose-6-phosphate dehydrogenase (G6PD) deficiency: A deficiency of an enzyme in the pentose pathway associated with hepatomegaly, hypoglycemia, acidosis, decreased serum haptoglobin, and failure to thrive.

glycophorin A: A sialoglycoprotein produced by the *MN* gene.

glycophorin B: A sialoglycoprotein produced by the *Ss* gene.

glycosylated: Chemically linked with glycosyl (sugar) groups.

graft rejection: An immune response against an engrafted organ or tissue resulting in failure of the graft to survive.

graft-versus-host disease (GVHD): A disease that results when transplanted immunocompetent cells mount an immune response against the recipient. The disease can be either acute or chronic and most often affects the skin, gastrointestinal tract, and liver.

granulocyte colony-stimulating factor (G-CSF): A growth factor used to mobilize granulocytes thereby increasing the yield of stem cells in peripheral blood progenitor cell collection.

Granulocytes: Leukocyte concentrates prepared from a single donor by apheresis techniques. The component contains granulocytes, variable amounts of lymphocytes, platelets, and red cells suspended in approximately 250 mL of plasma.

granulopoietic factors: Naturally occurring glycoproteins that stimulate the development of granulocytes (granulocytopoiesis).

haploid: The condition of having one set of chromosomes (maternal or paternal). The sex cells (gametes) of higher organisms are haploid.

haplotype: A set of alleles from a group of closely linked genes that are inherited together and are responsible for the production of a number of blood group antigens.

haptoglobin: A mucoprotein that binds hemoglobin which has been released from lysed red cells. Haptoglobin is decreased in hemolytic disorders.

Hazard Communication Standard: An OSHA regulation that requires employers to identify workplace hazards and have written policies for documentation of employee hazard training.

Health Insurance Portability and Accountability Act (HIPAA): Legislation passed in 1996 intended to ensure confidentiality of medical information and to prevent discrimination based on health status. HIPAA training of employees is required in all health care institutions.

hematopoiesis: The formation of blood cells.

hematopoietic progenitor cells (HPCs): Cells capable of differentiation into all blood cell lineages.

hemizygous: Used to describe the genetic material on the X chromosome of the male for which there is not equivalent material on the Y chromosome.

hemochromacytosis: A disease characterized by the deposition of hemosiderin in parenchymal cells. Acquired and secondary forms of the disease exist.

hemodilution (acute normovolemic hemodilution): A perioperative procedure whereby blood is drawn from a patient immediately before surgery and volume is replaced by fluids such as normal saline. Blood is held for reinfusion at the end of the procedure or earlier if indicated.

hemoglobinemia: The presence of free hemoglobin in the plasma.

hemoglobinuria: The presence of hemoglobin in the urine.

hemolysis: The disruption of the red cell membrane with the subsequent loss of cellular contents. Immune hemolysis is the result of the binding of complement on the cell membrane in conjunction with the binding of antibody to a red cell antigen.

hemolytic anemia: Anemia associated with the destruction (hemolysis) of red blood cells.

hemolytic disease of the newborn (HDN): A disease characterized by the destruction of fetal/newborn red cells resulting from the placental transfer of maternal alloantibody.

hemophilia B: An inherited (sex-linked) disorder associated with a deficiency of factor IX.

hemorrhagic shock: Serious derangement of the circulatory system resulting from the loss of fluid of sufficient quantity to overcome the ability of the vasculature to compensate by vessel constriction. Symptoms of shock include hypotension, coldness of the skin, tachycardia, and insufficient tissue perfusion. Immediate resuscitation is aimed at the restoration of volume.

hemosiderosis: Deposition of iron in tissues and organs which may result from the long-term administration of blood to patients with chronic anemia.

hepatitis: Inflammation of the liver.

hepatitis A virus: Virus that is generally transmitted by the fecal-oral route; transmission by transfusion is extremely rare.

hepatitis B vaccine: A formalin-inactivated vaccine derived from the surface antigen of the hepatitis B virus. The vaccination is indicated for immunization against all subgroups of hepatitis B but does not protect against hepatitis A, C, or non-A, non-B, non-C. The immunization is required for all laboratory professionals. The vaccine is administered intramuscularly in three doses: initial, 1 month, and 6 months.

hepatitis B virus: Virus that is transmitted by transfusion, but the incidence has decreased with the advent of sensitive donor screening for the surface antigen (Hb_SAg) and antibody to core antigen (anti-HBc).

hepatitis C virus: Before the viral genome was discovered, this disease was referred to as non-A, non-B (NANB) hepatitis. The implementation of nucleic acid testing in 1999 has decreased the incidence of transfusion-transmitted infection.

hepatitis D virus: Virus that is capable of causing disease only in the presence of HBV. Screening of blood for HBV results in a low risk of transfusion-associated hepatitis D infection.

hepatocellular damage: Damage to cells of the liver.

hepatosplenomegaly: Enlargement of the liver and spleen.

hereditary spherocytosis: An inherited disorder characterized by hemolysis, spherocytosis, anemia, jaundice, and splenomegaly.

Heterozygous: pertaining to the condition that exists when two alleles for a given trait are different.

high-incidence antigens: Antigens that occur in greater than 99% of the population.

high-protein reagents: Reagents that are enhanced by the addition of significant amounts of protein such as albumin. Such reagents are useful in the detection of IgG antibodies that may not agglutinate in saline media.

histamine: A substance produced from the amino acid histidine, the release of which results in increased gastric secretion, dilation of capillaries, and contraction of bronchial smooth muscle.

HLA: human leukocyte antigen.

homeostasis: That function of the immune system which removes effete or damaged self-components, such as aged red cells.

homozygous: Pertaining to the condition that exists when the two alleles for a given trait are the same.

human immunodeficiency virus types 1 and 2 (HIV-1/2); human T-cell lymphotropic virus types I and II (HTLV-I/II): Viruses that have been documented to be transmitted by blood transfusion.

human leukocyte antigens: Glycoprotein antigens found on the surface of all nucleated cells of the body, including most circulating blood cells: lymphocytes, monocytes, granulocytes, and platelets.

humoral immunity: Immunity mediated by antibodies.

hybrid glycophorins: Abnormal glycophorins resulting from a crossover between the genes for GPA and GPB, which results in the production of a number of unique low-incidence antigens in the MNSs system.

hydatid cyst fluid: Fluid from a cyst formed from the larval form of the dog tapeworm.

hydrops fetalis: A clinical condition in infants characterized by cardiac insufficiency with resultant edema and respiratory distress.

hydroxyethyl starch (HES): A red cell sedimenting agent used in apheresis procedures. HES is also useful as a cryoprotective agent.

hyperacute rejection: Rapid and extensive graft rejection associated with preformed HLA or ABO antibodies.

hyperammonemia: Excess ammonia in the blood.

hyperinsulinemia: Excess insulin in the blood.

hyperkalemia: Elevated levels of potassium in the blood, which can result from the transfusion of large amounts of potassium in units of stored bank blood.

hypernatremia: Increased blood sodium.

hyperphosphatemia: An excess of phosphate in the blood.

hypersplenism: Enlargement of the spleen.

hypervolemia: Increased blood volume.

hypoalbuminemia: Decreased serum albumin levels.

hypoglycemia: Decreased blood glucose.

hypoperfusion: Inadequate supply of blood to an organ or tissue.

hypoperfusion injury: Tissue/organ injury resulting from inadequate blood flow.

hypoproteinemic: Referring to an abnormal decrease in the concentration of protein in the blood.

hypothermia: Decreased body temperature (core temperature less than 35° C).

hypovolemia: Decreased blood volume.

hypoxemia: Insufficient oxygenation of the blood.

hypoxia: Insufficient delivery of oxygen to the tissues.

iatrogenic anemia: Anemia resulting from treatment, for example, anemia in newborns resulting from the collection of blood samples for laboratory testing.

iatrogenic blood loss: Because the sampling of blood for laboratory procedures is the major factor leading to the need for transfusion in low birth weight infants, every attempt is made to reduce the quantity and frequency of blood drawing from these patients. Pediatric institutions use micro samples whenever feasible.

icterus gravis neonatorum: Jaundice of the newborn resulting from accelerated red cell destruction.

idiopathic hemochromatosis: The infiltration of iron into the tissues.

idiopathic thrombocytopenic purpura: Abnormally low numbers of circulating platelets of unknown origin.

Ig subclass: Heavy-chain structural differences that result in distinctive functional differences in the Ig class. IgG, for example, has four distinctive subclasses.

immunodominant group: The portion of the epitope or antigenic determinant that binds most strongly with the antibody. The immunodominant group gives the antigen its specificity.

immunodominant sugar: The terminal sugar that confers ABO antigen specificity.

immunogenicity: The degree to which an antigen is capable of eliciting an immune response; also called antigenicity.

immunoglobulins: Any of the structurally related glycoproteins that function as antibodies. Immunoglobulins are divided into five classes based on their structure and function.

incomplete dominance: The condition in which the products (traits) of both alleles are expressed but the effect of one allele is stronger than that of the other.

increased osmotic fragility: Abnormal sensitivity of red cells to lysis in various concentrations of saline.

indicators (monitors): Selected data collected as a measure of some significant quality outcome.

indirect antiglobulin technique: The use of antihuman globulin reagents to detect red cell–bound antibodies.

indirect antiglobulin test (IAT): A two-step test used to determine if antibody reacts with antigen on red blood cells in vitro.

infectious disease marker (IDM) testing: Testing performed to screen for markers such as antigens or antibodies present in donated blood to screen for risk of transfusion-transmitted diseases. This testing enhances blood safety but also increases the cost of blood and blood products.

inhibitor (circulating anticoagulant): An endogenous substance in the blood that directly inhibits the activity of plasma coagulation factors. Most Factor VIII inhibitors are IgG immunoglobulins.

innate immunity: Inborn immune system mechanisms that confer basic resistance to invasion by bacteria, fungi, viruses, and so on.

International Organization for Standardization (ISO): A nongovernmental organization that promulgates quality and safety standards for business and industry.

intraoperative salvage: The process of collecting blood-containing fluid from the surgical site. Blood thus collected can be reinfused with or without subsequent processing.

intrauterine transfusion (IUT): Treatment of fetal anemia by the transfusion of blood to the fetus. Blood can be infused into the peritoneal cavity, from which it is absorbed by the fetus, or can be administered directly into the umbilical vein.

intravascular hemolysis: The destruction of transfused red cells within the vascular compartment due to either immunologic or nonimmunologic means. This type of hemolysis is associated with the transfusion of ABO-incompatible red cells.

intravenous immune globulin (IVIG): A plasma product produced by Cohn fractionation and treated to inactivate viruses. The IV preparation contains monomeric IgG molecules almost exclusively.

intron: Gene segment that is initially transcribed but is then removed from within the primary RNA transcript by splicing together the sequences (exons) on either side of it

ISBT 128: An adaptation of a conventional bar-coding system (system 128) used by blood banks throughout the world.

ischemic: Characterized by a local deficiency in the blood supply to a tissue or organ.

isotype switching: A change in isotype expression by B cells from IgM to IgG secretion with continuous antigen stimulation.

Joint Commission on Accreditation of Healthcare Organizations (JCAHO): An independent not-for-profit organization that seeks to improve the quality of health care through accreditation and related services.

K_0 ($Kell_{null}$) phenotype: Phenotype resulting from the inheritance of two rare *KEL* genes and associated with red cells that lack all Kell system antigens but express large amounts of Kx antigen.

kernicterus: A grave condition resulting from the passage of bilirubin into the brain and spinal cord.

Kleihauer-Betke stain: A technique used to quantitate fetal-maternal hemorrhage based on the fact that fetal hemoglobin is resistant to acid elution, whereas adult hemoglobin is not. Estimates of fetal bleed are made from counts of fetal cells per 1000 adult cells in a sample of maternal blood.

knockout gene: Gene that has been disrupted usually by recombinant DNA technology; used as a model for investigation of the function and interactions of the normal counterparts of the disrupted gene

L/S ratio: Levels of two phospholipid surfactants found in the amniotic fluid. As the fetal lung matures, the lecithin levels increase and the sphingomyelin remains constant. An L/S ratio of greater than 2.0 is a good predictor of fetal lung maturity.

laboratory safety program: A systematic laboratory plan that sets safety and health goals for the laboratory work environment. This plan must be described in a laboratory safety manual that provides program goals, policies, and procedures for all aspects of laboratory safety. The laboratory safety committee is generally the formal body responsible for the development, maintenance, and review of the safety program.

lacto-*N*-tetraose: The precursor substance for the Le^a antigen in the body fluids.

lacto-*N*-tetraosylceramide: The precursor substance for the Le^a antigen in the plasma.

lectin: Any of a group of plant substances capable of binding specifically with antigen substances (sugars) on the surface of red blood cells, resulting in agglutination. *Dolichos bifloris,* for example, is a lectin with anti-A$_1$ specificity.

leishmaniasis: A parasitic disease spread by the bite of infected sand flies.

leukoagglutinins: Antibodies to antigens on the surface of white cells that can be identified by their ability to agglutinate antigen-positive cells.

leukotrienes: A series of compounds that function as regulators of allergic and inflammatory responses. They can cause bronchial constriction.

Lewis antigens: Soluble antigens that are adsorbed onto the red cell surface and are not an integral part of the red cell membrane.

linkage: The tendency of genes that are located in close proximity on a chromosome to be associated in inheritance.

linkage disequilibrium: The occurrence of a haplotype in the population more frequently than would be expected based on probability.

LISS-polybrene: The combination of low ionic strength saline and polybrene, a polymer that brings about the agglutination of red cells.

low birth weight: Infants weighing less than 1500 g.

low ionic polycation tests: The combination of red cell antibody uptake in a low ionic strength, low pH medium and the use of a chemical red cell aggregating agent. If antibody has coated the cells, the aggregation does not disperse.

low ionic strength saline (LISS): A blood banking reagent that potentiates some antigen-antibody reactions by lowering the ionic strength and thus decreasing the net charge of red cells.

low-incidence antigens: Antigens that occur in less than 1% of the population.

low-protein reagents: Reagents that are not enhanced by the addition of protein. Monoclonal reagents are examples of low-protein reagents.

lymphokines: A general term for those soluble mediators of the immune response, other than complement and antibody, that are secreted by sensitized lymphocytes on contact with antibody.

macrophage clearance: The ability of macrophages to remove antibody-coated cells via the Fc receptor.

major crossmatch: A procedure used to determine compatibility between red cells of the donor and the serum (plasma) of the recipient.

malaria/babesiosis: Protozoan diseases transmitted by transfusion. Both are rare, and no donor testing is available.

material safety data sheets (MSDSs): Information regarding hazardous chemicals designed to reduce risk. MSDSs are required by OSHA as a part of the hazard communication standard.

maximum surgical blood order schedule (MSBOS): Criteria developed from institutional usage statistics providing a figure for the number of units to be crossmatched for any given surgical procedure.

McLeod phenotype: A phenotype associated with a decreased expression of Kell antigens on red cells.

McLeod syndrome: The pathologic process usually associated with the McLeod phenotype, which includes hematologic, cardiac, and neurologic defects.

meconium: The first stool produced by a newborn.

mefenamic acid: A nonsteroidal agent with antiinflammatory, antipyretic, and analgesic activity.

meiosis: Cell division and replication that result in the formation of haploid gametes (eggs and sperm), which carry either the maternal or paternal genetic information.

methyldopa/levodopa (Aldomet): An antihypertensive drug.

MHC molecules: Major histocompatibility complex molecules, either class I or class II. Also called histocompatibility locus antigens (HLAs).

MHC restriction: T cells respond to antigens presented in association with the same set of MHC molecules as expressed by the T cells themselves.

microaggregate filters: Screen- or depth-type filters that remove aggregates smaller than 170 μm. Microaggregate screen filters have pore sizes ranging from 20 to 40 μm and effectively remove 70% to 90% of the leukocytes.

microplate techniques: Serologic procedures that use micro well plates rather than test tubes.

minor crossmatch: A procedure used to determine compatibility between the serum (plasma) of the donor and the red cells of the recipient. This test is no longer used routinely but has historical significance.

mitosis: Cell division and replication that result in the formation of two diploid daughter cells with exactly the same genetic information as the parent cell.

monoclonal/polyclonal reagents: Reagents produced in part by hybridization techniques.

monocyte-macrophage: Monocytes are phagocytic leukocytes produced in the bone marrow. Monocytes are transported to the tissues, such as lung, liver, and spleen, where they develop into macrophages.

mosaic: A complex antigen, such as D, that has more than a single antigenic determinant.

multiparous: Having multiple pregnancies.

myeloablative: Therapy designed to eliminate marrow cells before HSC transplant.

narcolepsy: Intermittent attacks of sleepiness during the daytime.

National Committee for Clinical Laboratory Standards (NCCLS): A professional organization that develops consensus standards and best practices for clinical laboratory testing. Effective January, 2005, the new organizational name will be Clinical and Laboratory Standards Institute (CLSI).

National Fire Protection Association (NFPA): An organization that provides information regarding the risks associated with chemical exposure.

neocytes: A population of relatively young red cells. Larger and less dense younger red cells can be separated from older red cells that are smaller and more dense by differential centrifugation techniques. During automated cell washing the young cells are pushed out of the bag earlier and collected for transfusion.

neonate: An infant less than 4 months of age.

neutralization: Inactivation of an antibody resulting from binding with a soluble antigen. Blood group substances in saliva, for example, bind with their corresponding antibody, thus reducing the ability of the antibody to bind with particulate antigen (red cells).

neutropenia: A decrease in the number of circulating neutrophils in the peripheral blood.

NK cells: The population of lymphocytes that carry neither T-nor B-cell markers.

normal saline: A volume expander (0.9% saline) that is compatible with red blood cells.

Northern blotting: A technique analogous to Southern blotting for detection of RNA molecules by hybridization to a complementary DNA probe.

Occupational Safety and Health Administration (OSHA): The agency of the federal government that develops standards and regulations for safety and health in the workplace.

oncotic pressure: The pressure exerted by colloids in solution. This pressure affects the balance of fluid in the intravascular and extravascular spaces. Decreases in blood protein (colloid) result in the movement of water out of the vascular compartment and into the extravascular spaces, resulting in edema. Increases in intravascular oncotic pressure (as with the infusion of 25% albumin) results in the movement of water into the vascular compartment.

opsonic activity: Refers to the presence of substances in the serum that potentiate the phagocytosis of particles by macrophages and neutrophils.

optical aids: Devices that enhance the reading of test tube agglutination reactions.

orthopnea: Difficulty breathing in any but an erect position.

OSHA infectious risk categories: Classifications based on probable risk of exposure to blood-borne pathogens from I (routine exposure) to III (no risk of exposure).

oxygen-carrying capacity: The relative ability of red blood cells to combine with oxygen and release the bound oxygen to tissues.

oxygen dissociation curve: The sigmoid relationship between the partial pressure of O_2 (pO_2) and the $\%O_2$ saturation of hemoglobin. The P_{50} is the pO_2, under standard pH and temperature conditions, where hemoglobin is 50% saturated with O_2. The normal range for the P_{50} is 26 to 30 mm Hg.

pancytopenia: Decreased numbers of all blood cell lines.

parabens: Substances added to preserve reagents that may result in some discrepant serologic results.

pedigree chart: A diagrammatic method of illustrating the inheritance of genes within a given family.

permissible exposure limits: Levels of chemical exposure below which there have been no substantiated reports of adverse reaction.

personal protective equipment: Clothing and equipment designed to protect the laboratory worker from risk of infection or injury. Examples of personal protective equipment include chemical-resistant gloves, fluid-impervious garments, face shields, explosion-proof cabinets, hoods, and masks.

petechiae: Small purplish spots on the skin due to pinpoint hemorrhages often associated with platelet dysfunctional states.

phenacetin: An over-the-counter analgesic.

phenotype: The inherited traits that are expressed in an individual.

phototherapy: The use of light to degrade bilirubin in mildly jaundiced infants.

physiologic anemia: The progressive fall in hemoglobin during the first 3 to 18 months of life.

Plasma: The product prepared by the separation of plasma from whole blood before the fifth day after expiration. When stored in the frozen state at $-18°$ C, the product can be kept for up to 5 years.

Plasma and Plasma Cryoprecipitate Reduced: Plasma components that lack labile coagulation factors but do contain stable coagulation factors.

Plasma Protein Therapeutics Association: The professional association that develops standards of practice for the plasma industry.

platelet survival: Platelet posttransfusion increments can be affected by excessive destruction or utilization of transfused platelets by both immune and nonimmune mechanisms.

Platelets: Cellular elements separated by differential centrifugation from a single whole blood donation (random platelets) and used to treat patients with qualitative and quantitative platelet disorders.

Platelets Pheresis: A component separated by a pheresis technique allowing for large platelet yields from a single donor, which makes this product valuable for the patient who requires HLA-matched platelets.

pluripotential cell: A bone marrow cell capable of differentiation into many different cell types.

polyagglutinable cells: Cells that are agglutinated by most normal sera and not by cord sera.

polyagglutination: A condition in which red cells are agglutinated by a large percentage of human sera regardless of blood types but not agglutinated by autologous serum. Most forms of polyagglutination are due to the exposure of some hidden receptor on the surface of the red cell.

polychromasia (polychromatophilia): The bluish color of young erythrocytes in Wright-stained blood smears. These young cells are shown to be reticulocytes when stained with supravital stains.

polycythemia: An increase in red cell mass that may be a primary disorder (polycythemia vera) or a secondary response to sustained hypoxia.

polyethylene glycol (PEG): A commercially available enhancement reagent used for the detection and identification of weak IgG antibodies.

polyhydramnios: An excessive amount of amniotic fluid.

polymerase chain reaction (PCR): The molecular genetic technique by which a short DNA or RNA sequence is amplified enormously by means of two flanking oligonucleotide primers used in repeated cycles of primer extension and DNA synthesis with DNA polymerase.

polymorphic: Describes a population that contains two or more phenotypes.

polymorphism: The quality of having many different forms or states. In the science of genetics, this refers to many different phenotypes.

pooled products: Pooling of multiple units of components (e.g., Platelets or Cryoprecipitated AHF) into one bag for ease of transfusion.

portal hypertension: Increased pressure in the portal vein, which delivers blood to the liver. This is commonly due to some obstruction of blood flow through the liver.

posterior and anterior iliac crests: The superior portion of the hip bone.

postoperative blood salvage: The process of collecting blood-containing fluid from a closed site such as chest tube drainage.

postpartum: After delivery.

posttransfusion purpura: Red discoloration of the skin caused by hemorrhage resulting from immune destruction of transfused platelets by antiplatelet antibodies in the recipient.

postzone: The condition of antigen excess in which few agglutinates form.

prednisone: A synthetic corticosteroid used as an antiinflammatory agent.

preoperative/predeposit autologous donation (PAD): The donation of one or more units of blood by a donor for his or her own use for some anticipated future need such as pending surgery.

primary immune response: The characteristics of the immune response to the first or primary antigen presentation.

private epitopes: Antigenic determinants that are the product of a single gene.

proband/propositus: The individual being studied in a pedigree, such as the individual with a certain disease or other inherited trait of interest.

procainamide: A cardiac antiarrhythmic drug.

progenitor cells: Committed to a blood cell lineage and do not have the ability to differentiate into all blood cell lineages.

proteomics: A field of biochemistry encompassing the comprehensive analysis and cataloging of the structure and function of all the proteins present in a given cell or tissue (the proteome).

prozone: The condition of antibody excess in which few agglutinates form.

public epitopes: Antigenic determinants that are produced by more than one gene.

pulmonary edema: An accumulation of fluid in the lungs.

quality assessment plan: A written comprehensive plan for laboratory-wide assessment of quality outcomes.

quinine and quinidine: Quinine is a malarial suppressant. Quinidine sulfate and quinidine gluconate are antimalarial schizonticides and antiarrhythmic drugs.

Raynaud's syndrome: Pallor and cyanosis of the extremities (especially the fingers) during exposure to the cold. The syndrome is secondary to a number of diseases, including cold agglutinin syndrome.

recessiveness: Expression of inherited trait only when the allele is present in the homozygous form.

Red Blood Cells: The blood component prepared by removing most of the residual plasma (200 to 250 mL) from a unit of centrifuged or sedimented whole blood. Red blood cells have the same red cell volume and therefore the same oxygen-carrying capacity as whole blood but in a significantly reduced volume. Red cells are indicated for the treatment of anemia in normovolemic patients.

Red Blood Cells Deglycerolized: A component prepared by thawing and washing red cells that have been stored in a cryoprotective agent for up to 10 years. This freezing process is especially useful for rare blood storage.

Red Blood Cells Frozen: Red cells from a whole blood donation separated and frozen. Freezing allows for extended storage and is especially valuable for rare blood stockpiling.

Red Blood Cells Leukocytes Reduced: A red cell component from which white cells have been removed by one of a number of leukocyte-reduction methods. This component is useful for patients who have exhibited severe febrile reactions.

Red Blood Cells Rejuvenated: Red cells to which agents have been added that are capable of restoring concentrations of ATP and 2,3-DPG in stored red cell products. Adequate levels of ATP are necessary for red blood cell viability, and 2,3-DPG is necessary for satisfactory oxygen delivery to tissues.

Red Blood Cells Washed: Red cells that are washed with sterile saline.

refractory: A state of general unresponsiveness to therapy. Patients who do not respond to platelet transfusion with the expected increase in platelet number are termed refractory.

Reiter's syndrome: A syndrome that, in its full-blown picture, consists of urethritis, arthritis, and conjunctivitis. Urethritis usually occurs first. There are countless clinical symptoms, but the clinical picture is dominated by polyarthritis. There is pain, swelling, redness, and heat in the joints.

rejuvenation solutions: Can be added to stored blood up to 3 days after its initial outdate and extend the shelf life. After washing to remove the solution, blood can then be transfused within 24 hours if kept at 1° to 6° C, or it can be glycerolized and frozen.

responders: Individuals who produce antibody when stimulated by foreign antigen.

reticulocytosis: An abnormal increase of immature red cells (reticulocytes) in the circulation.

reticuloendothelial (RE) system or mononuclear phagocytic system (MPS): A system of phagocytic cells in the liver, spleen, and bone marrow that are involved in the destruction of antibody-coated cells in disorders such as hemolytic disease of the newborn.

reticulosis: A series of disorders characterized by an increase in cells derived from the reticuloendothelial (RE) system.

retinitis pigmentosa: An inherited condition associated with the progressive loss of retinal response.

reverse testing (typing): ABO testing that uses reagent red cells (A_1 and B cells) to identify antibodies in the serum.

Rh control reagent: The manufacturer's control that contains all of the components of the anti-D reagent except for the antibody. If required by the manufacturer, this reagent serves as a negative control for Rh typing.

Rh immune globulin (RhIG): A solution of gamma globulin containing anti-D. A 300 μg dose of RhIG, if administered within 72 hours of delivery, protects against alloimmunization of the mother to the D antigen of the fetus. Each vial of 300 μg of RhIG protects against 30 mL of fetal whole blood or 15 mL of packed cells.

Rh_{mod} phenotype: An inherited characteristic associated with a substantial decrease in Rh antigen expression.

Rh_{null} phenotype: An inherited characteristic in which none of the Rh antigens is expressed.

rosetting test: A screening test for fetal-maternal hemorrhage. The test is based on the principle that Rh-positive fetal cells coated with anti-D form rosettes with Rh-positive indicator cells, thus making them distinguishable from the Rh-negative maternal cell population.

rouleaux: red cell rolls that have the appearance of a stack of coins.

saline test system: An in vitro test procedure that uses a normal (0.9% NaCl) saline medium. This system is often used to detect IgM antibodies.

satellite bags: Additional bags attached to the main donor set by sterile tubing. These satellite bags are used for the removal of various blood components, avoiding nonsterile entry of the system.

secondary immune response (anamnestic): The characteristics of the immune response to a second or subsequent exposure to a specific antigen. This response varies from the primary response with regard to time, titer, antibody class, and antibody affinity and avidity.

secretor: An individual who has inherited at least one *Se(FUT2)* gene, which results in the secretion of ABH antigens into body fluids. These individuals make up approximately 80% of the random population.

sensitization: The binding of antibody or complement components to a red cell antigen, the first phase of the agglutination reaction.

septicemia: A serious condition marked by the presence of pathologic microorganisms in the blood.

serotonin: The chemical 5-hydroxytryptamine, which is a potent vasoconstrictor.

sex-linked (X-linked) inheritance: An allele that is carried on the X chromosome.

sickle cell trait: A condition that result when an individual is heterozygous for hemoglobin S, that is, inherits one gene for hemoglobin S and one for normal adult hemoglobin (A). Red cells of patients with sickle cell trait can become deformable under certain physiologic conditions such as hypoxia.

single-donor screening cells: Cells from individual group O donors selected for their antigen typing configuration. Two or three unpooled cells are selected to screen for most of the commonly encountered red cell alloantibodies and are used for routine antibody detection.

single-nucleotide polymorphism (SNP): A polymorphism in DNA sequence consisting of variation in a single base.

Southern blotting: A technique for preparation of a filter to which DNA has been transferred, following restriction enzyme digestion and gel electrophoresis to separate the DNA molecules by size; specific DNA molecules can then be detected on the filter by their hybridization to labeled probes.

specificity: The configuration of an antibody that results in its reaction only with the unique antigenic determinant that elicited its response.

sphygmomanometers: Blood pressure measurement devices with inflatable pressurized cuffs.

splanchnic: Refers to the large organs in any of the body cavities.

splenomegaly: An enlarged spleen.

splits/subtypes: HLA antigens may have additional epitopes that divide them into one or more subtypes (splits).

standard operating procedures (SOPs): An approved set of written procedures that delineate in detail the procedures, policies, and processes performed in a blood center or transfusion service.

standard precautions: Procedures and methods that reduce the risk of exposure to blood-borne infection. Standard precautions are based on the assumption that all body fluids are potentially infectious. Standard precautions in the donor phlebotomy setting are discussed in Chapter 8.

Standards for Blood Banks and Transfusion Services **(AABB Standards):** A publication of the AABB that provides voluntary standards for blood centers and transfusion services. The AABB offers an accreditation program through which institutions can be audited and subsequently accredited to demonstrate conformance to the quality principles that are the basis for the AABB Standards.

stem cells: Precursor cells that have the capacity to both self-perpetuate and differentiate into a vast array of specialized tissue types.

sterile connection (docking) device: Instruments capable of heat-welding plastic tubing in a sterile manner, often used when blood components are needed and satellite bags are not available.

stomatocytes: Red cells with a slit-shaped rather than a circular zone of central pallor.

storage lesion(s): Take place during blood storage and include changes in blood pH and the levels of 2,3-BPG, ATP, Na^+/K^+, plasma hemoglobin, NH_3, and several bioactive substances.

sulfhydryl reagents: Substances that cleave the disulfide bonds of IgM molecules, abolishing the ability of the molecule to agglutinate or bind complement. Thiol and sulfhydryl reagents (DTT and 2-ME) are useful in differentiating IgM antibodies from IgG antibodies.

suppressor gene: A gene that diminishes the effect of another independently inherited gene.

surveillance: That function of the immune system which detects and destroys mutant cells, thus providing protection from malignancy.

symptomatic anemia: A decrease in the number of circulating red cells, the amount of hemoglobin, or the volume of packed red cells per volume of blood. When anemia is severe enough, a patient has some or all of the following symptoms: pallor, weakness, vertigo, headache, sore tongue, drowsiness, malaise, dyspnea, tachycardia, palpitation, angina pectoris, gastrointestinal disturbances, amenorrhea, and slight fever.

syphilis: A sexually transmitted disease that is rarely transmitted by the transfusion of blood that has been stored more than 72 hours. Serologic testing for syphilis is performed on donor blood.

systolic pressure: That period of highest pressure in the arterial system which corresponds to the time in the heart cycle when the muscle contracts and expels its contents (systole).

task force: A small group of individuals usually selected for their expertise who gather to solve a focused problem in a relatively short time frame.

T-cell receptors: Highly variable antigen receptors of T cells usually consisting of α and β subunits.

thalassemia: An inherited anemia due to the production of abnormal hemoglobin molecules.

therapeutic apheresis: Application of apheresis procedures to the treatment of disease.

thermal range: The temperature range in which an antibody binds with its corresponding antigen. Thermal ranges are important predictors of the clinical significance of a blood group antibody. Cold autoantibodies can activate complement in vitro, especially in specimens that are stored at 4° C. To avoid this in vitro phenomenon, specimens can be collected in tubes containing chelating agents such as EDTA. In these specimens, calcium is bound and therefore complement cannot be fixed to red cells.

thiol reagents: Substances that cleave the disulfide bonds of IgM antibodies, abolishing the ability of the molecule to agglutinate or bind complement.

thrombocytopathy: Functionally abnormal platelets.

thrombocytopenia: Decreased platelet numbers.

thromboelastography (TEG): A mechanical-electrical whole blood clotting system that measures the kinetics of clot formation and the strength and dissolution of the clot.

thrombotic thrombocytopenic purpura: A disorder characterized by decreased platelet numbers, hemolytic anemia, and thrombosis.

titer: The highest dilution at which agglutination can be detected. Titration procedures in antibody identification are discussed in Chapter 12. Titers of maternal antibody are used as indicators of the course and severity of hemolytic disease of the newborn.

titration: A technique involving the serial dilution of an antiserum to determine the range of antibody activity (titer). In a mixture of antibodies, specificities can sometimes be distinguished by titration methods.

T lymphocytes (T cells): Thymus-dependent lymphocytes that originate from lymphoid stem cells, differentiate under the influence of thymus hormones, are characterized by cell-surface antigens, and are primarily responsible for cell-mediated immunity.

transferase: An enzyme that transfers chemical groups from one compound to another. *A* and *B* gene products are glycosyltransferases, meaning that they transfer sugars. These sugars are responsible for ABO blood group specificity.

transfusion-associated graft-versus-host disease: Proliferation of immunologically competent donor cells in an immunocompromised recipient. Also at risk are individuals who receive blood and components from blood relatives. Such reactions can be avoided by irradiation of blood and components that contain white cells.

transfusion committee: The process by which physicians and other transfusion service personnel review transfusion practice within the institution using a set of predetermined criteria. The goal of peer review is improvement in the quality of blood transfusion practice.

transfusion reaction: Any adverse outcome associated with the infusion of blood or blood components.

transfusion-related acute lung injury: Pulmonary edema, not associated with cardiac failure, that is usually due to the transfusion of preformed donor leukoagglutinins in the plasma of blood components.

transfusion service: A facility traditionally housed in the institution where transfusion takes place, usually a hospital. The role of the transfusion service is to provide the necessary testing and support to ensure the appropriate and safe transfusion of blood, blood components, and blood products. Typical roles of the transfusion service include pretransfusion testing, antibody identification, product selection, and monitoring of transfusion outcomes.

type 1 and type 2 structures: Precursor substances and antigens in the ABO system differentiated by the type of linkage between terminal carbohydrates.

type and screen: Abbreviated compatibility testing that does not include a cross-match. Such procedures are recommended for patients with a low probability of transfusion. Indications for type and screen are included in the institutional maximum surgical blood order schedule (MSBOS).

type 1 (insulin-dependent) diabetes mellitus (IDDM): A form of early-onset hyperglycemia resulting from pancreatic hypofunction.

type specific: Refers to the selection of blood/components of the identical type as the recipient's. When transfusing Whole Blood, type-specific blood must be used.

ultrasonography: Using high-frequency, inaudible sound (approximately 20,000 cycles per second) to produce an image of an organ or tissue based on the fact that ultrasound waves move at different velocities in tissues of differing elasticity and density.

unexpected antibodies: Red cell antibodies that, unlike the naturally occurring anti-A or anti-B, are not routinely present in the serum and are generally a result of red cell stimulation (transfusion or pregnancy).

Uniform Donor History Questionnaire (UDHQ): A recently revised questionnaire for the screening of donors of blood and blood components. The questionnaire has been approved by the FDA

urticaria: Hives.

urticarial transfusion reaction: An allergic reaction characterized by the development of hives.

validation: Testing whether the computer system does what it purports to do. Documentation of computer validation is required.

variant Creutzfeldt-Jakob disease (vCJD): A fatal human neurodegenerative condition transmitted by prions. As with Creutzfeldt-Jakob disease, vCJD is classified as a transmissible spongiform encephalopathy (TSE) because of characteristic spongy degeneration of the brain.

vasopressor: A substance that causes the contraction of the muscle fibers in capillaries and arteries, resulting in vasoconstriction and diminished blood flow.

vernix: The deposit that covers the fetus during intrauterine life.

von Willebrand's disease: An inherited disorder characterized by decreased levels of Factors VIII:C, VIII:vWF, and VIII:Ag.

warfarin sodium: The generic name for 3-(alpha-acetonylbenzyl)-4-hyroxy-coumarin, an anticoagulant drug that acts by inhibiting the synthesis of the vitamin K–dependent Factors (II, VII, IX, and X). Product names include Coumadin, Panwarfin, and Sofarin.

weak D: A weakened expression of the $Rh_o(D)$ antigen on red cells. For a complete discussion of weak D phenotypes, refer to Chapter 5.

Wharton's jelly: A gelatinous substance from the umbilical cord that is rich in hyaluronic acid. This substance can contaminate cord blood specimens and interfere with serologic testing.

Whole Blood: Blood collected (450 ± 45 mL) into anticoagulant/preservative solutions for the purpose of transfusion and/or component preparation. Whole blood is indicated for hypovolemic patients with clinical symptoms associated with poor oxygen-carrying capacity.

Whole Blood Modified: Whole blood from which cryoprecipitate and/or platelets have been removed.

window period: That period from the time an individual is infected with a disease until it is detectable by standard laboratory assays.

ZZAP: A mixture of cystine-activated papain and dithiothreitol. Treatment of cells with ZZAP removes the activity of a number of blood group antigens. The technique is useful for the preparation of artificial Ko cells.

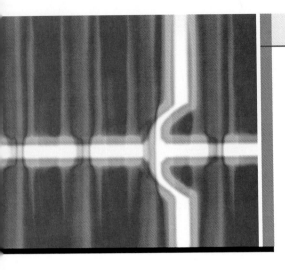

Index

A

A antigen, 71. *See also* ABO *entries.*
  immunodominant sugar for, 73
  structure of, 75
A gene, 72, 73–74. *See also* ABO *entries.*
  enzyme produced by, 72, 73t
A phenotype, 78t. *See also* ABO blood group
      (ABO blood group system).
  subgroups of, 77–79, 78t
    with anti-A₁ antibody, 77, 357
      and ABO typing discrepancies, 357, 358t
A₁ subgroup, 77, 78t. *See also* ABO blood group
      (ABO blood group system).
A₂ subgroup, 77, 78t. *See also* ABO blood group
      (ABO blood group system).
AABB (American Association of Blood Banks),
      181, 183, 183d
AABB (American Association of Blood Banks)
      Uniform Donor History Questionnaire, for
      donors of whole blood, 189–190, 194–195,
      195f–196f
AABB inspectors, 183
AABB Standards. *See also* Quality control.
  for antibody detection, 291, 292
  for apheresis performed as therapy, 464–465
  for blood product request forms, 284
  for blood warming, 453
  for hemoglobin level in whole blood
      donation, 196
  for human progenitor cells, 517
  for irradiation of blood products, 382
  for neonatal exchange transfusion, 437
  for record keeping, 311–312
  for record retention, 572, 573, 574
  for records of laboratory testing, 214
*AABB Standards for Blood Banks and Transfusion
      Services,* 184, 184d, 186b
A(B) phenotypes, ABO typing discrepancies
      and, 356
Abbreviated compatibility testing, for
      massive/emergency transfusion,
      299
Abbreviated crossmatch, in compatibility testing,
      295–296, 295d
Abbreviations
  for anticoagulant/preservative solutions, 237t
  in record keeping, 576

Page numbers followed by b indicate boxes; d,
definitions; f, figures; t, tables.

ABH antigens, 71, 86–99, 87–88. *See also* ABO
      entries and Antigen(s), H.
  diminished expression of, in newborn, 75
  presence of, in secretions, 71, 87–88, 88t
  of para-Bombay individuals, 80
  structure of, 75
ABO antibodies, 75–77. *See also* ABO blood
      group (ABO blood group system); Anti-A
      antibody; Anti-B antibody, etc.
  characteristics of, in serum of group O
      individuals, 76
  complement activation of, 76, 397
  IgA, IgG, and IgM components of, 76
  origin and development of, 75–76
  selection of blood for transfusion based
      on, 76–77
ABO antigen expression, 71. *See also* A antigen;
      ABH antigens; B antigen; H antigen.
  weak, acquired, ABO typing discrepancies
      and, 349–350
ABO blood group (ABO blood group system),
      70–84
  A phenotype in, 78t
    subgroups of, 77–79, 78t
      with anti-A₁ antibody, 77, 357, 358t
  antigen exposure effects on, 76
  antibody production and, 76. *See also* ABO
      antibodies; Anti-A antibody; Anti-B
      antibody; *etc.*
  antigen expression by, 71. *See also* A
      antigen; ABH antigens; B antigen;
      H antigen.
  B phenotype in
    acquired. *See* B antigen, acquired.
    subgroups of, 78, 79t
  blood sample testing for
    donor, 211
    in donor plasma selection for platelet
        transfusion, 381
    expected results of, 71t
    in granulocyte selection for transfusion, 383
    maternal, 427. *See also* Hemolytic disease of
        newborn (HDN).
    newborn infant, 477
    post-transfusion, 414
    recipient, 288–289, 379
    selection of blood for transfusion based on,
        76–77, 379
    typing discrepancies in. *See* ABO typing
        discrepancies.

ABO blood group (ABO blood group
      system) (*Continued*)
  Bombay (Oₕ) phenotype in, 71, 71d, 79–80,
      358–359, 359t
  genetics and biochemistry of, 72–75
    ABO locus in, 73–75. *See also* ABO genes
        and A gene; B gene, *etc.*
    H locus in, 72–73
    type I structures in, 72, 72d, 72f
    type II structures in, 72, 72d, 72f
  Landsteiner's description of, 69, 70–71
  mating of pheno- or genotypes in, possible
      pheno- or genotypes of offspring from, 74t
  O donor blood and, 76–77, 457
  Oₕ (Bombay) phenotype in, 71, 71d, 79–80,
      358–359, 359t
  presence of H antigen in
    range for. *See also* H antigen.
    variation in, 72f
  retyping of, after transfusion reaction, 414
  specificity in, sugars conferring, 71, 73
  transferases and, 71, 71d, 72
  subgroups of, 77–79, 78t, 79t
    typing discrepancies and, 81, 833
  typing of, 80–81, 288–289
    choice of blood for transfusion based on,
        76–77, 378–379, 379
    in donor plasma selection for platelet
        transfusion, 381
    expected results of, 71t
    in granulocyte selection for
        transfusion, 383
    inconsistent results of. *See* ABO typing
        discrepancies.
    maternal, 427. *See also* Hemolytic disease
        of newborn (HDN).
    post-transfusion vs. pretransfusion results
        of, 414
ABO genes, 73–74. *See also* ABO blood group
      (ABO blood group system) *and specific genes.*
  enzymes produced by, 71, 73
  interactions of, with other genes, in presence
      of *Le* or *lele,* 91–93, 93t
ABO-HDN, 439
ABO locus, 73–75. *See also* ABO blood group
      (ABO blood group system).
ABO reagents, 80–83
ABO subgroups, 77–79, 78t
    ABO typing discrepancies
        and, 81, 83, 349

ABO typing, 80–81, 288–289
  choice of blood for transfusion based on,
    76–77, 378–379, 379
  discordant results of. *See* ABO typing
    discrepancies.
  in donor plasma selection for platelet
    transfusion, 381
  expected results of, 71t
  in granulocyte selection for transfusion, 383
  maternal, 427. *See also* Hemolytic disease of
    newborn (HDN).
  post-transfusion vs. pretransfusion results
    of, 414
ABO typing discrepancies, 80–83, 81t, 344–359
  A subgroups with anti-A$_1$ antibody
    and, 357, 358t
  A(B) phenotypes and, 356
  ABO subgroups and, 81, 83, 349
  acquired B antigen and, 82, 356
  age of patient and, 79
  antibody-coated red blood cells and, 82
  B(A) phenotypes and, 356
  categorization of causes of, 348b
  chimerism and, 81–82, 356
  clerical errors and, 345t, 347
  cold alloantibodies and, 83, 355
  contaminating antibody in reagent
    and, 82, 357
  cord blood contamination (by Wharton's jelly)
    and, 82, 355, 355t, 436
  disease and, 83
  equipment dysfunction and, 345t, 346–347
  excess of blood group substances and, 82, 351
  glass fragments in tube and, 346
  human error and, 347
  missing or weak-reacting antibodies and,
    351–352, 351t
  mosaicism and, 81, 356
  overview of, 347–348
  passively acquired anti-A antibody and, 358
  patient with clotting deficiency and, 346
  polyagglutination and, 82, 353–354
  procedural errors and, 345t, 347
  reactions to drugs, dyes, and additives and, 359
  reagent dysfunction or contamination and, 82,
    83, 345t, 346, 357
  red blood cell-mediated, 81–82, 81t
  resolution of, 361–368
  room temperature-reactive alloantibodies
    and, 357–358
  rouleaux and, 83, 353, 353f, 358
  sample collection errors and, 345–346
  sample contamination and, 346
  serum-mediated, 81t, 83
  technical errors and, 345–347, 345t
  transfusion and, 83
  unexpected antibody reactions and, 357–359
  unexpected antigen reactions and, 352–357
  weak-reacting or missing antibodies and,
    351–352, 351t
  weak-reacting or missing antigens and, 348t,
    349–351
Acanthocytosis, 122d
  McLeod syndrome and, 122
Acceptance, of blood donors, 187. *See also*
    Donor(s).
Accident reporting, 542
Accrediting agencies
  with quality assessment requirements, 546

Accrediting agencies (*Continued*)
  quality control and, 184. *See also* Quality
    control *and* AABB *entries.*
ACD (acid-citrate-dextrose) anticoagulant/
    preservative solution, 261d
  development of, 261
3-α-*N*-Acetylgalactosaminyltransferase, 73,
    73d, 73t
Acid-base imbalances, massive transfusion and, 454
Acid-citrate-dextrose (ACD) anticoagulant/
    preservative solution, 261d
  development of, 261
Acidosis, 215d, 451d
  from massive transfusion, 451
  metabolic, from blood loss, 454
  oxygen-dissociation curve and, 266t
  sickle cell trait and, 215
Acquired anti-A antibodies, ABO typing
    discrepancies and, 358
Acquired B antigen, 356
  ABO typing discrepancies and, 82, 356
Acquired coagulation disorders, 390–391
Acquired immunodeficiency syndrome. *See*
    AIDS *entries.*
Activated C1s (activation phase, activation unit),
    in classic complement activation pathway,
    54–55, 54f
Acute inflammatory demyelinating
    polyradiculoneuropathy (AIDP), plasma
    exchange for, 461
Acute lung injury, transfusion-related, 172–173,
    403, 403d
Acute myelocytic leukemia (AML), therapeutic
    leukapheresis in, 463
Acute normovolemic hemodilution, 391
Acute transfusion reaction(s), 400–406
  hemolytic, 400–401, 407
    investigation of, 415–417
    signs and symptoms of, 400
  investigation of, 413–417
  nonimmunologic, 403–406
Adaptive immune response, 156, 156d
Adaptive immunity, 38, 38d, 39
Adaptive immunotherapy, cytapheresis in, 464
Additive-enhanced anticoagulant/preservative
    solution(s)
  content of, 454t
  red blood cells stored in, avoidance of use of,
    in neonatal transfusion, 477
Additive solutions (AS), 261d
  development of, 261
  in red blood cell preservation, 267–268, 268f,
    268t, 269t
  for red blood cells, 238
Adenine, 261d
  in anticoagulant/preservative
    solutions, 261
Adenosine triphosphate (ATP), in red blood
    cells, 268
  rejuvenated preparations of, 243
  stored, 268
Administration sets, for blood transfusion,
    305–307. *See also* Blood filter(s).
Adoptive cellular therapy for cancer, 518
Adrenal hyperplasia, congenital, 172, 172d
Adsorption, 76d, 492d
  for antibody identification, 319
  drug, immune hemolytic anemia due to,
    497–499, 499f

Adsorption studies
  for antibody identification, 319d
  in cold agglutinin syndrome, 496
  in paroxysmal cold hemoglobinuria, 496
  in warm autoimmune hemolytic anemia,
    492–493
AET (2-aminoethylisothiouronium
    bromide), 121d
Affinity, antibody, 45, 45d
Affinity maturation, 37
Age, ABO typing discrepancies and, 83
Agglutination, 59–60, 59d
  in antibody identification, direct vs. indirect,
    320–321
  antigen-antibody ratio and, 61
  antigen sites and, 62
  "clumping" phase of, 62
  detection of antibody-antigen reactions via,
    59–60
  electrostatic repulsion forces and, 62–63
  first stages of, 61–62
    variables affecting, 61–62
  formation of rouleaux vs., 63
  grading of, 321–322, 322t, 323f
    optical aids in, 321f, 322, 322d
  incubation time and, 62
  induction of, IgG vs. IgM in, 62
  ionic strength and, 61
  mixed-field, 321–322, 322t, 323f, 351, 351d,
    351t
  pH and, 61
  reading and interpreting, 63
  second stage of, 62–63
  sensitization phase of, 61, 61d
    variables affecting, 61
  stages of, 61–63
    variables affecting, 61–63
  strength of, grading of. *See* Agglutination,
    grading of.
  temperature and, 61–62
  time (incubation time) and, 62
Agglutination viewer, 321f, 322
Agglutinin, cold. *See also* Cold agglutinin
    syndrome (CAS).
  Rh typing discrepancies and, 360
AHF (antihemophilic factor). *See* Factor VIII
    entries.
AHG (antihuman globulin), 64
AHG (antihuman globulin) reagents, 64. *See also*
    Antiglobulin test(s).
AICC. *See* Anti-inhibitor coagulation complex
    (AICC).
AIDS (acquired immunodeficiency syndrome),
    transfusion-transmitted, 411
AIDS test, 212
  results of, biohazard labeling and, 221
Alarm systems, in monitoring of blood product
    storage temperatures, 271, 272
Albumin, 287d
  in blood sample evaluation, 287
  normal serum, 253
  preparations of, 252t, 386
  use of, in compatibility testing, 293
Aldomet (methyldopa), 500d
  autoimmune hemolytic anemia due to,
    500–501
  positive DAT from, 500–501
ALG (antilymphocyte globulin), 169
Alkalosis, metabolic, in massive transfusion, 454